Geriatric Nutrition
The Health Professional's Handbook
Third Edition

Ronni Chernoff, PhD, RD, FADA

Associate Director
Geriatric Research Education and Clinical Center
Central Arkansas Veterans Healthcare Center
Little Rock, AR

JONES AND BARTLETT PUBLISHERS
Sudbury, Massachusetts
BOSTON   TORONTO   LONDON   SINGAPORE

World Headquarters
Jones and Bartlett Publishers
40 Tall Pine Drive
Sudbury, MA 01776
978-443-5000
info@jbpub.com
www.jbpub.com

Jones and Bartlett Publishers Canada
6339 Ormindale Way
Mississauga, Ontario L5V 1J2
CANADA

Jones and Bartlett Publishers
International
Barb House, Barb Mews
London W6 7PA
UK

Jones and Bartlett's books and products are available through most bookstores and online booksellers. To contact Jones and Bartlett Publishers directly, call 800-832-0034, fax 978-443-8000, or visit our website www.jbpub.com.

Substantial discounts on bulk quantities of Jones and Bartlett's publications are available to corporations, professional associations, and other qualified organizations. For details and specific discount information, contact the special sales department at Jones and Bartlett via the above contact information or send an email to specialsales@jbpub.com.

Production Credits
Publisher: Michael Brown
Production Director: Amy Rose
Associate Production Editor: Dan Stone
Editorial Associate: Kylah Goodfellow McNeill
Director of Marketing: Alisha Weisman
Marketing Manager: Emily Ekle
Associate Marketing Manager: Wendy Thayer
Manufacturing and Inventory Coordinator: Therese Connell
Composition: Auburn Associates, Inc.
Cover Design: Anne Spencer
Printing and Binding: Malloy, Inc.
Cover Printing: Malloy, Inc.

Library of Congress Cataloging-in-Publication Data
Geriatric nutrition : the health professional's handbook / [edited by] Ronni Chernoff.— 3rd ed.
    p. ; cm.
  Includes bibliographical references and index.
  ISBN 0-7637-3181-1
1. Older people—Nutrition.
  [DNLM: 1. Aged. 2. Nutrition. 3. Aging—physiology. WT 115 G3699 2006] I. Chernoff, Ronni.
    RC952.5.G44342 2006
    613.2084'6—dc22

6048   2005034297

ISBN 13: 978-0-7637-3181-6
ISBN 10: 0-7637-3181-1

Printed in the United States of America
10 09 08 07 06   10 9 8 7 6 5 4 3 2 1

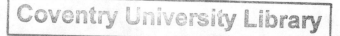

Contents

Preface

January 2006 marks the beginning of the post-world war II baby boom generation passing the threshold of age 60 years. It is a harbinger of things to come as the 76 million individuals born between 1946 and 1964 turn age 60 at the rate of 8000 a day and their demands for health care resources increase. The baby boomers are unique in that they are very different from previous generations: they are better educated, have a more sophisticated awareness of health care, are more invested in wellness and physical activity, expect accessible and affordable health care, and want to be a partner with their health care providers in making health care decisions. To meet the needs and expectations of this large cohort of elderly people, there is an obvious need to train health professionals to meet the challenges of caring for this very large group of older adults.

One dimension of health care that is important throughout the human life span is nutrition. Dietary intake must meet needs for growth and development, support successful reproduction, minimize risk factors for the development of chronic disease, and provide adequate substrate to heal injuries and wounds, fight infection, repair fractures, and recuperate from illness. All of this must be addressed within the context of aging organ systems, age-related physiologic changes, and the existence of chronic disease.

Aging successfully is dependent on a variety of factors including genetic inheritance, health habits, lifestyle, environmental factors, chronic and acute disease, and access to health care.

Relationships among these factors become clearer when continuing research is integrated into what knowledge presently exists. With the goals of all who work with elderly individuals to promote healthy aging and maximize life span, this book was revised and updated to integrate new research and information with knowledge already known. The contributors are all noted experts in their fields and provide new and updated information for all who would expand their understanding of the role of nutrition in aging, nutritional needs of aging adults, and nutrition and disease. Every chapter has been updated and new chapters have been added for this third edition.

The first chapter addresses some of the issues that we can expect to encounter as the population ages and demographics are shifted by changes in the population profile, immigration, and disease management. In this new edition, the chapters on nutrient requirements have been expanded by adding a chapter on protein requirements and including a new chapter on carbohydrate, fat, and fluid. Successive chapters on vitamin, mineral, and trace metal requirements have all been updated. Chapters on smell, taste and somatosensation, and oral health have been revised, and now are followed by a discussion of swallowing disorders in older adults.

Subsequent chapters have all been updated including revisions to chapters on the aging gastrointestinal tract and the cardiovascular, renal, hematopoietic, and endocrine systems; there is a completely new chapter on the aging skeleton.

Hopefully these chapters contribute to a greater understanding of human aging and the interrelationships with nutrition. A totally revised chapter on drugs and nutrient interactions gives new information on drugs, supplements, and herbal products.

Nutritional status and assessment, as well as aggressive nutrition interventions, are discussed in chapters on nutrition assessment and nutritional support. Additionally, our understanding of health promotion and secondary and tertiary disease prevention and management is deepened in the chapter on exercise, and a revised chapter on nutrition services for older adults (that integrates recently analyzed data from the Framingham study), and a revised and expanded chapter on health promotion and disease prevention in elderly adults.

The more information that is added to this text with each revision, the more we would like to add, but limited by time, publishers guidelines, and production requirements, this volume represents the basis of what will provide a primer in geriatric nutrition for the health professional. The hope is that the contents contribute to a greater understanding of aging and nutrition, to the reader's own successful aging, and will support any endeavor to enhance healthy aging for parents, patients, family, and friends.

Contributors

Chapter 2
Wayne W. Campbell, PhD
Associate Professor
Department of Foods and Nutrition
Purdue University
West Lafayette, IN

Nadine S. Carnell, MS, RD
Research Assistant and Dietitian
Department of Foods and Nutrition
Purdue University
West Lafayette, IN

Anna E. Thalacker, BS
Graduate Research Assistant
Department of Foods and Nutrition
Purdue University
West Lafayette, IN

Chapter 4
Paolo M. Suter, MD, MS
Medical Policlinic
University Hospital
Zürich, Switzerland

Chapter 5
Robert D. Lindeman, MD
Professor Emeritus of Medicine
Department of Internal Medicine
University of New Mexico
    Health Sciences Center
Albuquerque, NM

Chapter 6
Gary Fosmire, PhD
Associate Professor, Nutrition Sciences
College of Health & Human Development
The Pennsylvania State University
University Park, PA

Chapter 7
Valerie B. Duffy, PhD, RD
Dietetics Program
School of Allied Health
University of Connecticut,
Storrs, CT

Audrey K. Chapo, MS, RD
School of Medicine
Yale University School of Medicine
New Haven, CT

Chapter 8
Wendy E. Martin, DDS
Chief, Dental Service
Veterans Administration Medical Center
Albuquerque, NM

Michèle Saunders, DDS, MS, MPH
Associate Director, GRECC
South Central Texas Healthcare System
Director, South West & Panhandle Consortium
 Geriatric Education Center
Professor, Departments of Medicine, Dental
 Diagnostic Science, and Dental Hygiene
University of Texas Health Sciences Center
 San Antonio
San Antonio, TX

Susan P. Stattmiller
Associate Director, South, West & Panhandle
 Consortium Geriatric Education Center
Faculty Associate, Department of Medicine
University of Texas Health Sciences Center San
 Antonio
San Antonio, TX

Chapter 9
Joanne Robbins, PhD
Associate Director Research/GRECC
Wm. S. Middleton VA Hospital
Associate Professor, Dept. of Medicine
Sections of Geriatrics and Gastroenterology
University of Wisconsin-Madison
Madison, WI

Stephanie Kays, MS
Clinical Speech Language Pathologist,
 Dept. of Medicine
Sections of Geriatrics and Gastroenterology
University of Wisconsin-Madison
Madison, WI

Chapter 10
David N. Moskovitz, MD
Gastroenterology Fellow
Department of Medicine
University of Toronto

John Saltzman, MD

Young-In Kim, MD, FRCP (C)
Associate Professor
Departments of Medicine and
 Nutritional Sciences
University of Toronto
Staff Gastroenterologist
St. Michael's Hospital
Toronto

Chapter 11
Jeanne P. Goldberg, PhD
Tufts University
Boston, MA

Chapter 12
Robert D. Lindeman, MD
Professor Emeritus of Medicine
Department of Internal Medicine
University of New Mexico
 Health Sciences Center
Albuquerque, NM

Chapter 13
Gurkamal S. Chatta, MD
Associate Professor
Division of Hematology/Oncology
University of Pittsburgh
Co-Program Leader
Cancer and Aging Program
University of Pittsburgh Cancer Institute
Pittsburgh, PA

Linda Barry Robertson, RN, MSN
Associate Director for Patient Care Services
University of Pittsburgh Medical Center
 Cancer Centers
Adjunct Faculty
University of Pittsburgh School of Nursing
Pittsburgh, PA

Chapter 14
Gustavo Duque, MD, PhD
Assistant Professor
Division of Geriatric Medicine
Jewish General Hospital Bloomfield Centre for
 Studies in Aging
Lady Davis Institute for Medical Research
McGill University
Montreal, Canada

Bruce R. Troen, MD
Geriatric Research Education and
 Clinical Center
Miami Veterans Administration Medical Center
Associate Professor of Medicine
University of Miami School of Medicine
Miami, FL

Chapter 15
John E. Morley, MB, BCh
Dammert Professor of Gerontology and
    Director, Division of Geriatric Medicine
St. Louis University School of Medicine;
Director, Geriatric Research, Education and
    Clinical Center (GRECC)
Veterans Administration Medical Center
St. Louis, Missouri

Chapter 16
R. Rebecca Couris, PhD, RPh
Massachusetts College of Pharmacy and
    Health Sciences
Boston, MA

**Kathleen M. Gura, PharmD, BCNSP,
    FASHP**
Children's Hospital Boston
Boston, MA

Jeffrey Blumberg, PhD, FACN, CNS
Tufts University
Boston, MA

Chapter 17
Maria A. Fiatarone Singh, MD
Professor of Medicine,
    Faculty of Health Sciences
Professor, John Sutton Chair of Exercise and
    Sports Science
School of Exercise and Sport Science
University of Sydney
Australia

Chapter 18
Carol O. Mitchell-Eady, PhD, RD
Professor, Nutrition
Department of Health and Sport Sciences
The University of Memphis
Memphis, TN

Chapter 20
Barbara E. Millen, DPH, RD, FADA
Professor of Public Health
Boston University School of Public Health
    Professor of Socio-Medical Sciences and
    Community Medicine Chairman, Graduate
    Programs in Medical Nutrition Sciences
Boston University School of Medicine
Boston, MA

Lisa S. Brown MS, RD
Graduate Programs in Medical Nutrition
    Sciences Division of Graduate Medical
    Sciences
Boston University School of Medicine
Boston, MA

Elyse Levine, PhD, RD
Independent Consultant
Rockville, MD

Chapter 21
Beverly J McCabe, PhD, RD
USDA, Agricultural Research Service Lower
    Mississippi Delta
Nutrition Intervention Research Initiative
Little Rock, AR

Ruth E. Johnston, MS, RD
Assistant Director, Dietetic Internship
University of Arkansas for Medical
    Sciences/Central Arkansas Veterans
Healthcare System Dietetic Internship Program
Little Rock, AR

Dedication

To my mother Lynn who has set a high standard for successful and graceful aging and to Seth and Bret who will one day learn to age well from those of us who love them.

CHAPTER 1

Demographics of Aging

Ronni Chernoff, PhD, RD, FADA

All living organisms experience the process of aging as they approach the end of their predestined life span. Aging has been described as "intrinsic, deleterious, universal, progressive and irreversible."[1] It is likely that aging begins when growth and development cease, and that occurs on an individual timetable, affected by many factors that may not be regulated by any conscious effort; the process of aging may be referred to as "senescence." Senescence is considered to be the nonreversible, deteriorating changes that occur as cells and organisms age, increasing vulnerability to fatal disease, dysfunction, and ultimately, death.[2]

Geriatrics experts cannot predict prospectively how an individual will age and at what rate the changes associated with advancing age will become obvious or significant. Aging is a continuous process that occurs in the absence of disease. Aging cells do, however, become more susceptible to dysfunction or disease, and organisms may decrease in mass due to an inefficient replacement of cells. Despite the process that occurs in all living organisms, the life expectancy of humans continues to lengthen. At the beginning of the last century, it was not common for people to live much beyond the age of 50 years; average life expectancy in 1900 was approximately 42 years. Of children born today, 95% will live well past 50 years, probably into their 80s or older. In 1999, 24.7 million men and 30.6 million women were age 55 years or older.[3] Life expectancy has nearly doubled in the past century, and life ex-

pectancy has come close to tripling over human history.[4] One factor contributing to the gains in life expectancy in industrialized countries is a reduction in death rates among elderly people.[5] Death rates due to heart disease and cancer declined in the latter decades of the 20th century due to medical interventions and other factors.[4] There is a consequence to this increased longevity, which is the increases in health care costs anticipated to begin imminently with the aging of the baby boomers.[5]

An interesting artifact that has existed since the early 20th century is that the age of 65 is arbitrarily identified as a demarcation between middle age and old age, although there is no biological data to support this threshold. Biological aging occurs as a continuous process that varies among individuals. The selection of 65 as a marker of age was established in the late 19th century by Otto von Bismarck as the dividing line which, when crossed, allowed eligibility for retirement pensions; this was an interesting decision since so few people were expected to achieve this many years of life at that time in history.[1]

The advances in disease prevention and treatment that have been achieved during the last century have contributed to extending the human life span close to its predestined limits, but there is probably a limit to future extensions beyond many more years than have been already been added.[6]

Factors that may affect individual aging rates include such diverse occurrences as genetic profile,[7] food supply, social circumstances, political events, exposure to disease, climate and natural disasters, and other environmental events.[8] The impact of these factors and other life events is impossible to quantify and hard to interpret, especially since it is quite challenging and very expensive to conduct prospective studies on aging for the entire life span of a large enough group of people to draw conclusions about cause and effect of any factor and life span. It is noteworthy that individual aging and population aging, although related, are not the same.[9] For individuals, aging remains surviving into advanced years; for population groups, aging is related to an increase in its median age.[9] The premier study on aging in the United States is the Baltimore Longitudinal Study of Aging, which has been gathering data prospectively since 1958.

The most valuable information collected regarding human aging must be gathered prospectively so that events that occur throughout the life span of an individual can be linked to physiologic, physical, and psychological changes experienced in later life. It is certainly easier to conduct cross-sectional studies in which groups of individuals at various life stages and varying ages are examined and the differences among them at one point in time are measured; such studies do not yield much information about the events that preceded that point in time or what factors may have contributed to the differences observed.

This area of study is further complicated by the fact that humans are subject to an uncontrolled genetic pool; medical knowledge and interventions that change from one generation to the next; advances in science that affect quality of life, such as food supply and security, refrigeration and climate control; transportation systems; and advances in, and access to, new medications. Adding to the challenge is the lack of biological markers that measure true physiologic age. Although this issue has demanded attention and research resources, there are still no biological markers of aging and little progress in linking the impact of disease to expected life span. It is notable that the maximum human life span has been estimated at approximately 112 to 114 years, and this projection has not changed in 200 years.

DEMOGRAPHIC TRENDS

Until research provides us with a better definition of old age, people who have reached the age of 65 years or older will remain the reference group when the elderly population is discussed. Between 1950 and 1980, the population of those older than age 65 more than doubled so that one in every eight people fell into this age group; by 1997 one in six fell into this age group. Projections indicate that by 2030, 70 million people will be age 60 or older.[10,11]

What is truly significant about this increase is not the total size of this group, but rather that the greatest increases occur among the "old" and the "oldest old." Between 1997 and 2025, the percentage of individuals 75 years and older will increase from 5.8% to 7.9%. During the 1990s, the population age 85 years and older increased from 3.1 million to 4.2 million, a 38% growth.[12] This 85+ population is anticipated to grow from 4.2 million to 8.9 million by 2030.[11] The number of centenarians, people age 100 years or older, is projected to increase from 37,000 in 1990 to approximately 131,000 (middle estimate based on population projections) in 2020.[13] If these projections prove accurate, one out of 20 Americans will be 85 years or older by 2050.[14] (Figure 1–1.)

Death rates have been declining or remaining constant throughout the 20th century; however, declines in mortality rates vary by age, race, and sex.[15] Women have had a consistently greater decline in mortality rate, making the proportion of women in older age categories larger. (Figure 1–2.) Actually, more boys than girls are born, but since there is a higher death rate for males and an improvement in mortality rate for females, this ratio changes early in life. In 1980, there were 44 males to every 100 females over age 85. In 1996, there were 20 million older women and 13.9 million older men. The ratio of males to females declines with advancing age; this ratio is

Projected Numbers of Elderly People
1960–2040

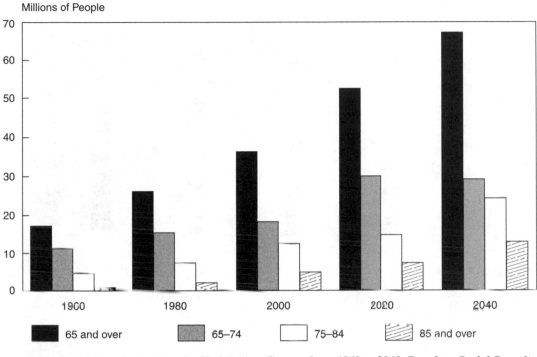

Figure 1–1 Population Projections for Various Age Groups from 1960 to 2040, Based on Social Security Administration Data

expected to fall to 36 males for every 100 females over age 85 by 2020.[16] The result will be an increasingly large group of women in the very old age group, and this is not expected to change.[17]

The impact of this trend is yet to be seen. Increased incidence of disability and severity of disability are associated with lower socioeconomic status, age, and gender.[18] Women live longer, but they also have more disabilities than do elderly men. Disability in men is usually related to heart disease and stroke; in women, disability is related to osteoporosis and associated fractures, arthritis, and circulatory diseases. Women tend to live longer with disability than do men and tend to be more economically dependent.[12] However, men with lower education levels

have a significantly greater loss of mobility than women who have the same income, age, and chronic conditions.[18] Disability is linked with increased health care expenditures in later years.[19] There seems to be a decreasing trend in disability in older persons in recent years associated with a more educated elderly cohort.[20]

There are differences in population demographics by race as well as by age and sex. By 2030, individuals who are in minority groups are projected to be 25% of the total older population.[11] In data published in 2002, non-Hispanic whites accounted for 80% of the over 65 population, 86% of those 75 to 84 years, and 87% of those 85 years and older.[21] American Indians and Alaska Natives represent 3.6%, Asians and Pacific Islanders are 2.9%, and Hispanics are 4.1% of the group 85

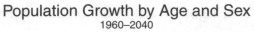

Population Growth by Age and Sex
1960–2040

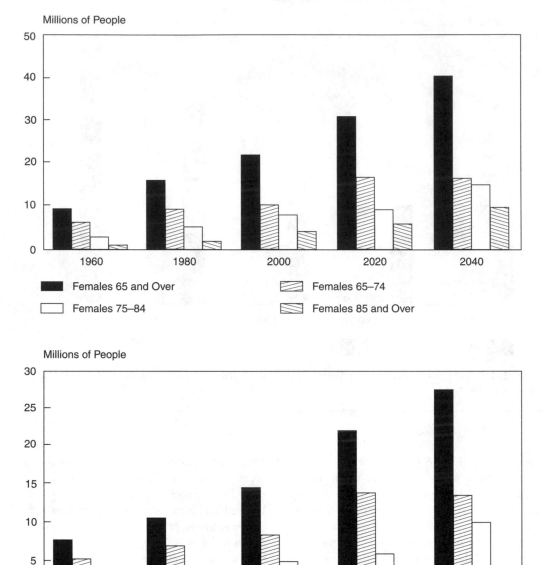

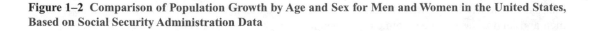

Figure 1–2 Comparison of Population Growth by Age and Sex for Men and Women in the United States, Based on Social Security Administration Data

years old and older.[21] Presently, there are many more elderly white people than there are elderly African Americans, despite a proportionately higher birth rate among African Americans. This discrepancy may be due to a higher mortality rate at younger ages for African Americans as well as increased mortality from hypertension, less access to preventive health care services, and delays in seeing physicians until the later stages of disease.[22,23] Although the early mortality rate for African Americans is expected to decrease, it is not expected to compensate for the gap between the races in the near future. Between 1990 and 2030, the elderly African American population is expected to grow by 159%.

The ethnic diversity of the older population, as well as the working-age population, will increase due to the larger families and higher birth rates of both African Americans and Hispanic Americans.[14] The number of Hispanic Americans is expected to increase by 570% between 1990 and 2030.

In 2001, there were about 3.4 million older adults living below the poverty line.[11] Compared with elders in other ethnic groups, Hispanic American elders are 2.5 times more likely to live with incomes below the poverty line; in 1989, 27% of Hispanic American women and 20% of Hispanic American men were classified as poor.[24] However, Hispanic Americans tend to spend a larger proportion of their disposable income on health care, despite a lower likelihood of having health insurance than other groups of elderly people.[25] Health care tends to be accessed through emergency departments, and hospital admissions are usually through the emergency department.

Along with the socioeconomic barriers to accessing health care, Hispanic American elderly also have cultural and language barriers to overcome. There appears to be a link between having English language skills and having a primary care provider. This may reflect a higher socioeconomic status or more successful acculturation among English speakers than those who speak only Spanish.[25]

Asian and Pacific Islander elders have different cultural traditions than other minority groups. They tend to form a more cohesive family group that offers support for elderly family members. Their cultural mores contribute to a unique approach to medical care, relying heavily on the customary view of mind and body linkages and the use of traditional medicines. Although this group of older adults represents a small proportion of the population, the number of elderly is expected to grow as the immigrants from the 1970s age.[26]

Life expectancy of Native Americans has increased dramatically during the past decade and is expected to increase by 294% by 2030. Data regarding the health status of elderly Native Americans are sparse, and their availability is highly variable among tribes. The Indian Health Service was elevated to agency status in the Public Health Service in 1988, and it can be anticipated that this will allow for greater awareness of the health needs of all Native Americans. It is well known that heart disease, diabetes mellitus, cancer, oral health, and nutrition problems exist among Native American groups.[27] Nutrition services and meals for Native Americans receiving care from the Indian Health Service are generally provided through Title III of the Older Americans Act.

The income of today's elderly populace is greater than that of similarly aged cohorts of previous generations. Social Security benefits represent the largest source of income for this group, followed by earnings and income from property, pensions, and investments. Although the current group of elderly people is less educated than are Americans of younger age groups, the gap is closing and is expected to change and the indicators for this shift are beginning.[20] The next generation of elderly, the World War II baby boom generation, is much better educated and more affluent than the current age cohort.[28] This fact will have an impact on income levels of future groups of older people, most likely making them more sophisticated and with greater expectations of social care systems and medical care options,[16] and may, therefore, lead to greater expenditures of health care resources. These factors will contribute to more of the future elderly adult population owning their own homes and wanting to stay in them for as long as they can manage.

Demographic trends are affected by many factors, including migration, immigration, and "new elderly births." New elderly births are the number of people who are newly classified as "elderly" because they have passed their 60th birthday. This effect has shifted the elderly population in the United States to make it appear to grow faster than the total population; the first wave of the "baby boom" generation, people born between 1946 and 1964, are moving into this group. Elderly births are making a noticeable impact on African American, Hispanic, and Asian populations where immigration occurred in large numbers in the years prior to World War II. For the future, the impact of this phenomenon will continue to be greater than the effect of migration and immigration.[29]

Another demographic factor that distinguishes the present cohort of elderly people from future generations of older people is their mobility. Older people tend to move geographically less often, and less far, than do younger people; they tend to settle in the geographic region where they were born and raised or where they settled when they married.[16] This is likely to change as the next generation ages; younger retirees are moving to locales different from where they raised their families.

As population demographics shift, population projections by the Census Bureau predict significant difference in rates of change in different regions of the United States. The regions that are growing most rapidly are the South and the West, while the north central region of the country will lose population.[12] Immigration per se has a minimal effect on the demographics of this age group except in four states: Hawaii, California, Florida, and New York. Internal migration has a more noticeable impact on states that tend to be magnets for retirees, led by Nevada, Florida, and Arizona.[29] These factors will influence the need for, and accessibility to, health care resources in the future.

IMPACT ON THE HEALTH CARE SYSTEM

One of the natural consequences that accompanies aging is an increase in the prevalence of disabilities and diseases. The incidence of concurrent illnesses and multiple disabilities rises sharply with age and is greatest in the very old segment of the population, those 85 years and older.[16] Perceptions of health status tend to be lower among older adults; 27% of older adults assessed their health as fair or poor compared to 9% for all other people. Older African Americans (42%) and older Hispanics (35%) were more likely to rate their health as fair or poor than were older Caucasians (26%).[11]

When an acute illness episode occurs, the consumption of health care resources is greater in this age group of patients because of the multiple chronic problems they may have that must be attended to along with their acute illnesses. Unfortunately, the health care system in the United States is becoming increasingly focused on the short-term delivery of acute care, allowing expensive and limited technologies to be used for the maximum number of patients. Complex, frail, very old patients require these expensive, lifesaving technologies, but concurrently they also require extended periods of skilled care for adequate recuperation and rehabilitation.[30] This increasingly large portion of the population will soon strain the resources of the existing health care system if that has not already occurred. Life expectancy and health status at age 70 predict health care expenditures in later years; elderly people in good health at age 70 have similar health expenditures when compared to those whose health status at age 70 is poor; however, individuals who are institutionalized by age 70 have much greater health care expenditures.[5]

Another important factor is having providers appropriately trained to care for frail elders. Primary care physicians find caring for older patients somewhat difficult due to their medical complexity and their chronicity of care needs, among other challenges.[31]

On the basis of relatively recent statistics, the population segment older than 65 years is approximately 35 million, which represents slightly over 12% of the total population.[12] These individuals account for more than 38% of all hospital stays,[32] use approximately 48% of acute care hospital bed days,[33,34] have longer in-hospital stays than younger adults (6.4 days vs. 4.6 days),[11] buy 25% of all the prescription drugs, spend 30% of the health care dollars in the United States (about $53 billion/year), and account for more than 50% of the federal health care budget (about $20 billion).[33] By 1993, the population older than 85 years of age represented 1.3% of the total population but accounted for 36% of all personal health expenditures, totaling approximately $162 billion.[35]

The incidence of disability increases with advancing age. Approximately 74% of individuals aged 80 years or older have at least one disability; almost 58% of those older than 80 had one or more severe disabilities and 35% required assistance associated with their disabilities.[11]

There is no doubt that health care managers and planners must assess the growth of the older segment of the population carefully and plan accordingly. For example, although only 5% of elderly people are in nursing homes at any one time, 90% of those are older than 65 years and 42% of those older than 85 years have experienced a nursing home admission, making the availability of nursing home beds and services an increasingly important part of planning for and allocating health care resources in the future.[35] The heaviest users of nursing home beds are women aged 85 years and older.[36] It is projected that the nursing home population will increase from 1.5 million in 1980 to 5.2 million in 2040. There is an increased shift in resources toward home health and community-based service providers; this will be a factor in future policy making and planning.[35]

When the "baby boomers" become the elderly generation between 2020 and 2040, a very large demand for resources and services will occur.[34] Other issues that will affect the utilization of and demand for services include the higher level of education of this generation compared to past generations; the level of medical sophistication they have; and the expanded expectations of the health care system compared to those displayed by their parents. Baby boomers want the health care system to keep them well, not just to take care of them when they are sick. They have had better childhood health and medical care and are generally healthier than previous generations. The next generation of older adults expects accessible, local, convenient, available, and cost-effective services.[28]

The issue of how health care services for the elderly will be paid for is a major policy problem that needs to be addressed now. As the baby boomers reach retirement age, starting in 2006, it is expected that there will be a major stress on Social Security and Medicare resources. Presently, Medicare pays for a notable percentage of the health care costs incurred by 41 million older adults when they reach the age of 65, become disabled, or are persons with end-stage renal disease; in fiscal year 2003, Medicare expenditures for older persons came to $278 billion.[37] Medicare Part A covers in-hospital costs as well as skilled nursing and hospice care; as health care costs rise, the likelihood that the funds paid in to Medicare will cover the projected health care demands is rapidly decreasing.[36] Medicare Part B (referred to as Supplementary Medical Insurance or SMI) covers physicians' and other practitioners' services, hospital outpatient department costs, and suppliers of medical equipment.[37]

Policy decisions to increase the retirement eligibility age will not address the problem with Medicare unless the eligibility age for Medicare changes too. Expenditures for acute and long-term care increase substantially with the increase in longevity. For individuals who die at age 65, approximately $31,000 is expended in health care costs; this may exceed $200,000 for those who die at age 90, in part due to nursing home care of the very old.[38]

One approach to saving Medicare Part A funds is to shift costs to Medicare Part B, which covers less costly outpatient services. Reducing acute care hospital lengths of stay and shifting health care delivery to outpatient clinics, day hospitals, and home-delivered services are potential options for saving money.[36]

Health care utilization is a very complex issue. The major factor in this complicated matrix of resource utilization is health status, whether it is based on a medical diagnosis or an individual's perception.[30,39–40] Utilization has been described utilizing a supply/demand model with some secondary factors that have a major effect on both supply and demand. These secondary factors are demographic (eg, age, gender, socioeconomics), sociopsychological (eg, attitudes, personality, health beliefs), sociocultural (eg, religion, norms and values, ethnicity), and financial-economic (eg, health insurance, disposable income).[39] On the demand side are age, sex, household composition, education, income, housing, social support system, medical technologies, and attitudes. On the supply side are health insurance and health care policy decisions, productivity of providers, efficiency, efficacy and technological developments, prescription drug costs, and suppliers' cooperation in the provision of services.

QUALITY OF LIFE AND HEALTH STATUS

It is well known that older people have more health problems than do younger individuals. However, a large percentage of the population over age 65 years is relatively healthy and vigorous. Good health status contributes to vitality and quality of life.

Quality of life is a difficult term to define well. Objective indicators of quality of life show only a weak relationship to individuals' perceptions of quality of life.[41] There are many subjective factors that contribute to quality of life, only one of which is health status. For example, general health and functional status represent one dimension of perceived quality of life, along with socioeconomic status, general life satisfaction,

and self-esteem.[41] One point of interest is that subjective estimates of health status by the individual do not correlate closely with objective assessment of health status as measured by laboratory tests and physical examinations.[41] The dimension that appears to correlate better when perceptions are compared with objective measures is functional status. *Functional status* is defined as that ability to perform activities related to self-care and daily living and can be measured by several instruments.[42] Frequently, poor health status and physical disability have an impact on functional ability; it is difficult to separate the two dimensions.[19,43]

Approximately 54% of all those older than age 65 report having at least one disability and approximately one-third have at least one severe disability. Over 4.4 million elders reported that their disability limits their ability to carry out the activities of daily living, and 6.5 million reported difficulties in attending to fulfilling the instrumental activities of daily living. Seventy-two percent of those 85 years of age or older need assistance with the activities of daily living.[19] As the population ages, there will be an increased need for assistive services to supplement family support.[14]

Quality of life takes on different meanings when applied to institutionalized elderly people. Since their health status is questionable, or they would not require institutionalization, factors that contribute to their perceptions of quality of life tend to relate to their immediate environment. The quality of their food; the ability to make choices and control some parts of their lives; participation in events in the institution, such as self-feeding or exercise programs; and the attitudes of the care providers and other residents all contribute to quality of life for chronically ill, elderly people cared for in institutions.[44] Certainly, satisfaction with one's life and surroundings contributes to perception of the overall quality of life. A positive outlook can contribute to better cooperation and compliance with health care regimens and perhaps help to maintain health status for a greater part of the latter years of life. All of these factors contribute to successful aging.

HEALTH CARE COSTS

As the elderly portion of the population expands, the consumption of health care resources may grow beyond their present availability. Efforts to curb expenditures have focused on acute care resources and have had an impact primarily on elderly, poor, and underprivileged patients. Many factors contribute to the large amounts of money spent on health care in the United States. Certainly, advances in medical technology, which result in the availability of expensive equipment needed to perform diagnostic tests and to provide technical treatment modalities, have contributed to rising costs. Another important contributing factor is that a large proportion of the population is living longer,[21,46] since the management of chronic disease has become easier and since technological advances have made the diagnosis and treatment of serious illnesses more effective.

Data from the National Center for Health Statistics support the proposal that one of the reasons the elderly segment of the population is getting larger is that their death rates are decreasing.[24] Because older people tend to have more disabilities and more chronic conditions, they require and use more health care resources.[47] There is no doubt that people older than 65 years require more acute care hospital days than do younger people, and this need increases in even older groups; individuals older than 85 years use 8300 days of acute care hospital resources per 1000 persons;[33] for chronic care resources, individuals over age 85 years use 8640 days per year per 1000 persons.[33] Medicare hospitalization study data reveal that African Americans, Hispanics, and Native Americans have higher hospitalization rates than do Causcasians, but Asian American Medicare beneficiaries are hospitalized less frequently.[22]

The need for health care services in the area of chronic care also requires an examination of the availability of appropriate providers. Models that analyze the requirements for physicians who are trained in geriatrics and are primary care providers indicate that there probably is not a compelling need for more physicians;[45] rather, the kind of health care and services needed can, and should, be provided by midlevel providers such as physician assistants (PAs) and advanced practice nurses (APNs).[48] It is estimated that if service delivery is shifted to ambulatory care practice with PAs and APNs, the number of patient visits can be increased by 12% to 37%, improving physician efficiency.[46]

The need for quality long-term care and the complexity of the issue are attracting the attention of policymakers. There are little demographic data to describe residents of long-term care facilities because they are often missed or overlooked in censuses or household surveys. However, as the population of frail, elderly people increases, interest in payment sources for their care has become greater. Currently, public or private insurance to help defray the costs of long-term care is limited, although more options are becoming available.[49] Skilled nursing services are expensive, and it is likely that in most cases public funds such as Medicare or Medicaid will not cover the costs of care.[50,51] Proprietary nursing homes are reluctant to accept patients who require skilled care; facilities that accept this type of patient may have staff inadequately skilled to care for ill patients. This limitation often creates a difficult situation when services are needed but are not affordable or available.[48]

Alternatives to nursing home care are being explored through experimental or demonstration projects. Home health services are one option that may prove to be a viable alternative to nursing home care. There are limitations to home care services, particularly the need for caregiver support required to make it work. In one model, a large portion of the care provided (about 72%) is delivered by family members, particularly if the patient's disabilities are not too great. Costs for home services increase with the level of patient disability.[21]

One alternative that has garnered some attention, and is becoming more popular among those who can afford it, is assisted living facilities. This option allows older individuals to live independently in their own space until they require assistance such as skilled nursing care; then, they can move within the facilities to living spaces that better meet their needs.[24]

Some physicians do not favor the home health care concept because they are concerned with malpractice issues, quality-of-care issues, loss of control over patient care, and loss of reimbursement, since the home health agencies take over managerial responsibilities.[52] Physicians have a limited role in the delivery of health care when the home care agencies become the primary providers, although recent trends indicate an increase in "house call" programs. The physician is involved only in approving forms that allow home care professionals to be reimbursed or in providing telephone consultations to the primary care provider. To be paid for patients' home health care, physicians must see the patients in the office or visit them in their homes; these activities are very time-consuming and not very cost-effective.

Hospitals are becoming involved in developing home health services because they are a viable option for extending services and marketing other hospital programs. These have become prime objectives because hospital reimbursement systems have contributed to the limited income in many facilities.[21] In fact, hospital-based home health care programs have grown faster than independent home health care agencies.[52]

Other models of home care have been developed by the Veterans Health Administration. For frail but medically stable elderly individuals who have able caregivers, the home-based primary care program is a successful alternative. The hospital-based staff members make home visits within a 50-mile radius of their base, and skilled health professionals (social workers, pharmacists, advanced practice nurses, dietitians, and physicians) track patients on a regular schedule and assess their home situations. This program provides continuity of care, which is an important dimension of caring for frail elderly people. There is regular contact by telephone so that problems can

be dealt with early in their course, and hospitalization arranged efficiently when needed.[53]

Another program alternative that may offer a feasible solution to the problems of providing health care to elderly patients is adult day health care.[54] Access to appropriate adult day health care facilities may enable frail elderly people to remain at home and maintain familiar surroundings and lifestyles. There are different types of adult day care models. The most common model is the social model. Social day care programs are designed to meet the needs of clients who may be disabled but are medically stable. The primary purpose of these programs is to maintain social and physical capacities through recreational and other social programs and to prevent or delay institutionalization.[54]

Medical model day care programs are designed to provide rehabilitative and support services, with the goal being the restoration of physical and functional abilities. One type of medical model adult day care has been under study through a multicenter health services research study of the Veterans Health Administration. In this program, elderly people can remain in their own homes yet receive health care through a day care center that provides therapeutic services. Family members, friends, or other support providers must arrange for transportation to the sites, or the program must provide transportation services. Patients can be enrolled in the program if they require rehabilitative care, such as physical or occupational therapy, medical treatment, or respite care. Patients can attend the center as needed, but usually they attend two or three times per week. They are brought in early in the morning and are picked up late in the afternoon, making it possible for care providers, spouses, or adult children to continue to participate in other activities, such as work, household, and child care responsibilities.[54]

Although there may not be ready-made answers to the problems of providing health care to older adults in the future, there are certainly options being explored.[37] It is obvious that something must be done to provide quality health care for this segment of the population. However, to develop the services and find the resources to pay for them, a great deal must be learned about aging, discases that are common in old age, and the maintenance of health in aging people.

CONCLUSION

There is no doubt that the expansion of the population segment older than 65 years will force health care providers to face problems associated with an aging society sooner than they may have liked. Many creative options have been proposed to provide appropriate quality health care to elderly people, but they need to be tested and evaluated before solutions can be found to the problems inherent in health care delivery to a large, distinct population of patients who have different income levels, unique medical problems and profiles, and diverse life experiences.

Within this context, health care providers must understand the role of nutrition in the maintenance of health, the management of chronic conditions, and the treatment of serious illness. The remainder of this text addresses the relationship among physiologic aging, nutrition, and disease. Comprehension of these important associations and the application of this knowledge will contribute to more effective health promotion, disease prevention, and disease management in elderly adults.

REFERENCES

1. Haynes SG, Feinleib M. *Second Conference on the Epidemiology of Aging*. Washington DC: US Public Health Service, 1980. US Dept of Health and Human Services publication NIH 80-969.

2. Vijg J, Wei JY. Understanding the biology of aging: the key to prevention and therapy. *J Amer Geriatr Soc* 1995; 43:426.

3. Smith D, Tillipman H. Current population reports, US Census Bureau, September 2000.

4. Wilmoth JR. Demography of longevity: past, present, and future trends. *Exp Gerontol* 2000;35(9–10): 1111–1119.

5. Rice DP, Fineman N. Economic implications of increased longevity in the United States. *Annu Rev Publ Health* 2004;25:457–473.

6. Olshansky SJ, Carnes BA, Grahn D. Confronting the boundaries of human longevity. *Amer Scientist* January/February 1998;86:52–61.

7. Yashin AI, DeBenedictis G, Vaupel JW, et al. Genes, demography, and life span: the contribution of demographic data in genetic studies on aging and longevity. *Am J Hum Genet* 1999;65(4):1178–1193.

8. Seeman TE, Crimmins E. Social environment effects on health and aging: integrating epidemiologic and demographic approaches and perspectives. *Annals N Y Academy Sciences* 2001;954:88–117.

9. Solomons NW. Demographic and nutritional trends among the elderly in developed and developing regions. *Eur J Clin Nutr* 2001;23(2):343–350.

10. US Bureau of the Census, International Programs Center, International Data Base, March 1997.

11. Administration on Aging. *A Profile of Older Americans: 2002*. Washington, DC: US Department of Health and Human Services; 2003.

12. US Census Bureau. *The 65 Years and Over Population. 2000*, October 2001.

13. US Census Bureau. *Current Population Reports: Special Studies, Centenarians in the United States, 1990*. July 1999.

14. Waite LJ. The demographic face of America's elderly. *Inquiry* 1996;33:220–224.

15. Anderson RN, Arias E. The effect of revised populations on mortality statistics for the United States, 2000. *Natl Vital Stat Rep* 2003;51(9):1–24.

16. Manton G. Demographic trends for the aging female population. *J Amer Womens Med Assoc* 1997;52(3):95–105.

17. Grundy E, Glaser K. Socio-demographic difference in the onset and progression of disability in early old age: a longitudinal study. *Age Aging* 2000,29(2):149–157.

18. Guralnick JM, LaCroix AZ, Abbott RD, et al. Maintaining mobility in late life. I. Demographic characteristics and chronic conditions. *Am J Epidemiol* 1993;137(8): 845–857.

19. Fried TR, Bradley EH, Williams CS, Tinetti ME. Functional disability and health care expenditures for older persons. *Arch Intern Med* 2001;161:2602–2607.

20. Waidmann TA, Liu K. Disability trends among elderly persons and implications for the future. *J Gerontol Series B: Psychological Sciences and Social Sciences* 2000;55: S298–S307.

21. US Census Bureau. *The Older Population in the United States: March 2002*, April 2003.

22. Eggers PW, Greenberg LG. Racial and ethnic differences in hospitalization rates among aged Medicare beneficiaries. *Health Care Financ Rev* 2000;21(4):91–105.

23. Niefeld MR, Kasper JD. Access to ambulatory medical and long-term care services among elderly Medicare and Medicaid beneficiaries: Organizational, financial, and geographic barriers. *Medical Care Research and Review* 2005;62(3):300–319.

24. Bureau of the Census Statistical Brief: *Sixty-Five Plus in the United States,* May 1995.

25. Pousada L. Hispanic American elders: implications for health-care providers. *Clinics in Geriatric Medicine* 1995;11(1):39–52.

26. Douglas KC, Fujimoto D. Asian Pacific elders: implications for health care providers. *Clinics in Geriatric Medicine* 1995;11(1):39–52.

27. Bernard MA, Lampley-Dallas V, Smith L. Common health problems among minority elders. *Journal of the American Dietetic Association* 1997;97(7):771–776.

28. Chernoff R. Baby boomers come of age: nutrition in the 21st century. *Journal of the American Dietetic Association* 1995;95(6):650–654.

29. Frey WH. Elderly demographic profiles of US states: impacts of "new elderly births", migration, and immigration. *Gerontologist* 1995;35:761–770.

30. O'Bryan D, Clow KE, Kurtz D. An empirical study of the influence of demographic variable on the choice criteria for assisted living facilities. *Health Mark Q* 1996; 14(2):3–18.

31. Adams WL, McIlavin HE, Lacy, NL, et al. Primary care for elderly people: Why do doctors find it so hard? *The Gerontologist* 2002;42:835–842.

32. *A Profile of Older Americans:1997.* Washington, DC; Program Resources Department, American Association of Retired Persons and the Administration on Aging, Department of Health and Human Services, 1998.

33. Hanson MJ. How we treat the elderly. *Hastings Center Report* 1994:24(5):4–6.

34. Pegels CC. *Health Care and the Older Citizen.* Gaithersburg, MD: Aspen Publishers, Inc, 1988.

35. Background materials.1995 White House conference on aging; May 2–5, 1995; Washington, DC.

36. Chen Y-P. "Equivalent retirement ages" and their implications for Social Security and Medicare financing. *Gerontologist* 1994;34:731–735.

37. The Long-Term Budget Outlook: Chapter 3: The Long-Term Outlook for Medicare and Medicaid, Congressional Budget Office, December 2003. www.cbo.gov/showdoc.cfm?index=4916&sequence=4

38. Spillman BC, Lubitz J. The effect of longevity on spending for acute and long-term care. *N Engl J Med* 2000; 342(19):1409–1415.

39. van der Berg Jeths A, Thorslund M. Will resources for elders be scarce? *Hastings Center Report* 1994;24(5): 6–10.

40. Lubitz J, Cai L, Kramarow E, Lentzner H. Health, life expectancy, and health care spending among the elderly. *New Engl J Med* 2003;349(11):1048–1055.

41. George L, Bearon L. *Quality of Life in Older Persons: Meaning and Measurement* New York, NY: Human Sciences Press, 1980.

42. Hills GA. Activities of daily living. In Lewis CB (ed): Aging: The Health Care Challenge, 4th edition, FA Davis Company: Philadelphia, PA: 2002, 27–47.

43. Covinsky KE, Palmer RM, Fortinsky RH, Counsell SR, Stewart AL, Kresevic D, Burant CJ, Landefeld CS. Loss of independence in activities of daily living in older adults hospitalized with medical illnesses: increased vulnerability with age. *J American Geriatr Soc* 2003;51(4): 451–458.

44. *A Profile of Older Americans:2000* Washington, DC; Administration on Aging, Department of Health and Human Services, 1998.

45. Reuben DB, Bradley TB, Zwanziger J, Beck JC. Projecting the need for physicians to care for older persons: effects of changes of demography, utilization patterns, and physician productivity. *Journal of the American Geriatrics Society* 1983;41:1033–1038.

46. Alemayehu B, Warner KE. The lifetime distribution of health care costs. *Health Services Research* 2004;39(3): 627–642.

47. Garber AM, MaGurdy TE, McClellan MC. Persistence of Medicare Expenditures among Elderly Beneficiaries, Working Paper 6249, National Bureau of Economic Research: Aging and Health Care, 1997. www.nber.org/papers/w6249

48. Beck C, Chumbler N. Planning for the future of long-term care: consumers, providers, and purchasers. *J Gerontological Nursing* 1997;23(8):6–13.

49. O'Bryan D, Clow KE, Kurtz D. An empirical study of the influence of demographic variable on the choice criteria for assisted living facilities. *Health Mark Q* 1996; 14(2):3–18.

50. Hoover DR, Crystal S, Kumar R, Sambamoorthi U, Cantor JC. Medical expenditures during the last year of life: Findings from the 1992–1996 Medicare Current Beneficiary Survey. *Health Services Research* 2002; 37(6):1625–1642.

51. Crystal S, Johnson RW, Harman J, Sambamoorthi U, Kumar R. Out-of-pocket health care costs among older Americans. *J Gerontol: Soc Sci* 2000;55B(1): S51–S62.

52. Moffa-Trotter ME, Anemat W. Home care. In Lewis CB, ed *Aging: The Health Care Challenge,* 4th ed. Philadelphia, PA: FA Davis Company; 2002: 368–378.

53. Dickerson GM. Non-institutional alternatives to long term care, Testimony before the Committee on Veterans Affairs, US Senate, April 25, 2002.

54. Hedrick SC, Rothman ML, Chapko M, et al. Summary and discussion of methods and results of the Adult Day Health Care Evaluation Study. *Med Care* 1993;31(9): SS94–SS103.

CHAPTER 2

Protein Metabolism and Requirements

Wayne W. Campbell, PhD, Nadine S. Carnell, MS, RD, and Anna E. Thalacker, BS

Adequate dietary protein intake is critical to maintain the integrity, function, and health of humans by providing amino acids that serve as precursors for essential molecules that are components of all cells in the body.[1] Human aging is a dynamic process that includes progressive changes in body composition, metabolism, physiological functional capacities, physical activities, food intake, the frequency of disease, and the ability of the body to respond to these changes.[2] It is important to recognize that these changes are both progressive and integrated. For example, sarcopenia, the age-associated loss of skeletal muscle mass, muscle strength, and muscle efficiency,[3,4] has been linked to declines in physical activity, motor neuron numbers and function, protein synthesis, hormones, insulin-like growth factors (IGF-1), testosterone, estrogen and growth hormones, and serum albumin concentration.[5]

Dietary protein and amino acids are also essential for the composition of the protein-dense bone structure.[6] The loss of bone has been associated with both excessive and inadequate dietary protein intakes.[7] The protein needs of an adult human might be expected to change in concert with these metabolic and physiological changes, and the Recommended Dietary Allowance (RDA) for protein should ideally be sufficient to preserve bodily functions throughout adulthood.[2] Despite the recognized importance of knowing the protein needs of all adults, surprisingly little data are available to firmly establish recommended protein intakes for elderly persons to maintain health.[1,8]

PROTEIN REQUIREMENTS

The average daily protein intake estimated to meet the requirement of one-half of healthy men and women age 19 years and older (ie, the Estimated Average Requirement, EAR) is 0.66 g protein/kg^{-1}/d^{-1}.[1] The average daily protein intake estimated to be sufficient to meet the need of nearly all (97.5 %) healthy men and women age 19 years and older (ie, the RDA) is 0.80 g protein/kg^{-1}/d^{-1}.[1] The EAR and RDA for protein are the same for 51- to 70-year-old men and women and those older than 70 years as for younger adults. For the reference 77 kg older male and 65 kg older female, the RDA for protein is 63 g/d and 50 g/d, respectively. Sarcopenia results in the apparent protein requirement of elderly persons being lower than for younger adults when expressed per kilogram body weight. However, the impact of sarcopenia on protein requirement is likely modest because muscle has a lower rate of protein turnover relative to most nonmuscle tissues, and the rate of whole-body protein turnover is not reduced with advancing age when expressed per kilogram fat-free mass.[9]

The EAR and RDA of protein for adults are based primarily on a large meta-analysis of nitrogen balance data.[1,10] Nitrogen balance is an assessment of the difference between dietary nitrogen intake and nitrogen excretion in urine, feces, and other miscellaneous losses, including sweat and skin. Unfortunately, there are a limited number of nitrogen balance studies in older persons.[11–16] The results and interpretations of these studies have been mixed, with some supporting the adequacy of the RDA for protein,[14,16] and some suggesting that it is inadequate.[11,13,15,17] The inconsistent results and interpretation of these studies[9,11,18] severely limit the confidence that the RDA is accurate and adequate for elderly persons.

Part of the confusion in interpreting these studies is that each study used a different nitrogen balance formula to calculate a mean protein requirement. To correct this inconsistency, Campbell et al.[11] recalculated the data from Cheng et al.,[16] Uauy et al.,[13] and Zanni et al.[14] using the nitrogen balance formula recommended by the 1985 WHO Consultation.[2] Combined, these data established a mean protein requirement of 0.91 g protein/kg^{-1}/d^{-1} for older people (a value that is 50% higher than the 0.6 g protein/kg^{-1}/d^{-1} established by the WHO and they suggest that the RDA for protein is higher in older people. More recently, Kurpad and Vas[19] have reaffirmed this interpretation, based on an independent evaluation of short-term nitrogen balance data. Millward et al.[9,18] have questioned the suitability of the available short-term nitrogen balance data to determine protein requirements of older people, based on issues that include study length, protein and energy intakes, propagation of errors of the nitrogen balance technique, and the apparent health of the research subjects. They have concluded that the RDA for protein is adequate for older people. The apparent differences in interpretation of the available short-term nitrogen balance data reemphasize the need for more data in older people.[1]

A recently completed short-term nitrogen balance study in older women[20] was unable to resolve the issue of whether the protein need of elderly women is the same or higher than the RDA and indicated that shorter-term nitrogen balance protocols may be insufficient to firmly establish the RDA for protein of older women;

further research is required using alternative criteria.

Nitrogen balance experiments with controlled dietary periods lasting more than two to three weeks are valuable when assessing protein adequacy and requirements.[21] Longer studies are desirable because they provide a longer time for metabolic adaptation to occur at a given protein intake, and they allow for quantitative assessment of changes in independent variables such as body composition and physiological or biochemical functions. Gersovitz et al.[15] conducted a controlled feeding study with seven older men and eight older women who had chronic but stable metabolic or physiological disorders. Each participant consumed weight-maintaining diets providing 0.8 g protein/kg^{-1}/d^{-1} for 4 weeks. During week 2, all seven men and four of eight women were in negative nitrogen balance. By week 4, mean nitrogen balance had moved toward equilibrium for both groups, but three men (43%) and four women (50%) were in negative nitrogen balance. Gersovitz et al. concluded that the RDA of 0.8 g protein/kg^{-1}/d^{-1} was not adequate for a majority of older men and women.

Castaneda et al.[12,22,23] conducted a 9-week nitrogen balance study in elderly women. Six women consumed diets providing 0.45 g protein/kg^{-1}/d^{-1} (56% of the RDA) and 6 women consumed 0.92 g protein/kg^{-1}/d^{-1} (115% of the RDA). Nitrogen balance, body composition, protein metabolism, muscle strength and function, and immune response were measured to see whether these older women successfully adapted (ie, adjusted without adverse consequences) or accommodated (ie, adjusted with simultaneous and significant losses of function)[24] to these levels of protein intake. Mean nitrogen balance was positive at week 3 and week 9 for the women provided 0.92 g protein/kg^{-1}/d^{-1}, an indication that nitrogen equilibrium was attained at this level of protein intake. Each of the six women who consumed 0.45 g protein/kg^{-1}/d^{-1} was in negative nitrogen balance during study week 3. Nitrogen balance moved significantly toward equilibrium at week 9, similar to the observations of Gersovitz et al.,[15] yet remained negative for five of these six women. The nitrogen balance shift toward equilibrium occurred as these older women accommodated with significant losses of lean body mass (8% decline in body cell mass and an 8% decline in muscle mass). Loss of muscle mass was also associated with reduced muscle strength and function. Thus, a protein intake higher than the current RDA was adequate, but the lower protein intake was clearly inadequate. Campbell et al.[25,26] documented that older men and women who consumed the RDA of 0.8 g protein/kg^{-1}/d^{-1} for 14 weeks accommodated with a decrease in skeletal muscle mass. The results from these long-term feeding studies suggest that the RDA for protein may not be adequate to completely meet the metabolic and physiological needs of older people and to maintain skeletal muscle mass. The public health implications of this accommodation response to the protein RDA in elderly people are largely unknown.

As the importance of nutrition as a tool to prevent and treat sarcopenia grows, knowledge of the protein requirement for older people is necessary. An accurate RDA for protein intake in older people is critical since the RDA serves as the foundation for "planning and procuring food supplies for population subgroups, for interpreting food consumption records for individuals and populations, for establishing the adequacy of food supplies in meeting national nutrition needs, for designing nutrition education programs, and for developing new products in industry."[8]

MARKERS OF PROTEIN METABOLISM AND NUTRITIONAL STATUS

The assessment of dietary protein requirements is limited by the availability of sensitive indicators of protein status.[1,8] Research has focused on several possible markers, including selected serum proteins, amino acid kinetics, and serum albumin and hepatic albumin synthesis. Several serum proteins were shown to be sensitive to changes in dietary protein intake and were thus suggested as possible indicators of visceral protein status, such as albumin, transferrin,

retinol-binding protein, thyroxine-binding prealbumin, and IGF-1 (somatomedin-C).[27] The usefulness of these serum proteins (other than albumin) to indicate inadequate protein intake by older people is largely unstudied. The usefulness of serum albumin concentration as a short-term marker of protein status, especially related to changes in protein intake, is limited.[28,29] The ability of the liver to increase the rate of albumin synthesis with increased dietary protein intake may be blunted in older people[30] and may provide insight into age-related changes in dietary protein needs. Several studies[24,31] indicate that 1-[^{13}C]leucine oxidation and postprandial and postabsorptive leucine balance studies are a useful addition to controlled nitrogen balance studies in the determination of protein requirements. Fereday et al[32] conducted 1-[^{13}C]leucine balance studies to determine leucine oxidation, utilization, and balance in young and older men and women. They concluded, "In this group of healthy older adults protein requirements as assessed from leucine balance studies were either similar to or less than those of younger adults."[32] The authors correctly cautioned, however, that "the present studies were not designed to assess a minimum protein requirement and define any influence of age."[32]

DIETARY PROTEIN INTAKE

The influence of age on protein intake depends on how the dietary data are reported. In quantitative terms, protein intake declines with advancing age in independent-living persons (Figure 2–1). Compared to adults in their 20s to 40s, protein intake was decreased by about 27% for men and 12% for women in their 70s. The age-associated decrease in protein intake occurred progressively over time. Starting at age 50–59 years, men had a 10% decrease in intake, another 6% decrease between age 60–69 years, and a further 13% decrease at age 70+ years. Older women had decreased protein intake by 2% at age 50–59 years, another 8% at 60–69 years, and a further 5% decrease for those 70 years and older.[33] The decline in protein intake is

Total Protein Intake of Adults

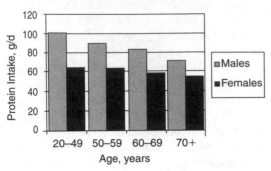

Figure 2–1 Total Protein Intake of Adults
Source: Adapted from: 1994–96 Continuing Survey of Food Intakes by Individuals and 1994–96 Diet and Health Knowledge Survey, Table Set 10. Report from the USDA Food Survey Research Group.

Relative Protein Intake of Adults

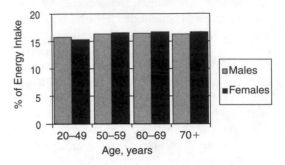

Figure 2–2 Relative Protein Intake of Adults
Source: Adapted from: Food and Nutrient Intakes by Individuals in the United States, by Race, 1994–96, Table Set 11. Report from the USDA Food Survey Research Group. Beltsville Human Nutrition Research Center.

likely due to a decrease in energy intake and not a change in the proportion of energy consumed as protein. Protein intake as a percentage of energy consumed remained constant in men and women across the age range of 20 to 70+ years (Figure 2–2). Both men and women consumed about 16% of energy as protein across all age groups.

With the amount of protein consumed by older persons progressively declining with advancing age, it is important to know how many older persons are consuming inadequate dietary protein. Using the RDA of 0.8 g protein/kg^{-1}/d^{-1} as the criteria for adequacy, results from the 1994–96 USDA Continuing Survey of Food Intakes (CSFI) by Individuals (Figure 2–3) indicate that 36% of men and 41% of women age 60 years and older did not habitually consume this minimum suggested intake, with 14% of men and 19% of women consuming less than 75% of the recommendation. The Salisbury Eye Evaluation,[34] a study of 2655 elderly men and women, aged 65 to 85 years from rural Maryland, reported the prevalence of inadequate protein intake as shown in Table 2–1. For the age and race groups combined, the prevalence of inadequate protein intake was 24% for older men and 31% for older

women. For the age and gender groups combined, blacks compared to whites had an 11% higher prevalence of inadequate protein intake. Based on data from all age groups combined, the prevalence of inadequate protein intake for Caucasian and African American women and men were as follows: 25% for Caucasian women, 37% for African American women, 20% for Caucasian men, and 28% for African American men. In general, the proportion of persons who consumed inadequate protein increased with advancing age, with 80- to 84-year-old African American women at greatest risk of inadequate protein intake (43% of this group). Collectively, the results from the CSFI survey[33] and the Salisbury Eye Evaluation study[34] suggest that 25–40% of elderly persons are at risk of consuming less than the RDA for protein. In 2002, there were about 35.6 million persons aged 65 years or older living in the United States (12.3% of the population), and the number of older persons is expected to double to about 70 million (20% of the population) by the year 2030.[35] Thus, the prevalence of inadequate protein intake among elderly persons currently may be estimated at 8.9–14.2 million and projected to be 17.5–28.0 million in the year 2030.

Protein Intake of Adults 60+ Years

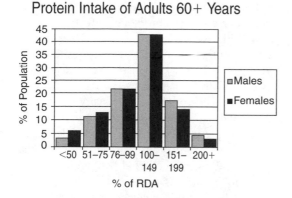

Figure 2–3 Protein Intake of Adults Aged 60+ Years
Source: Adapted from: Food and Nutrient Intakes by Individuals in the United States, by Race, 1994–96, Table Set 11. Report from the USDA Food Survey Research Group. Beltsville Human Nutrition Research Center.

DIETARY PROTEIN SOURCES

The Boston Nutrition Status Survey[36] reported food sources and the percentage of their contribution to protein intake, consumed by community living adults aged 60 years and older, as shown in Table 2–2. Red meat contributes the largest percentage (20%) of protein foods, with beef accounting for 13% and pork products accounting for 3%. The remaining 4% is from meat mixtures and other meats. Milk products contribute 18%, with 10% coming from milk and 6% from cheese. Poultry contributes 12% with

chicken supplying 10%. Grains, breads, and flours contribute 12%. Fish and shellfish contribute a total of 11% with 10% from fish and 1% shellfish. Vegetables make up 6% of total protein intake with 2% being derived from potatoes. Eggs and mixed dishes contributed 4% each. Fruits contributed 3% of protein intake with noncitrus fruits and citrus juices contributing 1.5% and 1%, respectively. The contribution of protein from cereals totaled 3% with ready-to-eat cereals at 2% and cooked cereal 1%. Legumes, nuts, and seeds contributed 2.5% to the total protein consumed.

EXERCISE EFFECTS ON PROTEIN REQUIREMENTS IN ELDERLY PERSONS

As stated previously, the RDA for protein is 0.8 $g/kg^{-1}/d^{-1}$ for all healthy adults. It may be of interest to question if circumstances would arise when a healthy older person might need more protein. This question may be appropriate for the older person who exercises regularly. In 2002, the Food and Nutrition Board Panel stated, "In view of the lack of compelling evidence to the contrary, no additional dietary protein is suggested for healthy adults undertaking resistance or endurance exercise."[1] This statement contrasts with the year 2000 conclusion from the American College of Sports Medicine (ACSM), American Dietetic Association (ADA), and Dietitians of

Table 2–1 Estimated Prevalence of Inadequate Protein Intake

| Age (y) | White | | Black | |
	Male (%)	Female (%)	Male (%)	Female (%)
66–69	14.3	18.7	27.0	31.1
70–74	21.1	26.1	28.3	38.2
75–79	24.8	28.8	35.5	36.8
80–84	19.6	25.4	21.9	43.4

Source: Adapted from Cid-Ruzafa J, Caulfield LE, et al. Nutrient intakes and adequacy among an older population on the eastern shore of Maryland: the Salisbury Eye Evaluation. *J Am Dietetic Assoc* 1999;99:564–571.

Table 2–2 Foods Contributing to Protein Intake

Major Food Groups	% ± SD
Meats	20±14
Milk/Milk Products	18±10
Poultry	12±12
Grain/Breads/Flours	12±6
Fish and Shellfish	11±12
Vegetables	6±3
Eggs	4±4
Mixed Dishes/Soups	4±6
Fruits/Fruit Juices	3±2
Breakfast Cereals	3±4
Legumes/Nuts/Seeds	2±4

Source: Adapted from the Boston Nutritional Status Survey, *Nutrition in the Elderly,* (1992) Smith-Gordon Company, Limited.

Canada (DC) committee that the need for protein of highly physically active persons is higher than for sedentary persons.[37] Specifically, strength-trained athletes may require as high as 1.6 to 1.7 g protein/kg^{-1}/d^{-1}, and endurance athletes may require 1.2 to 1.4 g protein/kg^{-1}/d^{-1}. The higher protein requirement of athletes was recommended to offset the increased use of protein for energy during exercise, provide substrate for muscle hypertrophy, and provide adequate amino acids for the repair of exercise-induced muscle damage. It may be appropriate to view the ACSM, ADA, and DC recommendations as the maximum protein requirements of highly trained athletes who routinely exercise at high intensity and long duration, training routines that most people do not attempt or maintain. It may also be appropriate to consider that the RDA for protein may be adequate for athletes to meet their basal needs, but be below that needed to enhance or optimize athletic performance,[38] although more research is required to resolve this issue. It is commonly thought that most athletes' customary diets provide enough protein to adequately meet need, especially when the diets contain sufficient energy and include high bioavailable sources of protein (eg, dairy, meats, eggs, and fish).[38] The protein intakes of older athletes are largely unknown.

It is difficult to establish the protein needs of the older athlete. Consistent with the general view of the RDA[1], Reaburn[39] suggests that older athletes might require less dietary protein than younger athletes because they have age-associated declines in fat-free and muscle masses and decreased volume and intensity of training. As stated earlier, the protein requirement for older people is not known with confidence, independent of exercise or training status. Research by Campbell et al.[25] suggests that the RDA for protein is a marginal intake, as evidenced by a significant decrease in midthigh muscle size of sedentary older persons who habitually consumed this amount of protein for 14 weeks. Campbell et al.[26] reported that older persons who performed strength training 3 days per week while consuming the RDA for protein achieved an offset of the muscle atrophy in the exercised muscle groups, but did not prevent the apparent loss of whole-body fat-free mass. A similar finding was shown in older men who apparently lost fat-free mass while consuming a lacto-ovo-vegetarian diet that contained the RDA for protein during a 12-week period of resistive training.[40] In contrast, fat-free mass and skeletal muscle hypertrophy occurred in older men who performed the same 12-week resistive exercise training program and consumed an omnivorous diet that provided 125% of the RDA for protein.[40] This differential body composition response with altered protein intakes was not observed in older men who consumed 129–144% of the RDA for protein from diets that contained either beef (omnivorous) or soy (lacto-ovo-vegetarian) foods during a 12-week period of resistive training.[41] Collectively, these results indicate that protein quantity, compared to protein source, had a greater effect on differential body composition and muscle hypertrophy responses to strength training in older men. These results also continue to draw into question whether the RDA for protein is sufficient for older persons to maximally hypertrophy muscle using strength training.

The older athlete should monitor protein intake and strive to consume about 1.2 to 1.4

g/kg^{-1}/d^{-1}. It is important to emphasize that currently, there are no data to suggest protein intakes above this range are more beneficial, and that this recommendation does not extend to persons with acute or chronic diseases that require therapeutic diets.

CONCLUSIONS

The RDA for protein is set at 0.8 g/kg^{-1}/d^{-1} for apparently healthy adults of all ages. It is estimated that 25–40% of persons aged 65 years and older consume less than this amount of protein. Chronological aging is associated with numerous changes that may impact dietary protein needs. These changes may include sarcopenia; increased body fat; decreased food intake; decreased physical activity; decreased physical functional capacity; and increased number and frequency of acute and chronic diseases. The loss of fat-free mass with advancing age theoretically results in a relatively lower protein requirement (per kg of body mass) compared to a younger adult. However, at present, there is not a consensus regarding the protein needs of elderly persons, with some research suggesting that the RDA should be higher than the current level. Short-term nitrogen balance studies are inconclusive, while the limited longer-term nitrogen balance studies suggest that the RDA is not sufficient to completely meet the metabolic and physiological needs of elderly persons, especially for persons who strive to offset sarcopenia and achieve muscle hypertrophy using strength training exercises. It is suggested that older sedentary persons consume at least 1.0 g protein/kg^{-1}/d^{-1}, and that older persons who habitually perform high-intensity exercise consume 1.2 to 1.4 g protein/kg^{-1}/d^{-1}.

REFERENCES

1. Institute of Medicine of the National Academies. *Dietary reference intakes for energy, carbohydrate, fiber, fat, fatty acids, cholesterol, protein, and amino acids (macronutrients)*. Washington, DC: National Academies Press; 2002.

2. FAO/WHO/UNU Expert Consultation. Energy and protein requirements. In: World Health Organization, Technical Report Series 724;1985:1–206.

3. Bales CW, Ritchie CS. Sarcopenia, weight loss, and nutritional frailty in the elderly. *Annu Rev Nutr* 2002;22: 309–323.

4. Roubenoff R. The pathophysiology of wasting in the elderly. *J Nutr* 1999;129:256S–259S.

5. Baumgartner RN, Waters DL, Gallagher D, Morley JE, Garry PJ. Predictors of skeletal muscle mass in elderly men and women. *Mech Aging Dev* 1999;107:123–136.

6. Heaney RP. Excess dietary protein may not adversely affect bone. *J Nutr* 1998;128:1054–1057.

7. Hannan MT, Tucker KL, Dawson-Hughes B, Cupples LA, Felson DT, Kiel DP. Effect of dietary protein on bone loss in elderly men and women: the Framingham Osteoporosis Study. *J Bone Miner Res* 2000;15: 2504–2512.

8. National Research Council Recommended Dietary Allowances. Washington, DC: National Academy Press, 1989.

9. Millward DJ, Fereday A, Gibson N, Pacy PJ. Aging, protein requirements, and protein turnover. *Am J Clin Nutr* 1997;66:774–786.

10. Rand WM, Pellett PL, Young VR. Meta-analysis of nitrogen balance studies for estimating protein requirements in healthy adults. *Am J Clin Nutr* 2003;77:109–127.

11. Campbell WW, Crim MC, Dallal GE, Young VR, Evans WJ. Increased protein requirements in elderly people: new data and retrospective reassessments. *Am J Clin Nutr* 1994;60:501–509.

12. Castaneda C, Charnley JM, Evans WJ, Crim MC. Elderly women accommodate to a low-protein diet with losses of body cell mass, muscle function, and immune response. *Am J Clin Nutr* 1995;62:30–39.

13. Uauy R, Scrimshaw NS, Young VR. Human protein requirements: nitrogen balance response to graded levels of egg protein in elderly men and women. *Am J Clin Nutr* 1978;31:779–785.

14. Zanni E, Calloway DH, Zezulka AY. Protein requirements of elderly men. *J Nutr* 1979;109:513–524.

15. Gersovitz M, Motil K, Munro HN, Scrimshaw NS, Young VR. Human protein requirements: assessment of the adequacy of the current Recommended Dietary Allowance for dietary protein in elderly men and women. *Am J Clin Nutr* 1982;35:6–14.

16. Cheng AH, Gomez A, Bergan JG, Lee TC, Monckeberg F, Chichester CO. Comparative nitrogen balance study between young and aged adults using three levels of protein intake from a combination wheat-soy-milk mixture. *Am J Clin Nutr* 1978;31:12–22.

17. Bunker VW, Lawson MS, Stansfield MF, Clayton BE. Nitrogen balance studies in apparently healthy elderly

people and those who are housebound. *Br J Nutr* 1987; 57:211–221.

18. Millward DJ, Roberts SB. Protein requirements of older individuals. *Nutr Res Rev* 1996;9:67–87.

19. Kurpad AV, Vaz M. Protein and amino acid requirements in the elderly. *Eur J Clin Nutr* 2000;54(suppl 3): S131–S142.

20. Morse MH, Haub MD, Evans WJ, Campbell WW. Protein requirement of elderly women: nitrogen balance responses to three levels of protein intake. *J Gerontol A Biol Sci Med Sci* 2001;56:M724–M730.

21. Rand WM, Scrimshaw NS. Conventional ("long-term") nitrogen balance studies for protein quality evaluation in adults: rationale and limitations. Protein quality in humans: assessment and in vitro estimation. Westport, CT: AVI Publishing Company, Inc; 1981.

22. Castaneda C, Dolnikowski GG, Dallal GE, Evans WJ, Crim MC. Protein turnover and energy metabolism of elderly women fed a low-protein diet. *Am J Clin Nutr* 1995;62:40–48.

23. Castaneda C, Gordon PL, Fielding RA, Evans WJ, Crim MC. Marginal protein intake results in reduced plasma IGF-I levels and skeletal muscle fiber atrophy in elderly women. *J Nutr Health Aging* 2000;4:85–90.

24. Young VR, Marchini JS. Mechanisms and nutritional significance of metabolic responses to altered intakes of protein and amino acids, with reference to nutritional adaptation in humans. *Am J Clin Nutr* 1990;51: 270–289.

25. Campbell WW, Trappe TA, Wolfe RR, Evans WJ. The recommended dietary allowance for protein may not be adequate for older people to maintain skeletal muscle. *J Gerontol A Biol Sci Med Sci* 2001;56:M373–M380.

26. Campbell WW, Trappe TA, Jozsi AC, Kruskall LJ, Wolfe RR, Evans WJ. Dietary protein adequacy and lower body versus whole body resistive training in older humans. *J Physiol* 2002;542:631–642.

27. Gibson RS. Assessment of protein status. *Principles of Nutritional Assessment*. New York, NY: Oxford University Press; 1990:307–348.

28. MacLennan WJ, Martin P, Mason BJ. Protein intake and serum albumin levels in the elderly. *Gerontology* 1977; 23:360–367.

29. Munro HN, McGandy RB, Hartz SC, Russell RM, Jacob RA, Otradovec CL. Protein nutriture of a group of free-living elderly. *Am J Clin Nutr* 1987;46:586–592.

30. Gersovitz M, Munro HN, Udall J, Young VR. Albumin synthesis in young and elderly subjects using a new sta-

ble isotope methodology: response to level of protein intake. *Metabolism* 1980;29:1075–1086.

31. Zello GA, Telch J, Clarke R, Ball RO, Pencharz PB. Reexamination of protein requirements in adult male humans by end-product measurements of leucine and lysine metabolism. *J Nutr* 1992;122:1000–1008.

32. Fereday A, Gibson NR, Cox M, Pacy PJ, Millward DJ. Protein requirements and aging: metabolic demand and efficiency of utilization. *Br J Nutr* 1997;77:685–702.

33. US Department of Agriculture. 1994–96 Continuing Survey of Food Intakes by Individuals and 1994–96 Diet and Health Knowledge Survey. Available at http://www.barc.usda.gov/bhnrc/foodsurvey/home.htm. Accessed December, 2003.

34. Cid-Ruzafa J, Caulfield LE, Barron Y, West SK. Nutrient intakes and adequacy among an older population on the eastern shore of Maryland: the Salisbury Eye Evaluation. *J Am Diet Assoc* 1999;99:564–571.

35. US Department of Health and Human Services. *Physical Activity and Health: A Report of the Surgeon General*. Atlanta, GA: US Department of Health and Human Services, Centers for Disease Control and Prevention, National Center for Chronic Disease Prevention and Health Promotion; 1996.

36. Hartz SC, Russell RM, Rosenberg IH, eds. *Nutrition in the Elderly; the Boston Nutritional Status Survey*. Gunter Grove, London: Smith-Gordon and Company Limited; 1992.

37. American College of Sports Medicine, American Dietetic Association, and Dietitians of Canada. Joint position statement: nutrition and athletic performance. *Med Sci Sports Exerc* 2000;32:2130–2145.

38. Lemon PW. Beyond the zone: protein needs of active individuals. *J Am Coll Nutr* 2000;19:513S–521S.

39. Reaburn P. Nutrition and the aging athlete. In: Burke L, Deakin V, eds. *Clinical Sports Nutrition*. Australia: McGraw-Hill; 2000:602–639.

40. Campbell WW, Barton ML Jr, Cyr-Campbell D, et al. Effects of an omnivorous diet compared with a lactoovovegetarian diet on resistance-training-induced changes in body composition and skeletal muscle in older men. *Am J Clin Nutr* 1999;70:1032–1039.

41. Haub MD, Wells AM, Tarnopolsky MA, Campbell WW. Effect of protein source on resistive-training-induced changes in body composition and muscle size in older men. *Am J Clin Nutr* 2002;76:511–517.

CHAPTER 3

Carbohydrate, Fat, and Fluid Requirements in Older Adults

Ronni Chernoff, PhD, RD, FADA

One of the features of human aging is the change in body composition that occurs with advancing age. In general, there is a decrease in lean body mass, a reduction in total body water, a loss of bone density, and an increase in the proportion of body fat. These changes are experienced by all living organisms; this has been previously described as senescence, the nonreversible deterioration of cells.[1] Body composition changes are difficult to quantify in elderly people due to the variability in the rate of aging among individuals.[2,3] These body composition alterations, which occur independent of declines in physical activity,[4] contribute to changes in nutrient requirements, metabolism, and physiologic function.[5]

ENERGY NEEDS IN OLD AGE

Most noticeable among the changes associated with body composition alterations is a decrease in energy required to maintain homeostasis, including body weight and function.[6] Accordingly, to avoid excess weight gain, caloric intake must be reduced. The Baltimore Longitudinal Study of Aging demonstrated a decrease in energy intake from 2700 kilocalories at age 30, to 2100 kilocalories by age 80 in male subjects.[6] As basal energy needs decrease and activity levels slow, less energy substrate is required to maintain lean body mass and support energy expenditure. However, reducing total caloric intake may place the individual at risk for deficiencies of intake of other nutrients.

The reduction in lean body mass, including both skeletal and visceral tissue, as well as other protein compartments such as blood components, antigens and antibodies, platelets, leukocytes, hormones, enzymes, cytokines, and other compounds, contributes to the reduction in calorie requirements.[7] The onset of serious chronic disease is associated with functional disability associated with diabetes, cardiovascular disease, renal and hepatic dysfunction, cancer, bone and joint diseases, autoimmune conditions, and dementias. This is a factor in decreased energy expenditure associated with increasingly sedentary behavior, although this effect may vary among older adults.[9–11] There is good evidence that there is a decrease in consumption of calories as well as a decrease in energy expenditure.[12] However, actual energy consumption must be measured accurately for a better sense of individual variability in both energy expenditure and energy needs.[13,14] This is particularly important when estimating needs to heal, fight infection, make new tissue, and address the demands of illness.

For older adults who do not reduce their caloric intake as they become more sedentary and reduce their basal energy requirements, weight gain may result. Obesity has been defined as body mass index ≥30; although specific guidelines for older adults are not in place, the prevalence of notable overweight continues to grow.[15]

Significant gain in weight may contribute to an additional reduction in activity level. Conversely, a decrease in physical activity associated with increasing disability may lead to weight gain, further exacerbating disabling conditions.

Most studies on energy requirements in adults often include a very small sample of elderly subjects, making extrapolation of current research data to clinical application in older adults unreliable. There are reports that elderly men do not respond similarly to young men after periods of energy restriction or overconsumption;[16,17] requirements for energy to maintain weight are often linked to energy consumption, but research indicates that this may not be reasonable in estimating energy needs for elderly individuals. Under any circumstances, prediction equations for energy requirements also do not give reliable estimates of energy requirements in elderly people, and indirect calorimetry should be employed when actual energy needs must be defined rather than grossly estimated.[18,19]

One approach that has been reported to estimate total energy expenditure is the use of doubly labeled water. When comparing results using doubly labeled water to measure total energy expenditure and resting energy expenditure measured using the same method, the total energy expenditure is slightly higher; this has been validated when direct measurements of energy expended are conducted.[20]

Using total body potassium, investigators have reported that this is the most accurate method to measure the decrease in lean body (fat-free) mass that best explains the reduction in resting energy expenditure with more accuracy than does doubly labeled water.[8] Regardless of the method used, it is clear that energy requirements decrease with advancing age. The clinical challenge is to continue to meet all nutrient requirements in a smaller caloric base of food consumed.

CARBOHYDRATE REQUIREMENTS

Carbohydrates are an essential component of a well-balanced diet. In its simplest form, glucose is an efficient energy substrate that can be used by all body tissues but is necessary for energy production in brain and red blood cells.[21,22] Requirements for dietary carbohydrate generally approximate 55–60% of total energy intake. The complexity of dietary carbohydrate may be as important as the percentage of calories contributed by carbohydrate-rich food.

Consumption of food that has had indigestible dietary fiber removed may contribute to gastrointestinal disorders commonly encountered in older adults, including constipation, diverticular disease, diabetes, and hyperlipidemia.[23] Dietary fiber is derived from structural components of plant cell walls and is mainly composed of plant polysaccharides and lignin, which are resistant to human digestive enzymes.[23] Hydroscopic particulate fiber with high pentosan content, such as wheat bran, increases fecal bulk and decreases gut transit time and intraluminal pressure within the colon.[23] These effects help to reduce the incidence of constipation and the formation of colonic diverticula. However, soluble fibers such as gums and pectins increase the viscosity of intestinal contents, increase gut transit time, and decrease the rate of small intestinal absorption.

Increased consumption of fibers such as guar, pectin, and tragacanth reduced insulin secretion following a test meal in normal subjects and increased carbohydrate tolerance in diabetics.[24] The mechanism of the positive effect seems to be related to delayed gastric emptying and reduced rate of absorption of carbohydrate in the small intestine. Recommendations from the American Diabetes Association as well as other national nutrition and diabetes organizations advise increased consumption of high-fiber carbohydrate-containing foods in the management of diabetes mellitus.[23]

Inclusion of purified fibers such as guar, pectin, and oat bran and high-fiber foods, including cereals, starchy vegetables, and beans, has been reported to lower serum lipids.[25] Decreases in total cholesterol, LDL cholesterol, and triglycerides without changes in HDL cholesterol have been reported.[26] The mechanism appears to be related to the decrease in gastric emptying and reduced intestinal absorption of cholesterol and triglycerides.

For the reasons described, it seems prudent to have a dietary fiber intake of 25–35 g/day and to include a variety of fibers from fresh fruits, vegetables, legumes, and whole-grain products. Every effort should be made to encourage a varied dietary intake of carbohydrate-containing foods daily in the diet of older adults.

FAT REQUIREMENTS

A desirable fat intake in elderly adults does not differ from that of younger adults. Fats and carbohydrates are the major macronutrient substrates that provide dietary energy, responsible for 85% to 95% of total caloric intake. Dietary fat is the most efficient source of energy, providing more than twice the energy of carbohydrate and protein per gram. As with younger adults, a minimum of 10% of total energy intake should be derived from fat to assure an adequate dietary intake of fat-soluble vitamins and essential fatty acids. Essential fatty acids are required for the synthesis of prostaglandins and cell membrane phosopholipids.[27]

Recommendations for dietary fat intake to be limited to 30% or less with saturated fats providing from 8% to 10%, polyunsaturated fats being approximately 10%, and monounsaturated fats making up the difference of 15% of total fat intake are the same for older versus younger adults.[28] Dietary cholesterol intake is recommended to be 300 mg/day or less. Although total cholesterol is generally considered an important risk factor for coronary heart disease, its impact in elderly people is unknown. In a 5-year prospective study that included 4066 men and women older than age 71 years, elevated total cholesterol levels were associated with a similar pattern of death from coronary heart disease as seen in younger adults (younger than age 70 years), but first adjustments for age, preexisting cardiovascular disease, risk factors, and general health status had to be made. Unexpectedly, the subject group with the lowest total cholesterol levels (<160 mg/dL) had the highest incidence

of preexisting cardiovascular disease, the highest risk factors for cardiovascular disease, the highest indices of poor health, and the highest crude coronary heart disease mortality.[29] It appears that elevated total cholesterol levels remain a risk factor for death from coronary artery disease in elderly persons. High-density lipoprotein cholesterol values less than 35 mg/dL predict coronary heart disease mortality and occurrence of new events in individuals older than 70 years.[30]

However, there are some contradictory outcomes associated with lowering dietary fat intake in older adults. In one study, a decrease in dietary fat intake was associated with an increased risk of ischemic stroke in middle-aged men.[31] Additionally, low cholesterol levels have been associated with short-term mortality after ischemic stroke in older patients.[32] However, in a 20-year follow-up study of men in the Framingham Heart Study, the risk of ischemic stroke declined as intake of saturated and monounsaturated, but not polyunsaturated, fat increased.[33] Specific recommendations for dietary fat modifications must be made on an individual basis based on a complete profile of cardiovascular and stroke risk factors.

The prevention of coronary heart disease in older adults deserves consideration, although this chronic condition develops over years. One approach to reducing risk in older adults is to reduce the intake of saturated fat and simultaneously increase the intake of polyunsaturated and monounsaturated fat, keeping the total fat intake about the same.[34] In another trial, subjects who had previously suffered a myocardial infarction were put on a Mediterranean-style diet with more complex carbohydrate; fruit; green vegetables; fish, with less beef, lamb, or pork; and monounsaturated cooking oils. The group on this type of diet had fewer cardiac events and deaths at 2-year follow-up than did a control group who made no dietary modifications.[35] Even on this modified diet, there was no change in total cholesterol or low-density lipoprotein cholesterol levels.

In another study of obese, postmenopausal women, subjects were put on an American Heart Association (AHA) Step 1 diet followed by a weight-loss diet. This combination of dietary modifications decreased triglyceride levels and total low-density and high-density lipoprotein levels in women who had hypercholesterolemia. However, this combination had no effect in women who had normal cholesterol levels or were mildly hypercholesterolemic. The authors' conclusion was that this dietary regimen of an AHA Step 1 diet and weight loss would help obese, postmenopausal women with elevated lipid profiles, but would have no impact on women with normal lipid profiles.[36] Nevertheless, reduction of dietary fat will reduce overall caloric intake and contribute to weight loss or the avoidance of obesity in older adults.

Diet is a major factor, although not the only factor, that influences total cholesterol and low-density lipoprotein cholesterol. In younger adults, lifestyle changes, including diet and exercise, are often recommended. These recommendations may contribute to weight loss and a slight reduction in cardiovascular disease risk factors in adults older than age 70 years.[37,38] Management of weight appears to be a significant factor in health status and cardiovascular health in older individuals.[39] More recently, use of statins has been shown to reduce cardiovascular events in adults aged 65–80 years.[40]

It is noteworthy that reduction of serum cholesterol levels in elderly, institutionalized individuals may not be beneficial. There has been a higher mortality rate in older men when cholesterol levels were depressed.[41,42]

FLUID REQUIREMENTS

Water is an essential nutrient that often does not receive the attention it needs in older adults. Total body water decreases with age and with the decrease in total lean body mass. In older adults, inadequate fluid intake may lead to rapid dehydration, which has its own potentially risky problems; these include hypotension, constipation, nausea and vomiting, mucosal dryness, decreased urinary output, elevated body temperature, and mental confusion.[43] Consequences of inadequate fluid intake may also include an inappropriate dosage of medications. The dose

level of many medications is calculated on body weight and an assumption that the drug will be distributed through the body to reach its intended organ or tissue with water serving as a diluent; a decrease in body water may lead to a greater concentration of a drug than intended, which may prove toxic.[43]

Water also has a role as a thermal buffer to protect the individual from hypo- or hyperthermia. In older adults, there is a decrease in sweating and other thermoregulatory responses, making a physiologic adjustment to periods of environmental shifts in temperature difficult to accommodate. The poor response to dehydration associated with extreme environmental temperature can lead to decreased plasma volume and osmolality and may result in death during periods of extreme environmental heat.[44]

In older adults, consuming adequate fluid intake, whether from water or other beverages, becomes a greater challenge than it is in younger adults. Thirst mechanisms and sensitivity are compromised in elderly people and there may also be external factors that affect adequate fluid intake.

Thirst sensitivity decreases with age and, in the aging kidney, there is a decreased urinary concentrating ability and a reduced ability to compensate for a high water load.[45] The decrease in fluid intake is due to alterations in mechanisms that control thirst sensitivity, particularly a decrease in osmoreceptors and baroreceptors and secretion of vasopressin.[45,46] The primary stimulus of thirst is increased plasma osmolality; this contributes to an increase in osmotic pressure, which stimulates vasopressin secretion and increased water intake.[45]

Another mechanism that stimulates thirst is hemodynamic factors, particularly hypovolemia and hypotension. The carotid artery and aortic arch are sites for baroreceptors that are responsive to changes in blood pressure. Increased blood pressure or blood volume will excite baroreceptors, turn off vasopressin release, and decrease thirst.[45] Additionally there is a variety of endocrine and environmental factors that also affect thirst. Endocrine factors include secretion of renal angiotensin and atrial natriuretic peptide secretion. Environmental factors include climate, temperature, humidity, and availability of water and food.[45] Other factors that may be more important in elderly adults include medical problems, diuretic abuse, polypharmacy, low levels of hormone production, and a voluntary decrease of fluid intake to manage mild incontinence.

Dehydration may be a serious problem for older adults. Along with disordered thirst control mechanisms and inadequate intake of adequate fluid for maintenance,[46,47] older adults who have fever, infection, institutionalization, immobility, dementia, coma, excess loss (hemorrhage, diarrhea, vomiting, diabetes insipidus), or acute illness may become chronically dehydrated.[43,48,49] With age, the kidneys' ability to concentrate urine or efficiently conserve water may also impact fluid balance.[50] Hypotonic dehydration results when sodium losses exceed water losses; this is usually diagnosed when serum sodium levels are less than 135 mmol/L and serum osmolality is less than 280 mmol/kg body weight.

There has been a series of studies that indicate that when compared to young men, older men who are water deprived for a period of time will not rehydrate to baseline levels as younger men will when ad lib access to water is allowed.[49,51]

There are indications that many elderly adults, particularly those who are institutionalized, are not consuming adequate amounts of fluid.[52,53] Although the usual stated requirement for fluid intake is eight 8-ounce glasses of fluid/day, data supporting this recommendation do not appear to exist. Actual need is probably in the range of six 8-ounce glasses of fluid/day. Fluid intake should be adequate to compensate for normal losses through the kidneys, bowel, lungs, and skin, as well as losses associated with fever, vomiting, diarrhea, or hemorrhage.

Diagnosis of dehydration is more difficult than it may seem because the signs of clinical dehydration can be confusing.[54,55] Dehydration is associated with increased morbidity and mortality; appropriate, aggressive rehydration can improve clinical outcomes. Dehydration may truly exist if serum osmolality is greater than 295 mOsm. Intravascular volume depletion is diagnosed with a BUN:creatinine ratio greater than 20 or serum sodium (Na) that is greater than 145 g/dL.[54] It is common for a clinical judgment of dehydration to be made without laboratory values to support the diagnosis.

Adequate fluid intake is often a problem in healthy, free-living elderly, but the challenge of adequate hydration in institutionalized elderly may be of greater concern. Chronically ill, functionally dependent elderly people may not meet their fluid needs voluntarily and may have to be strongly encouraged to drink sufficient fluids.[56] Individuals who are dependent on nutrition support, including both chronically and critically ill elderly people, may be underhydrated because they are receiving inadequate volumes of nutrient solutions or they are receiving hypertonic formulas without adequate solute-free water to compensate for the solid solute load of enteral feedings or the hypertonicity of parenteral solutions.[44]

Conversely, the possibility of water intoxication in older adults may present a similar, and possibly more challenging, problem in this population. This condition is not well recognized; symptoms may include hyponatremia, depression, mental confusion, and anorexia. When serum sodium concentrations are depressed (levels at 110 mEq/L or less), the individual may experience seizures, stupor, and central nervous system (CNS) damage.[43] Water intoxication may be due to decreased renal capacity to excrete excess water or hyponatremia due to oversecretion of arginine vasopressin associated with pulmonary and CNS disorders, stroke, pneumonia, tuberculosis, and other diagnoses. When decreased renal blood flow exists, treatment should focus on maximizing renal function; volume repletion if extracellular fluid depletion exists; and normalization of blood pressure.

Estimating actual fluid needs is challenging and there are several methods that may be used to gauge an individual's actual requirement. Methods commonly used to determine fluid needs in individuals include calculating 30 mL/kg body weight with a minimum of 1500 mL/day;

1 mL per kilocalorie consumed; or 100 mL/kg for the first 10 kg of actual weight, 50 mL/kg for the next 10 kg actual body weight, and 15 mL/kg for remaining weight. The first method (30 mL/kg body weight) approximates fluid needs most accurately in institutionalized elderly persons; additional research needs to be conducted to better estimate actual needs of older adults.[57] For individuals who are tube-feeding dependent, provision of free water at approximately 25% of the total formula volume is recommended.

To rehydrate individuals who are dehydrated, insensible losses of 600–1200 mL must be accounted for as baseline before adding fluid adequate to rehydrate any individual. Intravenous fluid repletion with a physiologic solution will work most rapidly. For acute rehydration in someone losing fluid rapidly such as from vomiting or diarrhea, 2.5–4.0 L of fluid may be needed to replace acute losses and restore normal hydration status. Strong and chronic encouragement for oral fluid intake may be necessary to maintain hydration status.[58]

CONCLUSIONS

For older adults, macronutrient recommendations may be somewhat altered. Encouragement of consumption of complex carbohydrates rather than simple carbohydrates may contribute to adequate dietary fiber intake. Reduction of saturated fat, with an increased emphasis on consumption of poly- and monounsaturated fats, and decreased overall fat intake will compensate for lower basal energy requirements and a decreased activity level often encountered in older adults. Meeting fluid needs in older adults is challenging because thirst mechanisms are not as sensitive in older adults as they are in younger individuals. Attention to overall fluid intake in healthy free-living, chronically ill, functionally dependent, or acutely ill elderly is key to maintaining optimal health in any person but particularly important for this age group. Needs for these macronutrients (carbohydrate, fat, fluid) can be met with awareness of individual requirements, imagination, and attention to daily intake.

REFERENCES

1. Vijg J, Wei JY. Understanding the biology of aging: the key to prevention and therapy. *J Amer Geriatr Soc* 1995; 43:426.

2. Dupler TL, Tolson H. Body composition prediction equations for elderly men. *J Gerontol: MED SCI* 2000; 55A(3):M180–M184.

3. Baumgartner RN, Stauber PM, McHugh D, Koehler KM, Garry PJ. Cross-sectional age differences in body composition in persons 60+ years of age. *J Gerontol: MED SCI* 1995;50A:M307–M316.

4. Rutherford O, Jones DA. The relationship of muscle and bone loss and activity levels with age in women. *Age and Aging* 1992;21:286–293.

5. Ritz P. Factors affecting energy and macronutrient requirements in elderly people. *Publ Health Nutr* 2001; 4(2B):561–568.

6. McGandy RB, Barrows CH, Spanias A, Meredith A, Stone JL, Norris AH. Nutrient intakes and energy expenditure in men of different ages. *J Gerontol* 1966;21: 581–587.

7. Young VR. Energy requirements in the elderly. *Nutr Revs* 1992;50(4):95–101.

8. Roubenoff R, Hughes VA, Dallal GE, Nelson ME, Morganti C, Kehayias JJ, Fiatarone Singh MA, Roberts S. The effect of gender and body composition method on the apparent decline in lean mass-adjusted resting metabolic rate with age. *J Gerontol: MED SCI* 2000; 55A(12):M757–M760.

9. Reilly JJ, Lord A, Bunker VW, Prentice AM, Coward WA, Thomas AJ, Briggs RS. Energy balance in healthy elderly women. *British J Nutr* 1993;69:21–27.

10. Voorrips LE, van Acker TM-CJ, Deurenberg P, van Staveren WA. Energy expenditure at rest and during standardized activities: a comparison between elderly and middle-aged women. *Am J Clin Nutr* 1993;58:15–20.

11. Campbell WW, Cyr-Campbell D, Weaver JA, Evans WJ. Energy requirement for long-term body weight maintenance in older women. *Metabolism* 1997;46(8):884–889.

12. Kannel WB, Gordon T. *The Framingham Diet Study: An Epidemiological Investigation of Cardiovascular Disease.* Washington DC: US Department of Health, Education and Welfare, Public Health Service; 1970.

13. Greteback RJ, Boileau RA. Self-reported energy intake and energy expenditure in elderly women. *J Am Dietet Assoc* 1998;98(5):574–576.

14. Deurenberg P, van der Kooij K, Evers P, Hulshof T. Assessment of body composition by bioelectrical impedance in a population aged >60 y. *Am J Clin Nutr* 1990;51:3–6.

15. Jensen GL, Rogers J. Obesity in older persons. *J Am Dietet Assoc* 1998;98(11):1308–1311.

16. Roberts S. Effects of aging on energy requirements and the control of food intake in men. *J Gerontol:MED SCI* 1995;50A:101–106.

17. Clarkston WK, Pantano MM, Morley JE, Horowitz M, Littlefield JM, Burton FR. Evidence for the anorexia of aging: gastrointestinal transit and hunger in healthy elderly vs young adults. *Am J Physiol* 1997;272.

18. Frankenfield D, Roth-Yousey L, Compher C. Comparison of predictive equations for resting metabolic rate in healthy, non-obese individuals: a systematic review. *J Am Dietet Assoc* 2005;105(5):775–789.

19. Blanc S, Schoeller DA, Bauer D, Danielson ME, Tylavsky F, Simonsick EM, Harris TB, Kritchevsky SB, Everhart JE. Energy requirements in the eighth decade of life. *Am J Clin Nutr* 2004;79(2):303–310.

20. Roberts SB. Energy requirements for older individuals. *Eur J Clin Nutr* 1996;50(suppl 1):S112–S118.

21. Kohlmeier M. Carbohydrates, alcohols, and organic acids. In Kohlmeierm: *Nutrient Metabolism.* Boston, MA: Academic Press; 2003.

22. Brodsky IG. Hormone, cytokine, and nutrient interactions. In Shils ME, Olson JA, Shike M, Ross AC, eds. *Modern Nutrition in Health and Disease,* 9th ed. Philadelphia, PA: Williams & Wilkins; 1999.

23. Jenkins DJA, Wolever TMS, Jenkins AL. Fiber and other dietary factors affecting nutrient absorption and metabolism. In Shils ME, Olson JA, Shike M, Ross AC, eds. *Modern Nutrition in Health and Disease,* 9th ed. Philadelphia, PA: Williams & Wilkins; 1999.

24. Vinik AI, Jenkins DJA. Dietary fiber in the management of diabetes. *Diabetes Care* 1988;11:160–173.

25. Ballesteros MN, Cabrera RM, Saucedo MS, Yepiz-Plascencia GM, Ortega MI, Valencia ME. Dietary fiber and lifestyle influence serum lipids in free living adult men. *J Am Coll Nutr* 2001;20(6):649–655.

26. Seim HC, Holtmeier KB. Effects of a six-week, low-fat diet on serum cholesterol, body weight, and body measurements. *Fam Pract Res J* 1992;12(4):411–419.

27. Ausman LM, Russell RM. Nutrition in the elderly. In Shils ME, Olson JA, Shike M, Ross AC, eds. *Modern Nutrition in Health and Disease,* 9th ed. Philadelphia, PA: Williams & Wilkins; 1999.

28. National Cholesterol Education Program. Second report of the expert panel on detection, evaluation, and treatment of high blood cholesterol in adults. *Circulation* 1994;89:1333–1432.

29. Corti MC, Guralnick JM, Salive ME, et al. Clarifying the direct relation between total cholesterol levels and death from coronary heart disease in older persons. *Ann Intern Med* 1997;126:753–760.

30. Corti MC, Guralnick JM, Salive ME, et al. HDL cholesterol predicts coronary heart disease mortality in older persons. *JAMA* 1995;274:539–544.

31. Gillman MW, Cupples LA, Millen BE, Ellison RC, Wolf PA. Inverse association of dietary fat with development of ischemic stroke in men. *JAMA* 1997; 278:2145–2150.

32. Zuliani G, Cherubini A, Atti AR, Blè A, Vavalle C, Di Todaro F, Bendetti C, Volpato S, Marinescu MG, Senin U, Fellini R. Low cholesterol levels are associated with short-term mortality in older patients with ischemic stroke. *J Gerontol:MED SCI* 2004;59A:M293–M297.

33. Siguel E. A new relationship between total/high density lipoprotein cholesterol and polyunsaturated fatty acids. *Lipids* 1996;31:S51–S56.

34. Oliver MF. It is more important to increase the intake of unsaturated fats than to decrease the intake of saturated fats: evidence from clinical trials relating to ischemic heart disease. *Am J Clin Nutr* 1997;66 (suppl):980S–986S.

35. de Loregil M, Renaud S, Mamelle N, et al. Mediterranean α-linolenic acid-rich diet in the secondary prevention of coronary heart disease. *Lancet* 1994;343:1454–1459.

36. Nicklas BJ, Katzel LI, Bunyard LB, Dennis KE, Goldberg AP. Effects of an American Heart Association diet and weight loss on lipoprotein lipids in obese, postmenopausal women. *Am J Clin Nutr* 1997;66: 853–859.

37. Law MR, Wald NJ, Thompson SC. By how much and how quickly does reduction in serum cholesterol concentration lower risk of ischemic heart disease? *Am J Public Health* 1994;308:367–372.

38. Fox AA, Thompson JL, Butterfield GE, Gylfadottir U, Moynihan S, Spiller G. Effects of diet and exercise on common cardiovascular disease risk factors in moderately obese older women. *Am J Clin Nutr* 1996;63: 225–233.

39. Harris TB, Sacage PJ, Tell GS, Haan M, Kumanyika S, Lynch JC. Carrying the burden of cardiovascular risk in old age: associations of weight and weight change with prevalent cardiovascular disease, risk factors, and health status in the Cardiovascular Health Study. *Am J Clin Nutr* 1997;66:837–844.

40. Aronow WS. Treatment of older persons with hypercholesterolemia with and without cardiovascular disease. *J Gerontol:MED SCI* 2001;56A:M138–M145.

41. Rudman D, Mattson DR, Nagraj HS, et al. Antecedents of death in the men of a VA nursing home. *JAGS* 1987; 35:496–502.

42. Rudman D, Mattson DE, Feller AG, Nagraf HS. A mortality risk index for men in a Veterans Administration extended care facility. *JPEN* 1989;13(2):189–195.

43. Chernoff R. Thirst and fluid requirements in the elderly. *Nutr Revs* 1994;52:132–136.

44. Miescher E, Fortney SM. Responses to dehydration and rehydration during heat exposure in young and older men. *Am J Physiol* 1989;257:R1050–1056.

45. Naitoh M, Burrell LM. Thirst in elderly subjects. *J Nutr Health Aging* 1998;2(3):172–177.

46. Rolls BJ, Phillips PA. Aging and disturbances of thirst and fluid balance. *Nutr Revs* 1990;48(3):137–144.

47. Ramsay DJ. The importance of thirst in maintenance of fluid balance. *Baillieres Clin Endocrinol Metabol* 1989; 3(2):371–391.

48. Armstrong-Esther CA, Browne KD, Armstrong-Esther DC, Sander L. The institutionalized elderly: dry to the bone! *Intl J Nurs Studies* 1996;33(6):619–628.

49. Phillips PA, Bretherton M, Johnston CI, Gray L. Reduced osmotic thirst in healthy elderly men. *Am J Physiol* 1991;261(1 Pt 2):R166–171.

50. McGee M, Jensen GL. Nutrition in the elderly. *J Clin Gastroenterol* 2000;30(4):372–380.

51. Phillips PA, Rolls BJ, Ledingham JG, et al. Reduced thirst after water deprivation in healthy elderly men. *N Engl J Med* 1984;311:753–759.

52. Haveman-Nies A, de Groot LC, Van Staveren WA. Fluid intake of elderly Europeans. *J Nutr Health Aging* 1997; 1(3):151–155.

53. Kleiner SM. Water: an essential but overlooked nutrient. *J Am Dietet Assoc* 1999;99(2):200–206.

54. Thomas DR, Tariq SH, Makhdomm S, Haddad R, Moinuddin A. Physician misdiagnosis of dehydration in older adults. *J Am Med Dir Assoc* 2004;5:S31–S34.

55. Robinson BE, Weber H. Dehydration despite drinking: beyond the BUN/creatinine ratio. *J Am Med Dir Assoc* 2004;suppl:S68–S71.

56. Holben DH, Hassell JT, Williams JL, Helle B. Fluid intake compared with established standards and symptoms of dehydration among elderly residents of a long-term care facility. *J Am Dietet Assoc* 1999;99(11):1447–1450.

57. Chidester JC, Spangler AA. Fluid intake in the institutionalized elderly. *J Am Dietet Assoc* 1997;97(1):23–28.

58. Bennett RG. Oral rehydration therapy for older adults. *Dietet Curr* 1992;19:15–18.

CHAPTER 4

Vitamin Metabolism and Requirements in the Elderly: Selected Aspects

Paolo M. Suter, MD, MS

In many areas of the world, aging of the population represents one of the major demographic shifts. The population strata of the 60+ group constitutes the fastest growing group in most Western countries and will soon also be the fastest growing group in many other societies (eg, India or People's Republic of China).[1] Many of these elderly people are enjoying good health, but for a large segment of them, aging is associated with continuing impairment of health and well being. The chronic diseases of aging are on the rise worldwide,[2,3] and more and more individuals are affected by these, potentially in part preventable, diseases. Evidence has accumulated that the roots for the development of the chronic diseases of aging are laid early in life and that the vitamin nutriture may be of special importance.[4]

During the last few years, important new functions of certain vitamins in the modulation of chronic disease risk have been found (eg, the role of homocysteine as a risk factor for several disease conditions).[5,6] In view of the aging of our society, the maintenance of an adequate intake of all essential nutrients, including all vitamins, becomes more important than ever, but the intake of the recommended amounts is not always easily achievable. Selected new aspects of vitamin metabolism will be discussed in relation to the aging process and chronic diseases.

The aim of any medical strategy in relation to aging should not only be that more people live longer, but also that they live well. This is a function not only of the vitamin nutrition, but of overall nutrition and other lifestyle factors that are not directly related to nutrition (ie, physical activity, smoking, and psychological factors). Nevertheless, in formulating recommendations for the nutriture of older adults, it should be remembered that a 50 to 60-year-old person is very different from a 70-year-old or person older than 70 years. The whole elderly population represents an extremely heterogeneous group as compared to younger population groups. This heterogeneity has been accounted for in the last Dietary Reference Intakes (DRI) by adding separate recommendations for the age group of those older than 70 years as compared to the "young old" (the age group 51–70 years).[7–9] This heterogeneity has important consequences for medical therapy, as well as for the formulation of dietary guidelines. The only common aspect in elderly people is that they share several factors putting them at increased risk of malnutrition and chronic diseases.

An adequate intake of the different vitamins is not only of importance for the prevention of the development of deficiency, but also the control of chronic disease risk.[10–12] During the last few years, new functions and health effects of vitamins have been identified.[13] Vitamins may play a role in prevention of the pathogenesis of most chronic diseases of aging such as decreased cognitive function, cardiovascular diseases, and cancer.[13–15] Some of these aspects will be discussed in the following sections.

VITAMIN A

The importance of vitamin A and the vitamin A precursors in the form of different carotenoids is well known, and the classical vitamin A deficiency signs were described a long time ago for the first time but are only very rarely encountered in modern society.[16,17] Vitamin A (retinol) plays an important role in growth, cell differentiation, vision, and maintenance of immune function.[17] The discovery of new functions of vitamin A, especially its role in the regulation of gene expression in the nuclear retinoid receptors,[18–21] constitutes what has been claimed to be the "retinoid revolution."[22] The present Recommended Dietary Allowance (RDA) for the age group of those older than 51 years is lower than in earlier editions of the recommendations: 900 μg of Retinol Activity Equivalents (RAE) for older men and 700 μg RAE for older women.[8] In view of the new equivalency factors for the bioconversion of different carotenoids to retinol it is recommended to use the "new units" of RAE instead of μg retinol equivalents (RE) or international units (IU). Vitamin A can also be obtained by the conversion of provitamin A carotenoids.[23] Covering vitamin A needs by an increased ingestion of carotenoids might actually be a good and safe strategy.[23]

Others, however, have recommended an even lower intake of 700 μg and 600 μg RAE for men and women, respectively.[24] In view of the evidence discussed by these authors, this recommendation may eventually be right. Epidemiological studies would support the lower figures of intake recommendations because the vitamin A intake of many elderly is below the recommendations, but their vitamin A levels remain well within the limits of normality.[25–33] In the follow-up analysis of the Euronut Survey in Europe on Nutrition and the Elderly, a Concerted Action (SENECA) study, retinal intake decreased over the period of 4 to 5 years, but the prevalence of biochemical vitamin A deficiency was nevertheless zero.[34] Vitamin A intakes vary widely, and up to 70% of elderly people, depending on their income, sex, and race, have been shown to have vitamin A intakes less than 660 μg RAE (corresponding to two-thirds of the 1989 RDA). These data must be interpreted with caution because the vitamin A content of food varies considerably and there are technical difficulties in analyzing the vitamin A content of food. Some elderly populations, however, may consume more than the recommendations.[30] Institutionalization is associated with an overall impairment of nutritional status, including lower vitamin A intakes than in free-living elderly.[31] Some studies describe a sex difference in plasma retinol levels and β-carotene levels that is in part attributable to differences in the plasma lipid levels, as well as changes in the concentration of retinol-binding protein.[31]

Plasma carotenoids are a very heterogeneous group of chemical substances, including lycopene, α-carotene, β-carotene, zeaxanthin, lutein, and β-cryptoxanthin.[17,23,35,36] The importance of these carotenoids varies considerably, but they may be of great importance in the pathogenesis of different age-related chronic conditions such as cardiovascular diesease or age-related macular degeneration and cataracts.[17,37] A recent study reported a direct association between lycopene status and functional capacity (including dependence in self-care) in women aged 77 to 98 years.[38] Whether this described relationship between functional parameters and lycopene is causal remains unclear. Low-density lipoprotein (LDL) cholesterol is the major carrier of lycopene in the blood.

The protective effects of antioxidants[23] in different disease processes are well known.[11,13,39–43] The increased intake of carotenoids from fruits and vegetables was found to be associated with a decreased cardiovascular mortality in an elderly population of Massachusetts residents.[44] Others described a similar finding but reported only a small effect of carotenoid *supplementation* on the reduction of cardiovascular risk.[45] The lower mortality in subjects with plasma carotenoids above the median in the latter study is probably caused, not only by improved carotenoid status, but probably also by other nutrients and phytochemicals. A colinearity of nutrients is very important and must be considered in any interpretation of the association between a single nutrient and a specific disease. An increase of vitamin C, vitamin E, or carotenoids is usually associated with a greater plasma concentration of one or both other vitamins[46] and is a marker of an overall healthier lifestyle.

Vitamin A may have considerable toxicity.[8,17,24] In view of the widespread vitamin A supplement use by the elderly, it has been suggested that the rather high intake in combination with the increased absorption of vitamin A with age could contribute to toxicity in elderly individuals (especially those who have high vitamin A intakes from supplements and/or fortified food).[47–50] There are two forms of hypervitaminosis A: chronic and acute. Acute hypervitaminosis A is rare in elderly people, but chronic toxicity can be seen in this group.[51]

Chronic diseases of old age may influence vitamin A nutriture at the level of intake, absorption, recycling, tissue utilization, and storage. Of special importance in the elderly are chronic liver diseases, often related to the chronic ingestion of alcohol, which impairs the storage of vitamin A in the liver as well as the ability of the liver to synthesize retinol-binding proteins.[52–56] In normal aging, defined as aging in the absence of any relevant disease, the liver hardly senesces, and constitutive liver functions are maintained, suggesting no alterations in vitamin A metabolism. In view of the widespread intake of drugs in the elderly, it must be remembered that several drugs (including ethanol and barbiturates) are capable of affecting the metabolism of vitamin A by accelerating hepatic retinol breakdown. Chronic toxicity is mainly due to the long-term intake of vitamin A supplements and is hardly due to excessive intakes of vitamin A from diet alone. Due to the availability of over-the-counter vitamin A capsules containing up to 20,000 IU of vitamin A, the risk of toxicity may be high. The supplemental intake of vitamin A may be associated with greater levels of circulating retinyl esters

in fasting blood. These high retinyl esters may be an indicator of vitamin A toxicity and liver damage.[51,57]

In a study using the relative dose response (RDR) for assessing vitamin A intake in the elderly, the maximum plasma retinol response occurred in elderly subjects 60 to 120 minutes later than in younger subjects.[58] Therefore, the procedures of the RDR should be modified when used with older adults. Unlike young people or children, elderly people should have their fasting vitamin A levels measured for correct assessment of vitamin A intake.[59]

The effects of vitamin A deficiency on immune functions in children are well known. In recent years, the effect of vitamin A and carotenoids on immune functions of elderly people have been evaluated in several studies.[20] The effects of this vitamin are of special interest because the immune system plays a crucial role in health maintenance and potentially also the aging process per se.

Santos et al[60] evaluated the effect of β-carotene on natural killer cell activity in a small sample of young old (aged 51–64 years) and older old (age range 65–86 years) participants of the Physician's Health Study. In this placebo-controlled study, the subjects received 50 mg of β-carotene every second day. With increasing age, natural killer cell activity declined only in the placebo group. In the younger subjects, however, β-carotene had no effect on natural killer cell activity.[60] Other nutrients such as vitamins C and E have also been shown to have the potential to modulate immune function in aging. In this context, the effect of vitamin A on pulmonary function in patients with chronic obstructive pulmonary disease (COPD) is interesting. This disease becomes more prevalent with age, and it is estimated that up to 20% of the elderly are afflicted to some degree with COPD. Several epidemiologic studies have shown an inverse association between COPD and vitamin A nutriture. Lower plasma vitamin A levels have been described in subjects with COPD, and supplementation with vitamin A may result in improved lung function tests.[61] Future studies will show whether this association is of clinical relevance. Because breathing is impaired, functional abnormalities due to COPD are often complicated by miscellaneous nutritional deficiencies, especially during food intake. This leads to higher energy requirements and reduced food intake to avoid breathing difficulties during eating. A recent study in younger subjects accumulated evidence suggesting that the different antioxidants may play an important role in bronchial reactivity and thus the prevalence and incidence of asthma and other allergic diseases.[62] Vitamin A deficiency results in an impairment of the response to viral and bacterial infection at several stages of the immune response.[63] Data from the Scotland health survey reported that the most beneficial combination of dietary components for respiratory health is found in natural foodstuffs, especially fresh fruits.[64] In this study, a dose/response relationship was found between fruit consumption and pulmonary function.[64] Again, as for other nutrients, potential health benefits are hardly obtained from a single nutrient but from an ideal combination found in natural foodstuffs.

The safety of β-carotene *supplements* is a matter of dispute (β-carotene from food sources alone does not bear any toxicity).[23] In view of current knowledge, a recommendation of β-carotene supplements is warranted only after a careful evaluation of the clinical constellation of a patient. Several large trials reported a higher mortality in subjects receiving β-carotene.[65–67] Data from the Finnish study and the Carotene and Retinol Efficiency Test (CARET) trial reported an association with alcohol intake.[66,67] The negative β-carotene effects became stronger in subjects consuming more than 11 g of alcohol per day. In view of this, the intake of fruits and vegetables should be increasingly promoted, particularly in the elderly. The promotion of β-carotene supplements for everyone should be reconsidered critically.

As discussed, vitamin A deficiency is rare in the elderly segment of our society. Nevertheless, it may have a higher occurrence in elderly with bizzare eating habits,[68] which is not that uncommon in some elderly people.

There is no consistent relationship between vitamin A status and mortality in elderly people. In the Medical Research Council Trial of Assessment and Management of Older People in the community, no evidence for an influence of β-carotene or retinol on total mortality was found.[69] The same was found also for α-tocopherol.[69]

The intake of vitamin A varies widely; in a recent study from Korea a high prevalence of inadequate vitamin A intake was reported.[70] In the United States and most European countries the ingestion of fortified milk products represents an important source of vitamin A, β-carotene, and other nutrients for elderly people. In a recent Spanish study it was reported that the consumption of three standard portions of dairy products per day would provide about 16% and 3% of the Spanish RDI for vitamins A (1000 μg/d) and E.[71] The same consumption using fortified/supplemented milk and yogurt would increase the dietary contribution up to 39% for vitamin A and up to 24% for vitamin E of the RDI for elderly subjects. In view of the ideal composition of milk products in regards to micronutrient and protein, the ingestion of this food group should be promoted in all population strata, especially in the elderly.

Compared to other nutrients in the United States and other Western countries, the intake of vitamin A is comparatively high because many supplements do contain vitamin A and different foods are fortified with vitamin A. In view of the physiologic alterations with age, where a higher absorption rate is found with hardly any biochemical deficiency, the concern for toxicity is more appropriate. Indeed during the last few years several publications reported a consistent relationship between the intake of vitamin A and the risk of osteoporotic fractures.[72,73] High plasma levels of vitamin A, even in the high normal range, are associated with a higher fracture risk.[74] Many multivitamin supplements for the elderly contain rather high amounts of vitamin A, which, when taken over longer time periods, will have adverse effects. Multivitamin supplements for the elderly should contain only small amounts of vitamin A, if at all, and any oversupplementation should be avoided.[75] Vitamin A antagonizes effects of calcium and vitamin D.[76] However, a higher intake, or even excess, of β-carotene is not likely to result in serious toxicity at the level of the bone or at the level of other organs[17] as long as the intake comes from foods.

Different vitamins do play important roles in bone formation. For example, vitamin C acts in the hydroxylation of proline and formation of collagen. The balanced supply of all essential nutrients is accordingly of major importance. For example, vitamin nutriture of osteoporotic women is often not optimal. Maggio et al.[42] reported that the antioxidant vitamin nutriture and antioxidant defense are markedly impaired in osteoporotic women. In the latter study, osteoporotic women showed significantly lower vitamin A plasma levels than normal controls, although not in the range of deficiency. This constellation shows the importance of focusing on a normal nutritional status, avoiding any excess as well as deficiency. High levels of vitamin A seem to be consistently associated with an increased risk for osteoporotic fractures. On the other hand, low levels in this population are probably only a reflection of the overall impaired nutritional status, including minerals and vitamin D.

In view of the antioxidant potential of vitamin A, β-carotene, and other carotenoids (eg, lutein), these compounds might also become more important for the maintenance of cognitive function and the prevention of dementia. The corresponding data are, however, at present not yet very convincing and a better carotenoid status may just be a proxy marker for other protective factors.[23] The increased consumption of these carotenoids, especially of lutein, is associated with a reduction of the risk of macular degeneration.[77]

Healthy elderly persons are able to maintain adequate body stores of vitamin A and normal vitamin A plasma/serum levels despite intakes below the RDA. It can be concluded that the vitamin A status of healthy elderly individuals does not require special attention; however, the risk for toxicity does require attention, even in the presence of a lower RDA for elderly persons.

VITAMIN D

Vitamin D and the vitamin D endocrine system are involved not only in the regulation of bone mass and bone mineral metabolism, but also in the modulation of several fundamental cellular processes.[78–81] The latter is illustrated in the very wide distribution of nuclear $1,25(OH)_2$-D_3 receptors[82] in adipose tissue, cartilage, certain cancer cells, and the retina. The current adequate intake (AI) for vitamin D in elderly subjects is 10 μg/d for women and men aged 51–70 years (1 μg cholecalciferol = 40 IU vitamin D). For elderly men and women older than 70 years the AI is 15 μg/d.[83] Accordingly, the AIs have been increased slightly for the older old (>70 years). Vitamin D can be obtained either from dietary sources or by synthesis in the skin upon exposure to the sun.[79] It seems that synthesis in the skin is of major importance as compared to the intake from food sources. Between 80% and 100% of the vitamin D content of the body is provided by cutaneous synthesis. It has been suggested that with adequate sun exposure, dietary sources of the vitamin become unnecessary.[84,85] This is probably correct because the vitamin D content of unfortified food is very small and comparatively of small importance for the maintenance of adequate vitamin D status. The best dietary sources are deep-sea fish such as salmon, herring, sardines, and mackerel. Plant foods are negligible sources of vitamin D, except certain wild mushrooms, which may contain up to 10 μg of vitamin D_2 per 100 g.[86] Fortified food, such as milk, contains considerable amounts of vitamin D, which could meet the needs in elderly people. Fortification is a good strategy for the improvement of the vitamin D nutriture of the whole population; however, fortification may bear the risk of toxicity and/or insufficiency due to inadequate fortification technologies.[87–89] A recent study analyzing samples from New York State reported that nearly half of the milk samples were underfortified.[89] In this study, overfortification of milk was less frequent (6% of samples). Nevertheless, in view of the common occurrence of vitamin D deficiency, underfortification is a cause for concern as is overfortification. Considering the food pattern of older adults, it is controversial which of the two possible sources of vitamin D is more important for maintaining adequate vitamin D nutriture in elderly people. As discussed later, elderly individuals should focus on both sources.

Vitamin D nutriture depends on the cutaneous synthesis of the vitamin and diet.[79] Food is, however, a rather bad source for vitamin D, except for certain selected foods such as deep-sea fish and vitamin D–fortified food products as mentioned earlier. Thus, up to 75% of elderly people consume less than 150 μg/d of vitamin D. McKenna[90] reviewed the vitamin D intakes in 31 studies. In many studies, there was no difference in the vitamin D intake of young and elderly subjects. In the northern countries of Europe, the intake of vitamin D in the elderly is a little higher due to the ingestion of more oily deep-sea fish. The intake of vitamin D from supplements varies according to the geographic region.[90] The latter differences are mainly due to differences in the consumption of fortified foods. Low intake of vitamin D is very prevalent and dietary vitamin D intake is not able to prevent vitamin D insufficiency especially during the winter months with low sun exposure.[91] The prevalence of elderly subjects taking supplements is higher in the northern European countries and North America than in other parts of Europe.[90] There are hardly any elderly people ingesting more than 5 μg of vitamin D per day. In most countries and populations, the intake of vitamin D is below the recommended intake.[92] In view of the low vitamin D content of natural food products, this is not surprising. It seems that especially the elderly (and other high-risk groups vulnerable for vitamin D deficiency) are not able to cover their needs by food.

The assessment of nutritional vitamin D status is defined by the amount of circulating 25(OH) vitamin D[79,93] alone and/or in combination with the parathormone (PTH) levels. Plasma and serum levels of 25-hydroxyvitamin D_3 (25(OH)D_3), the marker for vitamin D nutriture, decline with age in all populations.[29,83,90,94–97]

Plasma vitamin D levels in the elderly are more than 50% lower than those of younger controls. Blood levels of 25(OH)D_3 below 10 ng/mL have been reported in up to 50% of the free-living elderly.[98–100] In institutionalized elderly, this proportion may be as high as 90%.[101–104] Besides the low intakes, other mechanisms may contribute to the lower and decreasing plasma 25(OH)D_3 levels with aging (eg, decreased synthesis in the skin, decreased 1-α-hydroxylation in the kidney, decreased sunlight exposure, decreased plasma-binding capacity for vitamin D and vitamin D metabolites, and drug-nutrient interaction). Some evidence exists that a high intake of vitamin D is needed to assure an adequate biochemical vitamin D status. Decreased plasma levels of 1,25(OH)$_2$ vitamin D, the most active form for vitamin D, may parallel the decreased levels of the precursor (ie, 25(OH)D_3). This decrease is caused not only by a lack of the precursor molecule (25(OH)D_3) but by an age-related decline in 1-α-hydroxylase activity.[105,106] Even at the level of the bone itself, an age-related decline of 1, 25(OH)$_2$D$_3$ levels has been found.[107]

Vitamin D absorption and the hydroxylation in the liver are not affected during the normal aging process.[108] The capacity to hydroxylate the vitamin D molecule in the 21-position is, however, decreased due to age-specific changes.[109,110] The exact mechanisms of the latter phenomenon are not known, but parathormone (PTH) resistance may be of causal importance. Specific age-related effects at the level of the end organs (intestine and bone) may lead to a resistance to the effects of the activated form of the vitamin (ie, 1,25(OH)$_2$D).[111,112] The decline in estrogen levels with age may also play a central role in the modulation of end-organ responsiveness to vitamin D,[113] along with alterations of locally synthesized estrogens as a function of differences of the expression of vitamin D receptors.[114] Recently, particular steroid hormone receptors for vitamin D have been identified and studied intensively. At present it is controversial whether polymorphisms of vitamin D receptors may account for the genetic variations in bone mass or are also part of the age-related decline of bone mass.[115] Despite these changes it seems that vitamin D deficiency in the 21st century is nevertheless an unnecessary pandemic.[116] At least 50% of the house-bound elderly have impaired vitamin D status.[116]

Hypovitaminosis D is very common in people in all age ranges. For instance, in the National Health and Nutrition Examination Survey III (NHANES), the prevalence of hypovitaminosis D was more than 40% in African American women of reproductive age[117] but only a little more than 4% in Caucasian women. These high prevalence rates in dark-skinned individuals underline the importance of adequate sun exposure for all age groups, especially the elderly, independent of skin color.

Casual sun exposure can meet the vitamin D requirements of elderly people.[118] Many different factors can influence the synthesis of vitamin D in the skin. Geographical latitude may contribute to a large seasonal variation in the capacity of the skin to synthesize vitamin D. At high latitudes, there may be no vitamin D synthesis in the skin for up to 6 months of the year.[119,120] Sunlight exposure may help meet most vitamin D requirements, but the capacity to synthesize vitamin D in the skin upon sunlight exposure decreases with age. Elderly individuals do show a decline in the precursor for vitamin D synthesis, 7-dehydrocholesterol in the skin, and the conversion of the provitamin after exposure to ultraviolet light decreases in the skin of elderly people, leading to suboptimal endogenous vitamin D synthesis.[120] This is also reflected in less markedly expressed seasonal variations in 25(OH)D$_3$ plasma levels in the elderly compared to younger adults. Living in the south with a potential for much more sun exposure does not ensure adequate vitamin D nutriture. In the Euronut SENECA study, elderly from southern European countries had the lowest mean plasma 25(OH) vitamin D concentrations.[98] This study shows that sun exposure per se is not enough and that the factors of intensity and duration of sun exposure should also be accounted for. Elderly individuals should expose themselves regularly to sunlight, especially during the summer months. Exposure of suberythemal duration seems to be "safe" from the dermatologist's point of view regarding the development of skin cancer.[121] Suberythemal sun

exposure whenever possible should be recommended for the elderly, especially around noon time when the sun is in the highest position. However, in the absence of sun exposure it should be remembered that the recommended dietary intake is probably higher (in the range of 600–1000 IU) than the present recommendation.[84] Based on experiments with whole-body exposure to an artificial UV source and follow-up of the serum vitamin D$_3$ concentration, the serum response of elderly subjects was only about $1/4$ of the response of young control subjects.[122] This means that the elderly either have to stay longer in the sun (which bears the risk of erythema) or expose a larger skin surface to the sun (which would allow a shorter sun exposure with no cutaneous risk).

Dietary fortification and enrichment of food and the ingestion of vitamin D supplements have a high potential for improving vitamin D status as well as preventing bone loss and associated fracture risk. Also, in the elderly, the ingestion of vitamin D supplements will lead to an increase in the plasma/serum concentration of 25(OH) vitamin D. The change in 25(OH) vitamin D levels is accompanied by changes in the plasma concentration of other calcium-regulating hormones such as parathormone (PTH) or $1, 25(OH)_2$ vitamin D.[79,123] Despite many studies, the ideal amount of vitamin D intake to maintain adequate vitamin D nutriture is still a matter of controversy. Krall and colleagues[124] reported that at least 5.5 µg of vitamin D per day was needed to maintain stable (25)OH vitamin D serum levels and normal PTH concentrations, which is still low in view of the evidence presented here (5.5 µg corresponds to the AI for young adults). As discussed earlier, hardly any elderly people are receiving this amount of vitamin D from their diet. Several studies have reported a reduction of bone loss in elderly subjects due to the ingestion of vitamin D supplementation alone or in combination with calcium supplements.[125–127] Vitamin D supplementation is not necessarily associated with an increase in $1, 25(OH)_2$ vitamin D levels,[128] but other biochemical parameters of bone formation and resorption may be changed favorably. Osteocalcin, a bone matrix protein, is increased in vitamin D–deficient elderly but can be lowered upon vitamin D supplementation.[129,130]

Muscle weakness represents a central symptom of vitamin D deficiency. Muscle tissue is a nontraditional target tissue for the action of vitamin D and its metabolites.[81] Advancing age is associated with an altered muscle metabolism as well as muscle mass (sarcopenia) with impaired physical functioning and thus increased disability. Several studies reported a positive effect of vitamin D on physical functioning and a reduction of muscle deterioration. These data are very promising, however still controversial, and further studies need to clarify the role of vitamin D at the level of the skeletal muscle.[131–133]

The vitamin D requirements in elderly adults are higher than in younger individuals; this has been considered in the formulation of the present adequate intake (AI) recommendations. Nevertheless, it seems possible that requirements in older adults might even be higher than presently suggested. This is especially supported by the findings that young individuals often show a vitamin D insufficiency and that this cannot be compensated by dietary vitamin D intake from the usual diet[91] especially during the winter months. In elderly people, the correction of vitamin D status is needed due to specific age-related changes in vitamin D metabolism (see earlier). Accordingly, elderly people should consume the presently suggested recommended AI. Increased sun exposure during the summer months, as well as the consumption of vitamin D–fortified food, may help to improve overall vitamin D nutriture. Elderly people with a low degree of sun exposure should be motivated to increase their suberythemal sun exposure and, in addition, may qualify for low-dose vitamin D supplementation in the range of 400 IU to 600 IU (especially during the winter months), alone or in combination with calcium supplements. It should be remembered that vitamin D deficiency in the 21st century is an unnecessary pandemic.[116]

VITAMIN K

During the past few years, new functions of vitamin K have been elucidated that may be of spe-cial importance for elderly people. One of the most important roles of vitamin K is to support the posttranslational carboxylation of glutamate residues, which are involved in the formation of the modified amino acid γ-carboxyglutamate.[134,135] Despite the new discoveries concerning the function of vitamin K and its metabolites, only incomplete information is available on the vitamin K requirements of the elderly. Reasons for this are the limited knowledge of the amount of vitamin K in food sources as well as the difficulties in assessing biochemical vitamin K status correctly. In 1989, an RDA for vitamin K was formulated for the first time.[136] On the basis of a few studies, it is assumed that a dietary intake of 1 μg/kg of body weight per day should be sufficient to maintain normal blood clotting in adults. Accordingly, the adequate intake (AI) for vitamin K was set at 90 μg/d for elderly women and at 120 μg/d for elderly men, respectively.[8] The AI for vitamin K is identical for all adults. These recommendations are based on the maintenance and function of normal clotting mechanisms, but it is not known whether more vitamin K is needed for optimal functioning of other vitamin K–dependent proteins containing γ-carboxyglutamyl residues. Not only diet but also the bacterial flora in the jejunum and ileum contribute to the maintenance of vitamin K status. The relative contribution of the intestinal source of vitamin K depends on many factors, mainly the composition and the amount of the gut microflora. New evidence based on the induction of vitamin K deficiency in normal healthy subjects by dietary restriction alone argues against the nutritional relevance of the intestinal bacteria as an important vitamin K source. Similarly, in elderly people with atrophic gastritis with a bacterial overgrowth of the upper gastrointestinal tract, vitamin K status is not affected as assessed by measuring the resistance to warfarin therapy.[137]

There are little data available on vitamin K nutriture in the elderly. In a market survey of a representative sample of older adults, the mean reported intakes of phylloquinone among them increased with age.[138] It is estimated that the average US diet provides a daily intake of about 150–500 μg vitamin K.[8,136] In view of newer data from the FDA Total Diet Study (TDS), these data seem to be overestimated. In the oldest groups of the TDS (ie, aged 60 years and older), the highest mean dietary intakes of vitamin K from the whole population were reported.[139] The estimated vitamin K intake in this age category ranged from 76 to 80 μg/d.[139] In the latter study, gender differences in the dietary sources of vitamin K were identified. It has been reported that the mean intake increases with age:[8,140] the average phylloquinone intake, based on data of 11 different studies, was, in individuals aged 45 years or older, around 150 μg/d, whereas in those younger than 45 years, the intake was around 80 μg/d. In NHANES III, the median vitamin K intake of adults was between 82 and 117 μg/d.[8] For adult women, green vegetables represented a more important source of vitamin K than they did for men. Nevertheless, green vegetables represent the major source of vitamin K in elderly men and women, followed by grain products, meat, and fats (in the form of dressings). The addition of fats and oils to mixed meals and desserts represents an important modifier of vitamin K intake (see also later). In view of the trend of low-fat meals and different weight-control strategies, this observation gains importance for elderly people. With increasing age, the contribution of vitamin K from mixed meals declined, especially in women. In agreement with the TDS, a cross-sectional study of 402 healthy postmenopausal women showed the mean total dietary intake of phylloquinone to be 89 μg/d.[141] In this study, there was a significant relationship ($r = 0.13, p = .01$) between dietary intake of phylloquinones and plasma levels. In the British National Diet and Nutrition Survey (1994–1995), the weighted geometric mean intake of phylloquinone of free-living elderly (aged 65 years or older) was estimated at 65 μg/d (95% CI 62, 67) based on all study participants.[142] The intakes were higher in elderly men than in elderly women (70 vs. 61 μg/d, respectively, $P < .01$) and the mean nutrient densities of phylloquinone intake were 9.3 and 10.5 μg/MJ for elderly men and women, respectively ($P < .01$). Fifty-nine percent of this aged population had phylloquinone intakes below the current guideline for adequacy of 1 μg/kg body weight per day.[142] In this survey, the intake declined with increasing age and the subjects aged 85 years and older had the lowest intakes.[142] There were large differences according to the geographical area, probably due to availability of vegetables as well as specific food choices.

These apparently adequate intakes in elderly subjects would agree with the observation that the elderly subjects had higher vitamin K plasma levels than did younger subjects.[143] The higher plasma levels in elderly subjects may, however, only represent higher vitamin K hepatic stores (as in the case of vitamin A). The reported mean plasma phylloquinone levels in elderly adults are in the range of 1.05 to 1.15 nmol/L.[139,143,144]

Whether vitamin K absorption and/or relative bioavailability changes with age is not exactly known. Selected measures of vitamin K status have been reported to be different according to age. Adults aged 60 years and older have higher plasma phylloquinone concentrations[144,145] and higher urinary gla-creatinine ratios as compared to adults aged 40 years and older.[146] Further, elderly people seem to be more resistant to dietary vitamin K deficiency as assessed by the urinary excretion of gla-proteins.[143] There is so far no clear-cut explanation for these observed differences and they cannot be explained by differences in absorption. There is no significant difference in the relative phylloquinone bioavailability.[147] In the latter study, diet (ie, dietary sources of vitamin K) as well as gender were important determinants of the relative bioavailability of different forms of the vitamin. The differences may be of importance in the explanation of differences between studies.[148] In the latter study, there was no difference in absorption between the different age groups independent of the dietary form of vitamin K. The phylloquinone absorption was significantly greater after the consumption of a phylloquinone-fortified *oil diet* as compared to a simple broccoli diet.[148] This observation supports the recommendation to add a little oil to a vegetable dish, not only for the sake of a better β-carotene absorption but also for the improvement of vitamin K nutriture. In animal data, age-related changes in the pattern of tissue distribution of phylloquinone and menaquinones have been reported.[149] Alcohol consumption was associated with decreased fasting levels of vitamin K.[144]

Vitamin K–dependent proteins could be used to assess vitamin K nutriture.[146] Several studies have reported a relationship between osteocalcin and vitamin K nutriture.[150,151] Osteocalcin is less carboxylated when vitamin K status is impaired. In a study of 263 subjects (age range 18–85 years), the urinary γ-carboxyglutamic acid (gla)-to-creatinine excretion ratios increased significantly with age in both genders ($r = 0.63$ and 0.68, $P < .001$ for females and males, respectively).[146] In the same study, with aging increased levels of total, carboxylated, and undercarboxylated osteocalcin levels were reported.[146]

The measurement of blood-clotting factors can be used to assess vitamin K nutriture. Newer methods (direct measurements of vitamin K and its metabolites or gla-proteins) are used today to assess vitamin K nutriture. Nevertheless, some older studies use measurements of clotting factors, which may be proxy markers for alterations in the vitamin K metabolism in elderly subjects. It was shown, with a test depending on all four vitamin K–dependent clotting factors, that 50% of a group of randomly selected older adults (age range 56–100 years) had an impairment suggestive of a vitamin K deficiency.[152] The subjects in this study were afflicted with various diseases and thus were not representative of the normal healthy aging process. In animals, experimental vitamin K deficiency is more easily induced in older animals than in younger.[153]

Further, despite the absence of significant age-related changes in warfarin pharmacokinetics, healthy elderly persons do have an increased sensitivity to warfarin.[154]

Vitamin K is usually associated with blood coagulation. Research during the last few years identified vitamin K as an important cofactor in bone metabolism and thus osteoporosis. Vitamin K_2 has been shown to enhance the γ-carboxylation of bone glutamic acid residues and the secretion of osteocalcin. A low dietary intake of vitamin K was associated with a low bone mineral density in women, but not in men.[155] In a re-cent study, a combined treatment of vitamin K_2 and bisphosphonates in postmenopausal women with osteoporosis showed that the combination treatment with vitamin K_2 and bisphosphonates is more efficacious in the prevention of new vertebral fractures than a single treatment with bisphosphonate alone.[156]

In view of the potential importance of vitamin K in bone metabolism, an adequate intake during the whole life should be assured. A recent vitamin K depletion and repletion study showed that the γ-carboxylation of prothrombin was restored to normal levels at a supplementation of 200 μg/d,[157] which is higher than the actual AI for this vitamin. However, it is of additional interest to note that other biochemical markers of vitamin K nutriture remain below normal after short-term supplementation of up to 450 μg/d of phylloquinone, suggestive for a higher requirement (the stepwise supplementation in this study lasted for 56 days). In this study, the presently recommended adequate intake (AI) did not lead to maximal osteocalcin γ-carboxylation so the authors conclude that the requirements of older adults might be higher than presently suggested.[157] In agreement, others reported that usual dietary practices in younger as well as older individuals does not assure adequate amounts of vitamin K for maximal osteocalcin carboxylation.[158,159] At present there is only insufficient evidence for a general recommendation of vitamin K supplements for osteoporosis prevention. Nevertheless, vitamin K administration to elderly patients receiving no anticoagulant therapy did not induce any adverse hemostatic activation, not even in the vitamin K–deficient subjects.[160]

Despite the increased interest in vitamin K metabolism due to new analytical methods for the determination of the vitamin's levels and the new roles of vitamin K in bone health, no statement regarding the adequacy of the present recommendations for vitamin K in elderly adults can be made. It seems that the present lack of knowledge of the metabolism of this vitamin may be inversely related to its importance in health maintenance, especially regarding issues of age and aging. At present the intake of vitamin K–rich foods should be recommended for elderly persons with intake levels at least as high as the present AI, and it may be wise to consume some fat with these foods to enhance bioavailability of vitamin K.

VITAMIN E

Antioxidants, especially vitamin E, seem to be of special importance in the modulation of certain age-related phenomena.[39] Many different theories of aging have been formulated, but most of them lack universality regarding different organ systems and functions. However, age-related changes due to oxidation are found in most organ systems and are, therefore, rather universally applicable. Accordingly, a potential role of vitamin E and other antioxidants in aging and the aging process seems to be suggested.[40,161]

The RDA for elderly men and women is 15 mg (34.9 μmol) of α-tocopherol.[23] Compared to the 1989 and 1980 RDAs, the present recommendation is 5 mg higher.[136] There is no evidence that aging affects vitamin E absorption and/or utilization,[23] which is also supported by the fact that higher vitamin E intakes from natural sources or supplements can modulate the plasma concentration in all age groups without any difficulties. In an animal study with rats using intestinal perfusion with ^{3}H-methyl-α-tocopherol, it was reported that animals 24 months old had an increase in vitamin E absorption up to 35% compared to young controls (aged 4 months).[162] There is no such evidence from human studies. Many different factors may influence the bioavailability of vitamin E, including intraluminal events but also the dosage and the form of vitamin E.[163] Concomitant fat intake is an important determinant of the absorption of all fat-soluble vitamins, especially vitamin E.[164] Further, there is some controversy whether the absorptive phenomena differ from species to species; therefore, it remains to be seen whether vitamin E bioavailability is increased in humans as they age.

Nevertheless present evidence suggests that there is no impairment of vitamin E absorption with aging. Most studies of elderly subjects have reported plasma/serum vitamin E levels well within the normal range. In a cross-sectional study of 206 institutionalized elderly (mean age for men and women 68.8 ± 15 and 76.4 ± 13.2 years, respectively), only 2 subjects had low α-tocopherol plasma levels by the Euronut SENECA criteria.[25,26] In a group of more than 200 institutionalized elderly in Wülflingen, Switzerland, there was an adequate vitamin E status noted in all patients. The mean plasma vitamin E concentration was 27.3 ± 6.97 μmol/L; only one patient had a plasma vitamin E level below 15 μmol/L (Suter et al.). These data are in agreement with those of other studies in elderly subjects that report an adequate plasma/serum vitamin E content.[34,165-174] There may be larger differences in the biochemical vitamin E status as a function of the overall dietary pattern (including fat intake), age, associated diseases, or geographical region.[175] A recent study from Greece reported that most elderly people from rural areas had an adequate vitamin E status, whereas nearly two-thirds of the elderly from urban areas showed a low plasma α-tocopherol level.[173] Schmuck et al.[176] reported a low intake of most antioxidants in a hospitalized geriatric population.

Institutionalization is an important risk factor for malnutrition, whereas vitamin E nutriture seems to be rather resistant to any immediate effects of institutionalization.[177] Some studies report a decline in plasma/serum vitamin E levels with aging. This can be explained by a decline in the LDL cholesterol levels with increasing age, especially in the very old, because the LDL molecule is the major carrier of vitamin E in the blood. It has even been suggested that cardiovascular aging in animals (rats) is associated with an increase in vitamin E, which is regarded as a compensatory mechanism attempting to counterbalance age-associated oxidative stress phenomena.[178]

The maintenance of adequate blood vitamin E levels suggests an adequate intake and absorption in most elderly people. Illness associated with low food intake, especially low fat intake,[164] is one of the major determinants of vitamin E nutriture. Data regarding changes in tissue levels of vitamin E with age are inconsistent. Low platelet vitamin E levels have been described in a small group of old subjects (aged 78–94 years) as compared to young controls (aged 25–35 years).[179] These authors conclude that the increased platelet aggregation in aging may be caused by this decreased vitamin E concentration at the level of the platelets. A group of elderly subjects on low intakes of eicosapentaenoic acid platelets showed a higher vitamin E concentration compared to a control group.[180] Several animal studies analyzing vitamin E tissue levels in the central nervous system in different age groups have been performed recently. Meydani and colleagues[181] reported a selective decrease in the tocopherol concentration in the cerebellum of the brainstem. This decline was especially due to a decrease in α-tocopherol content. The authors conclude that these changes may be caused by a higher vitamin E turnover in these brain areas and that these brain areas require more vitamin E to maintain an adequate concentration of α-tocopherol. Supporting this conclusion were marked differences in the response upon supplementation in old versus young animals as assessed by the measurement of lipid peroxidation products.[172]

A similar study measuring the effect of vitamin E deficiency in aging animals on the accumulation of age pigments in neuronal structures was performed by Koistinaho et al.[182] Animal studies, however, have reported that dietary vitamin E could affect lipofuscin accumulation only up to middle age, but not in old age.[183] Further animal data suggest that during cardiovascular aging, vitamin E increases as a compensatory mechanism to counterbalance the age-related increase in prooxidation.[178] A Japanese study investigated the pathophysiological significance in biomembranes of the redox dynamics of α-tocopherol during aging as well as in the setting of non-insulin-dependent diabetes mellitus.[184] The latter animal as well as human data showed that the utilization rate of α-tocopherol in the erythrocyte membrane increased with aging, while the α-tocopherol uptake in the erythrocyte membrane decreased. In addition, the authors describe a significant positive correlation between age and the utilization rate of α-tocopherol in the

erythrocyte membrane of healthy volunteers aged 23 to 103 years.[184] Chronic diseases may further affect the distribution of the different vitamin E species in the body. Accordingly, the α-tocopherol uptake in the erythrocyte membrane was significantly lower in elderly non-insulin-dependent diabetes mellitus patients (average 68.1 years old) than in healthy age-matched individuals.

These data suggest that the redox dynamics of α-tocopherol in biomembranes could be of importance in the onset, aggravation, and complications of chronic diseases[184] and that the requirements might be different according to the baseline disease pattern. These mechanisms may also be responsible for age-related changes in the tissue distribution of vitamin E.

In a Swedish study, human adipose tissue tocopherol concentrations showed large variability depending on the serum tocopherol content ($r = 0.24–0.31$), but there was, contrary to other studies, no age-associated increase in the adipose tissue tocopherol content.[185] These controversial data need to be clarified in future studies. At present it is not known whether changes in vitamin E metabolism with age in certain selected tissues are representative of other tissues and organs or even overall requirements. From these studies, no conclusions regarding the requirements of vitamin E in aging can be drawn.

In the present context, the potential importance of vitamin E and other antioxidants in the pathogenesis of atherosclerosis must be addressed briefly.[23,39,186–189] LDL cholesterol plays a central role in the induction and progression of atherosclerosis. Evidence suggests that oxidatively modified LDL cholesterol molecules bear a much higher pathophysiologic potential than native nonmodified LDL molecules because these particles do show functional changes leading to improved recognition by the scavenger receptor. Antioxidants may interfere basically at all pathophysiological steps of atherogenesis. Thus, the lipoproteins and the different structures of the vessel wall have to be protected from oxidative attack. The antioxidant hypothesis of atherosclerosis is very attractive, but causality needs to be proved. Most prospective clinical trials were disappointing and failed to confirm the attractive antioxidant hypothesis of atherosclerosis.[186,190,191] The development of atherosclerosis is probably a chronic lifelong process, so an adequate supply of antioxidants should be ensured during all periods of life and natural food-based sources should be preferred whenever feasible and possible. In addition, the control of all risk factors should be a primary aim.

In view of the antioxidative effects of vitamin E and its membrane-stabilizing properties, the effects of vitamin E on most chronic diseases of aging have been studied. Epidemiological and experimental studies suggest a potential role of this vitamin in the prevention of atherosclerosis, cancer, cataracts, central nervous system disorders such as Alzheimer's disease and Parkinson's disease, immune function, impaired glucose tolerance, and many more conditions.[23,39,192–198]

Despite all these potential relationships, which are, in most cases, *only associations* (compare cardiovascular diseases and vitamins), the intake of high doses of supplements cannot be recommended.[23] Furthermore, there is still a lack of knowledge regarding the safety of long-term ingestion of these vitamins in large dosages. The use of vitamin E and other supplements to control certain diseases in the elderly is disappointing. Also a recent controlled trial in elderly men who smoked (aged 50–69 years) failed to show an effect on the incidence of the risk of hospital-treated pneumonia.[199] This study clearly points to the importance of the control of the classical risk factors in the elderly, and a potent risk can hardly be antagonized by vitamin supplements. In addition the study showed that in a subgroup of subjects who initiated smoking at a later age, vitamin E decreased the risk of pneumonia (RR, 0.65; 95% CI, 0.49–0.86), whereas the supplementation with β-carotene increased the risk (RR, 1.42; 95% CI, 1.07–189).[199] Again, balance in the nutrient supply from food sources is the key issue in nutritional pevention.

As mentioned earlier, vitamin E includes different chemical forms.[39] In most human tissues, as well as in food supplements, α-tocopherol is the predominant form. On the other hand γ-tocopherol represents one of the major chemical forms in food sources. Recently it has been postulated that γ-tocopherol may be much more important in disease control than the commonly studied γ-tocopherol.[200,201] The role of these specific vitamin E compound in aging is not exactly known, however, one older study showed an age related decline in plasma γ-tocopherol but not of α-tocopherol;[202] in platelets, both compounds declined with aging. Further studies in this important field are surely warranted, especially in relation to chronic disease risk.

Normal aging, that is, disease-free aging, is associated with an adequate vitamin E status; present evidence suggests that the actual RDA seems to be adequate. Pharmacological effects of vitamins do not imply an *in vivo* advantage for disease risk and especially not for mortality risk. Vitamin E plays an important role in antioxidant defense, but it has to remembered that vitamin E is only one of many players in this field. Further, it should not be forgotten that the control of oxidative stress includes not only the supply of adequate amounts of antioxidants, but more so the control of pro-oxidative metabolic conditions (eg, smoking).

VITAMIN C

The vitamin C (ascorbic acid) deficiency disease of scurvy is rare in Western societies, but due to an increasing knowledge of the metabolic properties of vitamin C, an adequate supply of this vitamin remains the cornerstone for health maintenance,[203] especially in elderly adults. For prevention of scurvy, a daily intake of approximately 10 mg of ascorbic acid is needed; nevertheless, scurvy may still be found in our society in subjects consuming an inadequate diet.[203,204] The RDA for vitamin C for elderly men is 90 mg/d (511 μmol) and 75mg/d (426 μmol) for elderly women.[23] This recommendation is identical to the recommendation for younger adults (aged 19–50 years), but is higher than the 1989 RDA for which 60 mg of vitamin C was recommended.[136] There are no consistent age-related changes in absorption and metabolism at median vitamin C intakes.[23] Accordingly, any deficiency is mainly due to poor intakes in the elderly and there is no evidence for increased requirements compared to younger adults.

Despite the wide distribution of vitamin C in food, vitamin C intakes in elderly people vary widely, and in newer and older studies up to 60% of the elderly may have intakes below 30 mg/d.[29,49,205–209] Dietary vitamin C intakes vary mainly as a function of the presence of illness associated with overall poor nutrient intake, institutionalization, and age.[210] The variability in intake is nicely illustrated in the following studies from very different populations and geographical areas. In the Boston survey, the median vitamin C intakes for free-living elderly men and women were 132 mg and 128 mg, respectively.[211] In an Italian population of free-living elderly aged 70 to 75 years, 45% of the subjects had dietary intakes below 40 mg/d.[206] Similarly, a free-living population of elderly people on the Greek island of Crete and in Spain had vitamin C intakes well above the US recommendations.[212,213] The latter data support the concept of recommending to elderly individuals a diet rich in fruits and vegetables as consumed by most Mediterranean populations. During the last decade, the intake of different supplements, especially vitamin C supplements, has increased widely and contributes considerably to the nutrient intake of large segments of the elderly population.

With increasing age, there is a decrease in ascorbic acid levels in whole blood, serum/plasma, and leucocytes.[214,215] Because the vitamin C plasma/ serum levels depend mainly on vitamin C intake, there is very wide variability in plasma/serum vitamin C levels as also illustrated in the previously cited studies. Between 1% and 60% of the free-living elderly may have low vitamin C levels (ie, <11.4 µmol/L).[205,216–220] In up to 80% of the institutionalized elderly of the Wülflingen study in Switzerland, the mean plasma ascorbic acid concentration was 25.8 ± 19.6 µmol/L. The lowest plasma concentration was 5.7 µmol/L, and 72% of the men and 42% of the women had plasma levels below 20 µmol/L (Suter et al).

Institutionalization, hospitalization, and illness lead to a sharp decrease of vitamin C intakes and thus low plasma levels.[103,176] Most studies show lower ascorbic acid levels in elderly men than in elderly women; it has been suggested that the sex difference in plasma ascorbic acid concentration may be caused by lower tubular reabsorption of the vitamin in elderly men. Rhesus monkeys exhibit the same age-related decline in plasma ascorbic acid concentration as do humans.[221] Healthy centenarians had significantly lower vitamin C plasma concentrations (due to lower intakes), whereas vitamin A and vitamin E levels (due to changes in plasma lipid levels) were significantly higher in centenarians than in young old.[222]

Disease states may modulate the plasma concentration of vitamin C. However, in general this is due to low intakes and not to specific disease-related phenomena.[23] In NHANES III, the serum vitamin C concentration in persons with newly diagnosed diabetes were significantly lower than in nondiabetics, also due to lower intakes of this vitamin[223] and not any metabolic alteration. Other disease states, such as pressure sores, are also associated with lower vitamin C serum concentrations due to low intakes.[224] For daily practice this means that any disease state has a high probability of leading to an impairment of vitamin C nutriture and that this should be corrected by dietary means or short-term supplementation. A higher serum concentration of vitamin C may be desirable, especially in elderly adults.[43] The presence of any of the classical chronic diseases of aging might be used as an indicator for suspicion of vitamin C insufficiency.

Despite the high prevalence of low intakes and low biochemical status in elderly subjects, the pharmacokinetic properties of a large dose of vitamin C (500 mg p.o.) were not affected by age.[225] In a depletion/repletion study of elderly subjects (aged 66–74 years) as compared to young controls (aged 21–28 years), no age-related difference in the response pattern was found.[225] In this study, 10 mg of ascorbic acid was given per day over a prolonged time period, and there was no difference in the vitamin half-life during the depletion period. In one metabolic study, elderly persons (aged >65 years) needed a larger dose of vitamin C to maintain a plasma concentration at which the ascorbic acid body pools were saturated (in this study, 56.7 μmol/L).[226] To maintain saturated ascorbic acid pools, the elderly men had to ingest approximately 150 mg/d and the elderly women approximately 80 mg/d, an intake considerably higher than the present recommendations. Interestingly, at an ascorbic acid intake of 60 mg/d, some elderly men were not able to achieve an adequate plasma ascorbic acid concentration (ie, above 22.7 μmol/L). These data suggest that at least certain subsets of the elderly may indeed need higher vitamin C intakes to maintain adequate vitamin C nutriture. The reason for this behavior is not known. In view of their eating habits and eating patterns, many elderly may have difficulties ingesting the recommended amounts from dietary sources only and a targeted supplementation may be considered. Whether tissue vitamin C levels do change with age is controversial.[227] Pinto et al,[228] using a vitamin C–loading test, reported a small increase of the plasma vitamin C levels in elderly subjects, suggestive of low tissue levels. Probably, as a function of intake and/ or certain diseases (eg, diabetes), tissue vitamin C content may decrease in aging.[229,230] A recent study in rats showed tissue-specific declines in vitamin C content, which might have pathophysiologic relevance for the development of certain chronic diseases of aging where free radical reactions are involved.[231]

Low levels of vitamin C in the blood of healthy elderly people can be corrected easily by the administration of oral ascorbic acid supplements,[232] but upon withdrawal, a rapid decrease of blood levels might be seen. This supports the hypothesis that the low blood levels seen in elderly people are mainly attributable to low intakes and not to an age-related physiologic alteration at the level of absorption and/or other metabolic steps. Elderly persons with low vitamin C levels do not necessarily show clinical symptoms, so it has been concluded that there is no real need to raise blood ascorbic acid levels through supplementation. In view of the functions of vitamin C, this conclusion may be wrong because the health

consequences of marginal vitamin C deficiency and its pathophysiologic role in the development of different diseases[23] are not yet exactly known. Further, in view of the rapid changes in plasma concentration as a function of intake, an adequate *daily* intake should be assured.

Ascorbic acid may be of importance in the pathogenesis of most chronic diseases of aging.[23,233] Ascorbic acid has been found to be potentially important in the prevention of atherosclerosis, cancer, senile cataract, lung diseases, cognitive function, and degenerative diseases of miscellaneous organs.[15,23,41,188,233–240] Vitamin C supplements are often promoted as a way to lower lipids, thus reducing the risk of atherosclerosis. However, a recent study reported that a 5-year vitamin C supplementation had no markedly favorable effects on the serum lipids and lipoprotein profiles in an adult population.[241]

Further, ascorbic acid may be of great importance in immunomodulation in elderly people.[23,233] It is controversial which of the different antioxidative vitamins are of major importance. Present evidence suggests that an adequate supply of all the different active antioxidative vitamins is needed and that it may be wrong to stress the importance of the miscellaneous vitamins; this depends on many different factors, such as body compartment, type of tissue or organ, and biochemical function. In a study by Sahyoun et al.[242] looking at the association between mortality and different antioxidants (carotenoids, vitamin E, vitamin C) in 747 free-living elderly subjects, only high intakes of vitamin C and frequent consumption of vegetables were significantly protective against early mortality. These findings would suggest a special importance of vitamin C, but adequacy of all nutrients is central for health maintenance, and the adequate intake of vitamin C may be a proxy for a more protective overall diet.[238] Similar results were reported in other studies.[243,244]

Coronary artery disease and atherosclerosis are the leading causes of morbidity and mortality. The antioxidant hypothesis of atherosclerosis (see the section titled "Vitamin E") seems very attractive,[23] but the effects of vitamin E on oxidative processes at the level of the LDL cholesterol molecule have drawn more attention than the effects of ascorbic acid have. It must be noted that vitamin C may decrease the oxidation of LDL and play an important role in the regeneration of vitamin E.[245] It also must be considered that a large fraction of the free radicals develops, in the water phase of the different body compartments, where vitamin C is the major antioxidant. In addition, vitamin C may elicit a direct lipid-modifying effect.[246] It may also play a role in the pathogenesis of essential hypertension; several studies have reported an inverse relationship between vitamin C nutriture and blood pressure.[247–249] The blood pressure–lowering effects are comparatively small and it is important to remember that essential hypertension should be treated with antihypertensive medications and not with nutrient supplements.

Several modifiable factors, such as stress and smoking, influence vitamin C requirements.[23] Vitamin C requirements of smokers may be up to 60 mg higher than those of nonsmokers.[250] Low levels in smokers can be corrected by a higher dietary or supplemental intake of vitamin C, but the maintenance of high plasma levels cannot counteract and counterbalance the negative health effects of smoking. Smoking cessation without an additional nutritional intervention leads rapidly to an improvement of vitamin C status, reflected in higher plasma levels.[251] Quitting smoking represents an irreplaceable central preventive strategy that is more powerful and effective than ingestion of higher levels of nutrients, including vitamin C.[252] The intake of vitamin C supplements seems to be fairly safe, but there is as yet no convincing evidence to advocate the intake of vitamin C supplements in smokers as a general strategy.

Cognitive impairment and frank dementia increase exponentially with age. In view of the many different pathophysiological forms of dementia, the findings regarding the importance of certain nutrients (including vitamin C) and cognitive impairment are very conflicting and at present no recommendation can be made. Nevertheless, some data suggest that a potential impairment of the vitamin status may be similar in all forms of dementia.[253] In view of the patho-

physiologic basis of vascular dementia, nutrition may play a central role. Nevertheless the optimal control of the classical cardiovascular risk factors remains the cornerstone of any preventive strategy.[254] Evidence suggests that certain nutrients (antioxidants and other vitamins) may protect against vascular dementia and may lead to an improved cognitive function in old age (see the section titled "Folate").[255] A recent cross-sectional and prospective study of dementia in the elderly (aged 65 years and older) in Cache County (Utah) reported that the use of vitamins E and C (ascorbic acid) supplements in combination was associated with reduced Alzheimer's dementia prevalence (adjusted OR, 0.22; 95% CI, 0.05–0.60) and incidence (adjusted HR, 0.36; 95% CI, 0.09–0.99).[256] This study did not report an effect of single nutrients on the risk of dementia.[256] This underlines again the importance of the overall diet.

Present evidence suggests the absence of any specific age-related change in the metabolism of ascorbic acid. The current intake recommendation of ascorbic acid seems to be adequate for elderly adults, although some evidence suggests that for some individuals, it might be difficult to achieve this intake level from the diet alone. Nevertheless, intake should be optimized in certain substrata of the elderly (the institutionalized, the ill, and those of lower socioeconomic status), especially during the winter months. An increased consumption of fresh fruits and vegetables should be encouraged in elderly people.

VITAMIN B$_1$

The classical vitamin B$_1$ (thiamine hydrochloride) deficiency disease of beri-beri is hardly seen in Western populations, except in chronic alcoholics.[257] Vitamin B$_1$ plays an important role in carbohydrate metabolism, so the recommended dietary intake of this vitamin depends on the total carbohydrate and overall energy intake.[257] The present RDA for thiamine is 1.2 mg/d for elderly men and 1.1 mg/d for elderly women.[7] This intake recommendation is not different from that for younger adults, but it is lower than the 1989 RDA.[136] In the 1989 RDA, the suggested minimal requirement was set at 0.20 and 0.23 mg/1000 kcal. To be on the safe side, an intake of 0.5 mg/1000 kcal is recommended, even if energy consumption is below 2000 kcal/d. These ranges of intake might nevertheless be helpful for daily practice. Several studies suggest that there may be a higher requirement for vitamin B₁ in the elderly; however, in view of the lower energy requirement in the elderly, this suggested increased requirement will be compensated for.[7] These recommendations are the subject of some debate because in young subjects with an intake of 0.3 mg/1000 kcal, no biochemical signs of deficiency could be detected.[258,259] Despite this controversy, the present recommendation is probably adequate for all adults independent of age.

Up to 70% of older adults, depending on income, race, and socioeconomic status, have been shown to have low thiamine intakes.[26,205,206,216, 260–267] For thiamine, institutionalization, socioeconomic level, and illness are the major determinants of vitamin status.[206,260,267,268] Living alone represents an additional important risk factor for thiamine deficiency and other nutritional deficiencies.[266] Physical activity stimulates overall energy intake, which is also associated with improved overall nutriture, including better thiamine status. In the Wülflingen study, on the basis of the measurement of the thiamine transketolase activity, 82% of the elderly men and 74% of the women did show a thiamine deficiency. When the α–erythrocyte transketolase activity coefficient (ETKAC) was used, 14% of elderly people revealed a deficiency and 34% had a marginal status; about 50% had an adequate thiamine nutriture by this index (Suter et al., data on file). These data are in agreement with data from other studies.[265] However, there is, as for most water-soluble vitamins, a very wide variability in thiamine nutriture in the elderly; in an Irish study, up to 70% of elderly women showed a marginal and/or deficient thiamine status based upon the ETKAC[264] whereas in other studies (as cited earlier) only about 10% showed a vitamin B₁ deficiency. This variability

of intakes has also been reported in the Euronut SENECA study, where the median daily intakes of this vitamin ranged from 0.84 mg/d (Yverdon, Switzerland) to 1.59 mg/d (North Ireland).[216] In the same study, the longitudinal data revealed a median decline in the intakes of this vitamin during a 4- to 5-year period in the range of 0.00 to 0.20 mg/d. Looking at these data, it must be remembered that the assessment of nutrient intakes is a very difficult task, due not only to the incompleteness of the food tables, but also to the inadequacy of the reports of intake by the subjects. In a study by Nichols and Basu,[262] the average thiamine intake was 0.4 mg/1000 kcal, which is well above the recommendation, but up to 50% of the subjects had a thiamine pyrophosphate activity coefficient above 14%, suggestive of deficiency. This finding may be caused by either an inadequate dietary assessment or age-related changes in thiamine metabolism. Up to now, no specific age-related alterations in the metabolism of this vitamin have been identified. Wilkinson et al.[268] reported that, in elderly subjects, the impaired thiamine status is more related to age than to comorbidities.

Elderly subjects admitted for a medical or psychiatric hospitalization very often show a thiamine deficiency.[269–271] Aside from insufficient intake, excessive alcohol intake is the most important factor for an impaired thiamine status independent of age. Alcohol interferes with thiamine nutriture at basically all levels of metabolism.[272] Because alcohol (even in small to moderate quantities) blocks the active thiamine absorption, this may become clinically relevant, especially in elderly persons with low thiamine intakes who depend on the active mechanism of the vitamin's uptake.[273] From a theoretical point of view, the simultaneous ingestion of alcohol and thiamine-containing food should be separated accordingly.

Patients with cardiac failure may represent a high-risk population for thiamine deficiency due to the chronic ingestion of diuretics.[274,275] In a study by Pfitzenmeyer et al,[274] thiamine nutriture worsened as a function of the New York Heart Association (NYHA) functional class. Experimental evidence shows that chronic diuretic treatment leads to increased thiamine losses in urine as a function of the urinary flow.[276,277] In heart failure patients, supplementation with thiamine has further been shown to improve left ventricular function within a few days.[278,279] These data are very suggestive that particularly elderly patients with chronic diuretic therapy may be at higher risk for a thiamine deficiency and that low-dose thiamine supplementation (eg, initially 50 mg/d, a low-dose supplementation) may be helpful in these patients. In view of the risk of anaphylactic reactions after parenteral administration (except in emergency situations), this vitamin should given preferentially by the oral route.[280]

Hospital malnutrition is a widely discussed topic that might indeed be a real problem in long-term care. However, in the setting of acute medicine the patient usually has other (ie, medical) priorities than nutritional issues, and after treatment of an acute illness, food intake usually becomes normal. In a prospective study, we evaluated the effect of hospitalization, on the overall biochemical vitamin status in subjects older than 50 years ($n = 149$, mean $\pm$ SD age 70 $\pm$ 10 years).[275] Vitamin nutriture and other parameters were assessed at admission and discharge (duration of the hospitalization 19 $\pm$ 1 days). Only vitamin B_1 nutriture worsened during the hospitalization, and in a multivariate analysis, the only significant predictor of the change in the vitamin B_1 nutriture was the use of diuretics during the hospitalization ($F = 4.06$, $p < .001$).[275] The changes in the ETK (erythrocyte transketolase activity in whole blood) and alpha-ETK (ETK activity coefficient) during the hospital stay correlated with the cumulative dosage of furosemide adjusted for the duration of therapy ($r = 0.36$, $p < .001$ and $r = -0.28$, $p > .03$). Our data suggest that hospitalized elderly are at increased risk for vitamin B_1 deficiency especially when on a diuretic treatment.[275] This study shows that hospital malnutrition is not an important problem in our population and that thiamine may indeed represent a critical nutrient. The effect of diuretics can be counterbalanced by

oral vitamin B_1 supplements.[281] Supplementation in patients on diuretics should be handled very generously especially in the presence of heart failure. A subclinical thiamine deficiency is probably more common in elderly on diuretics (independent from the presence of heart failure). Further, the clinical picture may not always be typical so that the condition is usually missed.[267]

Oral supplementation with thiamine has been reported to improve cognitive function and overall well-being in the elderly.[264,268] The data about the role of vitamin B_1 in cognitive function and dementia (separate from the dramatic situation of the Wernicke-Korsakoff syndrome) are not yet clear but might be, as compared to other nutrients, of only minor importance.[282] Despite the role of thiamine in brain energy metabolism, as well as other effects such as modulation of free radical production or inflammation in vascular endothelium of brain vessels, which may be of importance in the development of cognitive impairment, these mechanisms are presently far from proven.[283] Animal data suggest that the aging brain shows an increased susceptibility to thiamine deficiency.[284]

In summary, there are no specific changes in thiamine nutriture due to aging alone. The high prevalence of thiamine deficiency in some groups of elderly is caused by poor intakes, excessive alcohol intake, or an increased loss due to chronic diuretic treatment.

VITAMIN B_2

Vitamin B_2 (riboflavin) acts with its coenzymes flavin mononucleotide (FMN) and flavin adenine dinucleotide (FAD) in many electron transfer reactions.[285] In view of the many different roles of the flavoenzymes in intermediary metabolism, the important role of riboflavin is often forgotten, for example, in antioxidant defense or in the modulation of homocysteine metabolism. The RDA[7] for riboflavin was set at 1.1 mg/d for all adult women independent of age and at 1.3 mg/d for men, which is lower than the 1989 RDA for this vitamin, which was set at 1.4 mg/d for men and 1.2 mg/d for women.[136] There are no studies available looking at the effect of energy intake on riboflavin requirements.[7] For practical reasons, the riboflavin allowance in the 1989 RDA has been computed as 0.6 mg/1000 kcal for people of all ages, and 0.5 mg/1000 kcal has been considered to be the minimal requirement for adults. The latter approach has not been used directly in the new guidelines;[7] however, for practical reasons and daily practice these numbers are nevertheless useful. The latter approach would also be useful for those with a high energy expenditure due to high levels of physical activity for which the requirements might be higher.[7]

The median riboflavin intake from food in the United States was estimated to be 2 mg/d for men and 1.5 mg/d for women.[7] Several studies, which were also important for the formulation of the present RDA, found in elderly individuals a rather high riboflavin intake and less than 5% had a riboflavin intake below the Estimated Average Requirement.[7] Nevertheless, depending on race, income, gender, age, and health status, up to 70% of elderly adults ingest less than 0.93 mg/d (men) or 0.8 mg/d (women) (these numbers correspond to two-thirds of the 1989 RDA).[26,205,212,260,263,286-293] Some of the older studies in which urinary riboflavin excretion was used as an index for the assessment of the riboflavin status need to be interpreted with caution only because earlier fluorescence-based assays detected other flavins incorrectly, thus reporting higher excretion values.

Intake is the major determinant of riboflavin status. The intake of dairy products and cereal products is one of the most important sources of riboflavin for elderly people.[7] The latter relationship is nicely reflected in the different populations within the Euronut SENECA study, where the median riboflavin intake in the Danish population was 2.0 mg/d,[26] whereas at study sites with a lower consumption of milk products, the riboflavin intake was found to be well below the lowest European intake recommendation of 1.0 mg/d. Nevertheless, the median intake in the latter study ranged from 1.24 mg/d (Hamme, Belgium) to 2.10 mg/d (North Ireland).[216] Despite the high median intake in several of the studies, there might be a variable percentage of elderly

people for which intakes are well below the RDA and lower than the present EAR. In a carefully performed study in Guatemala, the rather high prevalence of riboflavin deficiency was mainly caused by an inadequate intake of dairy products.[294] In the same study, it was also found that a lower fat-to-carbohydrate ratio in the diet can be associated with decreased dietary needs for riboflavin.[290] Although the riboflavin content of alcoholic beverages varies widely, wine was identified as an important riboflavin source in a sample of elderly in Italy (aged >60 years);[286] in contrast, in a survey of free-living elderly in the Boston area, high alcohol consumers were found to have the lowest blood levels of riboflavin and also vitamin B₁₂.[295]

Urinary riboflavin excretion is a good index of riboflavin nutriture. In elderly people, a riboflavin intake above 1.0–1.1 mg/d leads to a sharp increase in the urinary riboflavin excretion, suggestive of adequate riboflavin status.[290] Other studies report a similar constellation; these studies are among the basic rationale for the formulation of the requirements.[7]

In the recent British Diet and Nutrition Survey, individuals aged 65 years or older showed only in about 10% a low dietary intake of this vitamin, however, 41% of the free-living elderly and 35% of the institutionalized elderly showed a low biochemical status assessed with the erythrocyte glutathione reductase activity coefficient (EGRAC).[296] This apparent discrepancy cannot readily be explained and might reflect the variable intake in the elderly and/or a theoretical higher requirement of this vitamin with aging, which is probably not the case.[7]

Assessments of riboflavin nutriture by the EGRAC have reported a similarly high prevalence of suboptimal or even deficient nutriture. In the Wülflingen study, in which milk products were consumed daily by a group of institutionalized elderly, low levels of EGR activity (ie, <30 μkatal/L) were found only in 10% of the men and 2% of the elderly women. The lowest EGR was 20.1 μkatal/L. When the EGRAC was used, only 8% of the subjects were found to be deficient; when the reference range of 1.2 to 1.3 was used to define a marginal status, 10% of these elderly subjects were identified as having marginal riboflavin nutriture (Suter et al, data on file). A similarly low prevalence of impaired riboflavin status was found in other studies from Italy[263] and in the Boston survey.[291] In a poor group of elderly (aged >60 years) in Hong Kong, an EGRAC greater than 1.3 was found in about 70% of the surveyed population.[297] Recent data suggest that riboflavin deficiency is especially widespread in older adults in developing countries.[298,299] Riboflavin absorption seems to be unaffected by age, and there are probably no specific changes in vitamin B_2 tissue levels with age.[300,301]

Recent evidence suggests a role for riboflavin in the pathogenesis of age-related cataract because this vitamin may be important as a photosensitizing agent.[302] Biochemical analysis of human lens capsules and epithelium revealed a high prevalence (over 20%) of severe glutathione reductase deficiency, suggestive of a dietary riboflavin deficiency.[303] Others have reported a decrease of glutathione reductase in red blood cells with advancing age independent of riboflavin nutriture.[304] Although these data are contradictory, they may point to possible age-related changes in the glutathione redox system at the tissue level. Despite the potential involvement in some disease states (see later information) there is no evidence that this would be associated with a higher need during the aging process. In this context it should be mentioned that the lack of a higher requirement does not mean that the suggested intake should not be covered, as is often wrongly assumed!

Important data for the formulation of riboflavin requirements in elderly people stem from a depletion study in healthy elderly subjects aged 60 years or older in Guatemala, eating a Western-type diet. Using urinary excretion of riboflavin, the authors found the requirement for this vitamin to be in the range of 1.1 to 1.3 mg/d.[290] Also in this elderly population an increase in the riboflavin excretion occurred around an intake of 1 mg/d. These data are in agreement with older data in different younger age groups using similar techniques for the assessment of riboflavin nutriture.[305–308] Because these rather old data are

in good agreement with the new data from Boisvert et al.,[290] aging per se does not affect riboflavin metabolism and requirements.

Due to its important role in flavoenzymes, riboflavin has a high potential to interfere with the metabolism of other nutrients and other vitamins (folate, vitamin B_{12}, vitamin B_6).[309] Homocysteine has been identified as an important independent cardiovascular risk factor and a risk factor for atherogenesis as well as other chronic diseases in general (see also the sections on folate and vitamin B_6).[5,310,311] In view of the potential role of homocysteine in the modulation of chronic disease risk, especially cardiovascular disease, the interaction with folate is of special interest. Blood levels of folate are probably the most important determinant of plasma homocysteine levels.[312] Major vitamins modulating homocysteine metabolism and thus plasma concentration are folate, vitamin B_6, and vitamin B_{12} (see the section titled "Folate"). In view of the strong effect of folate on homocysteine levels, other nutrients with modulatory capacity have been forgotten. FAD is an important coenzyme for methylene-tetrahydrofolate reductase (EC 1.7.99.5). Only after the action of this enzyme can folate be used in the methylation reaction of homocysteine metabolism.[313] Many nutrients do show colinear behavior; accordingly, it is not surprising that in the setting of low folate, low riboflavin plasma concentrations are often found.[314] Even in the setting of the mutation of the MTHFR gene (677CT) lower riboflavin plasma concentration is associated with a higher homocysteine plasma concentration,[315] and a folic acid supplementation alone exacerbated the riboflavin deficiency. In such a setting, riboflavin has to be supplemented to overcome the metabolic handicap. This example underlines the potential importance of well-equilibrated supplements for general use.

In summary, at present there is no evidence suggesting age-related changes in the metabolism of riboflavin. The high variability of riboflavin nutriture in healthy elderly people is mainly due to low intakes, especially of milk products, and thus can be easily corrected.

NIACIN

Niacin plays an important role as a coenzyme in nicotinamide adenine dinucleotide (NAD) and nicotinamide adenine dinucleotide phosphate (NADP).[316] Because the amino acid tryptophan can be converted to niacin,[316] niacin requirements are expressed as niacin equivalents (NE).[7] The present niacin RDA is 14 mg/d of niacin equivalents (NE) for adult females independent of age and 16 mg/d NE for men. One NE corresponds to 60 mg tryptophan. Compared to the 1989 RDA (15 mg NE per day for men and 13 mg NE per day for women),[136] the new recommendations are slightly higher. The niacin deficiency disease pellagra is uncommon in Western societies,[316] except in association with chronic alcoholism.[56]

Analytical procedures for the measurement of the niacin content of food, as well as the biochemical assessment of niacin nutriture, are uncertain and very incomplete, therefore making them limited in practical value.[316] Accordingly, the data about the niacin nutriture in elderly adults are very limited. There is still much controversy regarding the ideal method for the assessment of niacin nutriture.

Niacin intake in elderly people varies widely as a function of socioeconomic background, race, age, health status, and institutionalization. In the Boston survey, around 25% of the elderly consumed less than 10 mg/d NE (men) or 8.66 mg NE/d (women).[211] In the Health and Nutrition Examination Survey I (HANES I), 53% of the surveyed African American elderly with incomes below the poverty level had intakes below 10 and 8.6 mg NE per day (corresponding to two-thirds of the 1989 RDA) for men and women, respectively.[209] However, only 54% of healthy free-living, middle-income elderly surveyed by Garry et al.[49] in New Mexico had intakes of less than 10 mg/d of NE. As in the case of most other nutrients, nutritional intake of niacin is related to mortality of elderly individuals.[317] When urinary excretion of N-methyl nicotinamide is used as a measure, 1% to 50% of elderly subjects are shown to be niacin deficient.[318–320] Different factors affect the bioavailability of this vitamin, but

on the basis of the present data, aging per se does not affect absorption.[321,322]

Niacin may be obtained from the conversion of tryptophan to this vitamin. Many different factors (such as hormonal factors, amino acids, or certain nutrients) may influence the conversion of tryptophan to niacin.[316,323,324] At present, it is not known whether there are age-related changes in the conversion of tryptophan to niacin. Age-related changes in hormonal balance or in vitamin nutriture may affect this conversion. Animal data suggest that the conversion rate may be highly dependent on the adequacy of vitamin B$_6$ nutriture (see the section titled "Vitamin B$_6$").[325]

VITAMIN B$_6$

Vitamin B$_6$ is of major importance as a cofactor in many reactions of intermediary metabolism.[326] The present RDA for elderly men (>50 y of age) is 1.7 mg/d, and for elderly women it is 1.5 mg/d, of vitamin B$_6$.[7] Compared to the 1980 and 1989 RDAs,[136] the most recent recommendation is again lower, but nevertheless higher for young adults, where the RDA has been set at 1.3 mg/d of vitamin B$_6$ for young men (19–50 years of age) and 1.1 mg/d for women.[7] The Estimated Average Requirement (EAR) increases with age and the increase is approximately 0.2–0.3 mg/d of food B$_6$.[7] The evidence for the latter comes from a few carefully performed metabolic depletion and repletion studies as well as functional tests using homocysteine and selected immunological markers.[7] It is assumed that an intake of 1 mg/d of vitamin B$_6$ is sufficient for most younger adults, but under a very high protein diet the requirements may be higher.[7] High protein intakes are associated with a higher requirement for this vitamin, and an intake of 0.016 mg of vitamin B$_6$ per gram of protein eaten has been recommended.[136]

The intake of vitamin B$_6$ varies widely among the elderly as a function of age, socioeconomic level, and state of health. Intakes below the RDA have been reported in up to 50% or even 90% of elderly populations.[25,34,206,209,211,216,260,327–334] Even in the healthy, free-living, upper-middle-class elderly surveyed by Garry et al.,[49] 61% of the women consumed less than 1 mg of vitamin B_6 per day, and 54% of the elderly men consumed less than 1.1 mg (corresponding to 55% of the 1989 RDA). In the Euronut SENECA study, all populations in the different study centers had a median vitamin B_6 intake below the present US RDA. Between 10% and 50% of the US population older than 51 years consumed less than the Estimated Average Requirement (EAR) of vitamin B_6 (ie, less than 1.4 mg/d and 1.3 mg/d for men and women, respectively).[7] The EAR corresponds to the daily nutrient intake that is estimated to meet the requirement of half the healthy population of the corresponding age group. When pyridoxal levels for the biochemical assessment of vitamin B_6 nutriture, with a cutoff of 20 nmol/L, close to 25% of the subjects must be classified as deficient.[26] In the Boston survey of free-living elderly, 56% of the subjects had intakes below the 1989 recommendations, but only 5% showed a biochemical deficiency by the index of aspartate aminotransferase activity coefficients (AST-AC).[211] A similarly low prevalence of deficiency (9%) by the same index was found in a nationwide survey in the Netherlands in which the surveyed elderly (aged 65–79 years) consumed around 0.016 mg of vitamin B_6 per gram of protein ingested.[333] On the basis of their data, the latter authors conclude that a normal AST-AC could be achieved with vitamin B_6 intakes of at least 0.020 mg/g of protein. The discrepancy between a high prevalence of low intakes and a rather low prevalence of deficiency in some of the cited studies may be caused in part by the use of only incomplete dietary databases for vitamin B_6.

The prevalence of diagnosed deficiency depends on the biochemical methods used for the assessment of the B_6 status. In the Wülflingen study of institutionalized elderly in Switzerland, we observed a deficiency in about 33% of the elderly when the erythrocyte aspartate aminotransferase activity (AST; former EGOT) was used as an index. Using the AST-AC with a cutoff of less than 1.8 to define deficiency, we found 85% of the subjects to be deficient. On the basis of pyridoxal-5-phosphate levels, 93% were found

to be deficient (Suter et al., data on file). Also in other studies, socioeconomic level, institutionalization, and health status were the major determinants of vitamin B_6 status.

Serum and plasma vitamin B_6 levels are subject to large variations, depending mainly on recent food intake, and thus do not reflect long-term vitamin B_6 nutritional status. Several studies have shown a decline in serum and plasma levels of pyridoxal phosphate (PLP, which represents the most active form of the vitamin) with age.[335–337] The reported decrease of plasma PLP was approximately 0.90 ng/mL and was associated with an increased prevalence of low plasma PLP levels (ie, <5 ng/mL) from around 3% in healthy younger subjects (aged <40 years) to about 12% in individuals aged 80 years and older. It has been suggested that the age-related increase of the activity of alkaline phosphatase, which is considered to be of major importance in the degradation of PLP, and low intakes are the major causes of the age-related decline in plasma PLP levels with aging.[338]

Animal data suggest, however, an impairment of the formation of PLP in different tissues.[339] It is not established whether the capacity to phosphorylate this vitamin changes with age in humans. Little evidence for an alteration in pyridoxine phosphorylation with age comes from a few clinical case reports of primary sideroachrestic anemias responsive solely to the administration of pyridoxal phosphate and not to pyridoxine.[340] In these diseases, there is a clear pathophysiologic basis. Using the tryptophan-loading test as an index of vitamin B_6 nutriture, several older studies found an age-related increase in abnormal loading tests.[335,337] These abnormalities of vitamin B_6 nutriture can be corrected by the ingestion of vitamin B_6 supplements in most elderly persons.[318,341–343] However, a few studies report the inability of some elderly (up to 20%) to correct their biochemical vitamin B_6 status upon supplement intakes.[344–346] The latter observations are very suggestive of age-related changes in vitamin B_6 requirements of elderly adults. Nevertheless, effects of diseases and unknown comorbidities in these studies could not be ruled out as a cause of this non-responsiveness to supplements.

Functional or dynamic tests may be better means to study potential age-related changes in the metabolism of most vitamins. Despite the possibility of age-related changes in vitamin B$_6$ metabolism (as outlined earlier), Kant et al.[346] were unable to detect a change of the urinary vitamin B$_6$ load as a function of age. However, it is not exactly known whether these excretion tests can reliably detect any age-related changes. Therefore, it has been recommended that more than one biochemical index be used for the optimal assessment of vitamin B$_6$ nutriture.

Interesting and important data about vitamin B$_6$ requirements of elderly people were obtained in a recent depletion/repletion study of elderly subjects (>60 years) in a metabolic unit.[347] This study consisted of several experimental periods with well-defined amounts of vitamin B$_6$ ranging from 0.003 to 0.03375 mg/kg of body weight per day. After the initial depletion, the subjects were repleted in a stepwise fashion; the tryptophan-loading test (ie, the measurement of urinary xanthurenic acid excretion) was used to assess B$_6$ nutriture. The major result of this study was that in elderly subjects consuming proteins approximately 1.5 times the recommendation, the estimated vitamin B$_6$ requirements are about 1.96 mg for elderly men and 1.90 mg for elderly women. These data from Ribaya-Mercado et al.[347] strongly suggest that the B$_6$ requirements are increased in the elderly. This study was important for the reformulation of the latest version of the recommendations.[7] Furthermore, it has to be considered that in this study, the repletion was done with a highly bioavailable pyridoxine hydrochloride supplement in addition to the vitamin B$_6$ from ingested food. The bioavailability of vitamin B$_6$ from food is much lower, so the RDA based upon the intake of the vitamin from food sources may be even higher than assumed. The newest recommendations do account for these alterations of the metabolism with aging.

Vitamin B$_6$ deficiency or suboptimal status may result in an enhancement of the pathogenesis of different diseases and/or impairment of specific organ functions. The depletion of vitamin B$_6$ in studies by Meydani et al resulted in an impairment of the immune function in the elderly.[348-350] Vitamin B$_6$ has an important function as a cofactor for the cystathionine synthase, and a lack of this vitamin may result in high homocysteine levels in the blood. Recent evidence suggests that elevated plasma homocysteine levels should be regarded as an independent cardiovascular risk factor.[312,351-353] Several nutrients (folate, vitamin B$_6$, vitamin B$_{12}$, and vitamin B$_2$) are important modulators of the plasma homocysteine levels.[312] Retrospective and prospective studies have described a relationship between the risk of coronary artery disease and myocardial infarction and the intake of vitamin B$_6$.[343,354-356] This relationship, however, is strongest for folic acid.[312] The relationship between the different vitamins and the risk of atherosclerosis, especially coronary artery disease, has a high potential to be of great pathophysiologic and public health importance, but needs to be proved in more prospective interventional studies. The importance of homocysteine and the potential relationship between nutrition and the pathogenesis of atherosclerosis will be discussed in the next section (see also the sections titled "Folate" and "Vitamin B$_{12}$").

Vitamin B$_6$ plays an important role in the synthesis of neurotransmitters and neural function in general. Accordingly, it is not surprising that vitamin B$_6$ supplementation in the elderly may be associated with an improvement of memory and mental performance.[357] However, a recent Cochrane review did not find any supportive evidence for short-term benefit from vitamin B$_6$ in improving mood (depression, fatigue, and tension symptoms) or cognitive functions in general; however, the authors concluded that there may be a possible role in older adults in the context of a disturbed homocysteine metabolism.[358] Patients with Alzheimer's disease probably have an impaired vitamin status due to low intakes[359] and not due to metabolic alterations in intermediary metabolism. Vitamin B$_6$, compared to folate and vitamin B$_{12}$, has a much lower efficacy in lowering plasma homocysteine levels;[360] but vitamin

B_6 might be of greater importance in the modulation of the postprandial clearance of homocysteine.

The prevalence of impaired vitamin B_6 nutriture in elderly people is variable; however, compared to other vitamins, it is rather high. A deficiency is consistently found in different populations and is mainly caused by low dietary intakes. Further, vitamin B_6 metabolism may be affected by aging, which is accounted for in the present RDA for this vitamin.

FOLATE

Folate corresponds to the generic technical term for this water-soluble vitamin from the B-complex group. One of the main functions of folate is the transport of single carbon atoms in intermediary metabolic processes.[361] The RDA for folate is 400 µg/d of dietary folate equivalents (DFE) for elderly women and men.[7] The DFE adjust for approximately half of the lower folate bioavailability from food sources as compared to folic acid (DFE: 1µg food folate = 0.6 µg folic acid from fortified food or as a supplement consumed with food = 0.5 µg of a supplement taken on an empty stomach).[7] Compared to the 1989 RDA, the recommended intakes have been increased for elderly women and men (the 1989 folate RDAs were the same for the elderly as they were for well young adults: 200 µg for men and 180 µg for women).[136]

Folate intakes in the elderly may vary considerably, but most elderly people ingest amounts close to the RDA. Nevertheless, according to the surveyed population, intake may be very variable, especially in elderly samples. Based on survey data before the fortification of cereal grains with folate (before January 1,1998), the prevalence of low folate intakes varied between 0% and 50%[49,94,216,362,363] and is influenced mainly by institutionalization and health status.[103,364] The median intake at the population level was, before the mandatory folate cereal fortification, 250 µg/d,[7] which is well below the present recommendation. It is assumed that the average folate intake increases by approximately 80–100 µg/d by the

fortification of cereals with folate.[7] In the Wülflingen study, 27% of the men and 14% of the women had folate plasma levels below 10 nmol/L. The lowest value was 7.5 nmol/L, so none of these surveyed elderly were below the level of 6.8 nmol/L, which is regarded as the threshold level for deficiency. Nevertheless, about 50% of these institutionalized elderly had a marginal biochemical status (ie, plasma levels between 6.8 and 13.4 nmol/L) (Suter et al., data on file). This marginal status may be of pathophysiological relevance regarding the relationship of folate and other compounds in many reactions of intermediary metabolism, such as homocysteine. Other studies reported a similarly low prevalence of biochemical deficiency in elderly subjects. The median dietary folate intake in the Boston survey was 254 µg/d for men and 216 µg/d for women.[211] In agreement with these intakes, only 2.5% of this group of elderly showed plasma concentrations below 7 nmol/L.[211] A similarly low rate of deficiency was reported in a study from New York City and a town in New Zealand.[365,366] As in the Wülflingen study and SENECA study, no elderly subjects had plasma folate levels below 6.8 nmol/L. In some studies, despite low intakes, hardly any elderly subjects had low plasma folate levels;[49] this discrepancy may in part be caused by an underestimation of folate intakes due to the incompleteness of the food tables used.

Folate is widely distributed in food, where it is found mainly in the form of polyglutamates. Before absorption, polyglutamates must be deconjugated by an intestinal folate conjugase (pteroylpolyglutamyl hydrolase) present in the brush border and intracellular fraction of the jejunal mucosa.[367] Whether the activity of this enzyme is subject to age-related alterations is controversial; however, present evidence suggests that folic acid absorption is not influenced by age alone.[208,368] The activity of the folate conjugase, and thus folate absorption per se, is highly pH dependent. Russell and colleagues[368] reported a diminished folic acid absorption in elderly subjects with atrophic gastritis, which is characterized by diminished gastric acid output and thus a higher proximal small intestinal pH, leading to bacterial overgrowth in the upper gastrointestinal tract. This malabsorption may be due to a high intra-luminal pH that negatively influences the pH-sensitive active uptake of folic acid by small intestinal epithelial cells. In this study, the folic acid malabsorption in subjects with atrophic gastritis was completely corrected (ie, normalized) by the oral administration of 0.1 N hydrochloric acid.

Despite this folate malabsorption in atrophic gastritis, these individuals had normal serum folate levels, which might have been due to folate synthesis by the bacteria that were overgrowing the upper intestinal tract.[368] Different modifiable factors may affect folate absorption. A high intake of alcohol alone or in combination with an inadequate diet is one of the most important factors contributing to a clinical folate deficiency.[56] Alcohol has the potential to block several metabolic pathways of folic acid. Animal experiments using rats chronically fed a low-folate diet suggest changes in methyl group metabolism with aging, independent of the amount of folate in the diet.[369]

In elderly people, the combination of low folate intakes and elevated plasma homocysteine levels represents a rather prevalent clinical situation. Several lines of evidence suggest that homocysteine may be a risk factor for coronary artery disease and atherosclerosis.[353,370,371] In view of the potential importance of folate as a modulator of the plasma homocysteine levels and therefore potentially a factor in cardiovascular risk, folate nutriture should be optimized in all age groups, and theoretical considerations suggest that folic acid fortification of the food supply may be beneficial for the elderly.[372]

In the original Framingham Study cohort of subjects aged 67 to 96 years, 29% showed high plasma homocysteine levels (hyperhomocysteinemia, defined as >14 μmol/L).[312] These elevated levels of plasma homocysteine are mainly attributable to an impairment of folate, vitamin B_6, and/or vitamin B_{12} nutriture. But in most people, folate seems to be the major determinant of plasma homocysteine levels.[312,372] Other studies reported the same findings.[6,373] Other nutrients,

including vitamin B_6 (see earlier), play central roles in the modulation of plasma homocysteine levels. A rather large number of studies reported that homocysteine is an independent graded risk factor for mortality, especially cardiovascular mortality. Nevertheless, the effect of a reduction of homocysteine on homocysteine-related mortality is, so far, disappointing. A recent study by Anderson et al[374] reported that the effect of the ingestion of folic acid–fortified foods on homocysteine-related mortality was modest (adjusted relative risk = 1.03 per μmol/L; 95% CI: 1.01–1.05, $p = .006$). The authors suggest that homocysteine should be lowered more aggressively but the more likely explanation for the modest effect is that other (risk) factors were of greater importance as modulators of mortality. Similarly, in the recent double-blind prospective VISP (Vitamin Intervention for Stroke Prevention) study[375] even aggressive lowering of homocysteine with a high-dosage regimen of a vitamin mix did not have an effect on vascular outcomes in patients after nondisabling cerebral infarction. Nevertheless, there was, at baseline (as in other studies), an association of homocysteine with vascular risk, which might hint at a potential direct or indirect role of homocysteine. The VISP trial and the study by Anderson et al are very important; it seems that homocysteine is indeed only a proxy marker for other risks and risk factors. Despite very promising evidence for other vitamins (eg, antioxidants) in the risk of atherogenesis, CAD mortality and morbidity in all large prospective trials have only disappointing (negative) results.[190] This is actually not surprising because the pathogenesis of chronic disease risk is so complex that it is hardly imaginable that by the administration of a single vitamin or a vitamin mix, or by modulation of one single metabolite (eg, homocysteine), a reversal of such a complex disease pathogenesis could be induced. For the moment, the most promising strategy to control any chronic disease risk is the consumption of a balanced diet according to the present guidelines and optimal control of the classical risk factors for chronic diseases. In view of the newest data, it can be assumed that ongoing large trials involving the administration of vitamins to lower homocysteine will also lead to overall disappointing results. In agreement with these newest findings, the committee for the formulation of the RDA concluded that the knowledge about the relationship between folate, homocysteine, and atherogenesis has been judged too weak to be used as a basis for the derivation of the present recommendations.[7] The new studies support this latter statement.

Folate deficiency is comparatively common in psychogeriatric patients.[376] An elevated plasma homocysteine is often associated with low folate status, especially in geriatric and psychogeriatric populations.[376,377] These associations are suggestive that folate might play a central role in cognitive function of the elderly as well as dementia. Although many reasons (eg, poor diet) may lead to an impaired folate status in elderly (especially psychogeriatric patients), folic acid plays an important role in the pathogenesis of many diseases of aging (eg, cancer, atherosclerosis, stroke, and neurodegenerative disorders), especially the impairment of cognition. A recent review summarized the effect of folate as follows:[378] folate has particular effects on mood and cognitive function, and an impairment in folate metabolism may lead to a pattern of cognitive dysfunction as during aging.[378] In a study of the noninstitutionalized elderly, a relationship between the Mini-Mental Test and biochemical folate status was described.[330] Further, it is possible that folic acid status may be of crucial importance in the pathogenesis and/or management of depression and other neuropsychiatric disturbances in the elderly.[378-381]

A lower folate status has further been identified to be associated with a higher risk of an adverse cerebrovascular event.[382] It has to be remembered that all of these studies represent *only associations* and not necessarily causality, and folate and/or elevated homocysteine might just represent a proxy marker for other organic, functional, or metabolic abnormalities.[383] Accordingly, in a prospective study, a relationship between folate, vitamin B_{12}, and cognition was almost absent, but elevated homocysteine concentrations were associated with lower cognitive performance in a normal aging population (30–80 years).[384] Similarly, in an elderly population, there was no correlation between plasma homocysteine concentration and atrophic gastritis,[385] although the latter is an important determinant of folate and vitamin B_{12} nutriture. However, there are many mechanisms leading to elevated homocysteine levels, which may be completely independent from nutritional factors (eg, smoking or physical inactivity). The central question whether the B vitamins' (including folate) inadequacies contribute to brain malfunctions or whether these changes result from aging and disease cannot be answered at present.[386,387] Nevertheless, an adequate intake of all essential nutrients should be assured any time.[373] If nutrients help to treat some symptoms of neurocognitive functions in already ill elderly, this would be helpful. However, in the long term, research should focus on the role of nutrients in the prevention of neurodegenerative diseases.[387,388]

The formulation of the dietary recommended allowances for most nutrients, including folate, is based on population studies about intake as well as biochemical status. Nevertheless, in view of the role of vitamins in health and disease, metabolic studies (such as depletion-repletion studies) and functional tests may help to clarify some of the controversies around the recommended allowances. In the case of folate, folate catabolite excretion may represent a useful tool to determine adequate intakes. A recent study by Wolfe et al[389] reported that the excretion of certain folate catabolites reflected total body folate pool size and that these catabolites may be a useful long-term indicator paralleling functional measures of folate status.[389] In the latter study, folate catabolite excretion changed similarly in young and old individuals upon change of intake, which is suggestive of no fundamental changes in folate turnover regarding catabolite production in low-intake situations over age.

In view of the potential role of folate in the development of chronic diseases and/or the potential to modulate different metabolic functions, the latest RDA for folate has been increased.

Adequate intakes based on present guidelines should be more strongly encouraged, and an increased intake (whenever possible from dietary sources), even above the present recommendations, could only be encouraged.

VITAMIN B$_{12}$

The Recommended Dietary Allowance (RDA) for elderly women and men is 2.4 μg/d of vitamin B$_{12}$.[7] The primary dietary sources of this vitamin are animal products, but as will be discussed later, the bioavailability of vitamin B$_{12}$ from food sources (ie, the protein-bound vitamin B$_{12}$) decreases with aging. It is recommended in the present RDA[7] that most of the RDA for older persons (ie, >51 years) of 2.4 μg/d of vitamin B$_{12}$ should be obtained by the consumption of vitamin B$_{12}$–fortified foods or vitamin B$_{12}$–containing supplements.[7] These two sources contain crystalline vitamin B$_{12}$; its absorption is not affected by aging. The present recommendation is higher than the 1989 RDA, which was set at 2.0 μg/d for men and 1.6 μg/d for women.[136]

Vitamin B$_{12}$ intake in free-living elderly persons varies widely, and approximately 0% to 50% of this group have been reported to have (dietary non-supplemental) intakes below the present recommendation.[49,94,207,390,391] In the study by Garry et al.[391] of middle-class elderly subjects in New Mexico, 24% of the men and 39% of the women had intakes below 2 μg/d (men) and 1.6 μg/d (women); up to 15% had intakes below 1.5 μg/d and 1.2 μg/d, respectively. The elderly males surveyed in the Boston study had a median vitamin B$_{12}$ dietary intake of 3.1 μg/d, and for the female elderly it was 2.6 μg/d.[211] Only 3% of the elderly men and 12% of the elderly women had intakes below 1.3 μg/d (men) or 1.05 μg/d (women). The prevalence of low blood vitamin B$_{12}$ levels varies between 0% and 30% of the surveyed elderly.[365,366,392–402] In the Wülflingen study (Suter et al, data on file), only 3.8% of the surveyed institutionalized elderly had plasma vitamin B$_{12}$ levels below 100 pmol/L. Despite this low prevalence of biochemical deficiency, 28.3% of the elderly had plasma levels below 200 pmol/L, and most of the elderly (ie, 85.3%) had levels below 400 pmol/L. The lowest detected value was 14 pmol/L, and 86% of the elderly had levels above 147 pmol/L. Using the Euronut criteria, 6.3% have to be judged as deficient. In the Euronut SENECA study, only 2.7% of the subjects had vitamin B$_{12}$ levels below 111 pmol/L. These data are further in good agreement with the Boston survey, in which only 5% of the elderly were found to have vitamin B$_{12}$ values below 74 pmol/L.[211]

Several studies have reported a gradual decline in the plasma vitamin B$_{12}$ levels with age; however, despite this decline, the values remain within the limits of normality in most studies. The cutoff value of the limit of normality is, however, controversial. In a longitudinal study by Nilsson-Ehle et al.,[403] an annual decline of the serum vitamin B$_{12}$ levels of 3.4 pmol/L for men and 3.2 pmol/L for women was observed. In agreement with this decline, the prevalence of low vitamin B$_{12}$ levels increases with age in most studies as well as the serum (plasma) concentration of methylmalonic acid.[404] It has been suggested that this age-related decline in plasma/serum vitamin B$_{12}$ levels might be related to the increased occurrence of atrophic gastritis with increasing age.[390,405]

The prevalence of atrophic gastritis increases with age to almost 40% to 50% in those aged 80 years or older. It has been shown that atrophic gastritis decreases the bioavailability of dietary vitamin B$_{12}$ (ie, protein-bound vitamin B$_{12}$).[406–408] In natural food sources, vitamin B$_{12}$ is bound to food proteins and must be released from protein binding before the absorptive process can be initiated. Several mechanisms may lead to the malabsorption of protein-bound vitamin B$_{12}$ in atrophic gastritis. Because of diminished or completely lacking gastric acid production, protein digestion is impaired, and vitamin B$_{12}$ cannot be released from its protein binding. Additionally, bacteria that overgrow the upper gastrointestinal tract may bind vitamin B$_{12}$ and/or convert it to vitamin B$_{12}$ analogues, rendering the vitamin B$_{12}$ unavailable. Some of the analogues may even inhibit normal vitamin B$_{12}$ absorption in the ileum terminal.

The decreased output of intrinsic factor in atrophic gastritis is probably of no clinical significance because usually the degree of parietal cell destruction is only partial. In a metabolic study, it was shown that the malabsorption of the protein-bound vitamin B_{12} in subjects with atrophic gastritis could be reversed by an antibiotic treatment with tetracycline.[408] In this study, the bacterial counts in the upper gastrointestinal tract could have been reduced by the antibiotic treatment, and this decrease was associated with a normalization of the absorption of the protein-bound vitamin B_{12}, suggesting that the malabsorption was mainly due to bacterial overgrowth. In this context, it should be mentioned that the absorption of crystalline vitamin B_{12} is not impaired in atrophic gastritis. This possibility (ie, normal crystalline vitamin B_{12} absorption) should be accounted for in the selection of the type of vitamin B_{12} absorption test (crystalline or protein bound) used in clinical practice. Age per se (ie, in the absence of atrophic gastritis) does not affect the absorption of vitamin B_{12}. Therefore, it must be remembered that a normal absorption of crystalline vitamin B_{12} is not equal to a normal absorption of protein-bound vitamin B_{12}, that is, food vitamin B_{12}.[409] Accordingly in the present RDA the intake of B_{12}-fortified foods or vitamin B_{12}–containing supplements is recommended for the elderly.[7]

It is controversial whether adequate plasma vitamin B_{12} levels always reflect adequacy of vitamin B_{12} status correctly. Recently it has been shown that vitamin B_{12} deficiency, diagnosed by the measurements of serum methylmalonic acid and total homocysteine, might be present even in the absence of hematologic abnormalities, a normal Schilling test, and normal or only minimally depressed serum/plasma cobalamin levels.[410,411] This suggests that vitamin B_{12} deficiency could be a major undetected problem in apparently healthy elderly.[397] In view of the importance of vitamin B_{12} in intermediary metabolism as a cofactor for the L-methylmalonyl-CoA mutase and the methionine synthase, the measurement of serum metabolites in the diagnosis of cobalamin deficiency may be indicated in certain cases.[412,413]

Some evidence even suggests that the measurement of serum cobalamin to detect deficiency is a rather insensitive tool.[393] This should be remembered in any discussion of the implementation of generous folate fortification and/or supplementation for the control of plasma homocysteine levels. Measurement of plasma homocysteine and methylmalonic acid levels may be helpful in the evaluation of the adequacy of vitamin B_{12} nutriture. But besides vitamin nutriture, other factors, especially kidney function, may represent important modulators of plasma homocysteine levels. These factors have to be considered in the formulation of "normal values," and the definition of reference intervals should be adjusted for different age groups separately.[414] The controversy regarding the lower limit of normal plasma levels of vitamin B_{12} continues, so elderly subjects with low plasma levels of vitamin B_{12} should be monitored more closely, and in view of the potential benefit, even a parenteral supplementation of this vitamin may be indicated in certain patients.

Because of the primary importance of folate for the regulation of homocysteine levels, folate supplementation has been recommended. In view of the high prevalence of abnormalities in vitamin B_{12} metabolism, supplementation with folate alone may be associated with some risk; therefore, only combined supplementation/fortification with folate *and* vitamin B_{12} should be considered.[372,414]

A vegetarian diet in combination with aging is a very unfavorable situation.[415] As such, for older adults, a generous intake of crystalline vitamin B_{12} from fortified foods and/or supplements should be assured.

"Pernicious dementia" and other changes in cognitive function due to a deficiency of vitamin B_{12} have been described in the literature.[416,417] Often patients with different forms of cognitive impairment do have an impaired vitamin B_{12} status;[418] however, this is mainly due to low intakes as well as the age-related changes in B_{12} metabolism (malabsorption of food vitamin B_{12}) as discussed earlier. A recent study in elderly subjects shows a clear relationship between the intake of crystalline vitamin B_{12} and serum gastrin levels,[419] supporting the notion that the adequate intake of crystalline vitamin B_{12} is especially crucial in the elderly. Accordingly, associations between vitamin B_{12} status and different forms of cognitive impairment are not surprising. A recent Cochrane systematic review concluded that the evidence of any efficacy of vitamin B_{12} in improving the cognitive function in individuals with dementia and low vitamin B_{12} levels is insufficient at present.[421]

During the last few years, a revival of oral vitamin B_{12} therapy in the conditions of severe B_{12} deficiency (pernicious megaloblastic anemia) was propagated.[422] In view of the severity and the detrimental potential of a severe vitamin B_{12} deficiency, an initial parenteral therapy is nevertheless recommended, especially in the elderly with impaired cognitive function and suboptimal drug compliance.

Evidence suggests that elderly individuals, even with plasma vitamin B_{12} levels within the lower limit of normality, may show metabolic disturbances indicative of a "subclinical" vitamin B_{12} deficiency. The new Dietary Reference Intakes have been increased as compared to earlier recommendations. Because a large fraction of elderly people may malabsorb vitamin B_{12} from food sources (ie, protein-bound vitamin B_{12}), it is recommended that individuals older than 50 years should consume foods fortified with B_{12} or even take B_{12} supplements to meet their requirements.

BIOTIN

Biotin plays a central role in carboxylation reactions.[423,424] Biotin deficiency seems to occur rarely, but has been reported in persons who have been on long-term total parenteral nutrition, who have ingested raw eggs excessively, or who have an inborn error of metabolism. The recommendation for adequate intakes (AI) for biotin has been set at 30 μg/d for all adults independent of age.[7] This is in agreement with the 1989 RDA edition; however, at that time an intake range of 30 to 100 μg/d was provisionally recommended

for adults.[136] There are hardly any recommendation data for elderly adults. The paucity of data is mainly due to the lack of analytic tools to quantitate biotin in body fluids as well as lack of good experimental validation of different indices of biotin status.[425–427] One of the few studies reporting biotin intake is based on NHANES II data in which the mean biotin intake in young women (aged 18–24 years) was 39.9 ± 26.0 μg/d (mean $\pm$ SD).[428] There are no data for older adults, but based on the NHANES II data with the rather larger variability, it can be expected that a large fraction of elderly adults might have insufficient intakes. Data from Great Britain reported similar mean intakes in the range of the present US recommendations for adequate intake (AI).[429] There are hardly any data available on biotin nutriture in the aged. One study reported lower biotin plasma levels in a small group of elderly as compared with young athletes, but others have reported no change in these levels with age.[430,431] In the Wülflingen study, only 20 patients (9.7%) had plasma biotin levels below 1 nmol/L; 21 patients (10.2%) showed a marginal biotin status (defined as plasma biotin levels between 0.5 and 1.0 nmol/L). The lowest biotin plasma level was 0.61 nmol/L. If deficiency is defined as a plasma biotin level below 0.5 nmol/L, none of our subjects were deficient. Several conditions such as aging and excessive alcohol consumption may be associated with alterations in biotin metabolism. Animal data suggest that chronic excessive alcohol consumption inhibits intestinal biotin transport and induces a biotin malabsorption.[432] However, other animal data suggest that aging may lead to improved biotin absorption and thus increased plasma concentration.[433] The present evidence, although scarce, suggests that biotin nutriture is not a major concern for elderly people, but there is a need for specific data.

PANTOTHENIC ACID

The adequate intake (AI) for pantothenic acid has been set at 5 mg/d for all adults.[7] The AI is identical for women and men. This AI is approximately just in the middle of the estimated safe and adequate intake of 4–7 mg/d as formulated in the 1989 RDA.[136] In a study in a nursing home, the daily pantothenic acid intake was 3.75 mg/d or 2.22 mg/1000 kcal, which is less than the recommended allowance for the elderly.[434] Srinivasan et al.[435] reported a range of biotin intake of 2.5 to 9.5 mg/d in a small sample of 65 institutionalized elderly (mean age 73 years). The average intake was 2.9 mg/1000 kcal and it is accordingly conceivable that a larger fraction of elderly might indeed have intakes below the present AI.

In view of the wide distribution of this vitamin in most plant and animal foods, very low intakes are probably not often encountered except in situations of extremely low energy intake.[436] In humans as well as in animals, a decrease in protein-bound pantothenic acid in blood has been reported; however, some investigators have failed to find an age-related decline in blood levels of this vitamin. Using urinary excretion as an index of pantothenic acid nutriture in elderly people is not conclusive and may be contradictory.[437,438] On

the basis of the present evidence,[436] no statement about the adequacy of pantothenic acid nutriture in elderly adults or the optimal intakes can be made.

CONCLUSIONS AND RECOMMENDATIONS

In this chapter, selected aspects of vitamin nutriture of the elderly have been reviewed. Elderly adults are a heterogenous group, so they vary widely in their health as well as nutritional status. Accordingly, in daily practice, a global medical and nutritional assessment of each single patient has to be made.

The evidence suggests that for vitamins D and B$_{12}$ elderly adults may be at special risk for deficiency because in the metabolism of these vitamins, age-related changes do occur. In the absence of specific diseases as well as no supplement intake, there is no concern for toxicity of any of the vitamins except for vitamin A for most elderly people. A chronic high intake of

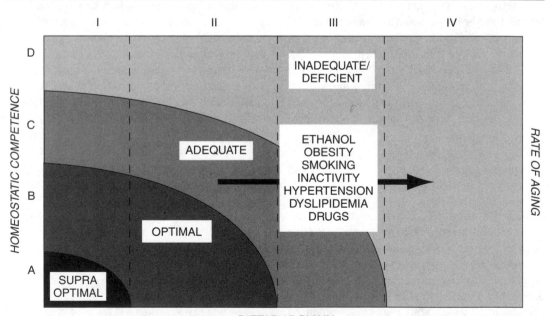

Figure 4–1 Relationship Among Nutrient Intake, Rate of Aging, and Homeostatic Competence
Control of Risk Factors Modulating the Nutrient Requirements may be of Primary Importance in Daily Life.

preformed vitamin A might have adverse health effects (eg, osteoporosis and fracture risk, see the section titled "Vitamin A") so that the intake of provitamin A in the form of β-carotene should be favored in all age groups, especially elderly adults. For several vitamins (vitamin K, niacin, biotin, and pantothenic acid), the database regarding vitamin nutriture in elderly people is very poor and more research is strongly needed; no definite statement about the nutritional requirements in the elderly can be made for these vitamins.

When discussing vitamin metabolism in the elderly, modifiable effects on the basic requirements of the different vitamins should be mentioned. Vitamins may play an important role in primary and secondary aging processes (Figure 4–1). The effect of overall lifestyle, including

nutrition, on the aging process and homeostatic competence (ie, the potential to develop diseases) are often forgotten until the age of retirement (Figure 4–2). Basically, it is never too late to improve one's lifestyle as well as nutrition. However, the aging process represents a continuum over the whole lifespan and accordingly optimal nutrition should be a central target during all periods of life. However, it should be remembered that it is not only the nutritional aspect that should be controlled, but also many modifiable factors with a potential to influence both vitamin and overall nutriture, increase risk of developing chronic diseases, and increase the rate of aging. These factors include smoking habits, body weight (obesity), physical activity, alcohol intake, and medications. The latter factors have to be controlled for during the whole

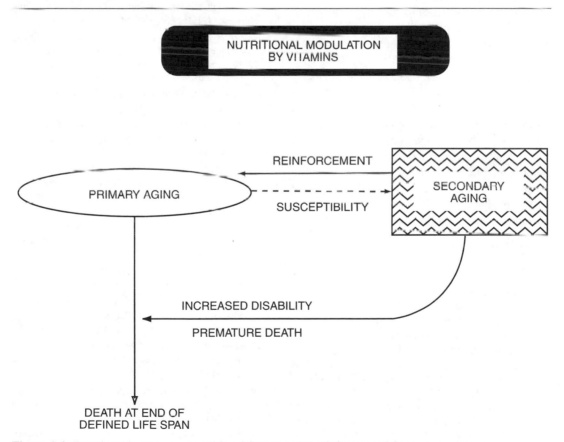

Figure 4–2 Relationship Between Nutritional Status and the Primary and Secondary Aging Processes

life. In the presence of these factors, an apparently adequate nutrient intake becomes inadequate, resulting in decreased functional homeostasis and an increased rate of aging and eventual deterioration of nutritional status. The primary aging process does not significantly affect the metabolism of most vitamins (except for vitamins D and B_{12}). However, many secondary aging phenomena (ie, the different chronic diseases of aging) may directly and indirectly affect nutrient requirements and especially nutrient status by the modification of food intake. Therefore, the maintenance of optimal vitamin nutriture includes the minimization of any secondary aging phenomena (ie, chronic disease risk) by the control of the well-known modifiable risk factors.

As mentioned in this review, there is still much controversy regarding vitamin nutriture and vitamin requirements in the elderly. The maintenance of an adequate supply of single vitamins remains essential for the assurance of an adequate status. Nutrient supplements may be indicated on an individual basis, however, rather than for all elderly people. The question "Who can profit from supplemental vitamin intake?" is still unsolved and controversial. Whenever possible, the requirements should be obtained from food sources. The vitamin nutrition for elderly people does not start when someone has reached retirement age; the optimization of daily nutrient supply at a young age probably remains the cornerstone for optimal vitamin nutriture at older age.

REFERENCES

1. Prakash IJ. Aging, disability, and disabled older people in India. *J Aging Soc Policy* 2003;15(2–3):85–108.

2. Forman DE, Rich MW. Heart failure in the elderly. *Congest Heart Fail* 2003;9:311–321.

3. Koelling TM, Chen RS, Lubwama RN, L'Italien GJ, Eagle KA. The expanding national burden of heart failure in the United States: the influence of heart failure in women. *Am Heart J* 2004;147:74–78.

4. Waterland RA, Jirtle RL. Early nutrition, epigenetic changes at transposons and imprinted genes, and enhanced susceptibility to adult chronic diseases. *Nutrition* 2004;20:63–68.

5. Haynes WG. Hyperhomocysteinemia, vascular function and atherosclerosis: effects of vitamins. *Cardiovasc Drugs Ther* 2002;16:391–399.

6. Mattson MP, Shea TB. Folate and homocysteine metabolism in neural plasticity and neurodegenerative disorders. *Trends Neurosci* 2003;26:137–146.

7. Institute of Medicine. *Dietary Reference Intakes for Thiamin, Riboflavin, Niacin, Vitamin B6, Folate, Vitamin B12, Pantothenic Acid, Biotin, and Choline.* Washington, DC: National Academy Press; 2001: 1–564.

8. Institute of Medicine. *Dietary Reference Intakes for Vitamin A, Vitamin K, Arsenic, Boron, Chromium, Copper, Iodine, Manganese, Molybdenum, Nickel, Silicone, Vanadium, and Zinc.* Washington, DC: National Academy Press; 2001.

9. Institute of Medicine. *Dietary Reference Intakes for Energy, Carbohydrates, Fiber, Fat, Fatty Acids, Cholesterol, Protein, and Amino Acids.* Washington, DC: National Academy Press; 2002:1–450.

10. Sauberlich HE, Machlin LJ. Beyond deficiency. New views on the function and health effects of vitamins. *Annals N Y Acad Sci* 1992;669:1–404.

11. Cutler RG, Packer L, Bertram J, Mori A. Oxidative stress and aging. In: Azzi A, Packer L, eds. *MCBU— Molecular and Cell Biology Updates* Basel, Switzerland: Birkhäuser Verlag; 1995:1–396.

12. Suter PM, Vetter W. The role of vitamins in aging and the aging process. *Age Nutrition* 1996;7:86–95.

13. Rucker RB, Suttie JW, McCormick DB, Machlin LJ. *Handbook of Vitamins.* New York, NY: Marcel Dekker Inc; 2001:1–600.

14. Grau MV, Baron JA, Sandler RS, et al. Vitamin D, calcium supplementation, and colorectal adenomas: results of a randomized trial. *J Natl Cancer Inst* 2003;95: 1765–1771.

15. Lee KW, Lee HJ, Surh YJ, Lee CY. Vitamin C and cancer chemoprevention: reappraisal. *Am J Clin Nutr* 2003; 8:1074–1078.

16. Wolf G. A history of vitamin A. *FASEB J* 1996;10: 1102–1107.

17. Olson JA. Vitamin A. In: Rucker RB, Suttie JW, McCormick DB, Machlin LJ, eds. *Handbook of Vitamins* New York, NY: Marcel Dekker Inc; 2001:1–50.

18. Oren T, Sher JA, Evans T. Hematopoiesis and retinoids: development and diseases. *Leuk Lymphoma* 2003;44: 1881–1891.

19. Ross AC, Zolfaghari R. Regulation of hepatic retinol metabolism: perspectives from studies on vitamin A metabolism. *J Nutr* 2004:269S–275S.

20. Chew BP, Park JS. Carotenoid action on the immune response. *J Nutr* 2004;134:257S–261S.

21. Mehta K. Retinoids as regulators of gene transcription. *J Biol Regul Homeost Agents* 2003;17:1–12.

22. Bollag W. The retinoid revolution. *FASEB J* 1996;10: 938–939.

23. Institute of Medicine. *Dietary Reference Intakes for Vitamin C, Vitamin E, Selenium, and Carotenoids.* Washington, DC: National Academy Press; 2000.

24. Olson JA. Recommended dietary intakes (RDI) of vitamin A in humans. *Am J Clin Nutr* 1987;45:704–716.

25. Euronut SENECA Investigators. Nutritional status: blood vitamins A, E, B$_6$, B$_{12}$, folic acid and carotene. *Eur J Clin Nutr* 1991;45(suppl 3):63–82.

26. Euronut SENECA Investigators. Intake of vitamins and minerals. *Eur J Clin Nutr* 1991;45(suppl 3):121–138.

27. Johnson EJ, Krall EA, Dawson-Hughes B, Dallal GE, Russell RM. Lack of an effect of multivitamins containing vitamin A on serum retinyl esters and liver function tests in healthy women. *J Am Coll Nutr* 1992;11: 682–686.

28. Saito M, Itoh R. Nutritional status of vitamin A in a healthy elderly population in Japan. *Int J Vitam Nutr Res* 1991;61:105–109.

29. Russell RM, Suter PM. Vitamin requirements of the elderly: an update. *Am J Clin Nutr* 1993;58:4–11.

30. Mino M, Tamai H, Tanabe T, et al. Nutritional status of antioxidant vitamins (A, E, and beta-carotene) in elderly Japanese. *J Nutr Sci Vitaminol (Tokyo)* 1993;39 (suppl):S67–S74.

31. Lipski PS, Torrance A, Kelly PJ, James OF. A study of nutritional deficits of long-stay geriatric patients. *Age Aging* 1994;22:244–255.

32. Haller J, Lowik MR, Ferry M, Ferro-Luzzi A. Nutritional status: blood vitamin A, E, B$_6$, folic acid and carotene. Euronut SENECA investigators. *Eur J Clin Nutr* 1991;45(suppl 3):63–82.

33. Monget AL, Galan P, Preziosi P, et al. Micronutrient status in elderly people. *Int J Vitam Nutr Res* 1996;66: 71–76.

34. Haller J, Weggemans RM, Lammi-Keefe CJ, Ferry M. Changes in the vitamin status of elderly Europeans: plasma vitamins A, E, B$_6$, B$_{12}$, folic acid and carotenoids. *Eur J Clin Nutr* 1996;50(suppl 2):S32–S46.

35. Granado F, Olmedilla B, Blanco I. Nutritional and clinical relevance of lutein in human health. *Br J Nutr* 2003;90:487–502.

36. Mayne ST. Beta-carotene, carotenoids, and disease prevention in humans. *FASEB J* 1996;10:690–701.

37. Cooper DA. Carotenoids in health and disease: recent scientific evaluations, research recommendations and the consumer. *J Nutr* 2004;134:221S–224S.

38. Snowdon DA, Gross MD, Butler SM. Antioxidants and reduced functional capacity in the elderly: findings from the Nun Study. *J Gerontol A Biol Sci Med Sci* 1996;51:M10–M16.

39. Packer L, Fuchs J. *Vitamin E in Health and Disease.* New York, NY: Marcel Dekker Inc; 1993:1–1000.

40. Bonnefoy M, Drai J, Kostka T. Antioxidants to slow aging, facts and perspectives. *Presse Med* 2002;31:1174–1184.

41. Carr A, Frei B. The role of natural antioxidants in preserving the biological activity of endothelium-derived nitric oxide. *Free Radic Biol Med* 2000;28:1806–1814.

42. Maggio D, Barabani M, Pierandrei M, et al. Marked decrease in plasma antioxidants in aged osteoporotic women: results of a cross-sectional study. *J Clin Endocrinol Metab* 2003;88:1523–1527.

43. Quinn J, Suh J, Moore MM, Kaye J, Frei B. Antioxidants in Alzheimer's disease—vitamin C delivery to a demanding brain. *J Alzheimers Dis* 2003;5(4): 309–313.

44. Gaziano JM, Manson JE, Branch LG, Colditz GA, Willett WC, Buring JE. A prospective study of consumption of carotenoids in fruits and vegetables and decreased mortality in the elderly. *Ann Epidemiol* 1995;5:255–260.

45. Greenberg ER, Baron JA, Karagas MR, et al. Mortality associated with low plasma concentration of beta carotene and the effect of oral supplements. *JAMA* 1996;275:699–703.

46. Jacques PF, Halpner AD, Blumberg JB. Influence of combined antioxidant nutrient intakes on their plasma concentration in an elderly population. *Am J Clin Nutr* 1995;62:1228–1233.

47. Anonymous. Processing of dietary retinoids is slowed in the elderly. *Nutr Rev* 1991; 49:116–118.

48. Chevalier S, Ferland, G, Tuchweber B. Lymphatic absorption of retinol in young, mature, and old rats: influence of dietary restriction. *FASEB J* 1996;10: 1085–1090.

49. Garry PJ, Goodwin JS, Hunt WC, Hooper EM, Leonard AG. Nutritional status in a healthy elderly population: dietary and supplemental intakes. *Am J Clin Nutr* 1982; 36:319–331.

50. Garry PJ, Hunt WC, Bandrofchak JL, VanderJagt D, Goodwin JS. Vitamin A intake and plasma retinol in healthy men and women. *Am J Clin Nutr* 1987;46: 989–994.

51. Krasinski SD, Russell RM, Otradovec CL, et al. Relationship of vitamin A and vitamin E intake to fasting plasma retinol, retinol binding protein, retinyl esters, carotene, alpha-tocopherol, and cholesterol among elderly people and young adults: increased plasma retinyl esters among vitamin A supplement users. *Am J Clin Nutr* 1989;49:112–120.

52. Leo MA, Lieber CS. Hepatic vitamin A depletion in alcoholic liver injury. *N Engl J Med* 1982;307:597–601.

53. Leo MA, Lieber CS. Hypervitaminosis A: a liver lovers lament. *Hepatology* 1988;8:412–417.

54. Sato M, Lieber CS. Hepatic vitamin A depletion after chronic ethanol consumption. *J Nutr* 1981;111: 2015–2023.

55. Mobarhan S, Seitz HK, Russell RM, et al. Age related effects of chronic ethanol intake on vitamin A status in Fisher 344 rats. *J Nutr* 1991;121:510–517.

56. Seitz HK, Suter PM. Ethanol toxicity and the nutritional status. In: Kotsonis FN, Mackey M, Hjelle J, eds. *Nutritional Toxicology* New York, NY: Raven Press; 1994: 95–116.

57. Krasinski SD, Cohn JS, Schaefer EJ, Russell RM. Postprandial plasma retinyl ester response is greater in older subjects compared with younger subjects. *J Clin Invest* 1990;85:883–892.

58. Bulux J, Carranza E, Castaneda C, et al. Studies on the application of the relative dose response test for assessing vitamin A status in older adults. *Am J Clin Nutr* 1992;56:543–547.

59. Rasmussen HM, Dallal GE, Phelan E, Russell RM. Serum concentrations of retinol and retinyl esters in adults in response to mixed vitamin A and carotenoid containing meals. *J Am Coll Nutr* 1991;10:460–465.

60. Santos MS, Meydani SN, Leka L, Wu D, Fotouhi N, Meydani M, Hennekens CH, Gaziano JM. Natural killer cell activity in elderly men is enhanced by β-carotene supplementation. *Am J Clin Nutr* 1996;64: 772–777.

61. Paiva SAR, Godoy I, Vannucchi H, Favaro RMD, Geraldo RRC, Campana AO. Assessment of vitamin A status in chronic pulmonary disease patients and healthy smokers. *Am J Clin Nutr* 1996;64:928–934.

62. Soutar A, Seaton A, Brown K. Bronchial reactivity and dietary antioxidants. *Thorax* 1997;52:166–170.

63. Ross AC, Stephensen CB. Vitamin A and retinoids in antiviral responses. *FASEB J* 1996;10:979–985.

64. Kelly Y, Sacker A, Marmot M. Nutrition and respiratory health: findings from the health survey for Scotland. *Eur Respir J* 2003;21:664–671.

65. Albanes D, Heinonen OP, Taylor PR, et al. α-Tocopherol and β-carotene supplements and lung cancer incidence in the Alpha-Tocopherol, Beta-Carotene Cancer Prevention Study: effects of base-line characteristics and study compliance. *J Natl Cancer Inst* 1996;88: 1560–1570.

66. Omenn GS, Goodman GE, Thornquist MD, et al. Risk factors for lung cancer and for intervention effects in CARET, the beta-carotene and retinol efficacy trial. *J Natl Cancer Inst* 1996;88:1550–1559.

67. Omenn GS, Goodman GE, Thornquist MD, et al. Effects of a combination of beta carotene and vitamin A on lung cancer and cardiovascular disease. *N Engl J Med* 1996;334:1150–1155.

68. Qureshi SH, Selva-Nayagam DN, Crompton JL. Hypovitaminosis A in metropolitan Adelaide. *Clin Experiment Ophthalmol* 2000;28(1):62–64.

69. Fletcher AE, Breeze E, Shetty PS. Antioxidant vitamins and mortality in older persons: findings from the nutrition add-on study to the Medical Research Council Trial of Assessment and Management of Older People in the Community. *Am J Clin Nutr* 2003;78:999–1010.

70. Park YH, de-Groot LC, van-Staveren WA. Dietary intake and anthropometry of Korean elderly people: a literature review. *Asia Pac J Clin Nutr* 2003;12:234–242.

71. Herrero C, Granado F, Blanco I, Olmedilla B. Vitamin A and E content in dairy products: their contribution to the recommended dietary allowances (RDA) for elderly people. *J Nutr Health Aging* 2003;6:57–59.

72. Michaelsson K, Lithell H, Vessby B, Melhus H. Serum retinol levels and the risk of fracture. *N Engl J Med* 2003;348:287–294.

73. Feskanich D, Singh V, Willett WC, Colditz GA. Vitamin A intake and hip fractures among postmenopausal women. *JAMA* 2002;287:47–54.

74. Lips P. Hypervitaminosis A and fractures. *N Engl J Med* 2003;348:347–349.

75. Anderson JJ. Oversupplementation of vitamin A and osteoporotic fractures in the elderly: to supplement or not to supplement with vitamin A. *J Bone Miner Res* 2002; 17:1359–1362.

76. Johansson S, Melhus H. Vitamin A antagonizes calcium response to vitamin D in man. *J Bone Miner Res* 2001; 16:1899–1905.

77. Sies H, Stahl W. Non-nutritive bioactive constituents of plants: lycopene, lutein and zeaxanthin. *Int J Vitam Nutr Res* 2003;73:95–100.

78. Lin R, White JH. The pleiotropic actions of vitamin D. *Bioessays* 2004;26:21–28.

79. Collins ED, Norman AW. Vitamin D. In: Rucker RB, Suttie JW, McCormick DB, Machlin LJ, eds. *Handbook of Vitamins,* 3rd ed. New York, NY: Marcel Dekker Inc; 2001:51–113.

80. Peleg S, Posner GH. Vitamin D analogs as modulators of vitamin D receptor action. *Curr Top Med Chem* 2003;3:1555–1572.

81. Demay M. Muscle: a nontraditional 1,25-dihydroxyvitamin D target tissue exhibiting classic hormone-dependent vitamin D receptor actions. *Endocrinology* 2003;144:5135–5137.

82. Yamada S, Shimizu M, Yamamoto K. Vitamin D receptor. *Endocr Dev* 2003;6:50–68.

83. Institute of Medicine. *Dietary Reference Intakes for Calcium, Phosphorus, Magnesium, Vitamin D, and Fluoride.* Washington, DC: National Academy Press; 1997:1–560.

84. Holick MF. Vitamin D: the underappreciated D-lightful hormone that is important for skeletal and cellular health. *Curr Opin Endocrinol Diabetes* 2002;9:87–98.

85. Holick M. Sunlight "D"ilemma: risk of skin cancer or bone disease and muscle weakness. *Lancet* 2001;357: 4–6.

86. Ovesen L, Brot C, Jakobsen J. Food contents and biological activity of 25-hydroxyvitamin D: a vitamin D metabolite to be reckoned with? *Ann Nutr Metab* 2003; 47:107–113.

87. Holick MF, Shao Q, Liu WW, Chen TC. The vitamin D content of fortified milk and infant formula. *N Engl J Med* 1992;326:1178–1181.

88. Faulkner H, Hussein A, Foran M, Szijarto L. A survey of vitamin A and D contents of fortified fluid milk in Ontario. *J Dairy Sci* 2000;83:1210–1216.

89. Murphy SC, Whited LJ, Rosenberry LC, Hammond BH, Bandler DK, Boor KJ. Fluid milk vitamin fortification compliance in New York State. *J Dairy Sci* 2001; 84:2813–2820.

90. McKenna MJ. Differences in vitamin D status between countries in young adults and the elderly. *Am J Med* 1992;93:69–77.

91. Vieth R, Cole DE, Hawker GA, Trang HM, Rubin LA. Wintertime vitamin D insufficiency is common in young Canadian women, and their vitamin D intake does not prevent it. *Eur J Clin Nutr* 2001;55:1091–1097.

92. Nowson CA, Margerison C. Vitamin D intake and vitamin D status of Australians. *Med J Aus* 2002;177: 149–152.

93. Hollis BW. Assessment of vitamin D nutritional and hormonal status: what to measure and how to do it. *Calcif Tissue Int* 1996;58(1):4–5.

94. Suter PM, Russell RM. Vitamin nutriture and requirements of the elderly. In: Munro HN, Danford DE, eds. *Nutrition, Aging and the Elderly* Vol. 6. New York: Plenum Press; 1989:245–291.

95. Baker MR, Peacock M, Nordin BEC. The decline in vitamin D status with age. *Age Aging* 1980;9:249–252.

96. Boonen S, Aerssens J, Dequeker J. Age-related endocrine deficiencies and fractures of the proximal femur. II. Implications of vitamin D deficiency in the elderly. *J Endocrinol* 1996;149:13–17.

97. Gallagher JC. Vitamin D metabolism and therapy in elderly subjects. *South Med J* 1992;85:2S43–2S47.

98. van der Wielen RP, Löwik MRH, van-den-Berg H, et al. Serum vitamin D concentrations among elderly people in Europe. *Lancet* 1995;346:207–210.

99. Mäenpää P, Pirhonen A, Pirskanen A, et al. Biochemical indicators related to antioxidant status and bone metabolic activity in Finnish elderly men. *Int J Vitam Nutr Res* 1989;59:14–19.

100. Villareal DT, Civitelli R, Chines A, Avioli LV. Subclinical vitamin D deficiency in postmenopausal women with low vertebral bone mass. *J Clin Endocrinol Metab* 1991;72:628–634.

101. Gloth FM, Gundberg CM, Hollis BW, Haddad JG, Tobin JD. Vitamin D deficiency in homebound elderly persons. *JAMA* 1995;274:1683–1686.

102. Goldray D, Mizrahi-Sasson E, Merdler C, et al. Vitamin D deficiency in elderly patients in a general hospital. *J Am Geriatr Soc* 1989;37:589–592.

103. Löwik MRH, van den Berg H, Schrijver J, Odink J, Wedel M, van Houten P. Marginal nutritional status among institutionalized elderly women as compared to those living more independently (Dutch Nutrition Surveillance System). *J Am Coll Nutr* 1992;11:673–681.

104. Sem SW, Sjoen RJ, Trygg K, Pedersen JI. Vitamin D status of two groups of elderly in Oslo: living in old people's homes and living in own homes. *Compr Gerontol A* 1987;1:126–130.

105. Slovik DM, Adams JS, Neer RM, Holick MF, Potts JT. Deficient production of 1, 25-dihydroxyvitamin D in elderly. *New Engl J Med* 1981;13:372–374.

106. Quesada J, Coopmans W, Ruiz R, Aljama P, Jans I, Bouillon R. Influence of vitamin D on parathyroid function in the elderly. *J Clin Endocrinol Metabol* 1992;75: 494–501.

107. Sagiv P, Hallel T, Edelstein S. Decrease in bone level of 1-25-dihydroxyvitamin D in women over 45 years old. *Calcifi Tissue Internat* 1992;51:24–26.

108. Clemens TL, Zhou XY, Myles M, Endres D, Lindsay R. Serum vitamin D_2 and vitamin D_3 metabolite concentrations and absorption of vitamin D_2 in elderly subjects. *J Clin Endocrinol Metabol* 1986;63:656–660.

109. Silverberg SJ, Shane E, de la Cruz L, Segre GV, Clemens TL, Bilezikian JP. Abnormalities in parathyroid hormone secretion and 1,25-dihydroxyvitamin D_3 formation in women with osteoporosis. *N Engl J Med* 1989;320:277–281.

110. Dandona P, Menon RK, Shenoy R, Houlder S, Thomas M, Mallinson WJW. Low 1,25-dihydroxyvitamin D, secondary hyperparathyroidism, and normal osteocalcin in elderly subjects. *J Clin Endocrinol Metab* 1986; 63:459–462.

111. Eastell R, Yergey AL, Vieira NE, Cedel SL, Kumar R, Riggs BL. Interrelationship among vitamin D metabolism, true calcium absorption, parathyroid function, and age in women: evidence of an age-related intestinal resistance to 1,25-dihydroxyvitamin D action. *J Bone Miner Res* 1991;6:125–132.

112. Wood RJ, Fleet JC. The genetics of osteoporosis: vitamin D receptor polymorphisms. *Annu Rev Nutr* 1998; 18:233–258.

113. Gennari C, Agnusdei D, Nardi P, Civitelli R. Estrogen preserves a normal intestinal responsiveness to 1,25-hydroxyvitamin D_3 in oophorectomized women. *J Clin Endocrinol Metabol* 1990;71:1288–1293.

114. Tanaka S, Haji M, Takayanagi R, Tanaka S, Sugioka Y, Nawata H. 1,25-Dihydroxyvitamin D_3 enhances the enzymatic activity and expression of the messenger ribonucleic acid for aromatase cytochrome P450 synergistically with dexamethasone depending on the vita-

min D receptor level in cultured human osteoblasts. *Endocrinology* 1996;137:1860–1869.

115. Houston LA, Grant SF, Reid DM, Ralston SH. Vitamin D receptor polymorphism, bone mineral density, and osteoporotic vertebral fracture: studies in a UK population. *Bone* 1996; 18:249–259.

116. Plehwe WE. Vitamin D deficiency in the 21st century: an unnecessary pandemic? *Clin Endocrinol* 2003; 59:22–24.

117. Neshy O'Dell S, Scanlon KS, Cogswell ME, et al. Hypovitaminosis D prevalence and determinants among African American and white women of reproductive age: third National Health and Nutrition Examination Survey, 1988–1994. *Am J Clin Nutr* 2002; 76:178–192.

118. Holick MF. McCollum Award Lecture 1994: Vitamin D—new horizons for the 21st century. *Am J Clin Nutr* 1994;60:619–630.

119. Webb AR, Pilbeam C, Hanafin N, Holick MF. An evaluation of the relative contributions of exposure to sunlight and of diet to the circulating concentrations of 25-hydroxyvitamin D in an elderly nursing home population in Boston. *Am J Clin Nutr* 1990; 51:1075–1081.

120. Webb AR, Holick MF. The role of sunlight in the cutaneous production of vitamin D_3. *Annu Rev Nutr* 1988;8: 75–99.

121. Prystowsky JH. Photoprotection and the vitamin D status of the elderly. *Arch Dermatol* 1988;124:1844–1848.

122. Holick MF, Matsuoka LY, Wortsman J. Age, vitamin D and solar ultraviolet. *Lancet* 1989;2:1104–1105.

123. Brazier M, Kamel S, Maamer M, et al. Markers of bone remodeling in the elderly subject: effects of vitamin D insufficiency and its correction. *J Bone Miner Res* 1996;10:1753–1761.

124. Krall EA, Sahyoun N, Tannenbaum S, Dallal GE, Dawson-Hughes B. Effect of vitamin D intake on seasonal variations in parathyroid hormone secretion in postmenopausal women. *N Engl J Med* 1989;321: 1777–1783.

125. Chevalley T, Rizzoli R, Nydegger V, et al. Effects of calcium supplements on femoral bone mineral density and vertebral fracture rate in vitamin-D-replete elderly patients. *Osteoporos Int* 1994;4:245–252.

126. Ooms ME, Roos JC, Bezemer PD, van-der-Vijgh WJ, Bouter LM, Lips P. Prevention of bone loss by vitamin D supplementation in elderly women: a randomized double blind trial. *J Clin Endocrinol Metab* 1995;80: 1052–1058.

127. Dawson-Hughes B, Dallal GE, Krall EA, Harris S, Sokoll LJ, Falconer G. Effect of vitamin D supplementation on wintertime and overall bone loss in healthy postmenopausal women. *Ann Int Med* 1991;115: 505–512.

128. Himmelstein S, Clemens TL, Rubin A, Lindsay R. Vitamin D supplementation in elderly nursing home residents increases 25(OH)D but not 1,25(OH)$_2$D. *Am J Clin Nutr* 1990;52:701–706.

129. Douglas AS, Robins SP, Hutchison JD, Porter RW, Stewart A, Reid DM. Carboxylation of osteocalcin in post-menopausal women following vitamin K and D supplementation. *Bone* 1995;17:15–20.

130. Pietschmann P, Woloszczuk W, Pietschmann H. Increased serum osteocalcin levels in elderly females with vitamin D deficiency. *Exp Clin Endocrinol* 1990; 95:275–278.

131. Latham NK, Anderson CS, Lee A, Bennett DA, Moseley A, Cameron ID. A randomized, controlled trial of quadriceps resistance exercise and vitamin D in frail older people: the Frailty Interventions Trial in Elderly Subjects (FITNESS). *J Am Geriatr Soc* 2003;51:291–299.

132. Visser M, Deeg DJH, Lips P. Low vitamin D and high parathyroid hormone levels as determinants of loss of muscle strength and muscle mass (sarcopenia): the Longitudinal Aging Study Amsterdam. *J Clin Endocrinol Metab* 2003;88:5766–5772.

133. Kenny AM, Biskup B, Robbins B, Marcella G, Burleson JA. Effects of vitamin D supplementation on strength, physical function, and health perception in older, community-dwelling men. *J Am Geriatr Soc* 2003;51:1762–1767.

134. Hauschka PV, Lian JB, Cole DE, Gundberg CM. Osteocalcin and matrix gla protein: vitamin K–dependent proteins in bone. *Physiol Rev* 1989;69:990–1047.

135. Suttie JW. Vitamin K. In: Rucker RB, Suttie JW, McCormick DB, Machlin LJ, eds. *Handbook of Vitamins*. New York, NY: Marcel Dekker Inc; 2001:115–164.

136. National Research Council. *Recommended Dietary Allowances*. In: Subcommittee on the Tenth Edition of the RDAs, Food and Nutrition Board, Comission on Life Sciences, National Research Council. 10th ed. Washington, DC: National Academy Press, 1989.

137. Camilo ME, Paiva SA, O'Brien ME, et al. The interaction between vitamin K nutriture and warfarin administration in patients with bacterial overgrowth due to gastritis. *J Nutr Health Aging* 1998;2:73–78.

138. Booth SL, Webb DR, Peters JC. Assessment of phylloquinone and dihydrophylloquinone dietary intakes among a nationally representative sample of US consumers using 14-day food diaries. *J Am Diet Assoc* 1999;99:1072–1076.

139. Booth SL, Pennington JAT, Sadowski JA. Food sources and dietary intakes of vitamin K-1 (phylloquinone) in the American diet: data from the FDA Total Diet Study. *J Am Diet Assoc* 1996;96:149–154.

140. Booth SL, Suttie JW. Dietary intake and adequacy of vitamin K. *J Nutr* 1998;128:785–788.

141. Booth SL, Sokoll LJ, O'Brien ME, Dawson-Hughes B, Sadowski JA. Assessment of dietary phylloquinone intake and vitamin K status in postmenopausal women. *Eur J Clin Nutr* 1995;49:832–841.

142. Thane CW, Paul AA, Bates CJ, Bolton-Smith C, Prentice A, Shearer MJ. Intake and sources of phylloquinone (vitamin K1): variation with sociodemographic and lifestyle factors in a national sample of British elderly people. *Br J Nutr* 2002;87:605–613.

143. Ferland G, Sadowski JA, O'Brien ME. Dietary induced vitamin K deficiency in normal human subjects. *J Clin Invest* 1993;91:1761–1768.

144. Sadowski JA, Hood SJ, Dallal GE, Garry PJ. Phylloquinone in plasma from elderly and young adults: factors influencing its concentration. *Am J Clin Nutr* 1989; 50:100–108.

145. Booth SL, Tucker KL, McKeown NM, Davidson KW, Dallal GE, Sadowski JA. Relationship between dietary intakes and fasting plasma concentrations of fat soluble vitamins in humans. *J Nutr* 1997;127:587–592.

146. Sokoll LJ, Sadowski JA. Comparison of biochemical indexes for assessing vitamin K nutritional status in a healthy adult population. *Am J Clin Nutr* 1996;63: 566–573.

147. Booth SL, O'Brien-Morse ME, Dallal GE, Davidson KW, Gundberg CM. Response of vitamin K status to different intakes and sources of phylloquinone-rich foods: comparison of younger and older adults. *Am J Clin Nutr* 1999;70:368–377.

148. Booth SL, Lichtenstein AH, Dallal GE. Phylloquinone absorption from phylloquinone-fortified oil is greater than from a vegetable in younger and older men and women. *J Nutr* 2002;132:2609–2612.

149. Huber AM, Davidson KW, O'Brien-Morse ME, Sadowski JA. Tissue phylloquinone and menaquinones in rats are affected by age and gender. *J Nutr* 1999; 129:1039–1044.

150. Koshihara Y, Hoshi K, Ishibashi H, Shiraki M. Vitamin K₂ promotes 1α-25(OH)₂ Vitamin D₃-induced mineralization in human periosteal osteoblasts. *Calcif Tissue Int* 1996;59:466–473.

151. Jie KSG, Bots ML, Witteman JCM, Grobbee DE. Vitamin K status and bone mass in women with and without aortic atherosclerosis: a population based study. *Clacif Tissue Int* 1996;59:352–356.

152. Hazell K, Baloch KH. Vitamin K deficiency in the elderly. *Gerontol Clin* 1970;12:10–17.

153. Doisy EA. Nutritional hypoprothrombinemia and metabolism of vitamin K. *Fed Proc* 1961;20:989–994.

154. Shepherd AM, Hewick DS, Moreland TA, Stevenson IH. Age as a determinant of sensitivity to warfarin. *Br J Clin Pharmacol* 1977;4:315–320.

155. Booth SL, Broe KE, Gagnon DR, et al. Vitamin K intake and bone mineral density in women and men. *Am J Clin Nutr* 2003;77:512–516.

156. Iwamoto J, Takeda T, Ichimura S. Combined treatment with vitamin K2 and bisphosphonate in postmenopausal women with osteoporosis. *Yonsei Med J* 2003; 44:751–756.

157. Booth SL, Martini L, Peterson JW, Saltzman E, Dallal GE, Wood RJ. Dietary phylloquinone depletion and repletion in older women. *J Nutr* 2003;133:2565–2569.

158. Binkley NC, Krueger DC, Engelke JA, Foley AL, Suttie JW. Vitamin K supplementation reduces serum concentrations of under-carboxylated osteocalcin in healthy young and elderly adults. *Am J Clin Nutr* 2000;72: 1523–1528.

159. Binkley NC, Krueger DC, Kawahara TN, Engelke JA, Chappell RJ, Suttie JW. A high phylloquinone intake is required to achieve maximal osteocalcin gamma-carboxylation. *Am J Clin Nutr* 2002;76(5):1055–1060.

160. Asakura H, Myou S, Ontachi Y, et al. Vitamin K administration to elderly patients with osteoporosis induces no hemostatic activation, even in those with suspected vitamin K deficiency. *Osteoporos Int* 2001; 12(12):996–1000.

161. Meydani M. The Boyd Orr lecture: Nutrition interventions in aging and age associated disease. *Proc Nutr Soc* 2002;61:165–171.

162. Hollander D, Dadufalza V. Lymphatic and portal absorption of vitamin E in aging rats. *Dig Dis Sci* 1989; 34:768–772.

163. Traber MG, Cohn W, Muller DPR. Absorption, transport and delivery to tissues. In: Packer L, Fuchs J, eds. *Vitamin E in Health and Disease*. New York, NY: Marcel Dekker Inc; 1993:35–51.

164. Roodenburg AJ, Leenen R, van-het-Hof KH, Weststrate JA, Tijburg LB. Amount of fat in the diet affects bioavailability of lutein esters but not of alpha-carotene, beta-carotene, and vitamin E in humans. *Am J Clin Nutr* 2000;71:1187–1193.

165. Vandewoude MFJ, Vandewoude MG. Vitamin E status in a normal population: the influence of age. *J Am Coll Nutr* 1987;6:307–311.

166. Morinobu T, Tamai H, Tanabe T, et al. Plasma alpha-tocopherol, beta-carotene, and retinol levels in the institutionalized elderly individuals and in young adults. *Int J Vit Nutr Res* 1994;64:104–108.

167. Heseker H, Schneider R. Requirement and supply of vitamin C, vitamin E and beta-carotene for elderly men and women. *Eur J Clin Nutr* 1994;48:118–127.

168. Birlouez-Aragon I, Girard F, Ravelontseheno L, Bourgeois C, Belliot JP, Abitbol G. Comparison of two levels of vitamin C supplementation on antioxidant

vitamin status in elderly institutionalized subjects. *Int J Vit Nutr Res* 1995;65:261–266.

169. Hallfrisch J, Muller DC, Singh VN. Vitamin A and E intakes and plasma concentrations of retinol, beta-carotene and alpha-tocopherol in men and women of the Baltimore longitudinal study of aging. *Am J Clin Nutr* 1994;60:176–182.

170. Campbell D, Bunker VW, Thomas AJ, Clayton BE. Selenium and vitamin E status of healthy institutionalized elderly subjects: an analysis of plasma, erythrocytes and platelets. *Br J Nutr* 1989;62:221–227.

171. Pokorn D, Accetto B, Prevorcnik A. Vitamin E status in men and women aged 60–90 years. *Acta Med Iugosl* 1990;44(3):223–232.

172. Meydani M, Verdon CP, Blumberg JB. Effect of vitamin E, selenium and age on lipid peroxidation events in rat cerebrum. *Nutr Res* 1985;5:1227–1236.

173. Leotsinidis M, Alexopoulos A, Schinas V, Kardara M, Kondakis X. Plasma retinol and tocopherol levels in Greek elderly population from an urban and a rural area: associations with the dietary habits. *Eur J Epidemiol* 2000;16:1009–1016.

174. Requejo AM, Andres P, Redondo MR, et al. Vitamin E status in a group of elderly people from Madrid. *J Nutr Health Aging* 2002;6:72–74.

175. Papas A, Stacewicz-Sapuntzakis M, Lagiou P, Bamia C, Chloptsios Y, Trichopoulou A. Plasma retinol and tocopherol levels in relation to demographic, lifestyle and nutritional factors of plant origin in Greece. *Br J Nutr* 2003;89:83–87.

176. Schmuck A, Ravel A, Coudray C, Alary J, Franco A, Roussel AM. Antioxidant vitamins in hospitalized elderly patients: analysed dietary intakes and biochemical status. *Eur J Clin Nutr* 1996;50:473–478.

177. Essama-Tjani JC, Guilland JC, Fuchs F, Lombard M, Richard D. Changes in thiamin, riboflavin, niacin, beta-carotene, vitamins C, A, D and E status of French elderly subjects during the first year of institutionalization. *Int J Vit Nutr Res* 2000;70:54–64.

178. van der Loo B, Labugger R, Aebischer CP, et al. Cardiovascular aging is associated with vitamin E increase. *Circulation* 2002;105:1635–1638.

179. Vericel E, Croset M, Sedivy P, Courpron P, Dechavanne M, Lagarde M. Platelets and aging, I-aggregation, arachidonate metabolism and antioxidant status. *Thromb Res* 1988; 49:331–342.

180. Croset M, Vericel E, Rigaud M, et al. Functions and tocopherol content of blood platelets from elderly people after low intake of purified eicosapentaenoic acid. *Thromb Res* 1990;57:1–12.

181. Meydani M, Macauley JB, Blumberg J. Influence of dietary vitamin E, selenium, and age on regional distribution of α-tocopherol in the rat brain. *Lipids* 1989; 21:786–791.

182. Koistinaho J, Alho H, Hervonen A. Effect of vitamin E and selenium supplement on aging peripheral neurons of the Sprague-Dawley rat. *Mech Aging Dev* 1990; 51:63–72.

183. Monji A, Morimoto N, Okuyama I, Yamashita N, Tashiro N. Effect of dietary vitamin E on lipofuscin accumulation with age in the rat brain. *Brain Res* 1994; 634:62–68.

184. Takasaki M, Yanagawa K, Shinozaki K, et al. Relationship between aging and vitamin E (article in Japanese, English abstract). *Nippon Ronen Igakkai Zasshi* 2002;39:495–500.

185. Ohrvall M, Tengblad S, Vessby B. Tocopherol concentration in adipose tissue—relationships of tocopherol concentrations and fatty acid composition in serum in a reference population of Swedish men and women. *Eur J Clin Nutr* 1994;48:212–218.

186. Meagher EA. Treatment of atherosclerosis in the new millennium: is there a role for vitamin E? *Prev Cardiol* 2003;6:85–90.

187. Dutta A, Dutta SK. Vitamin E and its role in the prevention of atherosclerosis and carcinogenesis: a review. *J Am Coll Nutr* 2003;22:258–268.

188. Antoniades C, Tousoulis D, Tentolouris C, Toutouzas P, Stefanadis C. Oxidative stress, antioxidant vitamins, and atherosclerosis. From basic research to clinical practice. *Herz* 2003;28:628–638.

189. Reznick AZ, Rappaport B, Landvik SV, Simon-Schnass I, Packer L. Vitamin E and the aging process. In: Packer L, Fuchs J, eds. *Vitamin E in Health and Disease.* New York, NY: Marcel Dekker Inc; 1993:435–454.

190. Heart Protection Study Collaborative Group. MRC/BHF Heart Protection Study of antioxidant vitamin supplementation in 20,536 high-risk individuals: a randomised placebo-controlled trial. *Lancet* 2002;360: 23–33.

191. Clarke R, Armitage J. Antioxidant vitamins and risk of cardiovascular disease. Review of large-scale randomised trials. *Cardiovasc Drug Ther* 2002;16: 411–415.

192. Fariss MW, Zhang JG. Vitamin E therapy in Parkinson's disease. *Toxicology* 2003;189:129–146.

193. Rimbach G, Minihane AM, Majewicz J, et al. Regulation of cell signalling by vitamin E. *Proc Nutr Soc* 2002;61:415–425.

194. Hasanain B, Mooradian AD. Antioxidant vitamins and their influence in diabetes mellitus. *Curr Diab Rep* 2002;2:448–456.

195. Sung L, Greenberg ML, Koren G, et al. Vitamin E: the evidence for multiple roles in cancer. *Nutr Cancer* 2003;46:1–14.

196. Meydani M. Effect of functional food ingredients: vitamin E modulation of cardiovascular diseases and

immune status in the elderly. *Am J Clin Nutr* 2000;71 (suppl 6):1665S–1668S.

197. Gale CR, Ashurst HE, Powers HJ, Martyn CN. Antioxidant vitamin status and carotid atherosclerosis in the elderly. *Am J Clin Nutr* 2001;74:402–408.

198. Khodr B, Howard J, Watson K, Khalil Z. Effect of short-term and long-term antioxidant therapy on primary and secondary aging neurovascular processes. *J Gerontol A Biol Sci Med Sci* 2003;58:698–708.

199. Hemila H, Virtamo J, Albanes D, Kaprio J. Vitamin E and beta-carotene supplementation and hospital-treated pneumonia incidence in male smokers. *Chest* 2004; 125:557–565.

200. Jiang Q, Christen S, Shigenaga MK, Ames BN. Gamma-tocopherol, the major form of vitamin E in the US diet, deserves more attention. *Am J Clin Nutr* 2001; 74:714–722.

201. Hensley K, Benaksas EJ, Bolli R, et al. New perspectives on vitamin E: gamma-tocopherol and carboxyelthylhydroxychroman metabolites in biology and medicine. *Free Radic Biol Med* 2004;36:1–15.

202. Vatassery GT, Johnson GJ, Krezowski AM. Changes in vitamin E concentrations in human plasma and platelets with age. *J Am Coll Nutr* 1983;2:369–375.

203. Johnston CS, Steinberg MF, Rucker RB. Vitamin C. In: Rucker RB, Suttie JW, McCormick DB, Machlin LJ, eds. *Handbook of Vitamins*. New York, NY: Marcel Dekker Inc; 2001:529–568.

204. Connelly TJ, Becker DOA, McDonald JW. Bachelor scurvy. *Int J Dermatol* 1982;21:209–211.

205. Woo J, Ho SC, Mak YT, et al. Nutritional status of the water-soluble vitamins in an active Chinese elderly population in Hong Kong. *Eur J Clin Nutr* 1988;42: 415–424.

206. Bianchetti A, Rozzini R, Carabellese C, Zanetti O, Trabucchi M. Nutritional intake, socioeconomic conditions, and health status in a large elderly population. *J Am Geriatr Soc* 1990;38:521–526.

207. Suter PM, Russell RM. Vitamin requirements of the elderly. *Am J Clin Nutr* 1987;45:501–512.

208. Yearik ES, Wang MSL, Pisias SJ. Nutritional status of the elderly: dietary and biochemical findings. *J Gerontol* 1980;5:663–671.

209. Bowmann BB, Rosenberg IH. Assessment of the nutritional status of the elderly. *Am J Clin Nutr* 1982;35: 1142–1451.

210. Lowik MR, Hulshof KF, Schneijder P, Schrijver J, Colen AA, van-Houten P. Vitamin C status in elderly women: a comparison between women living in a nursing home and women living independently. *J Am Diet Assoc* 1993;93(2):167–172.

211. Sahyoun N. Nutrient intake by the NSS elderly population. In: Hartz S, Rosenberg IH, Russell RM, eds. *Nu-trition in the Elderly. The Boston Nutritional Status Survey*. London: Smith-Gordon & Co Ltd; 1992: 31–44.

212. Kafatos A, Diacatou A, Labadarios D, et al. Nutrition status of elderly in Anogia, Crete, Greece. *J Am Coll Nutr* 1993;12:685–692.

213. Garcia-Arias MT, Villarino Rodriguez A, Garcia-Linares MC, Rocandio AM, Garcia-Fernandez MC. Iron, folate and vitamins B12 and C dietary intake of an elderly institutionalized population in Leon, Spain. *Nutr Hosp* 2003;18(4):222–225.

214. Loh HS. The relationship between dietary ascorbic acid intake and buffy coat and plasma ascorbic acid concentration at different ages. *Int J Vit Nutr Res* 1972; 42:80–85.

215. Kirk JE, Chieffi M. Vitamin studies in middle-aged and old individuals. XI. The concentration of total ascorbic acid in whole blood. *J Gerontol* 1953;8:301–304.

216. Cruz JAA, Moreiras O, Brzozowska A. Longitudinal changes in the intake of vitamins and minerals of elderly Europeans. *Eur J Clin Nutr* 1996;50(suppl. 2): S77–S85.

217. Porrini M, Simonetti P, Ciappellano S, Testolin G. Vitamin A, E and C nutriture of elderly people in North Italy. *Int J Vit Nutr Res* 1987;57:349–355.

218. Mandal SK, Ray AK. Vitamin C status of elderly patients on admission into an assessment geriatric ward. *J Int Med Res* 1987;15:96–98.

219. Marazzi MC, Mancinelli S, Palombi L, et al. Vitamin C and nutritional status of institutionalized and noninstitutionalized elderly women in Rome. *Int J Vit Nutr Res* 1990;60:351–359.

220. Chavance M, Herbeth B, Fournier C, Janot C, Vernhes G. Vitamin status, immunity and infections in an elderly population. *Eur J Clin Nutr* 1989;43: 827–835.

221. Preston AM, Bercovitch FB, Rodriguez CA, Lebron MR, Rivera CE. Plasma ascorbic acid concentrations in a population of rhesus monkeys (*Macaca mulatta*). *Contemp Top Lab Anim Sci* 2001;40:30–32.

222. Mecocci P, Polidori MC, Troiano L, et al. Plasma antioxidants and longevity: a study on healthy centenarians. *Free Radic Biol Med* 2000;28:1243–1248.

223. Will JC, Ford ES, Bowman BA. Serum vitamin C concentrations and diabetes: findings from the Third National Health and Nutrition Examination Survey, 1988–1994. *Am J Clin Nutr* 1999;70:49–52.

224. Selvaag E, Bohmer T, Benkestock K. Reduced serum concentrations of riboflavin and ascorbic acid, and blood thiamine pyrophosphate and pyridoxal-5-phosphate in geriatric patients with and without pressure sores. *J Nutr Health Aging* 2002;6(1):275–77.

225. Blanchard J. Depletion and repletion kinetics of vitamin C in humans. *J Nutr* 1991;121:170–176.

226. VanderJagt DJ, Garry PJ, Bhagavan HN. Ascorbic acid intake and plasma levels in healthy elderly people. *Am J Clin Nutr* 1987;46:290–294.

227. Schaus R. The ascorbic acid content of pituitary, cerebral cortex, heart and skeletal muscle and its relation to age. *Am J Clin Nutr* 1957;5:39–42.

228. Pinto RM, Unamuno MdR, Rodrigues MM, dos-Santos JE, Marchini JS, de-Oliveira JE. Vitamin C load test in elderly subjects. *Arch Latinoam Nutr* 1993;43:20–22.

229. Leveque N, Muret P, Mary S, et al. Decrease in skin ascorbic acid concentration with age. *Eur J Dermatol* 2002;12:XXI–XXII.

230. Sun F, Iwaguchi K, Shudo R, et al. Change in tissue concentrations of lipid hydroperoxides, vitamin C and vitamin E in rats with streptozotocin-induced diabetes. *Clin Sci (Lond)* 1999;96:185–190.

231. van-der-Loo B, Bachschmid M, Spitzer V, Brey L, Ullrich V, Luscher TF. Decreased plasma and tissue levels of vitamin C in a rat model of aging: implications for antioxidative defense. *Biochem Biophys Res Commun* 2003;303:483–487.

232. Bendich A, Langseth L. Health effects of vitamin C supplementation: a review. *J Am Coll Nutr* 1995;4:124–136.

233. Brown LAS, Jones DP. The biology of ascorbic acid. In: Cadenas E, Packer, L., eds. New York, NY: Marcel Dekker Inc; 1996:117–154.

234. Ely JJ. Inadequate levels of essential nutrients in developed nations as a risk factor for disease: a review. *Rev Environ Health* 2003;18:111–129.

235. Erbs S, Gielen S, Linke A, et al. Improvement of peripheral endothelial dysfunction by acute vitamin C application: different effects in patients with coronary artery disease, ischemic, and dilated cardiomyopathy. *Am Heart J* 2003;146:280–285.

236. Mayne ST. Antioxidant nutrients and chronic disease: use of biomarkers of exposure and oxidative stress status in epidemiologic research. *J Nutr* 2003;133(suppl 3):933S–940S.

237. Jacob RA, Sotoudeh G. Vitamin C function and status in chronic disease. *Nutr Clin Care* 2002;5:66–74.

238. Fairfield KM, Fletcher RH. Vitamins for chronic disease prevention in adults: scientific review. *JAMA* 2002;287:3116–3126.

239. Gotto AM. Antioxidants, statins, and atherosclerosis. *J Am Coll Cardiol* 2003;41:1205–1210.

240. Taylor A, Hobbs M. 2001 assessment of nutritional influences on risk for cataract. *Nutrition* 2001;17:845–857.

241. Kim MK, Sasaki S, Sasazuki S, Okubo S, Hayashi M, Tsugane S. Long-term vitamin C supplementation has no markedly favourable effect on serum lipids in middle-aged Japanese subjects. *Br J Nutr* 2004;91:81–90.

242. Sahyoun NR, Jacques PF, Russell RM. Carotenoids, vitamin C and E, and mortality in an elderly population. *Am J Epidemiol* 1996;144:501–511.

243. Gale CR, Martyn CN, Winter PD, Cooper C. Vitamin C and risk of death from stroke and coronary artery disease in a cohort of elderly people. *Br Med J* 1995;310:1563–1566.

244. Losonczy KG, Harris TB, Havlik RJ. Vitamin E and vitamin C supplement use and risk of all-cause and coronary heart disease mortality in older persons: the Established Populations for Epidemiologic Studies of the Elderly. *Am J Clin Nutr* 1996;64:190–196.

245. Jialal I, Fuller CJ. Effect of vitamin E, vitamin C and beta-carotene on LDL oxidation and atherosclerosis. *Can J Cardiol* 1995;11 (suppl. G):97G–103G.

246. Howard PA, Meyers DG. Effect of vitamin C on plasma lipids. *Ann Pharmacother* 1995;29:1129–1136.

247. Jacques PF. A cross-sectional study of vitamin C intake and blood pressure in the elderly. *Int J Vitam Nutr Res* 1992;62:252–255.

248. Ness AR, Khaw KT, Bingham S, Day NE. Vitamin C status and blood pressure. *J Hypertens* 1996;14:503–508.

249. Fotherby MD, Williams JC, Forster LA, Craner P, Ferns GA. Effect of vitamin C on ambulatory blood pressure and plasma lipids in older persons. *J Hypertens* 2000;18:411–415.

250. Weber P, Bendich A, Schalch W. Vitamin C and human health—a review of recent data relevant to human health. *Int J Vitam Nutr Res* 1996;66:19–30.

251. Lykkesfeldt J, Priem H, Loft S, Poulsen HE. Effect of smoking cessation on plasma ascorbic acid concentration. *Brit Med J* 1996;313:91.

252. Polidori MC, Mecocci P, Stahl W, Sies H. Cigarette smoking cessation increases plasma levels of several antioxidant micronutrients and improves resistance towards oxidative challenge. *Br J Nutr* 2003;90:147–150.

253. Rinaldi P, Polidori MC, Metastasio A, et al. Plasma antioxidants are similarly depleted in mild cognitive impairment and in Alzheimer's disease. *Neurobiol Aging* 2003;24:915–919.

254. Ravona-Springer R, Davidson M, Noy S. The role of cardiovascular risk factors in Alzheimer's disease. *CNS Spectr* 2003;8:824–833.

255. Solfrizzi V, Panza F, Capurso A. The role of diet in cognitive decline. *J Neural Transm* 2003;110:95–110.

256. Zandi PP, Anthony JC, Khachaturian AS, et al. Reduced risk of Alzheimer disease in users of antioxidant vitamin supplements: the Cache County Study. *Arch Neurol* 2004;61:82–88.

257. Tanphaichitr V. Thiamine. In: Rucker RB, Suttie JW, McCormick DB, Machlin LJ, eds. *Handbook of Vitamins,* 3rd ed. New York, NY: Marcel Dekker Inc; 2001: 275–316.

258. Rosenberg IH. Nutritional needs of the elderly. In: Bianchi L, Holt P, James OFW, eds. *Aging in Liver and Gastrointestinal Tract.* Lancaster, England: MTP Press; 1988.

259. Iber FL, Blass JP, Brin M, Leevy CM. Thiamin in the elderly—relation to alcoholism and to neurological degenerative disease. *Am J Clin Nutr* 1982;36: 1067–1082.

260. van der Wielen RP, de Wild GM, de Groot LC, Hoefnagels WH, van-Staveren WA. Dietary intakes of energy and water soluble vitamins in different categories of aging. *J Gerontol A Biol Sci Med Sci* 1996; 51:B100–B107.

261. Ben-Hur T, Wolff E, River Y. Thiamin deficieny is common in Israel. *Harefuah* 1992;123:382–384.

262. Nichols HK, Basu TK. Thiamine status of the elderly: dietary intake and thiamin pyrophosphate response. *J Am Coll Nutr* 1994;13:57–61.

263. Porrini M, Testolin G, Simonetti P, Moneta A, Rovati P, Aguzzi F. Nutritional status of non institutionalized elderly people in North Italy. *Int J Vitam Nutr Res* 1987; 57:203–216.

264. Smidt LJ, Cremin FM, Grivetti LE, Clifford AJ. Influence of thiamin supplementation on the health and general well-being of an elderly Irish population with marginal thiamin deficiency. *J Gerontol* 1991;46: M16–M22.

265. Sokoll LJ, Morrow FD. Thiamin. In: Hartz SC, Rosenberg IH, Russell RM, eds. *Nutrition in the Elderly. The Boston Nutritional Status Survey.* London: Smith-Gordon & Co Ltd; 1992:111–117.

266. Yamagami M, Noyama O, Nishimura I. Vitamin A, B1 and C status of elderly living alone (Article in Japanese, English abstract). *Nippon Koshu Eisei Zasshi* 1998;45: 213–224.

267. O'Keeffe ST. Thiamine deficiency in elderly people. *Age Aging* 2000;29:99–101.

268. Wilkinson TJ, Hanger HC, George PM, Sainsbury, R. Is thiamine deficiency in elderly people related to age or co-morbidity? *Age Aging* 2000;29:111–116.

269. Sumner AD, Simons RJ. Delirium in the hospitalized elderly. *Cleve Clin Med J* 1994; 61:258–262.

270. Kwok T, Falconer-Smith JF, Potter JF, Ives DR. Thiamine status of elderly patients with cardiac failure. *Age Aging* 1992;21:67–71.

271. Mookhoek EJ, Colon EJ. Nutritional status of elderly patients at admission to a general psychiatric hospital. An inventory. *Tijdschr Gerontol Geriatr* 1992;23:127–131.

272. Suter PM. Alcohol: its role in health and disease. In: Baumann BB, Russell RM, eds. *Present Knowledge in Nutrition.* Washington, DC: ILSI Press; 2001:497–507.

273. Baum RA, Iber FL. Thiamin: the interaction of aging, alcoholism and malabsorption in various populations. *World Rev Nutr Diet* 1984;44:85–116.

274. Pfitzenmeyer P, Guilland JC, d'Athis P, Petit-Marnier C, Gaudet M. Thiamine status of elderly patients with cardiac failure including the effects of supplementation. *Int J Vitam Nutr Res* 1994;64:113–118.

275. Suter PM, Haller J, Hany A, Vetter W. Diuretic use: a risk factor for subclinical thiamine deficiency in elderly patients. *J Nutr Health Aging* 2000;4:69–71.

276. Lubetsky A, Winaver J, Seligmann H, et al. Urinary thiamine excretion in the rat: effects of furosemide, other diuretics, and volume load. *J Lab Clin Med* 1999;134: 232–237.

277. Rieck J, Halkin H, Almog S, et al. Urinary loss of thiamine is increased by low doses of furosemide in healthy volunteers. *J Lab Clin Med* 1999;134:238–243.

278. Brady JA, Rock CL, Horneffer MR. Thiamine status, diuretic medications, and the management of congestive heart failure. *J Am Diet Assoc* 1995;95:541–544.

279. Shimon I, Almog S, Vered Z, et al. Improved left ventricular function after thiamine supplementation in patients with congestive heart failure receiving long-term furosemide therapy. *Am J Med* 1995;98:485–490.

280. Johri S, Shetty S, Soni A, Kumar S. Anaphylaxis from intravenous thiamine—long forgotten? *Am J Emerg Med* 2000;18:642–643.

281. Suter PM, Vetter W. Diuretics and vitamin B1: are diuretics a risk factor for thiamin malnutrition? *Nutr Rev* 2000;58:319–323.

282. Rodriguez-Martin JL, Qizilbash N, Lopez-Arrieta JM. Thiamine for Alzheimer's disease. *Cochrane Database Syst Rev* 2001;(2):CD001498.

283. Calingasan NY, Gibson GE. Vascular endothelium is a site of free radical production and inflammation in areas of neuronal loss in thiamine-deficient brain. *Ann N Y Acad Sci* 2000;903:353–356.

284. Pitkin SR, Savage LM. Age-related vulnerability to diencephalic amnesia produced by thiamine deficiency: the role of time of insult. *Behav Brain Res* 2004;148: 93–105.

285. Rivlin RS, Pinto JT. Riboflavin (vitamin B2). In: Rucker RB, Suttie JW, McCormick DB, Machlin LJ, eds. *Handbook of Vitamins*, 3rd ed. New York, NY: Marcel Dekker Inc; 2001.

286. Krogh V, Freudenheim JL, D'Amicis A, et al. Food sources of nutrients of the diet of elderly Italians: II. Micronutrients. *Int J Epidemiol* 1993;22:869–877.

287. Toh SY, Thompson GW, Basu TK. Riboflavin status of the elderly: dietary intake and FAD-stimulating effect

on erythrocyte glutathione reductase coefficients. *Eur J Clin Nutr* 1994;48:654–659.

288. Lowik MR, van den Berg H, Kistemaker C, Brants HA, Brussaard JH. Interrelationships between riboflavin and vitamin B6 among elderly people (Dutch Nutrition Surveillance System). *Int J Vitam Nutr Res* 1994;64: 198–203.

289. Mares-Perlman JA, Klein BE, Klein R, Ritter LL, Freudenheim JL, Luby MH. Nutrient supplements contribute to the dietary intake of middle- and older-aged adult residents of Beaver Dam, Wisconsin. *J Nutr* 1993; 123:176–188.

290. Boisvert WA, Mendoza J, Castaneda C, et al. Riboflavin requirement of healthy elderly and its relationship to macronutrient composition of the diet. *J Nutr* 1993;123: 915–925.

291. Sadowski JA. Riboflavin. In: Hartz SC, Rosenberg IH, Russell RM, eds. *Nutrition in the Elderly. The Boston Nutritional Status Survey*. London: Smith-Gordon & Co Ltd; 1992:119–125.

292. Garry PJ, Goodwin JS, Hunt WC. Nutritional status in a healthy elderly population: riboflavin. *Am J Clin Nutr* 1982;36:902–909.

293. Beauchenne RE, Davis TA. The nutritional status of the aged in the USA. *Age* 1979;2:23–28.

294. Boisvert WA, Castaneda C, Mendoza J, et al. Prevalence of riboflavin deficiency among Guatemalan elderly people and its relationship to milk intake. *Am J Clin Nutr* 1993;85:85–90.

295. Tucker KL, Dallal GE, Rush D. Dietary pattern of elderly Boston-area residents defined by cluster analysis. *J Am Diet Assoc* 1992;92:1487–1491.

296. Bates CJ, Prentice A, Cole TJ, et al. Micronutrients: highlights and research challenges from the 1994–5 National Diet and Nutrition Survey of people aged 65 years and over. *Br J Nutr* 1999;82:7–15.

297. Olson JA, Hodges RE. Recommended dietary intakes (RDI) of vitamin C in humans. *Am J Clin Nutr* 1987;45: 693–703.

298. Pongpaew P, Tungtrongchitr R, Lertchavanakul A, et al. Anthropometry, lipid and vitamin status of 215 health-conscious Thai elderly. *Int J Vitam Nutr Res* 1991;61: 215–223.

299. Bates CJ, Powers HJ, Downes R, Brubacher D, Sutcliffe V, Thurnhill A. Riboflavin status of adolescent vs elderly Gambian subjects before and during supplementation. *Am J Clin Nutr* 1989;50:825–829.

300. Schaus R, Kirk JE. The riboflavin concentration of brain, heart, and skeletal muscle in individuals of various ages. *J Gerontol* 1957;11:147–150.

301. Said HM, Hollander D. Does aging affect the intestinal transport of riboflavin? *Life Sci* 1985;36:69–73.

302. Ugarte R, Edwards AM, Diez MS, Valenzuela A, Silva E. Riboflavin-photosensitized anaerobic modification of rat lens proteins. A correlation with age-related changes. *J Photochem Photobiol B* 1992;13:161–168.

303. Straatsma BR, Lightfood DO, Barke RM, Horwitz J. Lens capsule and epithelium in age-related cataract. *Am J Ophthalmol* 1991;112:283–296.

304. Matsubara LS, Machado PE. Age-related changes of glutathione content, glutathione reductase and glutathione peroxidase activity of human erythrocytes. *Braz J Med Biol Res* 1991;24:449–454.

305. Williams RD, Mason HL, Cusick PL, Wilder RM. Observations on induced riboflavin deficiency and the riboflavin requirement of man. *J Nutr* 1943;25: 361–377.

306. Davis MV, Oldham HG, Roberts LJ. Riboflavin excretions of young women on diets containing various levels of the B vitamins. *J Nutr* 1946;32:143–161.

307. Friedmann TE, Ivy AC, Jung FT, Sheft BB, Kinney VM. Utilization of thiamin and riboflavin at low and high dietary intake. *Quart Bull Northwest School (Chicago)* 1949;23:177–189.

308. Horwitt MK, Harvey CC, Hill OW, Liebert E. Correlation of urinary excretion with dietary intake and symptoms of ariboflavinosis. *J Nutr* 1950;41:247–264.

309. Powers HJ. Riboflavin (vitamin B2) and health. *Am J Clin Nutr* 2003;77:1352–60.

310. Mangoni AA, Jackson SH. Homocysteine and cardiovascular disease: current evidence and future prospects. *Am J Med* 2002;112:556–565.

311. Morris MS. Homocysteine and Alzheimer's disease. *Lancet Neurol* 2003;2:425–428.

312. Selhub J, Jacques PF, Wilson PW, Rush D, Rosenberg IH. Vitamin status and intake as primary determinants of homocysteinemia in an elderly population. *JAMA* 1993;270:2693–2698.

313. Lathrop-Stern L, Shane B, Bagley PJ, Nadeau M, Shih V, Selhub J. Combined marginal folate and riboflavin status affect homocysteine methylation in cultured immortalized lymphocytes from persons homozygous for the MTHFR C677T mutation. *J Nutr* 2003;133: 2716–2720.

314. Apeland T, Mansoor MA, Pentieva K, McNulty H, Strandjord RE. Fasting and post-methionine loading concentrations of homocysteine, vitamin B$_2$, and vitamin B$_6$ in patients on antiepileptic drugs. *Clinical Chemistry* 2003;49(6 pt 1):1005–1008.

315. Moat SJ, Ashfield-Watt PA, Powers HJ, Newcombe RG, McDowell IF. Effect of riboflavin status on the homocysteine-lowering effect of folate in relation to the MTHFR (C677T) genotype. *Clin Chem* 2003;49: 295–302.

316. Kirkland JB, Rawling JM. Niacin. In: Rucker RB, Suttie JW, McCormick DB, Machlin LJ, eds. *Handbook of Vitamins*. New York, NY: Marcel Dekker Inc; 2001: 213–254.

317. Magni E, Bianchetti A, Rozzini R, Trabucchi M. Influence of nutritional intake on 6-year mortality in an Italian elderly population. *J Nutr Elder* 1994;13: 25–34.

318. Harrill I, Cervone V. Vitamin status of older women. *Am J Clin Nutr* 1977;30:431–440.

319. Bonati B, Nani S, Rancati GB. Eliminazione urinaria di vitamine del complesso B nei vecchi. *Acta Vitaminol* 1956;10:241–244.

320. Morgan AG, Kelleher J, Walker BE, et al. A nutritional survey in the elderly: blood and urine vitamin levels. *Int J Vitam Nutr Res* 1975;45:448–462.

321. Fleming BB, Barrows CH. The influence of aging on intestinal absorption of vitamin B_{12} and niacin in rats. *Exp Gerontol* 1982;17:121–126.

322. Rose RC. Intestinal absorption of water-soluble vitamins. *Proc Soc Exp Biol Med* 1996;212:191–198.

323. Peters JC. Tryptophan nutrition and metabolism: an overview. *Adv Exp Med Biol* 1991;294:345–358.

324. Oduho GW, Han Y, Baker DH. Iron deficiency reduces the efficacy of tryptophan as a niacin precursor. *J Nutr* 1994;124:444–450.

325. Shibata K, Mushiage M, Kondo T, Hayakawa T, Tsuge H. Effects of vitamin B_6 deficiency on the conversion ratio of tryptophan to niacin. *Biosci Biotechnol Biochem* 1995;59:2060–2063.

326. Leklem JE. Vitamin B6. In: Rucker RB, Suttie JW, McCormick DB, Machlin LJ, eds. *Handbook of Vitamins.* New York, NY: Marcel Dekker Inc; 2001:339–396.

327. Driskel JA. The vitamin B_6 status of the elderly. In: Sciences NAo, ed. *Human Vitamin B6 Requirements.* Washington, DC: National Academy of Sciences; 1978.

328. Osler M, Schroll M. A dietary study of elderly in the city of Roskilde 1988/1989 (II). A nutritional risk assessment. *Dan Med Bull* 1991;38:410–413.

329. Mantero-Atienza E, Beach RS, Sotomayor MG, Christakis G, Baum MK. Nutritional status of institutionalized elderly in south Florida. *Arch Latinam Nutr* 1992;42:242–249.

330. Ortega RM, Manas LR, Andres P, et al. Functional and psychic deterioration in elderly people may be aggravated by folate deficiency. *J Nutr* 1996;126:1992–1999.

331. Ribaya-Mercado JD. Vitamin B_6. In: Hartz SC, Rosenberg IH, Russell RM, eds. *Nutrition in the Elderly. The Boston Nutritional Status Survey.* London: Smith-Gordon & Co Ltd; 1992:127–134.

332. Manore MM, Vaughan LA, Carroll SS, Leklem JE. Plasma pyridoxal 5′-phosphate concentration and dietary vitamin B-6 intake in free-living, low-income elderly people. *Am J Clin Nutr* 1989;50:339–345.

333. Löwik MRH, van den Berg H, Westenbrink S, Wedel M, Schrijver J, Ockhuizen T. Dose-response relationships regarding vitamin B_6 in elderly people: a nationwide nutritional survey (Dutch Nutritional Surveillance System). *Am J Clin Nutr* 1989;50:391–399.

334. Kant AK, Block G. Dietary vitamin B_6 intake and food sources in the US population: NHANES II, 1976–1980. *Am J Clin Nutr* 1990;52:707–716.

335. Hamfelt A. Age variation of vitamin B_6 metabolism in men. *Clin Chim Acta* 1964;10:48–54.

336. Rose CS, Gyorgy P, Butler M, et al. Age difference in vitamin B_6 status of 617 men. *Am J Clin Nutr* 1976;29: 847–853.

337. Driskell JA. Vitamin B6. In: Machlin LJ, ed. *Handbook of Vitamins. Nutritional, Biochemical, and Clinical Aspects.* New York, NY: Marcel Dekker, Inc; 1984: 379–401.

338. Reynolds RD, Moser-Veilon PB, Kant AK. Effect of age on status and metabolism of vitamin B6 in man. In: Leklem JE, Reynolds RE, eds. *Current Topics in Nutrition and Disease: Clinical and Physiological Applications of Vitamin B_6.* New York, NY: Alan R. Liss Inc; 1988: 19–30.

339. Fonda ML, Eggers DK, Auerbach S, Fritsch L. Vitamin B-6 metabolism in the brains of young adult and senescent mice. *Exp Gerontol* 1980;15:473–478.

340. Mason DY, Emerson PM. Primary acquired sideroblastic anemia: response to treatment with pyridoxal-5-phosphate. *Br Med J* 1973;1:389–390.

341. Darnton-Hill I, Sriskandarajah N, Stewart PM, Craig G, Truswell AS. Vitamin supplementation and nutritional status in homeless men. *Aust J Public Health* 1993;17: 246–251.

342. Woo J, Ho SC, Mak YT, Law LK, Cheung A. Nutritional status of elderly patients during recovery from chest infection and the role of nutritional supplementation assessed by a prospective randomized single blind trial. *Age Aging* 1994;23:40–48.

343. Naurath HJ, Joosten E, Riezler R, Stabler SP, Allen RH, Lindenbaum J. Effects of vitamin B_{12}, folate, and vitamin B_6 supplements in elderly people with normal vitamin concentrations. *Lancet* 1995;346:85–89.

344. Hoorn RKJ, Flikweert JP, Westerink D. Vitamin B_1, B_2, and B_6 deficiencies in geriatric patients, measured by coenzyme stimulation of enzyme activities. *Clin Chim Acta* 1975;61:151–162.

345. Vir SC, Love AHG. Vitamin B_6 status of hospitalized aged. *Am J Clin Nutr* 1978;31:1383–1391.

346. Kant AK, Moser-Veillon PB, Reynolds RD. Effect of age on changes in plasma, erythrocyte, and urinary B_6 vitamers after an oral vitamin B_6 load. *Am J Clin Nutr* 1988;48:1284–1290.

347. Ribaya-Mercado JD, Russell RM, Sahyoun N, Morrow FD, Gershoff SN. Vitamin B_6 requirements of elderly men and women. *J Nutr* 1991;121:1062–1074.

348. Meydani SN, Ribaya-Mercado JD, Russell RM, Sahyoun N, Morrow FD, Gershoff SN. The effect of vitamin B_6 on immune response of healthy elderly. *Ann NY Acad Sci* 1990;587:303–306.

349. Meydani SN, Barklund MP, Liu S, et al. Vitamin E supplementation enhances cell mediated immunity in healthy elderly subjects. *Am J Clin Nutr* 1990;52: 557–563.

350. Meydani SN, Ribaya-Mercado JD, Russell RM, Sahyoun N, Morrow FD, Gershoff SN. Vitamin B_6 deficiency impairs interleukin 2 production and lymphocyte proliferation in elderly adults. *Am J Clin Nutr* 1991;53:1275–1280.

351. Mudd SH, Skovby F, Levy HL, et al. The natural history of homocystinuria due to cystathionine beta-synthase deficiency. *Am J Hum Genet* 1985;37:1–31.

352. Serfontein WJ, Ubbink JB, De-Villiers LS, Rapley CH, Becker PJ. Plasma pyridoxal-5-phosphate level as risk index for coronary artery disease. *Atherosclerosis* 1985; 55:357–361.

353. McCully KS. Homocysteine and vascular disease. *Nature Medicine* 1996;2:386–389.

354. Robinson K, Meyer E, Miller DP, et al. Hyperhomocysteinemia and low pyridoxal phosphate. Common and independent reversible risk factors for coronary artery disease. *Circulation* 1995;92:2825–2830.

355. Ellis JM, McCully KS. Prevention of myocardial infarction by vitamin B_6. *Res Commun Mol Pathol Pharmacol* 1995;89:208–220.

356. Chasan-Taber L, Selhub J, Rosenberg IH, et al. A prospective study of folate and vitamin B_6 and risk of myocardial infarction in US physicians. *J Am Coll Nutr* 1996;15:136–143.

357. Deijen JB, van-der-Beek BJ, Orlebeke JF, van-den-Berg H. Vitamin B-6 supplementation in elderly men: effects on mood, memory, performance and mental effort. *Psychopharmacology (Berl)* 1992;109:489–496.

358. Malouf R, Grimley EJ. The effect of vitamin B_6 on cognition. *Cochrane Database Syst Rev* 2003:CD004393.

359. Mizrahi EH, Jacobsen DW, Debanne SM, et al. Plasma total homocysteine levels, dietary vitamin B_6 and folate intake in AD and healthy aging. *J Nutr Health Aging* 2003;7:160–105.

360. Lee BJ, Huang MC, Chung LJ, et al. Folic acid and vitamin B_{12} are more effective than vitamin B_6 in lowering fasting plasma homocysteine concentration in patients with coronary artery disease. *Eur J Clin Nutr* 2004;58:481–487.

361. Brody T, Shane B. Folic acid. In: Rucker RB, Suttie JW, McCormick DB, Machlin LJ, eds. *Handbook of Vitamins* New York, NY: Marcel Dekker Inc; 2001:427–462.

362. Rosenberg IH, Bowman BB, Cooper BA, et al.. Folate nutrition in the elderly. *Am J Clin Nutr* 1982;36: 1060–1066.

363. Rosenberg IH. Folate. In: Hartz SC, Rosenberg IH, Russell RM, eds. *Nutrition in the Elderly. The Boston Nutritional Status Survey.* London: Smith-Gordon & Co Ltd; 1992:135–139.

364. Infante-Rivard C, Krieger M, Gascon-Barre M, Rivard GE. Folate deficiency among institutionalized elderly. *J Am Geriatr Soc* 1986;34:211–214.

365. Grinblat J, Marcus DL, Hernandez F, Freedman ML. Folate and vitamin B_{12} levels in an urban elderly population with chronic diseases. Assessment of two laboratory folate assays: microbiologic and radioassay. *J Am Geriatr Soc* 1986;34:627–632.

366. Hanger HC, Sainsbury R, Gilchrist NL, Beard MEJ, Duncan JM. A community study of vitamin B_{12} and folate levels in the elderly. *J Am Geriatr Soc* 1991;39: 1155–1159.

367. Davis RE, Nichol DJ. Folic acid. *Int J Biochem* 1988; 20:133–139.

368. Russell RM, Krasinski SD, Samloff IM, Jacob RA, Hartz SC, Brovender SR. Folic acid malabsorption in atrophic gastritis: compensation by bacterial folate synthesis. *Gastroenterology* 1986;91:1476–1482.

369. Varela-Moreiras G, Perez-Olleros L, Garcia-Cuevas M, Ruiz-Roso B. Effects of aging on folate metabolism in rats fed a long term folate deficient diet. *Int J Vitam Nutr Res* 1994;64:294–299.

370. Selhub J, Jacques PF, Bostom AG, et al. Association between plasma homocysteine concentrations and extracranial carotid artery stenosis. *N Eng J Med* 1995; 332:286–291.

371. Kang SS, Wong PWK, Cook HY, Norusis M, Messer JV. Protein-bound homocyst(e)ine. A possible risk factor for coronary artery disease. *J Clin Invest* 1986;77: 1482–1486.

372. Tucker KL, Mahnken B, Wilson PWF, Jacques P, Selhub J. Folic acid fortification of the food supply. Potential benefits and risks for the elderly. *JAMA* 1996;276:1879–1885.

373. Mattson MP, Kruman II, Duan W. Folic acid and homocysteine in age-related disease. *Aging Res Rev* 2002;1:95–111.

374. Anderson JL, Jensen KR, Carlquist JF, Bair TL, Horne BD, Muhlestein JB. Effect of folic acid fortification of food on homocysteine-related mortality. *Am J Med* 2004;116:158–164.

375. Toole JF, Malinow MR, Chambless LE, et al. Lowering homocysteine in patients with ischemic stroke to prevent recurrent stroke, myocardial infarction, and death: the Vitamin Intervention for Stroke Prevention (VISP) randomized controlled trial. *JAMA* 2004;291:565–575.

376. Hultberg B, Nilsson K, Isaksson A, Gustafson L. Folate deficiency is a common finding in psychogeriatric patients. *Aging Clin Exp Res* 2002;14:479–484

377. Nilsson K, Gustafson L, Hultberg B. Folate and cobalamin levels as determinants of plasma homocysteine in different age groups of healthy controls and psychogeriatric patients. *Clin Chem Lab Med* 2003;41:681–685.

378. Reynolds EH. Folic acid, aging, depression and dementia. *BMJ* 2002;324:1512–1515.

379. Nilsson K, Gustafson L, Faldt R, Andersson A, Hultberg B. Plasma homocysteine in relation to serum cobalamin and blood folate in a psychiatric population. *Eur J Clin Invest* 1994;24:600–606.

380. Santhosh-Kumar CR, Hassell KL, Deutsch JC, Kolhouse JF. Are neuropsychiatric manifestions of folate, cobalamin and pyridoxine deficiency mediated through imbalances in excitatory sulfur amino acids? *Med Hypotheses* 1994;43:239–244.

381. Guaraldi G, Fava M, Mazzi F, et al. An open trial of methyltetrahydrofolate (MTHF) in elderly depressed patients. *Ann Clin Psychiatry* 1993;5:101–106.

382. Maxwell CJ, Hogan DB, Ebly EM. Serum folate levels and subsequent adverse cerebrovascular outcomes in elderly persons. *Dement Geriatr Cogn Disord* 2002;13(4):225–234.

383. Mattson MO. Will caloric restriction and folate protect against AD and PD? *Neurology* 2003;60:690–695.

384. Teunissen CE, Blom AH, Van-Boxtel MP, et al. Homocysteine: a marker for cognitive performance? A longitudinal follow-up study. *J Nutr Health Aging* 2003; 7:153–159.

385. Salles-Montaudon N, Parrot F, Balas D, Bouzigon E, Rainfray M, Emeriau JP. Prevalence and mechanisms of hyperhomocysteinemia in elderly hospitalized patients. *J Nutr Health Aging* 2003;7(2):111–116.

386. Selhub J, Bagley LC, Miller J, Rosenberg IH. B vitamins, homocysteine, and neurocognitive function in the elderly. *Am J Clin Nutr* 2000;71:614S–620S.

387. Morris MS. Homocysteine and Alzheimer's disease. *Lancet Neurol* 2003;2:425–428.

388. Rampersaud GC, Kauwell GP, Bailey LB. Folate: a key to optimizing health and reducing disease risk in the elderly. *J Am Coll Nutr* 2003;22:1–8.

389. Wolfe JM, Bailey LB, Herrlinger-Garcia K, Theriaque DW, Gregory JF, Kauwell GP. Folate catabolite excretion is responsive to changes in dietary folate intake in elderly women. *Am J Clin Nutr* 2003;77: 919–923.

390. Prothro J, Mickles M, Tolbert B. Nutritional status of a population sample in Macon County, Alabama. *Am J Clin Nutr* 1976;29:94–104.

391. Garry PJ, Goodwin JS, Hunt WC. Folate and vitamin B_{12} status in a healthy elderly population. *J Am Geriatr Soc* 1984;32:719–726.

392. Meuleman JR, Hoffman NB, Conlin MM, Lowenthal DT, Delafuente JC, Graves JE. Health status of the aged: medical profile of a group of functional elderly. *South Med J* 1992;85:464–468.

393. Pennypacker LC, Allen RH, Kelly JP, et al. High prevalence of cobalamin deficiency in elderly outpatients. *J Am Geriatr Soc* 1992;40:1197–1204.

394. Basu TK, Donald EA, Hargreaves JA, et al. Vitamin B_{12} and folate status of a selected group of free living older persons. *J Nutr Elder* 1992;11:5–19.

395. Crystal HA, Ortof E, Frishman WH, Gruber A, Hershman D, Aronson M. Serum vitamin B_{12} levels and incidence of dementia in a healthy elderly population: a report from the Bronx Longitudinal Aging Study. *J Am Geriatr Soc* 1994;42:933–936.

396. Cals MJ, Bories PN, Devanlay M, et al. Extensive laboratory assessment of nutritional status in fit, health-conscious, elderly people living in the Paris area (Research Group on Aging). *J Am Coll Nutr* 1994;13: 646–657.

397. Matthews JH. Cobalamin and folate deficiency in the elderly. *Baillieres Clin Haematol* 1995;8:679–697.

398. Quinn K, Basu TK. Folate and vitamin B_{12} status of the elderly. *Eur J Clin Nutr* 1996;50:340–342.

399. Bunting RW, Bitzer AM, Kenney RM, Ellman L. Prevalence of intrinsic factor antibodies and vitamin B_{12} malabsorption in older patients admitted to a rehabilitation hospital. *J Am Geriatr Soc* 1990;38:743–747.

400. Marcus DL, Shadick N, Crantz J, Gray M, Hernandez F, Freedman ML. Low serum B_{12} levels in a hematologically normal elderly subpopulation. *J Am Geriatr Soc* 1987;35:635–638.

401. Nilsson-Ehle II, Jagenburg R, Landahl S, Lindstedt G, Swolin B, Westin J. Cyanocobalamin absorption in the elderly: results for healthy subjects and for subjects with low serum cobalamin concentration. *Clin Chem* 1986; 32:1368–1371.

402. Figlin E, Chetrit A, Shahar A, et al. High prevalences of vitamin B_{12} and folic acid deficiency in elderly subjects in Israel. *Br J Haematol* 2003;123:696–701.

403. Nilsson-Ehle H, Jagenburg R, Landahl S, Lindstedt S, Svanborg A, Westin J. Serum cobalamins in the elderly: a longitudinal study of a representative population sample from age 70 to 81. *Eur J Haematol* 1991; 47:10–16.

404. Morris MS, Jacques PF, Rosenberg IH, Selhub J. Elevated serum methylmalonic acid concentrations are common among elderly Americans. *J Nutr* 2002; 132(9):2799–2803.

405. Tauber S, Goodhart RS, Hsu JM, et al. Vitamin B_{12} deficiency in the aged. *Geriatrics* 1957;12:368–374.

406. King CE, Leibach J, Toskes PP. Clinically significant vitamin B_{12} deficiency secondary to malabsorption of protein-bound vitamin B_{12}. *Dig Dis Sci* 1979;24: 397–402.

407. Doscherholmen A, Ripley D, Chang S, et al. Influence of age and stomach function on serum vitamin B_{12} concentration. *Scand J Gastroenterol* 1977;12:313–319.

408. Suter PM, Golner BB, Goldin BR, Morrow FD, Russell RM. Reversal of protein-bound vitamin B_{12} malabsorption with antibiotics in atrophic gastritis. *Gastroenterology* 1991;101:1039–1045.

409. Lucas MH, Elgazzar AH. Detection of protein bound vitamin B_{12} malabsorption. A case report and review of the literature. *Clin Nucl Med* 1994;19:1001–1003.

410. Lindenbaum J, Healton EB, Savage DG, et al. Neuropsychiatric disorders caused by cobalamin deficiency in the absence of anemia or macrocytosis. *N Engl J Med* 1988;318:1720–1728.

411. Lorenzl S, Vogeser M, Muller-Schunk S, Pfister HW. Clinically and MRI documented funicular myelosis in a patient with metabolical vitamin B_{12} deficiency but normal vitamin B_{12} serum level. *J Neurol* 2003;250:1010–1011.

412. Joosten E, Pelemans W, Devos P, et al. Cobalamin absorption and serum homocysteine and methylmalonic acid in elderly subjects with low serum cobalamin. *Eur J Haematol* 1993;51:25–30.

413. Allen RH, Stabler SP, Savage DG, Lindenbaum J. Metabolic abnormalities in cobalamin (vitamin B_{12}) and folate deficiency. *FASEB J* 1993;7:1344–1353.

414. Joosten E, Lesaffre E, Riezler R. Are different reference intervals for methylmalonic acid and total homocysteine necessary in the elderly people? *Eur J Haematol* 1996;57:222–226.

415. Herrmann W, Geisel J. Vegetarian lifestyle and monitoring of vitamin B-12 status. *Clinica Chimica Acta* 2002;326:47–59.

416. Beck WS. Neuropsychiatric consequences of cobalamin deficiency. *Adv Int Med* 1991;36:33–56.

417. Nilsson K, Gustafson L, Hultberg B. Optimal use of markers for cobalamin and folate status in a psychogeriatric population. *Int J Geriatr Psychiatry* 2002;17(10):915–925.

418. Refsum H, Smith AD. Low vitamin B-12 status in confirmed Alzheimer's disease as revealed by serum holotranscobalamin. *J Neurol Neurosurg Psychiatry* 2003;74:959–961.

419. Campbell AK, Miller JW, Green R, Haan MN, Allen LH. Plasma vitamin B-12 concentrations in an elderly Latino population are predicted by serum gastrin concentrations and crystalline vitamin B-12 intake. *J Nutr* 2003;133:2770–2776.

420. Nagga K, Rajani R, Mardh E, Borch K, Mardh S, Marcusson J. Cobalamin, folate, methylmalonic acid, homocysteine, and gastritis markers in dementia. *Dement Geriatr Cogn Disord* 2003:269–275.

421. Malouf R, Areosa-Sastre A. Vitamin B12 for cognition. *Cochrane Database Syst Rev* 2003:CD004326.

422. Sharabi A, Cohen E, Sulkes J, Garty M. Replacement therapy for vitamin B12 deficiency: comparison between the sublingual and oral route. *Br J Clin Pharmacol* 2003;56:635–638.

423. Mock DM. Biotin. In: Rucker RB, Suttie JW, McCormick DB, Machlin LJ, eds *Handbook of Vitamins*. New York: Marcel Dekker Inc; 2001:397–426.

424. McMahon RJ. Biotin in metabolism and molecular biology. *Annu Rev Nutr* 2002;22:221–239.

425. Said HM. Biotin: the forgotten vitamin. *Am J Clin Nutr* 2002;75:179–180.

426. Mock DM. Biotin status: which are valid indicators and how do we know? *J Nutr* 1999;129 (suppl 2S):498S–503S.

427. Mock DM, Henrich-Shell CL, Carnell N, Stumbo P, Mock NI. 3-Hydroxypropionic acid and methylcitric acid are not reliable indicators of marginal biotin deficiency in humans. *J Nutr* 2004;134:317–320.

428. Murphy SP, Colloway DH. Nutrient intake of women in NHANES II, emphasizing trace minerals, fiber and phytate. *J Am Diet Assoc* 1986;86:1366–1372.

429. Bull NL, Buss DH. Biotin, pantothenic acid and vitamin E in British household food supply. *Hum Nutr Appl Nutr* 1982;36:190–196.

430. Bonjour JP. Biotin. In: Machlin LJ, ed. *Handbook of Vitamins: Nutritional, Biochemical and Clinical Aspects.* New York, NY: Marcel Dekker Inc; 1984.

431. Markkanen T, Mustakallio E. Absorption and excretion of biotin after feeding minced liver in achlorhydria and after partial gastrectomy. *Scand J Clin Lab Invest* 1963;15:57–61.

432. Said HM, Sharifian A, Bagherzadeh A, Mock D. Chronic ethanol feeding and acute ethanol exposure in vitro: effect on intestinal transport of biotin. *Am J Clin Nutr* 1990;52:1983–1086.

433. Said HM, Horne DW, Mock DM. Effect of aging on intestinal biotin transport in the rat. *Exp Gerontol* 1990;25:67–73.

434. Walsh JH, Wyse BW, Hansen RG. Pantothenic acid content of a nursing home diet. *Ann Nutr Metab* 1981;25:178–181.

435. Srinivasan V, Christensen N, Wyse BW, Hansen RG. Pantothenic acid nutritional status in the elderly—institutionalized and noninstitutionalized. *Am J Clin Nutr* 1981;119:1973–1983.

436. Plesofsky NS. Pantothenic acid. In: Rucker RB, Suttie JW, McCormick DB, Machlin LJ, eds. *Handbook of Vitamins*. New York, NY: Marcel Dekker Inc; 2001:317–337.

437. Sugarman B, Munroe HN. [C-14]-Pantothenate accumulation by isolated adipocytes from adult rats of different age. *J Nutr* 1980;110:2297–2301.

438. Ishiguro K. Aging effect of blood pantothenic acid content in females. *Tohoku J Exp Med* 1972;107:367–372.

CHAPTER 5

Mineral Requirements

Robert D. Lindeman, MD

Sodium, potassium, calcium, and magnesium are considered the bulk minerals in the human body; all other minerals are considered trace minerals (Chapter 6). The approximate quantity of each bulk mineral in a 70 kg man is 1000 g of calcium, 140 g of potassium, 110 g of sodium, and 20 g of magnesium.[1] Whereas specific recommendations for calcium and magnesium intakes have evolved over recent years (ie, Recommended Dietary Allowances [RDA]; Dietary Reference Intakes [DRI]), there are no similar recommendations for sodium or potassium.

With the development of accurate, inexpensive techniques for quantifying these minerals in biologic fluids, a vast literature has been generated documenting that deficits and excesses of these minerals in many pathophysiological conditions create many clinical challenges for practitioners. The ability of elderly people to maintain concentrations of these minerals within normal limits is often impaired by the frequently observed decrease in renal function (Chapter 12) and by aberrations in other homeostatic mechanisms designed to conserve or excrete excessive amounts of these minerals. For calcium and magnesium intakes, what is of most concern to the nutritionist is the failure to consume amounts adequate to meet known nutritional needs.

SODIUM

Essentially all of the body's sodium is located in the extracellular fluid volume or space (ECFV), so that total body sodium can be estimated by multiplying serum sodium concentration by ECFV. Sodium is the primary cation in the ECFV and is hydrophilic, attracting osmotically obligated water, which, in turn, maintains extracellular volume. The serum sodium concentration can be accurately and precisely measured, and this can be routinely performed in any clinical laboratory. It can then be used to determine whether or not an individual has a normal serum sodium concentration or is hyponatremic or hypernatremic. Water balance is judged by the clinical assessment of ECFV, which is much more subjective than the measure of serum sodium concentration. Indications of fluid deficit include postural hypotension, decreased skin turgor, and decreased mucous membrane moisture, while fluid excess results eventually in the retention of excess water (edema formation). Figure 5–1 demonstrates the relationships between sodium and water in various deficit and excess states.

Dehydration means a decrease in total body water, but the pathophysiology will be different depending upon whether the etiology is a primary salt loss with loss of obligated water or primary water

SALT and WATER IMBALANCES

SERUM SODIUM CONCENTRATION	LOW	DEHYDRATION (Primary Salt Loss) Na^+ Loss $>$ H_2O Loss	REDISTRIBUTION Hyperglycemia DISPLACEMENT Hyperlipemia Hyperproteinemia SYNDROME OF INAPPROPRIATE ADH WATER INTOXICATION	DILUTIONAL HYPONATREMIA H_2O Retention $>$ Na^+ Retention
	NORMAL	DEHYDRATION Na^+ Loss $=$ H_2O Loss	NORMAL	UNCOMPLICATED EDEMA H_2O Retention $=$ Na^+ Retention
	HIGH	DEHYDRATION (Primary Water Loss) H_2O Loss $>$ Na^+ Loss	HYPERALDOSTERONISM HYPERCORTISONISM	STEROID EXCESS SALT INTOXICATION Na^+ Retention $>$ H_2O Retention
		LOW	NORMAL	HIGH
		EXTRACELLULAR FLUID VOLUME		

Figure 5–1 Salt and Water Imbalances. ADH, Antidiuretic Hormone

loss. Water loss without proportionate sodium loss results in an increase in serum sodium concentration. Since water shifts out of the cell along an osmotic gradient, the increase in serum sodium concentration is directly proportionate to the decrease in total body water rather than ECFV. With free access to water, normal thirst mechanisms usually ensure that the patient maintains an adequate fluid intake. Patients with primary salt depletion first become volume depleted (dehydrated), but maintain normal serum sodium concentrations. When the volume depletion becomes sufficient to stimulate the release of antidiuretic hormone (ADH), the kidney concentrates the urine, water is provided to replace losses, and hyponatremia begins to develop.

The excessive retention of body fluids (overhydration) may result from primary salt retention with osmotically obligated water (simple edema) or from retention of water in excess of salt (dilutional hyponatremia). Simple edema may be local or generalized depending upon the etiology. Generalized edema occurs with in-

creasing frequency as one ages and those disease states, especially congestive heart failure, that are associated with edema occur more commonly in elderly people.

Hyponatremia

A low serum sodium concentration may result from (1) a loss of sodium in excess of osmotically obligated water (primary salt depletion), (2) a retention of water in excess of sodium (dilutional hyponatremia), or (3) a combination of both as seen in the syndrome of inappropriate ADH (SIADH) (Table 5–1). The initial pathology of SIADH is the retention of water, resulting in an expanded ECFV. This then increases urinary sodium excretion, resulting in the loss of osmotically obligated water so that ECFV moves toward the normal range.

A reduction in serum sodium concentration to less than 120 mEq/L, regardless of etiology, may produce symptoms ranging from mild, nonspecific complaints, such as malaise, irritability,

Table 5–1 Hypnoatremic Syndromes

I. Hyponatremia with contracted extracellular volume (ECFV)
   A. Urinary sodium <10 mEq/L
      1. Inadequate intake
      2. Excessive sweating
      3. Excessive gastrointestinal loss (diarrhea, bowel and biliary fistulas)
   B. Urinary sodium >10 mEq/L
      1. Severe metabolic alkalosis due to vomiting
      2. Excessive urinary losses (salt wasting)
         (a) Adrenal insufficiency (Addison's disease, hypoaldosteronism)
         (b) Renal disease (renal tubular acidosis, interstitial nephritis)
         (c) Diuretic-induced
II. Hyponatremia with normal ECFV
   A. Displacement syndromes (hyperglycemia, hyperlipidemia, hyperproteinemia)
   B. Syndrome of inappropriate antidiuretic hormone (SIADH)
      1. Malignancies, esp. small cell carcinoma of lung
      2. Pulmonary diseases, including positive pressure breathing
      3. Cerebral conditions (trauma, infection, tumor, stroke)
      4. Drugs (sulfonylureas, thiazides, antitumor agents, psychotropics, antidepressants)
      5. Other (myxedema, porphyria, idiopathic)
   C. Water intoxication (schizophrenia)
III. Hyponatremia with expanded ECFV (dilutional hyponatremia)
   A. Congestive heart failure
   B. Cirrhosis
   C. Nephrotic syndrome (hypoalbuminemia)
   D. Renal failure

muscle weakness, and change in personality, to marked central nervous system (CNS) impairment. Serious CNS impairment results from a shift of fluid along osmotic gradients from the hypotonic ECFV into the isotonic brain cells, thereby increasing brain volume and intracranial pressure. Depending on the severity of the hyponatremia and the state of hydration, a spectrum of alterations in consciousness ranging from confusion to coma may appear. Seizures are often the manifestations that prompt attention.

Hyponatremia with Contracted ECFV (Primary Salt Depletion)

In conditions where primary salt depletion with dehydration is suspected, a measure of urinary sodium concentration may be helpful in the differential diagnosis. If it is less than 10 mEq/L, suspected etiologies would include inadequate salt intake, excessive sweating, or gastrointesti-nal losses. If urinary sodium concentration is greater than 10 mEq/L, inappropriate renal losses of salt and water could be due to excessive use of diuretics, adrenal or pituitary insufficiency, or intrinsic renal disease (eg, renal tubular acidosis, salt-losing nephritis, or renal insufficiency). In severe vomiting with a metabolic alkalosis and bicarbonaturia, urinary sodium and bicarbonate may be increased despite hypovolemia and hyponatremia.

Epstein and Hollenberg[2] have shown that there is a reduction in the ability of the older person to conserve sodium when placed on a salt-restricted diet (Chapter 12). This may make the elderly more susceptible to development of salt depletion hyponatremia during episodes of acute illness.

Generally, treatment is best accomplished using isotonic saline as replacement; however, in patients with severe symptomatic conditions, small amounts of hypertonic saline can be used initially. Often it remains unclear whether one is dealing with a primary salt loss syndrome or SIADH; urinary sodium excretion may be high in both situations. In the elderly, ECFV is hard to assess, skin turgor appears poor due to loss of subcutaneous fat, and other signs may not be reliable. An important clue to making the differential diagnosis may be the serum urea nitrogen (SUN) because this becomes elevated in primary salt depletion and is subnormal in SIADH, that is, assuming there was no preexisting renal impairment. If all else fails, a central venous catheter may be placed to monitor pressure (CVP), so that normal saline can be slowly infused. If the patient has left ventricular failure or pulmonary hypertension, a Swan-Ganz catheter to monitor left ventricular pressure would be required.

Hyponatremia with Expanded ECFV (Dilutional Hyponatremia)

Impairment in water excretion occurs commonly in conditions in which salt excretion also is severely impaired. Patients with advanced cardiac, hepatic, or renal disease and generalized edema often are placed on diets that sharply restrict salt intake without placing limitations on fluid intake. Once hyponatremia begins to develop, restriction of water intake may become necessary.

Although total ECFV in these patients is increased, the blood volume returning to the heart and in the arterial vascular system tends to be decreased, stimulating baroreceptors in the right atrium and arterial system to retain sodium and baroreceptors in the left atrium and arterial system to stimulate ADH release and retain water. A decrease in glomerular filtration rate and/or an increase in sodium reabsorption in the proximal tubule limits water excretion by decreasing delivery of sodium and water to the distal nephron where dilution of urine below isotonic levels takes place. Because the relative intakes of salt and water represent an intake of hypotonic solutions whereas urinary concentration is near isotonic, the dilution of serum creates the hyponatremia. Treatment consists of administration

of a diuretic active in the loop of Henle, such as furosemide, which promotes excretion of sodium and a slightly hypotonic to isotonic urine even in the presence of ADH, along with fluid replacement with isotonic or hypertonic salt solutions if volume depletion becomes apparent.

It is very difficult for a normal person to ingest sufficient water to develop symptomatic hyponatremia (water intoxication). Some patients with schizophrenic illnesses, however, have been reported to be capable of ingesting sufficient fluid to lower their serum sodium concentrations into the symptomatic range.

Hyponatremia with Normal ECFV (Syndrome of Inappropriate ADH)

A diagnosis of SIADH is made after other causes of hyponatremia have been excluded. The following criteria must be met: (1) the extracellular fluid osmolality and sodium concentration must be decreased; (2) the urine must be hypertonic to serum; (3) urinary sodium excretion exceeds 10 mEq/L; (4) adrenal, renal, cardiac, and hepatic functions are normal; and (5) the hyponatremia can be corrected by water restriction. Persistence of circulating ADH is considered inappropriate when neither hyperosmolality nor volume depletion is present. The inability to excrete water because of high ADH levels leads to volume expansion that, in turn, promotes urinary salt loss. SIADH is seen in patients with a number of neoplasms, most commonly oat cell carcinoma of the lung. Any condition impairing blood flow through the pulmonary circulation, such as positive pressure breathing, creates a decreased filling of the left atrium that stimulates ADH release. The reported causes of this syndrome, especially those related to drug therapy, continue to grow as shown in Table 5–1. Recent reports have raised concerns about the association between the selective serotonin reuptake inhibitor antidepressants (SSRIs) and hyponatremia, with the elderly again at highest risk.[3]

Normovolemic hyponatremia also may result from the addition of an uncharged solute, such as glucose or mannitol, which increases serum osmotic pressure and draws water from inside the cell to expand and dilute the ECFV. This promotes an increased loss of sodium in the urine, reducing total body stores of this cation. Normovolemic hyponatremia (pseudohyponatremia) also can result from a displacement of water in a serum sample with abnormal amounts of large molecular weight solute, such as protein or lipids, so that there may be a false perception of the amount of serum water originally present when it is further diluted in the process of quantifying serum sodium concentration.

Hyponatremia in the Elderly

Surveys of older persons in both acute and chronic care facilities show a high prevalence of hyponatremia. Kleinfeld et al.[4] reported that 36 of 160 patients (23%) in a nursing home had serum sodium concentrations chronically below 132 mEq/L (mean 120 mEq/L). In most patients, the low serum sodium concentration was not explained except by the presence of chronic debilitating disease and old age. Miller et al.[5] later reported that more than half of their nursing home patients had been hyponatremic (serum sodium <135 mEq/L) on at least one occasion over the preceding year (monthly determinations). Hyponatremic patients had an impaired response to water loading, excreting only 56% as much water as comparable elders with normal serum sodium concentrations. The hyponatremic patients achieved a mean minimum urine osmolality of 195 mOsm/L compared to 84 mOsm/L in the normonatremic patients. Miller et al.,[6] using a similar definition for hyponatremia, also found that 11% of an ambulatory geriatric clinic population had hyponatremia. SIADH appeared to be the cause in nearly 60% of the cases of hyponatremia, with a quarter of these (7 cases) having no apparent underlying etiology other than age. Others[7] have found a similar high incidence of "idiopathic" SIADH (60%) in hospitalized elderly patients. However, they were asymptomatic unless the sodium concentration fell below 110 mEq/L and the subsequent course was benign, not requiring treatment.

Anderson et al[8] prospectively evaluated the prevalence, cause, and outcome of patients with hyponatremia in an acute care facility. The prevalence of hyponatremia was 2.5% with the mean age of the patients being 60 years. Two-thirds of the hyponatremic cases were iatrogenic. The most frequent cause was SIADH (normovolemic hyponatremia), accounting for 34% of cases; hypovolemia (dehydration), hypervolemia (dilutional hyponatremia), and hyperglycemia each accounted for another 16% to 19% of cases; renal failure (overhydration) and error accounted for the remainder. Nonosmotic (baroreceptor) stimulation of ADH release was a major factor in all cases.

Elderly persons appear to be more susceptible to the development of SIADH-like hyponatremia. The antidiuresis and hyponatremia observed postoperatively have been observed primarily in elders, as has been the hyponatremia observed with such drugs as sulfonylureas, SSRI antidepressants, and thiazide diuretics. Observations by Helderman et al[9] may help to explain this increased susceptibility of older patients to the development of hyponatremia. These investigators observed a greater increase (twofold) in serum arginine vasopressin (AVP) concentrations in older persons after infusion of a standardized hypertonic saline solution designed to raise serum osmolality to 306 mmol/L compared to younger persons, despite comparable baseline AVP concentrations. In contrast, ethanol infusions, known to inhibit ADH secretion, produced a more prolonged depression in serum AVP concentrations in young rather than old subjects. These two observations suggest an increasing osmoreceptor sensitivity with age, that is, a greater release of AVP and therefore water retention in response to any given stimulus.

Rowe et al.[10] subsequently reported on studies designed to determine whether this increase in AVP release in older subjects in response to hyperosmolality similarly occurred with other stimuli, specifically a change in baroreceptor responsiveness produced by quiet standing. They observed that older subjects, after 8 minutes of quiet standing, often failed to increase their serum AVP as much as did younger subjects. They could divide their subjects into those who released AVP (responders) and those who did not (nonresponders). Nearly half of the older subjects were nonresponders compared to only 10% of younger subjects. Because nonresponders still had a normal norepinephrine response to orthostasis, the authors proposed that the age-related defect was distal to the vasomotor center in the afferent limb of the baroreceptor reflex arc. They further speculated that the altered response to volume-pressure stimuli in elderly subjects might be related to impaired baroreceptor input to the supraoptic nucleus. This then would cause an up-regulated response to osmotic stimuli in older subjects. Subsequent studies have provided some supporting and some conflicting evidence as to whether AVP responses are really different in elderly compared to younger subjects as nicely summarized in a review by Epstein.[11]

The urinary excretion of aquaporin-2 (AQP-2) reflects the activity of AVP on the collecting ducts in producing channels through which water can be absorbed back into the medullary portion of the kidney. Presumably, increased levels of AQP-2 would facilitate an antidiuresis in the presence of AVP and might also explain why patients with SIADH might be retaining more water with resultant hyponatremia than do comparable patients with normal urinary excretions of AQP-2. Ishikawa et al.[12] examined this hypothesis recently and found an increased urinary excretion of AQP-2 in their elderly patients with hyponatremia due to SIADH. Furthermore, an antidiuresis with high AVP and AQP-2 levels persisted after a water load.

Hypernatremia

An increase in serum sodium concentration generally is a result of a loss of body water in excess of salt (dehydration), although it also can result from ingestion or administration of large amounts of salt without sufficient water or from excessive amounts of adrenal steroids (cortisone, aldosterone). Elderly persons have a diminished thirst sensation that is further impaired by cen-

tral nervous system dysfunction. Hypernatremia often occurs in elderly who are bedfast or physically handicapped so that they are not provided enough water to satisfy an already impaired thirst response. A net deficit of water also can be associated with vomiting and/or diarrhea, pituitary or nephrogenic diabetes insipidus, an osmotic diuresis such as hyperosmolar nonketotic diabetic acidosis, and hyperpyrexia (excessive sweating).

Older persons appear to be more predisposed to the development of hypernatremic dehydration than do younger ones. Snyder et al.[13] reported that more than 1% of all hospital admissions were patients older than 60 years who had or developed hypernatremia (serum sodium concentration >148 mEq/L). More than half developed their hypernatremia while in the hospital. Surgery, febrile illness, infirmity, and diabetes mellitus were responsible for two-thirds of these cases. Hypernatremia was a marker for associated severe illness, carrying a mortality rate of 42% in this group of patients. Rapid fluid replacement appeared to contribute to the increased mortality rates. Lavisso-Mourey et al.,[14] in a systematic evaluation of factors leading to dehydration in hospitalized nursing home patients, found a constellation of important risk factors that included advanced age, female gender, several chronic diseases, number of medications (especially laxatives), and decreased functional status.

Phillips et al[15] compared thirst perceptions in response to water restriction in young and old subjects. All subjects were deprived of water for 24 hours, after which free access to water was allowed. Even though older subjects ended the period of water restriction with higher serum sodium concentrations and osmolalities, they were less thirsty and drank less water during the recovery period, suggesting an impaired thirst response. Furthermore, the decline in renal concentrating ability observed with age (Chapter 12) might increase the potential for hypernatremia by augmenting urinary losses of water.

Hypernatremia reflects an increase in serum osmolality, which results in a shift of water from intracellular to extracellular spaces. One consequence of this shift is a shrinkage of brain cells, causing intracranial injury to blood vessels with venous thrombosis, infarction, and/or hemorrhage. The earliest manifestation of hypernatremia is thirst, followed by confusion and lethargy, and, ultimately, delirium, stupor, and coma. Because intravascular volume is preserved at the expense of cell water, changes in blood pressure and pulse rate are not prominent features of hypernatremic dehydration.

Once hypernatremia has occurred, restoration of fluids becomes necessary. The amount of water (or dextrose and water if given parenterally) needed can be estimated using this formula: observed serum sodium minus 140 divided by 140 times the total body water (60% of body weight). Total body water is used rather than ECFV (20% of body weight) because, as water is given, the osmolality in the ECFV falls, resulting in a shift of water along osmotic gradients back into the cell. To avoid a recurrence in individuals with demonstrated impaired thirst, a fluid prescription establishing the quantity of fluid to be ingested daily may become an important part of preventative management.

POTASSIUM

Potassium is the primary intracellular cation, with less than 2% of the total body potassium contained in the extracellular fluid compartment. Therefore, the serum concentration of potassium may not accurately reflect total body potassium stores. Flux of potassium into cells occurs with cell growth, intracellular nitrogen and potassium deposition, and increases in extracellular pH; potassium leaves the cell with cell destruction, glucose utilization, and decreases in extracellular pH. When one is interpreting serum potassium concentrations, factors that affect the ratio of intracellular to extracellular concentration must be kept in mind because normally a steep concentration gradient is maintained. For example, the patient with diabetic ketoacidosis has a high serum potassium concentration. However, rehydration, correction of the acidosis with sodium bicarbonate, and treatment of the hyperglycemia with insulin combine to produce a dra-

matic decrease in serum potassium concentration. Age alone does not appear to affect the ability to maintain this concentration gradient. Isotopic dilution studies and muscle biopsies, however, have been used to demonstrate that intracellular potassium stores can be depleted in a variety of clinical conditions commonly seen in elderly patients, such as metabolic and respiratory acidosis, congestive heart failure, cirrhosis, and uremia, with serum potassium concentrations remaining within normal limits.

Hypokalemia

The causes of hypokalemia are listed in Table 5–2. The most frequent cause of hypokalemia is the use of loop and thiazide diuretics to treat hypertension and/or edema. A frequently overlooked cause of hypokalemia in the elderly is the excessive use of enemas and purgatives, behavior that should be suspected whenever unexplained hypokalemic alkalosis is observed.

Although the normal kidney is not as efficient in conserving potassium as it is sodium, when intake is restricted or losses are excessive, it can reduce urinary excretions below 20 mEq/day. Because little potassium normally is lost through the gastrointestinal tract, it takes 2 to 3 weeks on a virtually potassium-free diet for a normal person to reduce his or her serum potassium concentration to 3.0 mEq/L. A reasonable criterion for establishing a diagnosis of urinary potassium wasting when the serum potassium concentration falls below 3.5 mEq/L would be the daily excretion of more than 20 mEq. The etiologies of excessive urinary potassium loss can be divided into four categories: (1) pituitary-adrenal disturbances, (2) renal defects, (3) drug-induced losses, and (4) idiopathic and miscellaneous.

Multiple pathophysiologic mechanisms occur in many, if not most, cases to explain the development of hypokalemia. As an example, a patient with vomiting not only has a reduction in potassium intake and some loss of potassium in the vomitus, he or she is losing hydrogen ions, which will produce a metabolic alkalosis. This, in turn, shifts potassium intracellularly and augments

Table 5–2 Causes of Hypokalemia

I. Inadequate intake
II. Excessive sweating
III. Dilution of extracellular fluid volume (ECFV)
IV. Shift of potassium intracellularly
    A. Increase in blood pH (alkalosis)
    B. Glucose and insulin
    C. Familial hypokalemic periodic paralysis
V. Excessive gastrointestinal losses
    A. Vomiting
    B. Biliary, pancreatic, and intestinal drainage from fistulas and ostomies
    C. Chronic diarrhea (chronic infections and inflammatory lesions, malabsorption, villous adenomas of colon and rectum, catechol-secreting neural tumors, abdominal lymphomas, islet cell tumors of pancreas, excessive use of enemas and purgatives)
VI. Increased urinary losses (potassium wasting)
    A. Pituitary-adrenal disturbances (primary aldosteronism; secondary aldosteronism due to renal artery stenosis; Cushing syndrome due to adrenal adenomas, carcinomas, and/or hyperplasia; pituitary corticotropin hypersecretion; ectopic corticotropin secretion secondary to tumor; 11 β-hydroxysteroid dehydrogenase deficiency due to Barter's syndrome or licorice ingestion [glycyrrhizic acid inhibits the enzyme responsible for the conversion of cortisol to cortisone])
    B. Renal disorders (distal or proximal renal tubular acidosis, renin-secreting renal tumor, salt-losing nephritis, diuretic phase of acute tubular necrosis, postobstructive diuresis)
    C. Drug induced (thiazide and loop diuretics; large nonabsorbable anions such as carbenicillin, cisplatin, aminoglycosides, amphotericin B; respiratory alkalosis due to acetylsalicylic acid; adrenergic agonists used to treat bronchospasm)
    D. Idiopathic, familial, and other pathologies (Liddle's and Gitelman's syndromes, hypomagnesemia, lysozymuria due to leukemia)

---

urinary potassium losses. The contracted extracellular volume then increases proximal tubular sodium and bicarbonate reabsorption that further enhances the metabolic alkalosis and induces a secondary hyperaldosteronism that increases urinary potassium losses.

The structural and functional defects associated with potassium deficiency are listed in Table 5–3. These involve the kidney, the myocardium and the cardiovascular system, the neuromuscular and central nervous system, and the gastrointestinal tract. The characteristic electrocardiographic changes are shown in Figure 5–2. Potassium deficiency can also contribute to impairments in carbohydrate metabolism and protein synthesis.

Because an alkalosis (chloride depletion) usually accompanies hypokalemia, replacement therapy should be instituted with potassium chloride rather than with the alkaline salts of potassium (the exception would be the patient with renal tubular acidosis). Foods rich in potassium (citrus and tomato juices, bananas, meats, and vegetables) provide the safest way to administer potassium. When additional oral replacement therapy is needed, commercial preparations come in liquid, tablet, and powder forms, usually in 20 mEq doses. Intravenous potassium repletion may become necessary but can be hazardous if infusion rates exceed 20 mEq/hour or if concentrations exceed 40 mEq/L. Urine output should be demonstrated, and electrocardiographic monitoring should be a requirement before potassium infusions are pushed above these levels.

Concern has been generated over patients receiving loop or thiazide diuretics that development of hypokalemia, especially in patients receiving digitalis for cardiac disorders or with acute myocardial infarction, might make them

Table 5–3 Manifestations of Hypokalemia

I. Myocardial and cardiovascular
   A. Focal myocardial necrosis
   B. Electrocardiographic changes (depressed ST segments, inversion of T waves, accentuated U waves, arrhythmias) (Figure 5-2)
   C. Other (potentiation of digitalis toxicity, salt retention, hypotension)
II. Neuromuscular and psychiatric
   A. Muscle weakness to flaccid paralysis
   B. Muscle pain and tenderness (rhabdomyolysis)
   C. Depressive reaction (anorexia, constipation, weakness, lethargy, apathy, fatigue, depressed mood)
   D. Acute brain syndrome (memory impairment, disorientation, confusion)
III. Renal
   A. Defect in urine concentrating ability (polyuria)
   B. Paradoxical aciduria
   C. Sodium retention
IV. Gastrointestinal
   A. Decreased motility and propulsive activity of intestine
   B. Paralytic ileus
V. Metabolic
   A. Carbohydrate intolerance delayed insulin release
   B. Growth failure due to impaired protein synthesis

more susceptible to cardiac arrhythmias and/or sudden death. Controlled trials with patients receiving either supplements or no supplements suggest that the additional potassium fails to affect outcome. In patients that have been made hypokalemic by diuretics, intracellular potassium concentrations are decreased more in patients with edematous or acidotic conditions than in hypertensive patients. Hypertensive patients maintain normal intracellular potassium concentrations, even in the presence of mild hypokalemia. Routine replacement potassium therapy, at least in hypertensive patients undergoing diuretic therapy with normal serum potassium levels, is not necessary. Rather it is better to monitor serum potassium levels because an occasional patient will develop hypokalemia that does potentiate the possibility of ventricular arrythmias.[16] A significant incidence of life-threatening hyperkalemia in patients receiving supplements means that the potential for benefit must be weighed against the risks.[17]

Hyperkalemia

The causes of hyperkalemia are outlined in Table 5–4. Hyperkalemia is most commonly observed in patients with impaired renal function. However, patients with chronic renal failure who maintain good urine flow rates do not develop significant hyperkalemia until the azotemia becomes life threatening. Because the distal nephron has such a large capacity for secretion of potassium, hyperkalemia develops only when there is some associated factor present, such as (1) oliguria (acute renal failure), (2) excessive endogenous or exogenous potassium load (supplements, medication, catabolism), (3) metabolic or respiratory acidosis, (4) spironolactone, triamterene, or amiloride therapy, (5) a deficiency of endogenous steroid (aldosterone, cortisol), or (6) administration of a drug that inhibits potassium secretion in the distal nephron such as an angiotensin converting enzyme (ACE) inhibitor, a beta-adrenergic antagonist (blocker), or a nonsteroidal anti-inflammatory drug (NSAID).

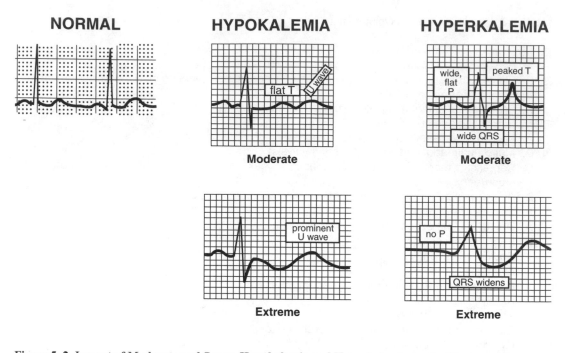

Figure 5–2 **Impact of Moderate and Severe Hypokalemia and Hyperkalemia on the Electrocardiogram**

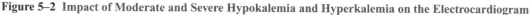

Poorly monitored potassium supplementation in patients on diuretic therapy can lead to potentially lethal hyperkalemia. In one study,[17] two significant risk factors were identified. Azotemia was predictable, but age was not. In patients under age 50 years, the frequency of incident hyperkalemia was 0.8% compared to 4.2% to 6.0% with advancing age in age groups older than that. Older individuals under all conditions (normal and restricted salt intakes, supine vs. upright) have much lower plasma renin activities and urinary aldosterone secretions that explain this observation.[18,19] This failure of the renin-aldosterone system in older patients, especially diabetics with interstitial nephritis, produces a type IV renal tubular acidosis with hyperkalemia.

The clinical manifestations of hyperkalemia often are subtle and may occur only shortly before death occurs from cardiac arrhythmia. Anxiety, restlessness, apprehension, weakness, stupor, and hyporeflexia should alert the clinician to the potential existence of this imbalance in patients at risk. Characteristic electrocardiographic changes are peaking of T waves followed by widening and loss of P waves and ultimately widening of the QRS complex (Figure 5–2).

Therapy should be started when the serum potassium concentration exceeds 5.5 mEq/L; a true medical emergency exists when it exceeds 7.0 mEq/L. Acute treatment is with glucose, insulin, and sodium bicarbonate to shift potassium intracellularly, and with calcium and sodium salts that act as physiologic antagonists. Sodium polystyrene sulfonate (Kayexalate) resins are used to remove excess potassium from the body and can be given orally or in enema form. To avoid constipation and fecal impaction with oral administration of these resins, sorbitol can be given, titrating the dose. When hyperkalemia is due to a mineralocorticoid deficiency, 9-fluorohydrocortisone (Florinef) can be given. Dialysis is rarely used as a last resort.

CALCIUM

A finely tuned endocrine system exists to maintain serum ionized calcium concentrations within a narrow normal range by controlling in-

Table 5–4 Causes of Hyperkalemia

I. Hyperkalemia caused by
  A. Decreased urinary excretion of potassium
  B. Increased exogenous or endogenous potassium
  C. Both
II. Decreased urinary excretion
  A. Renal insufficiency
  B. Potassium-retaining diuretics (spironolactone, triamterene)
  C. ACE-inhibitors, NSAIDs, β-adrenergic antagonists
  D. Adrenal hypofunction (Addison's disease, hyporeninemic hypoaldosterone)
III. Increased exogenous or endogenous load
  A. Supplemental potassium (with diuretics)
  B. Potassium-containing drugs (e.g., penicillin)
  C. Tissue catabolism (starvation, crush injury)
  D. Metabolic acidosis

testinal absorption, bone exchange, and renal excretion of calcium (Chapter 12). When serum ionized calcium concentrations decrease, parathyroid hormone (PTH) secretion increases, causing mobilization of calcium from bone, a decrease in renal tubular phosphate reabsorption, and a resultant decrease in serum phosphate concentration. This latter change facilitates bone resorption of calcium, increases renal tubular calcium resorption, and increases intestinal calcium absorption, either directly or by enhancing the effects of vitamin D. Vitamin D is converted by the liver to the carrier metabolite 25-hydroxycholecalciferol and by the kidney to the active metabolite 1,25-dihydroxycholecalciferol. This active form acts primarily to increase calcium absorption in the intestine, but it also increases bone resorption of calcium and decreases urinary calcium and phosphate excretion. PTH produces its effect on the intestine by accelerating the conversion of vitamin D from its carrier form to its active form. When the serum calcium concentration increases, the serum thyrocalcitonin concentration increases, producing an effect counter to that of PTH.

Serum calcium exists in both the ionized and bound states, but only the ionized calcium is physiologically active. The remaining calcium is either bound to serum proteins (albumin) or bound in a complex with various anions, such as citrate. Binding of calcium is dependent upon the concentration of serum proteins (albumin) and the blood pH, with calcium binding increasing as the pH increases. Because most clinical laboratories report only serum total calcium concentrations, these factors must be recognized in evaluating a specific serum calcium concentration.

Both hypocalcemia and hypercalcemia occur with increasing frequency in the elderly, primarily because specific disease entities causing these imbalances are more common in elderly persons. Of more importance is the age-related loss of bone calcium that occurs in both sexes, but more severely in women. This loss leads to the development of osteoporosis, with increased risk of fractures (Chapter 14).

Dietary factors play an important role in the age-related loss of bone calcium. In older persons, calcium intake is generally low and is associated with reduced absorption of calcium.[20] In addition, lack of vitamin D (hypovitaminosis D) is often associated with increasing age because older persons tend to avoid dairy products (source of vitamin D), have intestinal malabsorption of fat-soluble vitamin D, avoid exposure to sunlight (which aids conversion of precursors to vitamin D), and have a decreased ability in the skin to produce previtamin D.[21] Because vitamin D is the major regulator of intestinal calcium absorption, the cumulative effect of a deficit of calcium intake and an inadequate intake and generation of active vitamin D is a negative calcium balance. This stimulates PTH release, increasing bone calcium resorption and risk for osteoporotic fractures, a major cause of morbidity and mortality in the elderly.[22]

The nutritional requirements for calcium, especially in older persons, continue to generate controversy. Calcium differs from most other minerals in that the serum calcium concentration is not an adequate guide to the individual's calcium nutriture. Because there are 1000 grams of calcium in the skeleton and only 1 gram in extracellular fluid, serum calcium concentration does not reflect calcium stores in the body. It is not possible to discriminate between individuals in positive and negative calcium balance by measurement of serum calcium concentration alone. The fine regulation of serum calcium concentration is mediated by the parathyroid glands. Problems exist in trying to use either increased PTH or $1,25\text{-}(OH)_2$ cholecalciferol as indicators of calcium deficiency. The most practical definition of calcium requirement then is to determine the amount of calcium needed to maintain calcium balance, that is, the mean intake at which intake and output are equal. These kinds of balance studies are extremely time-consuming and laborious, and therefore not readily available, especially in postmenopausal women where they are most needed.

From available data, a RDA of 800 mg/day was proposed for the United States in 1980 with the recognition that pregnant and lactating women and postmenopausal women had higher requirements (1500 mg/day). These recommendations were not changed in the 1989 revisions made by the Food and Nutrition Board of the National Academy of Sciences and the National Research Council.[23] However, a NIH Consensus Conference held in 1993 concluded these recommendations were too low and recommended an intake of 1000 mg/day for adult men and estrogen-sufficient women (this would include postmenopausal women on estrogen therapy).[24] They recommended 1500 mg/day for postmenopausal women not on estrogen therapy. Furthermore, after recognizing that more research was needed on older persons, they felt

that, until more data are available, a daily intake of 1500 mg/day for persons over age 65 years should be recommended. Wood et al.,[25] after a comprehensive review of available information, also felt the current RDAs for calcium might be too low and warranted reevaluation. Then in 1997, the Food and Nutrition Board of the National Academy of Sciences published new Dietary Reference Intakes (DRI) to replace the RDA that established minimal amounts of nutrients needed to be protective against possible deficiency.[26–28] The new DRI were designed to reflect the latest understanding about nutrient requirements directed at optimizing health in individuals and groups. The DRI for calcium for adults was raised to 1200 mg/day, recognizing that the majority of adults, especially older persons, do not consume these levels of calcium without taking calcium supplements. One study of older individuals[29] reported that 62% of their subjects had an intake of less than 500 mg/day and that 21% had less than 300 mg/day.

New guidelines as to an adequate intake of vitamin D also were established.[26,27] The recommendation was made that for persons 51 to 70 years of age, an intake of 10 micrograms of vitamin D (400 IU) per day was appropriate; for persons over 70 years of age, this should increase to 15 micrograms (600 IU) per day.

Hypocalcemia

The causes of hypocalcemia are listed in Table 5–5. The majority of cases of hypocalcemia can be attributed to disturbances in the metabolism, production, or tissue responsiveness to PTH and/or vitamin D metabolites. In patients with unexplained hypocalcemia, and/or hypokalemia, hypomagnesemia as an underlying cause should be considered because it produces a peripheral resistance to PTH and decreases the release of PTH in response to the hypocalcemic stimulus.

The symptomatology associated with hypocalcemia is primarily related to increased neuromuscular excitability, such as tetany, paresthesias, muscle weakness and spasm, and movement disorders. Chronic manifestations include cataracts;

Table 5–5 Causes of Hypocalcemia

I. Hypoalbuminemia
II. Disturbances in parathyroid hormone (PTH) metabolism
   A. Decreased PTH production (surgical, infiltrative, or idiopathic hypoparathyroidism)
   B. End organ unresponsiveness to PTH (pseudohypoparathyroidism due to production of ineffective PTH or PTH receptor-G protein coupling disturbance)
III. Disturbances in vitamin D intake and metabolism
   A. Inadequate intake of vitamin D (dietary deficiency, malabsorption, postgastric surgery)
   B. Decreased 25-OH vitamin D production (parenchymal liver disease)
   C. Accelerated 25-OH vitamin D catabolism (anticonvulsant therapy, nephrotic syndrome)
   D. Decreased $1,25\text{-}(OH)_2$ vitamin D production (renal failure)
   E. End organ resistance to $1,25\text{-}(OH)_2$ vitamin D (vitamin D–resistant rickets)
IV. Hypomagnesemia (decreased PTH secretion, diminished skeletal response to PTH, reduced $1,25\text{-}(OH)_2$ response to PTH)
V. Hyperphosphatemia (renal insufficiency)
VI. Acute pancreatitis
VII. Calcitonin-producing tumors (medullary carcinoma of thyroid)

abnormalities of nails, skin, and teeth; and mental retardation.

Correction of acute symptomatic hypocalcemia can be accomplished with parenteral calcium gluconate. Oral calcium salts (carbonate, gluconate, or lactate) can be used to treat mild or latent hypocalcemia. Vitamin D or its more active metabolite, $1,25\text{-}(OH)_2$ cholecalciferol (Calcitriol), will increase intestinal absorption of calcium.

Hypercalcemia

The two most common causes of hypercalcemia are malignancy and hyperparathyroidism, which together are responsible for 80% to 90% of all cases[30] (Table 5–6). In hospitalized patients, malignancies are the most common cause of hypercalcemia, whereas in ambulatory patients, hypoparathyroidism is. Malignancy-associated hypercalcemia is the most common paraneoplastic syndrome, occurring in up to 10% of all patients with breast, renal cell, and lung cancers, squamous cell carcinomas of the head and neck, and multiple myeloma. In most cases, the onset of hypercalcemia is a poor prognostic sign. The exception is multiple myeloma where hypercalcemia may be responsible for the presenting manifestations of the disease. In patients with tumor cells metastatic to bone, release of bone-resorbing cytokines and growth factors results in osteolysis. In most patients without bony metastases, there is production by the tumor of a PTH-related protein (PTH-related protein or PTHrP). This protein acts like PTH in that it stimulates bone resorption and increases calcium reabsorption by the kidney. The development of precise assays for this protein has made it possible to establish the cause in the majority of patients with malignancy-associated hypercalcemia. Some tumors associated with hypercalcemia, however, have been shown to synthesize $1,25\text{-}(OH)_2$ vitamin D and, in rare instances, authentic PTH.

The early signs and symptoms associated with hypercalcemia are vague and nonspecific and include fatigue, anorexia, nausea, vomiting, constipation, somnolence, weakness, apathy, depression, and psychiatric disturbances. More severe hypercalcemia can lead to arrhythmias, seizures, or coma. Polyuria with dehydration and azotemia may complicate treatment, worsening the hypercalcemia. More chronic manifestations include osteopenia with fractures, nephrolithiasis, and nephrocalcinosis. Patients with hypercalcemia have an increased incidence of pancreatitis and peptic ulcer disease.

The initial therapy for hypercalcemia is rehydration with normal saline and administration of

Table 5–6 Causes of Hypercalcemia

I. Malignancies
   A. Bone metastases (release of bone-resorbing cytokines and growth factors by tumor cells metastatic to bone with resultant osteolysis)
   B. Humoral causes (production of PTH-related proteins, ectopic production of PTH by tumors, production of 1,25-$(OH)_2$ vitamin D by tumors)
   C. Multiple myeloma
II. Primary hyperparathyroidism (adenoma, hyperplasia, familial, multiple endocrine neoplasias, carcinomas)
III. Endocrine disorders (hyperthyroidism, pheochromocytoma, adrenal insufficiency)
IV. Granulomatous disease (sarcoidosis, tuberculosis, histoplasmosis, coccidiomycosis, berylliosis)
V. Miscellaneous (familial hypocalciuric hypercalcemia, immobilization, Paget's disease, milk alkali syndrome, hypervitaminosis A or D, thiazide or lithium administration)

a loop diuretic (furosemide). This decreases calcium concentration by hemodilution and increases urinary calcium excretion. Thiazide diuretics, in contrast, decrease urinary calcium excretion and potentiate hypercalcemia. Prednisone in high doses is effective when the mechanism of the hypercalcemia is increased vitamin D–mediated calcium absorption from the intestine (sarcoidosis, multiple myeloma, vitamin D intoxication), but is ineffective in malignancies with metastatic bone disease and hyperparathyroidism. Nonsteroidal anti-inflammatory drugs (NSAIDs) may be helpful in some malignancies without bone metastases in which prostaglandin E is the mediator of excessive bone breakdown, such as renal cell carcinoma. Inhibition of bone resorption can be accomplished with mithramycin, calcitonin, gallium, and the biphosphonates, such as etidronate, pamidronate, incadronate, clodronate, and a new third generation, nitrogen-containing biphosphonate, zoledronic acid (Zometa). One recent double-blind trial suggests zoledronic acid, which was shown to be safe and more effective than pamidronate, may become the drug of choice in the treatment of the hypercalcemia of malignancy due to a wide variety of tumors.[31]

MAGNESIUM

Magnesium is the second most important intracellular cation with about 60% of body magnesium located in bone, about 40% in the intracellular spaces (half of this in skeletal muscle), and only 1% located extracellularly. The normal serum magnesium concentration ranges from 1.4 mEq/L to 2.2 mEq/L and correlates poorly with intracellular magnesium. About 30% of serum magnesium is protein bound, with most of the remainder in ionized form, making it ultrafilterable through the kidney. Most of the intracellular magnesium is bound to protein and energy-rich phosphates. Magnesium is important in more than 300 different enzyme systems, being indispensable to the metabolism of adenosine triphosphate (ATP). Therefore, it affects glucose utilization; synthesis of fat, protein, and nucleic acids; muscle contraction; and several membrane transport systems.

The earlier RDA for magnesium of 350 mg/day for adult men and 280 mg/day for adult women, made using available balance data, were not changed in the 1989 revisions made by the Food and Nutrition Board of the National Academy of Sciences and the National Research Council.[23] Wood et al.,[25] however, presented arguments that these recommendations may be too high. In 1996, a working group on magnesium came up with recommendations based on energy expenditure.[32] Because older persons have more fat and less muscle, the working group concluded recommendations based on weight alone would make recommendations for elderly needs too high. They came up with recommendations of 161 mg/day for men over age 50 years and 133 mg/day for women over 50 years old. The new DRI recommended by the Food and Nutrition

Board in 1997 are 420 mg/day for men over 50 and 320 mg/day for women over 50.[26,27] Studies by Pao and Mickle[33] conducted on 37,000 healthy adults showed that the mean intakes for men and women were 266 and 228 mg/day, respectively. One can assume that for elderly persons, a deficiency of magnesium becomes a real concern, especially for those persons with chronic conditions that might affect food intake, gastrointestinal absorption, or urinary excretion of magnesium.

Magnesium Deficiency

The causes of magnesium deficiency are listed in Table 5–7. The first two entities are the most commonly encountered in the elderly. Gitelman's syndrome is an interesting, familial autosomal dominant inherited condition characterized by hypomagnesemia and hypocalciuria (which distinguish it from Barter's syndrome) and sodium depletion due to mutations of the gene encoding the thiazide-sensitive sodium-chloride cotransporter (NCCT) in the distal convoluted tubule. In its homogeneous form, it occurs early in life, but in its heterogeneous form, it may remain asymptomatic into later life when it is picked up by routine laboratory procedures or in evaluation of vague symptoms such as salt craving, nocturia, cramps, and fatigue.[34]

Serum magnesium concentrations do not decrease with advancing age, and magnesium depletion is not more common in older than younger persons. Hypomagnesemia produces neuromuscular and psychiatric symptoms, including neuromuscular hyperirritability, tetany, hyperacusis, seizures, muscle weakness, vertigo, gross tremors, and mental changes (eg, irritability and aggressiveness). Individuals with hypomagnesemia also develop polyuria and other electrolyte disturbances (hypocalcemia, hypokalemia, hypophosphatemia). Significant depletion of intracellular magnesium can occur before the serum magnesium concentration falls below the normal range.[35] Because symptoms appear related to intracellular concentrations of magnesium, the concern then arises as to how best to measure intracellular magnesium. Most methods are invasive, requiring tissue (muscle) biopsy, which is not practical for routine studies. One method for determining an intracellular deficit is to determine the amount of magnesium retained or excreted in a 24-hour period after infusion of a standardized quantity of magnesium.[36] This procedure has been useful in evaluation of patients with suspected symptomatology of magnesium depletion despite normal serum magnesium concentrations.

Hypermagnesemia

The earliest manifestations of hypermagnesemia are somnolence and hypotension, and an electrocardiogram may show prolongation of the PR interval and QRS duration with peaking of the T waves. Hypocalcemia frequently occurs as

---

Table 5–7 Causes of Hypomagnesemia

I. Gastrointestinal disorders with malabsorption and/or diarrhea
II. Chronic alcoholism
III. Diabetes mellitus, including therapy for diabetic ketoacidosis
IV. Acute pancreatitis
V. Protein-calorie malnutrition
VI. Renal magnesium wasting
   A. Diuretic states, including diuretic therapy (furosemide, thiazides)
   B. Endocrine and metabolic disorders (hyperthyroidism, hyperparathyroidism, hyperaldosteronism, hypercalcemia, hypophosphatemia)
   C. Nephrotoxic drugs (aminoglycoside antibiotics, cisplatin, cyclosporine, amphotericin B, pentamidine)
   D. Familial or isolated (Gitelman's syndrome)

a result of suppression of PTH secretion. Later, respiratory depression (respiratory acidosis) or paralysis and cardiac events can be terminal events. Life-threatening hypermagnesemia usually is seen only in patients with renal insufficiency taking magnesium-containing antacids or cathartics, but it also has been observed in elderly nonazotemic patients with bowel disorders (eg, active ulcer disease, gastritis, colitis, where there is enhanced absorption of magnesium given in excessive quantities).[37]

CONCLUSIONS

Elderly persons are more susceptible to the development of both hyponatremia and hypernatremia. There appears to be an increasing osmoreceptor responsiveness and decreasing baroreceptor responsiveness in elderly persons, which may make them more prone to the development of SIADH. Elderly individuals also develop a defect in their thirst responses, especially those with cerebral diseases, which make them more susceptible to the development of hypernatremia from dehydration (primary water depletion).

Both hypo- and hyperkalemia are more common in elderly persons. Hypokalemia occurs more frequently in the elderly primarily because of their increased use of medications, such as diuretics, purgatives, and enemas. Hyperkalemia is related to the loss of renal function and the lower renin and aldosterone levels in older individuals, making it more difficult to clear excess potassium via the kidneys.

A finely tuned endocrine system tends to insure that serum calcium concentrations are maintained within a narrow normal range, even when there is a negative calcium balance. Calcium and vitamin D intakes in the elderly generally are inadequate to prevent a negative calcium balance and bone demineralization. Calcium is lost from bone, resulting in bones more susceptible to fracture (osteoporosis). Hypercalcemia occurs more frequently in elderly persons, primarily because the malignancies responsible for hypercalcemia are more frequent.

Disorders of magnesium balance, even though not more common in the elderly, may be overlooked because serum magnesium concentrations are not routinely measured. Furthermore, intracellular magnesium depletion, responsible for the symptoms associated with magnesium depletion, can occur with serum magnesium concentrations still within the range of normal.

REFERENCES

1. Schroeder HA. Nutrition. In: Cowdry EV, Steinberg FU, eds. *The Care of the Geriatric Patient*. St. Louis, MO: CV Mosby; 1971:153.

2. Epstein M, Hollenberg N. Age as a determinant of renal sodium conservation in normal man. *J Lab Clin Med* 1976;87:411–417.

3. Kirchner V, Silver LE, Kelly CA. Selective serotonin reuptake inhibitors and hyponatremia: review and proposed mechanisms in the elderly. *J Psychopharmacol* 1998;12:396–400.

4. Kleinfeld M, Casimir M, Borra S. Hyponatremia as observed in a chronic disease facility. *J Am Geriatr Soc* 1979;27:156–161.

5. Miller M, Morley JE, Rubenstein LZ. Hyponatremia in a nursing home population. *J Am Geriatr Soc* 1995;43:1410–1413.

6. Miller M, Hecker MS, Friedlander DA, et al. Apparent idiopathic hyponatremia in an ambulatory geriatric population. *J Am Geriatr Soc* 1996;44:404–408.

7. Hirshberg R, Ben-Yehuda A. The syndrome of inappropriate antidiuretic hormone secretion in the elderly. *Am J Med* 1997;103:270–273.

8. Anderson RJ, Chung HM, Kluge R. Hyponatremia: a prospective analysis of its epidemiology and the pathogenetic role of vasopressin. *Ann Intern Med* 1978;102:164–168.

9. Helderman JH, Vestal RE, Rowe JW, et al. The response of arginine vasopressin to intravenous ethanol in man: the impact of aging. *J Gerontol* 1978;33:39–47.

10. Rowe JW, Minaker KL, Sparrow D, et al. Age related failure of volume-pressure mediated vasopressin release. *J Clin Endocrinol Metab* 1982;54:661–664.

11. Epstein M. Aging and the kidney. *J Am Soc Nephrol* 1996;7:1106–1122.

12. Ishakawa SE, Saito T, Fukagawa A, et al. Close association of urinary excretion of aquaporin-2 with appropriate and inappropriate arginine vasopressin-dependent antidiuresis in hyponatremia in elderly subjects. *J Clin Endocrinol Metab* 2001;86:1665–1671.

13. Snyder NA, Feigal DW, Arieff AI. Hypernatremia in elderly patients: a heterogeneous, morbid, and iatrogenic entity. *Ann Intern Med* 1987;107:309–319.

14. Lavizzo-Mourey R, Johnson J, Stolley P. Risk factors for dehydration among elderly nursing home residents. *J Am Geriatr Soc* 1988;36:213–218.

15. Phillips PA, Rolls BJ, Ledingham JG, et al. Reduced thirst after water deprivation in healthy elderly men. *N Engl J Med* 1984;311:753–759.

16. Siegal D, Hulley SB, Black DM, et al. Diuretics, serum and intracellular electrolyte levels, and ventricular arrhythmias in hypertensive men. *JAMA* 267;1083–1089.

17. Lawson DH. Adverse reactions to potassium chloride. *Q J Med* 1974;171:433–440.

18. Weideman P, DeMyttenaeu-Bursztein S, Maxwell MH, et al. Effect of aging on plasma renin and aldosterone in normal man. *Kidney Int* 1975;8:325–333.

19. Crane MG, Harris JJ. Effect of aging on renin activity and aldosterone excretion. *J Lab Clin Med* 1976;87: 947–959.

20. Gallagher JC, Riggs BL, Eisman J, et al. Intestinal calcium absorption and serum vitamin D in normal subjects and osteoporotic patients: effect of age and dietary calcium. *J Clin Invest* 1979;64:729–736.

21. MacLaughlin J, Holick MF. Aging decreases the capacity of the skin to produce vitamin D. *J Clin Invest* 1985;76:1536–1538.

22. McFayden IM, Nordin BEC, Smith DA, et al. Effect of variation in dietary calcium. *Brit Med J* 1985;1:161–164.

23. Food and Nutrition Board, National Research Council. *Recommended Dietary Allowances.* 10th ed., Washington, DC: National Academy Press; 1980.

24. NIH Consensus Conference. Optimal calcium intake. NIH Consensus Development Panel on Optimal Calcium Intake. *JAMA* 1994;272:1942–1948.

25. Wood RJ, Suter PM, Russell RM. Mineral requirements of elderly people. *Am J Clin Nutr* 1995;62:493–505.

26. Institute of Medicine, Food and Nutrition Board. *Dietary Reference Intakes for Calcium, Phosphorus, Magnesium, Vitamin D and Fluoride.* Washington, DC: National Academy Press; 1997.

27. Yates AA, Schlicker SA, Suitor CW. Dietary Reference Intakes: the new basis for recommendations for calcium and related nutrients, B vitamins, and choline. *J Am Dietet Assoc* 1998;98:699–706.

28. Bryant RJ, Cadogan J, Weaver CM. The new Dietary Reference Intakes for calcium: implications for osteoporosis. *J Am Coll Nutr* 1999;18(suppl):406S–412S.

29. Chapuy MC, Chapuy P, Meunier PJ. Calcium and vitamin D supplements: effects of calcium metabolism in elderly people. *Am J Clin Nutr* 1987;46:324–328.

30. Lafferty FW. Differential diagnosis of hypercalcemia. *J Bone Miner Res* 1991;6:S51–S59.

31. Major P, Lortholary A, Hon J, et al. Zoledronic acid is superior to pamidronate in the treatment of hypercalcemia of malignancy: a pooled analysis of two randomized, controlled clinical trials. *J Clin Oncol* 2000;19: 558–567.

32. Shils ME, Rude RK. Deliberations and evaluations of the approaches, endpoints and paradigms for magnesium dietary recommendations. *J Nutr* 1996;126(suppl 9): 2398S–2403S.

33. Pao EM, Mickle SJ. Problem nutrients in the United States. *Food Technol* 1981;35:58–69.

34. Cruz DN, Shaer AJ, Bia MJ, et al. Gitelman's syndrome revisited: an evaluation of symptoms and quality of life. *Kidney Int* 2001;59:710–717.

35. Reinhart RA. Magnesium metabolism: a review with special reference to the relationship between intracellular content and serum levels. *Arch Intern Med* 1988; 148:2415–2420.

36. Al-Ghandi SMG, Cameron EC, Sutton RAL. Magnesium deficiency: pathophysiologic and clinical overview. *Am J Kidney Dis* 1994;24:737–752.

37. Clark BA, Brown RS. Unsuspected morbid hypermagnesemia in elderly patients. *Am J Nephrol* 1992;12: 336–343.

CHAPTER 6

Trace Metal Requirements

Gary Fosmire, PhD

There is growing concern about the nutritional needs of the elderly, with increasing attention focused on various trace metals. Studies of dietary intake and status, both generally and in association with various disease states, have revealed that elderly people may be particularly vulnerable to developing deficiencies, or in some cases toxicities, of one or more of the trace metals. Reasons for this increased vulnerability include decreased energy intake without any increased density of trace metals in the diet, age-related physiologic changes that impair absorption, retention, or excretion; and various chronic and acute diseases experienced by the elderly and the medications used to treat them.

Several physiologic changes associated with aging[1] might be expected to affect the metabolism of most trace minerals. Changes in body composition, including a decline in lean body mass and a relative increase in adiposity, can be expected to alter body pool sizes of, or requirements for, most of the trace metals because they tend to be associated primarily with nonadipose tissues. The decline in basal metabolic rate associated with advancing age is usually accompanied by a decrease in energy intake, exacerbating problems of insufficient density of trace minerals in the diet. The impairment in kidney function observed with aging may result in less efficient elimination, with a concomitant retention of certain minerals, or less efficient reabsorption with

resultant increased losses (Chapter 12). The relative hypochlorhydria associated with aging adversely affects the solubility of the minerals and results in a decreased bioavailability or decreased absorption of various trace metals. The senescent changes in the intestine (Chapter 10) include a decreased mucosal surface area and decreased motility, potentially contributing to an impaired absorption of trace metals; such impairment with aging has not been a consistent finding, however, suggesting that in the absence of disease there is sufficient capacity for appropriate absorption.[2] The greater prevalence of disease states among the elderly may adversely affect nutritional status as a direct result of the disease processes or through drug–nutrient interactions (Chapter 16).

Dietary choices may also influence trace metal status. In an obvious way, selection of foods that do not contain substantial quantities of a particular trace mineral can result in a deficient state, but other dietary choices such as the incorporation of large amounts of fiber or foods containing phytate (myoinositol hexaphosphate), found in whole grains and legumes, can decrease the absorption or retention of various minerals.[3] The complexing of minerals by the fiber or phytate could impair absorption of exogenous sources as well as complex with those minerals, such as zinc, that are secreted into the intestine, thereby preventing their reabsorption. Although it may be difficult to generalize, many elderly people may restrict energy intake or have other restrictive dietary practices that would predispose them to developing deficiencies.[4]

ZINC

Zinc has been known to be an essential trace mineral for animals since the 1930s, and its importance for human health has been recognized for more than 40 years. A summary of the various roles that zinc is known to play in the body has been provided by Cousins.[5] These functions can be divided into three categories: catalytic, structural, and regulatory. Almost 100 enzymes are known to be zinc metalloproteins, enzymes, most requiring zinc for catalytic activity. In some proteins, zinc participates in specific folding of the protein to produce biologically active molecules (eg, "zinc fingers"). Zinc can also regulate gene expression. Knowledge about these biological roles has not as yet made it possible to fully understand the reasons for the various symptoms or signs of zinc deficiency. Explanations for depressed growth, immune dysfunction, diarrhea, altered cognition, reproductive teratogenesis, and numerous other clinical outcomes of marginal or severe zinc deficiency have not been conclusively established.[6] Given the important biological roles that zinc plays in the body, it is important to consider the dietary adequacy of zinc and other factors that may affect zinc status, particularly in the elderly.

Among factors affecting zinc status is the amount in the diet. Zinc is widely distributed in the food supply, although some foods are both richer and/or more bioavailable than are others (Table 6–1). A number of estimates of zinc intake from the diet have been done. For example, data from the Total Diet Study, 1982–1989, showed that intakes for individuals aged 60 to 65 years were 8.7 mg/d for women and 12.9 mg/d for men.[7] These values may be compared to the recently revised Estimated Average Requirement (EAR) and Recommended Dietary Allowances (RDA) of 9.4 mg/d for women and 11 mg/d for men, ages 19 to older than 70 years.[8] A review of 10 studies of elderly people revealed that mean intakes were between 7 and 10 mg/d.[9–11] In a recent commentary on dietary intakes of minerals,[12] Pennington states that dietary adequacy of zinc is of concern for a number of age and gender groups, including the elderly. Lower dietary intakes are, in part, a reflection of the density of zinc in the diet and the diminished energy intake associated with aging. Excellent sources of zinc include oysters, beef, poultry, and organ meats; whole grain products, legumes, and seeds are relatively rich, but bioavailability may be less than for products derived from animals.[13] If the elderly consume proportionately less of the foods that are richer in zinc, the density of zinc in their diets will decline and that, coupled with a diminishing energy intake, may result in intakes well less than the RDA.

Other factors than just the total amount of zinc in the diet can affect adequacy. Marginal zinc deficiency and suboptimal zinc status may be due to inadequate dietary intake, but inhibitors of zinc absorption are the mostly likely causes. Lonnerdal[14] has recently summarized these effects. For example, phytate, which is present in staple foods like cereals, corn, rice, and legumes, has a strong negative effect on zinc absorption from composite meals. Iron can also adversely affect zinc absorption, particularly if given as a supplement. Proteins typically improve zinc absorption, but casein will have a modest inhibitory effect on zinc absorption. Generally, zinc is less available from foods of vegetable origin than is the zinc from foods of animal origin.[3]

A great deal of research has been directed toward elucidating the mechanisms of zinc absorption and maintenance of zinc homeostasis.[5] Zinc absorption by the small intestine occurs by two processes, a saturable process that represents the process used to accomplish most of zinc absorption and a paracellular process that operates only at high intakes.[6] There is considerable endogenous secretion of zinc into the lumen of the intestine. Homeostatic regulation of zinc metabolism is achieved primarily by modulation of the rate of absorption and the rate of endogenous secretions. Conditions that interfere with these processes can adversely affect maintenance of appropriate levels of zinc in the body. Studies have shown that the efficiency of zinc absorption

Table 6–1 Zinc Content of Selected Foods

Food, Portion Size	Zinc Content (mg)
Beverages	
Carbonated, nonalcoholic, 12 fl oz	0.2–0.4
Coffee, 1 cup	trace
Tea, 1 cup	0.1
Wine, 4 fl oz	0.1
Beer, 12 fl oz	0.1
Bread, 1 slice	
White	0.2
Mixed grain	0.5
Rye	0.4
Whole wheat	0.6
Dairy products	
Milk, 1 cup	0.9–1.0
Cheese, 1 oz	0.9
Cottage cheese, 1 cup	0.7–1.0
Egg	0.6
Fish, 3.5 oz	
Bass	0.5
Cod	0.8
Tuna	0.9
Fruit, fresh, 1 each	
Apple	trace
Peach	0.1
Plum	0.1
Orange	0.1
Legumes, 1 cup, cooked	
Kidney beans	2.0
Soybeans	2.1
Dried peas	1.9
Meat, poultry	
Beef, cooked, 3 oz	5.1
Pork roast, 3 oz	2.2
Chicken, 1 cup	2.9
Beef liver, 3 oz	5.2
Chicken liver, 3 oz	3.6
Nuts, 1 cup	
Almonds	4.2
Cashews	7.7
Peanuts	4.8
Pecans	6.5
Shellfish, 3.5 oz	
Oysters, eastern	62.0
Oysters, western	48.0
Clams	2.7
Vegetables	
Green beans, 1 cup	0.5
Beets, $1/_2$ cup	0.2
Carrots, 1 each	0.1
Corn, 1 ear	0.4
Green peas, 1 cup	1.8
Potato, baked without skin, 1 each	0.5
Cabbage, raw, 1 cup	0.1

Source: Values from *Nutrition for Living* (pp. A12–A37) by JL Christian and JL Greger, Benjamin Cummings Publishing Company, San Francisco, CA1988.

is less in the elderly than in younger subjects.[15] Another study by Bales et al.[16] showed that elderly subjects failed to absorb as much zinc after a 25 mg zinc load as did younger subjects. Others have failed to observe such a decrease in efficiency of absorption with aging,[17] and a study by Turnlund et al.[18] found that elderly subjects could absorb zinc as well as young subjects when presented with a very low zinc diet. Reasons for the discrepancies in findings are not readily apparent. It has been reported[18] that the elderly can maintain zinc balance as well as younger subjects. Further studies will be required to resolve the questions of whether zinc efficiency declines with aging.

In addition to the amount of zinc in the diet, a number of other factors, called "conditioning-factors" by Sandstead and colleagues,[10] that impair the absorption or increase the excretion (or both) of zinc may influence requirements and lead to a deficient state. Chronic malabsorption syndromes, such as gluten-sensitive enteropathy, Crohn's disease, and sprue, can result in decreased zinc absorption and an impaired ability to control zinc homeostasis. Any physiological stress that results in substantially increased zinc losses into the urine will increase requirements. Examples of such stresses would include physical trauma, wounds (including surgery), thermal burns, starvation, and muscle wasting diseases. These all result in dramatic increases in urinary zinc losses. The consumption of alcohol results in increased urinary losses of zinc due to alcohol consumption, per se. If consumption has been prolonged enough to cause alcohol-induced cirrhosis, urinary losses of zinc will be high and the zinc content of the liver abnormally low. Many of the medications (both those sold over the counter and those sold by prescription) used by the elderly can affect zinc status. Diuretics, chelating agents, antacids, laxatives, and iron supplements may decrease absorption or increase excretion from the body.

Given the somewhat low intakes reported for the elderly and the likelihood of having one or more of the conditioning factors, it is reasonable to suppose that zinc deficiency would be preva-

lent in the elderly. The establishment of a zinc-deficient state is made more difficult owing to the absence of unambiguous indicators of zinc status.[6] The data that can be used to estimate prevalence rates for zinc deficiency are meager and clearly insufficient to allow confident estimates of such rates among the elderly as a whole. Data from a number of studies using relatively small subject population groups have been reviewed by Greger,[9] and data from several other studies[11,19–24] have been used to evaluate zinc nutriture among the elderly. Prevalence of deficient status, somewhat arbitrarily defined as plasma or serum zinc concentrations below 10.7 μmol/L or 70 μg/dL, ranged between 0% and 61%. Given the variability of plasma or serum measures unless time of day, infection, hormonal status, and so forth are controlled for and because the studies examined populations varying in age, socioeconomic class, and health status, such variability in prevalence is not unexpected. Studies that have examined larger population groups, such as the population sampled by the Health and Nutrition Examination Survey II (HANES II), showed that about 12% of men and women had zinc plasma or serum values below 70 μg/dL.[25] These findings suggest that a considerable number of elderly people have biochemical evidence of zinc deficiency; prevalence rates appear strikingly higher among those with poor health or low socioeconomic status.

Another approach to studying zinc status is to provide a zinc supplement and examine some biochemical or other response. Using a sample of 53 elderly subjects, Swanson et al.[26] did not observe improvements of circulating protein and immunoglobulin concentrations when zinc supplements were provided to those whose diets contained an average of 9.2 mg/d. However, dietary zinc was positively correlated with serum albumin in a group of elderly Canadians whose zinc intakes averaged 5.4 mg for women and 6.5 mg for men.[27] In a depletion study using elderly subjects, Bales et al.[28] showed a decline in the activity, of 5[1]-nucleotidase activity, which was reversed with zinc supplementation. Prasad et al.[29] showed that provision of a zinc supplement resulted in normalization of zinc in granulocytes and lymphocytes and improvement in various immune parameters.

Consequences of zinc deficiency may be serious and varied, depending in part on the severity of the deficiency. Manifestations of the deficiency have been reviewed by Prasad.[30] and may include growth retardation, impaired sexual development and performance, dermatitis, delayed wound healing, anorexia, altered taste acuity, and impaired immune function. A number of these symptoms only arise as a result of a severely deficient state, but even moderate or mild deficiency may adversely affect the health of an individual. A number of these deficiency symptoms resemble problems commonly observed in elderly individuals, and attempts have been made to relate zinc status to the occurrence of several of these symptoms. Most attention has been focused on taste acuity, wound healing, dermatitis, and immune function.

Taste acuity has been reported to decline with aging,[31] but it is unclear to what extent this can be attributed to zinc deficiency. It has been clearly shown that severe zinc deficiency will result in hypogeusia;[32] it is less clear that a less severely deficient state will result in diminished taste. Several studies have examined the interaction between zinc and taste acuity. Most studies of elderly subjects who did not have medical conditions that led to a severely deficient state have failed to observe such a relationship or see a positive change, that is, lower thresholds for the different tastes in response to zinc supplementation.[16,33–35] However, a study by Prasad et al.[36] reported that zinc supplementation (30 mg zinc/day for 6 months) improved taste acuity among elderly subjects who had normal plasma zinc but depressed granulocyte and lymphocyte values on entry into the study. For patients rendered severely zinc deficient due to medical conditions, zinc supplementation has been clearly shown to improve taste acuity.[37,38]

An essential role for zinc in wound healing is now well established.[39] It is apparent, however, that the increased rate of wound healing in response to zinc supplementation will occur only if the individual is in suboptimal zinc status; that is, there is no additional benefit obtained by supplementation once the deficiency has been corrected.[40] Initial poor zinc status, due to insufficient intake and/or losses associated with surgery or physical trauma, could limit the amount of zinc available for tissue repair and diminish the effectiveness of the healing process.

Severe zinc deficiency in humans may manifest as acrodermatitis of the extremities and in the oral, anal, and genital areas. The hypothesis that a portion of the dermatitis seen in the elderly is due to zinc deficiency has not been tested extensively. Wiesmann and colleagues[41] identified a number of elderly individuals who had skin problems similar to those described in zinc deficiency. A number of these subjects had subnormal plasma zinc concentrations, but supplementation with zinc for 4 weeks did not result in improvement in their skin lesions.

The hypothesis that zinc nutriture is related to the immune response in elderly people has attracted considerable attention. Elderly individuals are more susceptible to some infectious diseases, and the consequences of such infections may be more severe.[42] Data in humans indicate that the defect associated with aging is in the delayed immune mechanisms, expressed as deficits in delayed dermal hypersensitivity and a failure of T lymphocytes to respond to stimulation.[43] It is known that severe zinc deficiency markedly impairs cellular immunity,[44 46] but the effects of a less severely deficient state are not as well documented. Two studies have reported beneficial effects of zinc supplementation on cellular immunity in elderly subjects,[47,48] although neither study was conducted with a double-blind research design and the number of individuals examined was small. A double-blind zinc intervention trial by Bodgen et al.[24] was begun in 1987. Baseline data revealed that responses to seven skin test antigens were significantly associated with plasma zinc concentrations and that in vitro lymphocyte proliferative responses to various mitogens were related to various measures of cellular zinc levels. Zinc supplementation was eventually shown to improve immune status.[49] Others have reported that zinc supplementation for the elderly resulted in improvement in various measures of immunity,[36,50] Bogden[51] has recently summarized these findings. He states that severe zinc deficiency causes substantial impairment of cellular immunity, which can result in infection and possible death. Effects on immunity, of mild to moderate zinc deficiency are considerably less severe and may be subtle.

Given that dietary intakes of the elderly are frequently less than the RDA and that there are potential beneficial effects of normalizing suboptimal zinc status, it seems prudent to recommend that elderly people who are vulnerable to developing a deficient state routinely take a small supplement of zinc. It should be pointed out, however, that excessive use of zinc supplements can result in alterations in copper balance and may adversely affect lipoprotein profiles and may impair immune responses.[52] An Upper Limit (UL) has recently been established as 40 mg/d for adults.[8]

COPPER

Of the various trace minerals, copper was one of the first to be recognized as an essential nutrient. The concentration of copper in milk is very low.[53] Feeding a milk-based diet to rats resulted in a severe hypochromic, microcytic anemia that was unresponsive to iron but cured by copper administration.[54] Further research has identified many of the biological roles of copper, which are primarily as a component of various copper-containing enzymes. As reviewed by Harris,[55] important roles for the enzymes include the production of free energy by the electron transport chain of oxidative phosphorylation (cytochrome c oxidase), maintenance of antioxidant defenses (superoxide dismutase), posttranslational modification of amino acids needed for proper maturation of collagen and elastin, wound healing and maintenance of the integrity of blood vessels (lysyl oxidase), and production of melanin to protect the skin from ultraviolet light and for pigmentation of hair (tyrosinase).

Copper deficiency has been produced experimentally in a number of species and has been observed in livestock and occasionally in humans. Symptoms of the deficient state are somewhat species specific but are usually manifest in humans as hypochromic anemia and neutropenia, osteoporosis, myocardial disease, arterial disease, and neurological effects.[56] These manifestations of the deficiency can be largely explained by decreased activity of the various copper-containing enzymes or proteins.

Although there has been substantial uncertainty about the copper requirements for humans, a sufficient body of evidence has been gathered so that Estimated Average Requirements (EAR) and Recommended Dietary Allowances (RDA) have recently been set by the Food and Nutrition Board.[8] EAR values for both men and women ages 19 to older than 70 years are set at 700 μg Cu/d. RDA values for the same age brackets are 900 μg Cu/d. Two types of studies were used to establish these values. In the first type, the concentrations of various biochemical indicators of copper status (plasma copper, serum ceruloplasmin, erythrocyte superoxide dismutase, and platelet copper) were assessed in controlled depletion/repletion studies. In the second type, factorial studies were done to determine all copper losses from the body. Although both EAR and RDA values are given for older individuals, there is no appropriate data on which to base an EAR value for older adults and no evidence to suggest that the requirements would be different.[8]

Several studies have examined copper balance in elderly people. With mean intakes of 3.2 mg/day, copper balance was close to zero for elderly men in two studies conducted by Turnlund and colleagues.[57,58] Burke et al.[59] found that 8 or 10 elderly subjects were in positive balance at 2.33 mg/d. Healthy elderly subjects studied by Bunker and colleagues[20] were not able to maintain balance at intakes of 1.28 mg/d. For housebound elderly, intakes of 0.87 mg/d resulted in substantial negative balance.[21] These values are higher than the EAR and may reflect concerns about the use of balance studies to assess mineral requirements, as discussed by Mertz.[60]

Copper is widely distributed in foods, although some foods are not very rich sources (Table 6–2). Typically, organ meats, seafood, nuts, and seeds are major contributors to dietary copper.[61] An analysis of the contribution by food group to dietary intakes of copper by Pennington[62] showed that most of the copper was provided by grain products, meat, poultry, fish, vegetables, and legumes; relatively little came from dairy products, fruits, eggs, sugars and sweeteners, and fats and oils. Daily copper intakes averaged 1.0 mg for females and 1.3 mg for males.[62] These values may be compared with earlier studies designed to assess copper intake of elderly people directly. Gibson and colleagues[63] reported that vegetarian women (mean age 69 years) had copper intakes of 2.1 mg/d. In another study, average copper intake of elderly Canadian women was 1.2 mg/d.[19] A similar value of 1.28 mg/day was obtained for 24 healthy elderly people in England.[20] An earlier study by Pennington[7] for individuals 60 to 65 years of age estimated intakes of copper to be 0.86 for women and 1.18 mg for men. Evidence from the preceding studies would suggest that average copper intakes among older individuals would generally be adequate to meet the RDA. It is clear, however, that dietary choices can influence the adequacy of dietary copper. Dietary choices that limit those foods that are richer in copper can result in inadequate intakes.

Several factors may affect the adequacy of copper in the diet in addition to those food choices that affect density of copper. Among these are dietary components that may increase or impair the absorption of copper by the intestine.[64] The bioavailability of copper is influenced markedly by the amount of copper in the diet.[65] Among factors that facilitate copper absorption are protein and amino acids, citric acid, phosphate, and gluconate. Factors that decrease the bioavailability of copper include zinc, cadmium, fiber, unabsorbed fat, bile, and vitamin C. Individuals who supplement their diet with large quantities of zinc or vitamin C have an added risk of copper deficiency.

The essentiality of copper for humans is well established. Severe deficiencies have been reported in premature infants, children with severe malnutrition, patients with severe malabsorption syndromes, and individuals receiving parenteral nutrition without adequate copper supplementation. The deficiency is usually manifest as severe anemia, neutropenia, and osteoporosis, and, if uncorrected, may result in death. Such severe copper deficiency is relatively rare and does not usually occur in the absence of other medical problems that impair absorption or increase the rate of copper lost from the body. The more common state, although the prevalence rate cannot be accurately established, is probably that of a mild, chronic copper deficiency. The question of whether mild copper deficiency is a significant nutritional problem in humans has been addressed by Danks.[66] Possible features of chronic copper deficiency proposed by Danks are anemia and neutropenia refractory to other treatments, osteoporosis, arthritis, arterial and myocardial disease, loss of pigmentation, and neurological effects.

Although none of the preceding features are proven consequences of a mild, chronic copper deficiency, each has a biochemical or observational rationale that supports its inclusion in this list of suspected outcomes. As examples of these, the anemia seen in copper deficiency has been

Table 6–2 Copper Content of Common Foods

Food, Portion Size	Copper Content (mg)
Oyster, 3 oz	3.7
Crab, 3 oz	1.0
Rye flour, 1 cup	0.96
Beans, black, 1 cup	0.5
Almonds, 1 oz	0.3
Peanuts, 1 oz	0.2
Beef, ground, 3.5 oz	0.07
Codfish, 3 oz	0.03
Broccoli, $1/2$ cup	0.03
Milk, 8 fl oz	0.02

Source: Data from J. Pennington, *Bowes and Church's Food Values of Portions Commonly Used.* 17th ed. Philadelphia, PA: Lippincott; 1998:3-319.

related to decreased levels of ceruloplasmin, a copper-containing protein in plasma with ferroxidase activity and essential to convert iron from a ferrous to a ferric state so that it can be transported by transferring to the bone marrow for erythropoiesis. Copper's role in bone metabolism and in the prevention of skeletal abnormalities is primarily related to the maintenance of the activity of lysyl oxidase. This copper-containing enzyme is involved in posttranslational modification of lysine residues in collagen so that crosslinking of collagen to form mature, stable collagen fibrils is possible, ensuring the structural integrity of bone. The role of copper in arterial and myocardial diseases is partially related to its function in lysyl oxidase. The formation of the elastic cross-linkages of desmosine and isodesmosine in elastin requires lysyl oxidase; failure to form these cross-linkages results in less elasticity and weakening of the major blood vessels. Copper deficiency has been shown to result in hypercholesterolemia, glucose intolerance, and hypertension—all risk factors for cardiovascular disease.[67]

Because many of the problems observed with substantial frequency in elderly individuals are similar to those listed as possible features of chronic copper deficiency, it seems important to obtain better estimates of the prevalence of suboptimal copper intake and status in this group. Although assessment of copper nutriture in adult humans has not been perfected,[68] several methods are useful in the diagnosis of copper deficiency. These include the concentrations of plasma or serum copper and ceruloplasmin as well as the activities of superoxide dismutase, ceruloplasmin, and cytochrome c oxidase. Older individuals might be encouraged to include some of the richer sources of copper in their diets, including such things as legumes, chocolate, seeds, nuts, peanut butter, and oysters.

CHROMIUM

The essentiality of chromium for mammals was discovered in 1959 by Schwarz and Mertz,[69] who observed an impaired glucose tolerance in rats that could be corrected by supplementation with chromium. Observations in other species, including humans, have confirmed this alteration in glucose metabolism in chromium deficiency.[70] Chromium is now thought to potentiate the action of insulin in some fashion, perhaps by activating an insulin receptor by a low molecular weight chromium-binding substance, as proposed by Vincent.[71] Despite its acceptance as an essential trace mineral, information about the biological function of chromium is limited, perhaps because of the many technologic difficulties in chromium analyses and uncertainty about the validity of much of the early work.[72] It is clear, however, that chromium deficiency manifests with many of the symptoms of diabetes, especially those of impaired glucose tolerance, altered plasma lipids, and peripheral neuropathy.[72]

A number of factors can impair the chromium status of an individual.[73] The first is the amount of chromium in the diet. Chromium is widely distributed in the food supply although in small amounts. Despite limitations on the information about chromium content of foods, Anderson and colleagues[74] have shown that whole grains and cereals contain higher concentrations of chromium than do fruits and vegetables and that dairy products are poor sources of chromium. They also showed that the mean chromium content of 22 well-balanced daily diets, designed by nutritionists, was 13.4 ± 1.1 μg/1000 kcal (range of 8.4 to 23.7 μg/1000 kcal). Foods believed to be particularly rich in chromium include mushrooms, brewer's yeast, prunes, raisins, nuts, asparagus, and wine.[73] Analyses of various foodstuffs have been provided by Anderson and colleagues[74] and are the basis for Table 6–3.

Actual intakes of chromium have been determined in a few studies in which the methodology is adequate to trust the validity of the data. Chromium intakes have recently been estimated using the values of Anderson et al.[74] cited earlier and energy estimates of Briefel et al.[75] from the Third National Health and Nutrition Examination Survey, 1988–1991. Values of 30 μg for men and 20 μg for women of individuals 51 to older than 70 years of age were reported. These were then used to establish the current Adequate Intake (AI) values.[8] Anderson and Kozlovsky,[76]

Table 6–3 Chromium Content of Selected Foods

Food, Portion size	Chromium Content (μg)
Whole milk, 1 cup	<0.12
Egg, 1 ea	0.20
Beef cubes, 3 oz	2.0
Chicken breast, 3 oz	0.5
Haddock, 3 oz	0.6
Bread, whole wheat, 1 slice	0.98
Dinner roll, 1 each	0.62
Spaghetti, 1 cup	0.28
Rice, white, 1 cup	1.2
Apple, peeled, 1 med	0.4
Orange juice, 1 cup	2.2
Green beans, 1 cup	2.2
Carrots, raw, 1 each	0.29
Sugar, 1 pkt	0.03
Peanut butter, 1 tbsp	0.61

Source: Anderson R, Bryden N, Polansky M. Dietary chromium intake. Freely chosen diets, institutional diets, and individual foods. *Biol Trace Elem Res* 1992;32:117–121.

using analysis of duplicate daily composites of all food and beverages, reported mean intakes of 28 ± 1 μg for both men and women aged 25 to 65 years; intakes were somewhat greater for men (33 ± 3 μg) than they were for women (25 ± 1 μg). Analysis of diets of two different groups of elderly subjects revealed intakes of 37 μg/d and 25 μg.[77] Evaluation of a number of diets from the United States,[78] showed a chromium density of between 20 and 25 μg/1000 kcal, substantially greater than the density (13.4 ± 1.1 μg/1000 kcal) provided by Anderson et al.[74] These differences are likely due to improvements in analytic technique. From a study by Bunker et al.[77] intakes of 25 μg/d resulted in an estimated slightly negative balance if dermal and miscellaneous losses were considered. It seems clear that chromium intakes of the elderly may be insufficient to maintain optimal chromium status, especially as energy intakes decline.

In addition to insufficient dietary intakes, several other factors can influence chromium requirements. One of these factors is the body's ability, through presently unknown mechanisms, to improve the efficiency of absorption to compensate for low intakes.[76] It is important to note that the percentages of absorption are low (ie, from <0.3% to 1.9%), although they reflect more than a sixfold improvement in absorption efficiency with quite low intakes. Whether there is an equivalent response in absorption efficiency with aging is not a question that has been addressed.

Factors that may act to impair chromium utilization or increase chromium loss from the body include other dietary components, such as fiber, simple sugars or refined carbohydrates, and medication usage. It has been shown that consuming a diet high in simple sugars enhanced the urinary excretion of chromium when compared with subjects fed a diet higher in complex carbohydrates.[79] Bunker et al.[77] reported a severely negative chromium balance among elderly subjects when fed a diet high in fiber. Some currently used medications can affect chromium absorption. By using animal models, it has been shown that antacids such as calcium carbonate or magnesium hydroxide reduce absorption of chromium.[78,80] Aspirin and indomethacin administration increased chromium absorption.[81] It has also been shown that coadministration of ascorbic acid increases chromium absorption.[78]

Proven, relatively severe chromium deficiency has been demonstrated in humans. A patient receiving total parenteral nutrition without chromium for 3 years developed hyperglycemia, weight loss, ataxia, and peripheral neuropathy.[70] Symptoms did not respond to insulin, but addition of chromium resulted in normal glucose tolerance and neurologic function. Similar findings of diabetic-like symptoms refractory to insulin but reversed by supplemental chromium have been reported.[82] Because of the difficulty of assessing a chromium-deficient state, most studies of chromium status are conducted by giving a supplement to a group or individual thought to be at risk, and the effects are monitored before and after supplementation. Putative evidence of deficiency has been observed in malnourished children from a chromium-poor area, diabetics, elderly people, and individuals with hyper- and hypoglycemia.[83] Because of difficulties in assessment of chromium status and because investigators have given different amounts and forms of chromium supplements, it is difficult to compare studies. However, there does appear to be improvement in glucose tolerance and blood lipid profiles if individuals were chromium deficient prior to treatment. This latter point, that normalizing an individual's chromium status will likely improve glucose, insulin, and lipid levels, is important. Certainly as important is the fact that not all impaired glucose tolerance, hyperinsulinemia, or hyperlipidemia are due to chromium deficiency; further benefits of giving chromium supplements to individuals in good chromium status should not be expected.

Several studies have examined chromium status and response to supplementation in elderly people. Among those studies using elderly subjects, Urberg and Zemel[84] observed improved glucose tolerance with supplementation of 200 μg of chromium per day, and a study by Martinez et al.[85] found that about half of their subjects showed improved glucose tolerance with supplementation. Abraham and colleagues[86] did not report lower fasting glucose concentrations among subjects given chromium supplements, but did find an improvement in lipid profiles. Anderson et al.[87] studied subjects with type 2 diabetes given supplements of 200 or 1000 μg chromium for 4 months. At 2 months, fasting and 2-hour glucose concentrations were reduced in the group given the 1000 μg supplement; at 4 months, reductions in glucose, insulin, and glycosylated hemoglobin concentrations were observed in both groups.

It would seem that some elderly people, as well as those in younger age groups and especially those with type 2 diabetes, may have marginal or suboptimal chromium status. These are individuals who would likely respond to supplementation by normalizing insulin levels, show improved glucose tolerance, and have improved lipid profiles. Given the increased prevalence of impaired glucose tolerance in the population[88] and that chromium status declines with aging,[89] this issue takes on greater importance. Because there is currently no practical way to identify individuals

who are suspected to have poor chromium status, the only practical way to identify those with suboptimal chromium status is to try a course of supplementation at levels near the AI and see whether symptoms of hyperinsulinemia, hyperglycemia, and hyperlipoproteinemia improve.

SELENIUM

Selenium is recognized as one of the essential trace minerals.[90] A number of diseases are caused by simultaneous deficiencies of selenium and vitamin E. For example, liver necrosis in rats, exudative diathesis in chicks, mulberry heart in swine, and some forms of muscular dystrophy (white muscle disease) in lambs and calves can be prevented or cured by supplementation with either selenium or vitamin E. These examples demonstrate the interacting biochemical roles of selenium as a component of glutathione peroxidase and vitamin E, both acting as antioxidants in the detoxification of peroxides and free radicals that have their most damaging effects on cell membranes in blood, liver, and other tissues.

Roles for selenium independent of vitamin E status have been demonstrated. For example, rats fed a selenium-deficient diet with adequate vitamin E for two generations showed hair loss, growth retardation, and reproductive failure.[91] In humans, selenium deficiency has been implicated in Keshan disease, an endemic cardiomyopathy in parts of China.[92] The acute form is characterized by sudden onset of heart insufficiency; the chronic form shows moderate to severe heart enlargement with varying degrees of heart insufficiency. Selenium has been shown to prevent the disease, although selenium cannot reverse cardiac failure once it occurs. Another disease found in China, Siberia, and North Korea associated with selenium is Kashin-Beck disease, an endemic osteoarthropathy that causes joint deformation and limited joint mobility.[93] Both Keshan disease and Kashin-Beck disease undoubtedly are multifactorial in nature, perhaps having a viral or other nutrient component, but both are clearly associated with deficient selenium status.

Numerous studies have examined the relationship between selenium status and cancer. Selenium has been shown to act as an anticancer agent in various animal models.[94] With humans, a recent study[95] reported that a 200 μg selenium supplement was associated with a 37% reduction in total cancer incidence, a 63% reduction in the incidence of prostate cancer, a 58% reduction in colorectal cancer, a 46% decline in lung cancer, and a 50% reduction in cancer mortality. Several other studies of humans suggest that selenium status does play a role in protecting against the development of several cancers.[96–99] These studies suggest that selenium, through its function as an antioxidant, has a role in cancer prevention and that suboptimal selenium status is associated with increased risk of developing cancer. It has also been suggested that selenium may have a role in slowing some of the changes seen as part of the aging process, especially in the reduction in the levels of lipofuscin pigments and peroxidative damage to the cellular membranes and subcellular components.[100]

Biochemical roles of selenium are associated with 11 selenoproteins.[101] There are several glutathione peroxidase enzymes found in different tissues or subcellular locations. These enzymes use reducing equivalents from glutathione to catabolize hydroperoxides, thus providing protection from oxidant molecules. Three iodothyronine deiodinases are selenoproteins. These enzymes catalyze the deiodination of the thyroid hormones thyroxine and triiodothyronine and reverse triiodothyronine and thereby regulate the activity of the active hormone triiodothyronine. Thioredoxin reductase regenerates ascorbic acid from dehydroascorbic acid. Selenoprotein P has recently been shown to deliver selenium to the brain.[102] Selenophosphate synthetases are likely involved in the conversion of selenium to selenocysteine, the active form of selenium in enzymes. The function of the last of the selenoproteins, selenoprotein W, is unknown at present. The activity of all these enzymes and proteins decline in a selenium deficient state and the declines are likely responsible for the symptoms of the deficiency.

Dietary selenium intakes based on the Total Diet Study in the United States have been estimated at 87 μg/d.[103] Drinking water provides negligible amounts of selenium other than in those few areas in the United States that have high soil selenium concentrations.[104] Estimated Average Requirements (EAR) have recently been established as 45 μg Se/d for men and women 51 to older than 70 years and Recommended Dietary Allowances (RDA) at 55 μg/d for men and women in the same age ranges.[105] Data reporting selenium intakes and status in the elderly are quite limited. Selenium intakes of 77.6 ± 44.5 μg/d were reported for a population of elderly Canadian women, although 21% of women had intakes of less than 50 μg/d.[19] These values were similar to those reported for adults aged 60 years and older in the United States[106] and a bit lower than those reported by Lane et al.[107] At these levels of intake, most of the elderly subjects had serum selenium concentrations consistent with adequate status.[19]

Selenium deficiency is not likely to occur in free-living, healthy individuals in the United States. For individuals wishing to increase dietary selenium, richer sources of selenium include Brazil nuts, oysters and clams, pork, beef, lamb, chicken, breads, oatmeal, eggs, nuts and seeds; fruits and vegetables contain only small amounts.[13] Individuals choosing to take selenium supplements should be mindful of the Upper Limit (UL) established to be 400 μg selenium/day for both men and women 19 years and older.[105] Symptoms associated with selenium toxicity include nausea, vomiting, hair loss, nail changes, irritability, fatigue, and peripheral neuropathy.

ALUMINUM

Aluminum is not known to be required for any natural metabolic process and therefore is not thought to be an essential nutrient.[108] Although aluminum-containing compounds were considered to be essentially nonhazardous for many years, concerns about the potentially toxic effects of aluminum as it accumulates in tissues have been increasing during the last two decades.[109] These concerns have prompted examinations of dietary intakes of aluminum, responses to pharmaceutical-based exposure, and manifestations of toxicity.

Dietary exposure to aluminum includes that which is present naturally and that which comes from aluminum-containing food additives; other exposure arises from contact with aluminum used in food containers, cookware, utensils, and food wrapping. Most foods and beverages contain low concentrations of aluminum naturally, with the exception of tea, herbs, and spices.[110] Of the three factors affecting the aluminum content of foods, the aluminum-containing food additives have the greatest effects in increasing aluminum levels. For example, processed cheese contains 0.3 mg aluminum per gram, whereas cheddar cheese contains only 0.002 mg/g; white bread contains 0.003 mg/g, whereas baking powder biscuits contain 0.016 mg/g due to the inclusion of baking powder, which contains 2.3 mg/g.[111] The major sources of aluminum in daily diets are grain products with aluminum additives, processed cheese, tea, herbs, spices, and salt with aluminum additives. Little aluminum is contributed to the diet by meat, poultry, fish, fruit, vegetables, fats and oils, or sugar and sweeteners. A distribution of aluminum intakes among various food groups has been calculated for a mixed diet containing 2541 kcal (Table 6–4).

Aluminum can be transferred from aluminum food preparation equipment, particularly if the foods are acidic or exposure is prolonged. For example, the aluminum in tomato sauce increased from 0.1 mg/kg to 57.1 mg/kg after the sauce was cooked in an aluminum pan.[112] This route is not, however, a major or consistent source of dietary aluminum. Total intakes of aluminum are variable, primarily depending on the inclusion of aluminum-containing food additives in the diet, but they have been estimated to be about 9 mg/d for adult women and 12 to 14 mg/d for adult men.[110] A recent study from France estimated aluminum intake to be 2 mg/d.[113] Intakes in this range are not thought to pose a health risk.

The quantities of aluminum consumed in food and beverages are small when compared with

Table 6–4 Aluminum Intake in a Diet of 2541 kcal/day

Foods	Aluminum Intake	
	Mg/d	%
Milk, yogurt, cheese	3.69	27.0
Meat, poultry, fish	0.41	3.0
Grains and grain products	4.98	36.5
Vegetables	0.52	3.8
Fruits	0.02	0.1
Mixed dishes	0.69	5.1
Fats, sweets, condiments	0.23	1.7
Beverages	0.83	6.1
Desserts	2.26	16.1
Nuts and seeds	0.02	0.1
Total	13.65	100.0

Source: Values from *Journal of American Dietetic Association* (1989;89:659–664).

those that can be ingested in pharmaceutical products such as antacids, buffered analgesics, antidiarrheal medications, and certain antiulcer drugs. Lione[114] estimated that daily intakes of aluminum could be 800 to 5000 mg from antacids and 126 to 728 mg from buffered analgesics. Such high levels of intake may have adverse consequences, particularly when there is a preexisting medical condition such as uremia.

Consequences of aluminum toxicity have been reported for several clinical conditions. Uremic patients undergoing dialysis where the dialysis fluid was contaminated with aluminum and patients receiving aluminum-containing parenteral fluids have manifested aluminum toxicity.[115] Clinical signs of toxicity include osteodystrophy, encephalopathy, and anemia.[116] The osteodystrophy may be expressed as bone pain and an increased incidence of fractures. The symptoms of encephalopathy include dementia, speech difficulties, and motor abnormalities. The anemia is of the normochromic, normocytic type, most likely related to disturbances in heme synthesis and porphyrin metabolism. These symptoms are sometimes seen in uremic patients, especially children, who have not been exposed to aluminum-containing dialysis or intravenous fluids; the source of aluminum in these cases appears to be the aluminum-containing binder used to treat hyperphosphatemia.[117]

Most interest in aluminum toxicity as it relates to elderly people who are not on dialysis or parenteral feeding regimens is related to the putative connection between deposition of aluminum in the brain and the development of various senile dementias, including Alzheimer's disease.[118,119] There is no question that aluminum in a potent neurotoxin, both in experimental animals and in humans.[120] Reports of elevated aluminum in the brains of individuals with Alzheimer's disease and with amyotrophic lateral sclerosis (Lou Gehrig's disease) or with Parkinsonism dementia associated with regions that also contain neurofibrillary tangles have supported this putative association.[121] The hypothesis that aluminum is part of the etiology of various dementias remains controversial, however.[119] It is clear, however, that if aluminum does gain access to the central nervous system, it acts as a potent neurotoxin.[122]

Under normal physiological conditions, relatively little aluminum is absorbed by the gastrointestinal system after oral exposure, and, of the portion absorbed, only a much smaller amount is deposited in the central nervous system. It is therefore unlikely that under normal conditions, these natural barriers keep virtually all of the aluminum out of the central nervous system. However, Perl[121] has suggested that under conditions of advancing age, genetic predisposition, or possibly viral damage, these barriers may become impaired, allowing the element to gain access to the central nervous system, possibly inducing the neurofibrillary tangles. Supporting this hypothesis are reports that aluminum tends to accumulate in the brain with aging.[123,124] The body's ability to remove the aluminum that has been absorbed may be diminished in the older individual. The decline in renal function observed with aging[125] and the fact that the major excretory route of aluminum absorbed into the body is via the urine[126] suggests that aging might

promote accumulation of aluminum in the body. There has been very little research on the effects of aging on aluminum metabolism. Much of the concern about the potential hazards of aluminum exposure for older individuals remains unresolved.

MOLYBDENUM

The essentiality of molybdenum has been established for a number of species, including humans.[127] Molybdenum participates in a number of enzymatic reactions as an essential cofactor termed molybdopterin.[128] These enzymes are involved in the catabolism of sulfur amino acids and heterocyclic compounds, including purines and pyrimidines.[127] The importance of the molybdoenzymes, sulfite oxidase, is clearly shown by studies of individuals with an inborn error of metabolism involving this enzyme. Symptoms include severe brain damage, mental retardation, dislocation of the ocular lens, and eventual death.[129] In a report of a nutritional deficiency of molybdenum in a patient undergoing total parenteral nutrition,[130] clinical symptoms included mental disturbances that progressed to coma, tachycardia, tachypnea, and night blindness; symptoms were reversed by supplementation with 300 μg of ammonium molybdate/d. Changes were attributed to a loss of sulfite oxidase activity.

Molybdenum is widely distributed in soils, plants, and animal tissues. The richest sources of the element include legumes, cereal grains (and hence bread and baked products), leafy vegetables, milk, liver, and kidney. Fruits, stem and root vegetables, and muscle meats are among the poorest sources.[128] Data from the Total Diet Study[131] indicate that dietary intakes for women were 76 μg/d and for men 109 μg/d. These values are similar to those reported by Tsongas and colleagues;[132] older individuals had lower intakes, for example, 160 μg for men 65 to 74 years and 140 μg aged 75 years and older and 120 μg for women 65 years and older. These values for intake may be compared with the recently established Recommended Dietary Allowances of 34 μg for women and 45 μg for men.[8] Obviously, average intakes for both men and women are well able to meet the RDA for this essential nutrient. The use of molybdenum supplements is not advised. A Tolerable Upper Intake Level of 2 mg/d has been established.[8]

MANGANESE

Manganese is one of the essential trace minerals. Among various animal species, major manifestations of manganese deficiency include impaired growth, skeletal abnormalities, disturbed or depressed reproductive function, ataxia of the newborn, and defects in lipid and carbohydrate metabolism.[133] For a single human subject inadvertently rendered manganese deficient during an experimental study, the manifestations included hypocholesterolemia, weight loss, transient dermatitis, occasional nausea and vomiting, changes in hair and beard color, and slow growth of beard and hair.[134] In a manganese depletion study, 5 of 7 subjects developed a finely scaling, minimally erythematous rash that disappeared on repletion.[135] The authors also reported that there were changes in plasma calcium, phosphorus, and alkaline phosphatase concentrations consistent with alterations in bone remodeling; such changes have been proposed by Strause and colleagues[136] as a manifestation of manganese deficiency.

Manganese can function in the body both as an enzyme activator and as a constituent of metalloenzymes.[137] Arginase, the cytosolic enzyme responsible for urea synthesis; pyruvate carboxylase, a key enzyme in gluconeogenesis required for the synthesis of oxaloacetate from pyruvate; glutamine synthetase used for the synthesis of the amino acid glutamine; and manganese superoxide dismutase, which catalyzes the disproportionation of superoxide to hydrogen peroxide and oxygen, are all manganese metalloenzymes. Defects in carbohydrate metabolism and increased lipid peroxidation, especially after exposure to hyperbaric oxygen, ozone, or ethanol, may

be related to loss of enzymatic activity subsequent to development of manganese deficiency. Manganese can also activate various enzymes. Of particular importance is the manganese-specific activation of glycosyl transferases.[138] It is believed that the skeletal deformities and neonatal ataxia seen in manganese deficiency are due to impairment of cartilage synthesis as a result of decreased activity of the glycosyl transferases.

Common foods in human diets are highly variable in manganese concentrations. In general, the highest manganese levels occur in wheat germ, nuts and seeds, oatmeal, oysters, dark molasses, brown rice, sweet potatoes, chocolate, and brewed tea; dairy products, meat, fish, and poultry are poor sources.[13] Based on the Total Diet Study, grain products contributed 37% of dietary manganese; tea (a particularly rich source) and vegetables contributed 20% and 18%, respectively.[7] Average daily intakes of manganese for men and women 60 to 65 years of age were 2.60 mg and 2.66 mg/d, respectively.[62] Only a few studies have evaluated the manganese intake of older persons. A study of Canadian women by Gibson and colleagues[63] revealed that vegetarians (mean age 69 years) had greater dietary intakes than did nonvegetarian women (mean age 60 years) at 4.4 vs. 2.6 mg/d. In a subsequent study of Canadian women ranging in age from 58 to 89 years with a mean age of 66 years, the average intake was 3.8 mg/d.[139] These values for intakes may be compared with the recently revised Adequate Intake (AI) values of 1.8 mg for women and 2.3 mg for men.[8]

It should be recognized that a number of dietary components may limit manganese absorption or decrease manganese retention. Among these are fiber and phytate,[140,141] calcium,[142] iron,[143] and sugar.[144] Unrefined cereals, nuts, leafy vegetables, and tea are rich in manganese, while refined grains, meats (other than organ meats), and dairy products contain small amounts of this essential trace mineral. If elderly people shift dietary consumption toward those components less rich in manganese and if other dietary components limit absorption, adequacy of manganese status may be compromised. Decisions to include a manganese supplement should be informed by the Upper Limit (UL) of 11 mg/d.[8] Total dietary intakes at this level were not shown to be associated with adverse neurological or other outcomes.[145] Higher intakes may be associated with central nervous system pathology, similar to that seen in Parkinson's disease.[146] Individuals with chronic liver disease, especially involving impaired bile production and release, are at particular risk of developing toxicity.[147]

NICKEL

The essentiality of nickel for humans has not been established, although it is recognized as an essential nutrient for a number of other species.[127] The most prominent and consistent signs of the deficiency in rats and goats include depressed growth, reproductive performance, and plasma glucose and alterations in the distribution of other elements in the body. There is no firmly established biologic function for nickel in humans or animals, but it is thought that nickel functions as a cofactor or structural component in specific metalloenzymes as is the case for enzymes from a number of plants and microorganisms.[127]

There is no evidence for nickel deficiency in humans and intakes are therefore thought to be more than adequate to meet demands for this nutrient. Requirements are thought to be very low and may be met by the diets consumed or, in some cases, even by environmental pollution with nickel-containing dust.[148] Foods that contain generally high concentrations of nickel (more than 0.3 μg/g) include nuts, leguminous seeds, shellfish, cacao products, and hydrogenated shortenings; fish, milk, and eggs are generally low in nickel concentration (less than 0.1 μg/g).[149] Estimates of intakes of nickel in conventional diets are 150 to 700 μg/d.[149] The use of nickel supplements is not advisable. Oral nickel, in not particularly high doses, can adversely affect human health. For sensitive individuals, an oral dose of as little as 0.6 mg has been shown to produce adverse effects.[150]

CONCLUSION

It is clear that we do not know enough about the requirements for various trace minerals, particularly about the needs of older individuals. Many of the physiological changes that accompany aging probably interfere with optimal absorption, utilization, or retention of these minerals. Changes in dietary practices, both the decrease in food consumption that typically accompanies aging and changes in dietary choices, can be expected to adversely affect the trace mineral adequacy of the diet. When these changes are coupled with the effects of various chronic and acute disease processes and the medications used to treat these conditions, the potential for deficiency states is increased substantially. Evidence has been presented to indicate that the adequacies or status of zinc, copper, chromium, and manganese are of greatest concern. Intakes of selenium, molybdenum, and nickel are less likely to be deficient in other than unusual circumstances. Aluminum is of concern only as a toxic mineral; minimization of exposure is appropriate. It is clear that most of the trace minerals discussed are essential for normal health and well-being and it is important that optimal status be maintained. The theory that some of the deleterious effects of aging can be related to deficiencies in one or more of the essential nutrients remains to be proven.

REFERENCES

1. Timiras, PS. *Physiological Basis of Geriatrics*. New York, NY: Macmillan Publishing Co; 1988.
2. Mertz, W. Trace elements and the needs of the elderly. In: Hutchinson M, Munro H, eds. *Nutrition and Aging*. Orlando, FL: Academic Press, Inc; 1986.
3. Solomons, N. Biological availability of zinc in humans. *Am J Clin Nutr* 1982;35:1046–1075.
4. Smiciklas-Wright, H. Aging. In: Brown, M, ed. *Present Knowledge in Nutrition*. 6th ed. Washington, DC: International Life Sciences Institute-Nutrition Foundation; 1990.
5. Cousins R. Zinc. In: Filer LJ, Ziegler EE, eds. *Present Knowledge in Nutrition*. 7th ed. Washington, DC:

International Life Sciences Institute-Nutrition Foundation; 1996.

6. King, JC, Keen CL. Zinc. In: Shils ME, Olson JA, Shike M., Ross AC, eds. *Modern Nutrition in Health and Disease*. 9th ed. Baltimore, MD: Williams and Wilkins; 1999.

7. Pennington J, Young B. Total Diet Study nutritional elements, 1982–1989. *J Am Diet Assoc* 1991;91:179–183.

8. Food and Nutrition Board, Institute of Medicine. *Dietary Reference Intakes for Vitamin A, Vitamin K, Arsenic, Boron, Chromium, Copper, Iodine, Iron, Manganese, Molybdenum, Nickel, Silicon, Vanadium, and Zinc (2000)*. Washington, DC: National Academies Press; 2001.

9. Greger J. Trace minerals. In: Chen, L, ed. *Nutritional Aspects of Aging*. Boca Raton, FL: CRC Press; 1986.

10. Sandstead H, Hendrikson L, Greger J, et al. Zinc nutriture in the elderly in relation to taste acuity, immune response, and wound healing. *Am J Clin Nutr* 1982;36:1046–1059.

11. Fosmire G, Manuel P, Smiciklas-Wright H. Dietary intakes and zinc status of an elderly rural population. *J Nutr Elderly* 1984;4:19–30.

12. Pennington J. Intakes of minerals from diets and foods: is there a need for concern? *J Nutr* 1996;126: 2304S–2308S.

13. Hands E. *Nutrients in Foods*. Baltimore, MD: Lippincott, Williams and Wilkins; 2000.

14. Lonnerdal B. Dietary factors influencing zinc absorption. *J Nutr* 2000;130:1378S–1383S.

15. August D, Janghorbani M, Young V. Determination of zinc and copper absorption at three dietary Zn-Cu ratios by using stable isotope methods in young adult and elderly subjects. *Am J Clin Nutr* 1989;50:1457–1463.

16. Bales C, Steinman L, Freeland-Graves J, et al. The effect of age on plasma zinc, uptake, and taste acuity. *Am J Clin Nutr* 1986;44:664–669.

17. Couzy F, Kastenmayer P, Mansourian R, et al. Zinc absorption in healthy elderly humans and the effect of diet. *Am J Clin Nutr* 1993;58:690–694.

18. Turnlund J, Durkin N, Costa F, Margen S. Stable isotope studies of zinc absorption and retention in young and elderly men. *J Nutr* 1986;116:1239–1247.

19. Gibson R, Martinez O, MacDonald A. The zinc, copper, and selenium status of a selected sample of Canadian elderly women. *J Gerontol* 1985;40:296–302.

20. Bunker V, Hinks L, Lawson M, et al. Assessment of zinc and copper status of healthy elderly people using metabolic balance studies and measurement of leukocyte zinc concentrations. *Am J Clin Nutr* 1984;40: 1096–1102.

21. Bunker V, Hinks L, Stansfield M, et al. Metabolic balance studies for zinc and copper in housebound elderly people and the relationship between zinc balance and leukocyte zinc concentrations. *Am J Clin Nutr* 1987;46: 353–359.

22. Patterson P, Lee E, Christensen D, et al. Zinc levels of hospitalized elderly. *J Am Diet Assoc* 1985;85:186–191.

23. Sahyoun N, Otradovic C, Hartz S, et al. Dietary intakes and biochemical indicators of nutritional status in an elderly, institutionalized population. *Am J Clin Nutr* 1988;47:524–533.

24. Bogden J, Olesky I, Munves E, et al. Zinc and immunocompetence in the elderly: baseline data on zinc nutriture and immunity in unsupplemented subjects. *Am J Clin Nutr* 1987;46:101–109.

25. Fulwood R, Johnson C, Bryner I, et al. *Hematological and Nutritional Biochemistry Reference Data for Persons 6 Months–74 Years of Age: United States 1976–1980*. Washington, DC: Public Health Service; 1982. US Dept of Health and Human Services publication PHS 83-1628.

26. Swanson C, Mansourian R, Dirren H, Rapin C. Zinc status of healthy elderly adults: Response to supplementation. *Am J Clin Nutr* 1988;48:343–349.

27. Payette H, Gray-Donaldson K. Dietary intake and biochemical indices of nutritional status in an elderly population, with estimates of the precision of the 7-d food record. *Am J Clin Nutr* 1991;54:478–488.

28. Bales C, DiSilvestro R, Currie K, et al. Marginal zinc deficiency in older adults: responsiveness of zinc status indicators. *J Am Coll Nutr* 1994;13:455–462.

29. Prasad A, Fitzgerald J, Hess J, et al. Zinc deficiency in elderly patients. *Nutrition* 1993;12:344–348.

30. Prasad A. Clinical spectrum and diagnostic aspects of zinc deficiency. In: Prasad A, ed. *Essential and Toxic Trace Elements in Human Health and Disease*. New York, NY: Alan R Liss, Inc; 1988.

31. Weiffenbach I, Baum B, Burghauser R. Taste thresholds: quality specific variation with human aging. *J Gerontol* 1982;37:372–377.

32. Henkin R, Patten B, Re P, et al. Syndrome of acute zinc loss. *Arch Neurol* 1974;32:745–751.

33. Greger J, Geissler A. Effect of zinc supplementation on taste acuity of the elderly. *Am J Clin Nutr* 1978;31: 633–637.

34. Hutton C, Hayes-Davis R. Assessment of the zinc nutritional status of selected elderly subjects. *J Am Diet Assoc* 1983;82:148–153.

35. Greger J. Dietary intake and nutritional status in regard to zinc of institutionalized aged. *J Gerontol* 1977;32: 549–553.

36. Prasad A, Fitzgerald J, Hess J, et al. Zinc deficiency in elderly patients. *Nutrition* 1993;9:218–224.

37. Atkin-Thor E, Goddard B, O'Nion J, et al. Hypogeusia and zinc depletion in chronic dialysis patients. *Am J Clin Nutr* 1978;31:1948–1951.

38. Mahajan S, Prasad A, Lambujon J, et al. Improvement of uremic hypogeusia by zinc: a double blind study. *Am J Clin Nut* 1980;33:1517–1521.

39. Wacker W. Biochemistry of zinc: role in wound healing. In: Hambidge K, Nichols B, eds. *Zinc and Copper in Clinical Medicine*. New York, NY: Spectrum Publications; 1978.

40. Halbook T, Hedelin H. Zinc metabolism and surgical trauma. *Br J Surg* 1977;64:271–273.

41. Weismann K, Wanscher B, Krakaver R. Oral zinc therapy in geriatric patients with selected skin manifestations and a low plasma zinc level. *Acta Dermatol* (Stockholm) 1978;58:157.

42. Carder I. The effect of aging on susceptibility to infection. *Rev Infect Dis* 1980;2:801–810.

43. Fernandes G, West A, Good R. Nutrition, immunity and cancer: a review. III. Effects of diet on the disease of aging. *Clin Bio* 1979;9:91–106.

44. Allen J, Kay N, McClain C. Severe zinc deficiency in humans: association with a reversible T-lymphocyte dysfunction. *Ann Intern Med* 1981;95:154–157.

45. Oleski J, Westphal M, Shore S, et al. Zinc therapy of depressed cellular immunity in acrodermatitis enteropathica. *Am J Dis Child* 1979;133:915–918.

46. Pekarek R, Sandstead H, Jacob R, et al. Abnormal cellular immune responses during acquired zinc deficiency. *Am J Clin Nutr* 1979;32:1466–1471.

47. Duchateau J, Delepresse G, Vrigens R, et al. Beneficial effects of oral zinc supplementation on the immune response of old people. *Am J Med* 1981;70:1001–1004.

48. Wagner P, Jernigan J, Bailey L, et al. Zinc nutriture and cell-mediated immunity in the aged. *Int J Vitam Nutr Res* 1983;53:94–101.

49. Bogden J, Bendich A, Kemp F, et al. Daily micronutrient supplements enhance delayed-type hypersensitivity skin test responses in older people. *Am J Clin Nutr* 1994;60:437–447.

50. Doukaiba N, Flament C, Archer S, et al. A physiological amount of zinc supplementation: effects on nutritional, lipid, and thymic status in an elderly population. *Am J Clin Nutr* 1993;57:566–572.

51. Bogden J. Influence of zinc on immunity in the elderly. *J Nutr Health Aging* 2004;8:48–54.

52. Fosmire G. Zinc toxicity. *Am J Clin Nutr* 1990;51: 225–227.

53. Pennington J. *Bowes and Church's Food Values of Portions Commonly Used*. 17th ed. Philadelphia, PA: JB Lippincott; 1998.

54. Hart E, Steenbock H, Waddell J, et al. Iron in nutrition. VII: copper as a supplement to iron for hemoglobin building in the rat. *J Biol Chem* 1928;77:797–812.

55. Harris E. Copper. In: O'Dell B, Sunde R, eds. *Handbook of Nutritionally Essential Mineral Elements*. New York, NY: Marcel Dekker; 1997.

56. Linder M. Copper. In: Ziegler E, Filer L Jr, eds. *Present Knowledge in Nutrition*. 7th ed. Washington, DC: ILSI Press; 1996.

57. Turnlund J, Costa F, Margen S. Zinc, copper, and iron balance in elderly men. *Am J Clin Nutr* 1981;34:2642–2647.

58. Turnlund J, Reager R, Costa F. Iron and copper absorption in young and elderly men. *Nutr Res* 1988;8:333–343.

59. Burke D, DeMicco F, Taper L, et al. Copper and zinc utilization in elderly adults. *J Gerontol* 1981;36:558–563.

60. Mertz W. Use and misuse of balance studies. *J Nutr* 1987;117:1811–1813.

61. Pennington J, Schoen S, Salmon G, et al. Composition of core foods of the US food supply, 1982–1991. III. Copper, manganese, selenium, and iodine. *J Food Comp Anal* 1995;8:171–217.

62. Pennington J. Current dietary intakes of trace elements and minerals. In: Bogden J, Klevay L, eds. *Nutrition of the Essential Trace Elements and Minerals* Trenton, NJ: Humana Press, 2000.

63. Gibson R, Anderson B, Sabry J. The trace metal status of a group of post-menopausal vegetarians. *J Am Dietet Assoc* 1983;82:246–250.

64. Sandstead H. Copper bioavailability and requirements. *Am J Clin Nutr* 1982;35:809–814.

65. Turnlund J. Human whole-body copper metabolism. *Am J Clin Nutr* 1998;67:960S–964S.

66. Danks D. Copper deficiency in humans. *Annu Rev Nutr* 1988;8:235–257.

67. Klevay L, Madeiros D. Deliberations and evaluations of the approaches, end points and paradigms for dietary recommendations about copper. *J Nutr* 1996;124: 2419S–2426S.

68. Milne D. Assessment of copper nutritional status. *Clin Chem* 1994;40:1479–1484.

69. Schwarz K, Mertz W. Chromium (III) and the glucose tolerance factor. *Arch Biochem Biophys* 1959;85: 292–295.

70. Stoecker B. Chromium. In: Shils M, Olson J, Shike M, Ross AC, eds. *Modern Nutrition in Health and Disease*. 9th ed. Baltimore, MD: Williams and Wilkins; 1999.

71. Vincent J. Mechanism of chromium action: low molecular weight chromium-binding substance. *J Am Coll Nutr* 1999;18:6–12.

72. Stoecker B. Chromium. In: Ziegler E, Filer L Jr, eds. *Present Knowledge in Nutrition*. 7th ed. Washington, DC: ILSI Press; 1996.

73. Anderson R. Chromium requirements and needs of the elderly. In: Watson R, ed. *Handbook of Nutrition in the Aged*. Boca Raton, FL: CRC Press; 1985.

74. Anderson R, Bryden N, Polansky M. Dietary chromium intake. Freely chosen diets, institutional diets, and individual foods. *Biol Trace Elem Res* 1992;32:117–121.

75. Briefel R, McDowell M, Alaimo K, et al. Total energy intake of US populations: the third national health and nutrition examination survey, 1988–1991. *Am J Clin Nutr* 1995;62:1072S–1080S.

76. Anderson R, Kozlovsky A. Chromium intake, absorption and excretion of subjects consuming self-selected diets. *Am J Clin Nutr* 1985;41:1177–1183.

77. Bunker V, Lawson M, Delves H, et al. The uptake and excretion of chromium by the elderly. *Am J Clin Nutr* 1984;39:797–802.

78. Seaborn C, Stoecker B. Effects of antacid or ascorbic acid on tissue accumulation and urinary excretion of ^{51}chromium. *Nutr Res* 1990;10:1401–1407.

79. Kozlovsky A, Moser P, Reiser S, et al. Effects of diets high in simple sugars on urinary chromium losses. *Metabolism* 1986;35:515–518.

80. Davis M, Seaborn C, Stoecker B. Effects of over-the-counter drugs on ^{51}chromium retention and urinary excretion in rats. *Nutr Res* 1995;15:201–210.

81. Kamath S, Stoecker B, Davis-Whitenack ML, et al. Absorption, retention, and urinary excretion of chromium-51 in rats pretreated with indomethacin and dosed with dimethylprostaglandin E_2, misoprostol, or prostacyclin. *J Nutr* 1997;127:478–482.

82. Brown R, Forloines-Lynn S, Cross R, Heizer W. Chromium deficiency after long-term parenteral nutrition. *Dig Dis Sci* 1986;31:661–664.

83. Offenbacher E, Pi-Sunyer F. Chromium in human nutrition. *Annu Rev Nutr* 1980;8:543–563.

84. Urberg M, Zemel M. Evidence for synergism between chromium and nicotinic acid in the control of glucose tolerance in humans. *Metabolism* 1987;36:896–899.

85. Martinez O, MacDonald A, Gibson R, et al. Dietary chromium and effect of chromium supplementation on glucose tolerance of elderly Canadian women. *Nutr Res* 1985;5:609–620.

86. Abraham A, Brooks B, Eylath U. The effect of chromium supplementation on serum glucose and lipids in patients with and without non-insulin dependent diabetes. *Metabolism* 1992;41:768–771.

87. Anderson R, Cheng N, Bryden N, et al. Elevated intakes of supplemental chromium improve glucose and insulin variables in individuals with type II diabetes. *Diabetes* 1997;46:1786–1791.

88. Harris M, Flegal K, Cowie C, et al. Prevalence of diabetes, impaired fasting glucose, and impaired glucose tolerance in US adults. *Diabetes Care* 1998;21:518–524.

89. Davies S, McLaren H, Hunisett A, Howard M. Age-related decreases in chromium levels in 51,665 hair, sweat, and serum samples from 40, 872 patients— implications for the prevention of cardiovascular disease and type II diabetes mellitus. *Metabolism* 1997;46:469–473.

90. Combs G Jr, Levander O, Spallholz J, et al., eds. *Selenium in Biology and Medicine, Parts A and B.* New York, NY: Van Nostrand Reinhold Co; 1987.

91. McCoy K, Weswig P. Some selenium responses in the rat not related to vitamin E. *Euro J Nutr* 1969;98:383–389.

92. Ge K, Xue A, Bai J, Wang S. Keshan disease—an endemic cardiomyopathy in China. *Virchows Arch Pathol Anat Histopathol* 1983;401:1–15.

93. Moreno-Reyes R, Mathieu F, Boelaert M, et al. Selenium and iodine supplementation of rural Tibetan children affected by Kashin-Beck osteoarthropathy. *Am J Clin Nutr* 2003;78:137–144.

94. Milner J. The effects of selenium on virally induced and transplantable tumor models. *Fed Proc* 1985;44:2568–2572.

95. Clark L, Combs G Jr, Turnbull B, et al. Effects of selenium supplementation for cancer prevention in patients with carcinoma of the skin. *JAMA* 1996;276:1957–1963.

96. Schrauzer G, White D, Schneider C. Cancer mortality correlation studies. III. Statistical associations with dietary selenium intakes. *Bioinorg Chem* 1977;7:23–24.

97. Vogt T, Ziegler R, Graubard B, et al. Serum selenium and risk of prostate cancer in U.S. blacks and whites. *Int J Cancer* 2003;103:664–670.

98. Knekt P, Marniemi J, Teppo L, et al. Is low selenium status a risk factor for lung cancer? *Am J Epidemiol* 1998;148:975–982.

99. Clark L, Dalkin B, Krongrad A, et al. Decreased incidence of prostate cancer with selenium supplementation: results of a double-blind cancer prevention trial. *Br J Urol* 1998;81:730–734.

100. Yuncie A, Hsu I. Role of selenium in aging. In: Combs G Jr, Levander O, Spallholz J, et al., eds. *Selenium in Biology and Medicine, Parts A and B.* New York, NY: Van Nostrand Reinhold Co.; 1987.

101. Burk R, Levander O. Selenium. In: Shils M, Olson J, Shike M, Ross A, eds. *Modern Nutrition in Health and Disease.* 9th ed. Baltimore, MD: Williams and Wilkins; 1999.

102. Hill K, Zhou J, McMahan W, et al. Neurological dysfunction occurs in mice with targeted depletion of the selenoprotein P gene. *J Nutr* 2004;134:157–161.

103. Pennington J, Schoen S. Total Diet Study: estimated dietary intakes of nutritional elements, 1982–1991. *Int J Vitam Nutr Res* 1996;66:350–362.

104. NRC (National Research Council). *Selenium.* Washington, DC: National Academy of Sciences; 1976.

105. Food and Nutrition Board, Institute of Medicine. *Dietary Reference Intakes for Vitamin C, Vitamin E, Selenium, and Carotenoids.* Washington, DC: National Academies Press; 2000.

106. Thimaya S, Ganapathy S. Selenium in human hair in relation to age, diet, pathological condition, and serum levels. *Sci Total Environ* 1982;24:41–49.

107. Lane A, Warran D, Taylor B, et al. Blood selenium and glutathione peroxidase levels and dietary selenium of free-living and institutionalized elderly subjects. *Proc Soc Exp Biol Med* 1983;173:87–95.

108. Underwood E. *Trace Elements in Human and Animal Nutrition.* 4th ed. New York, NY: Academic Press; 1977.

109. Greger J. Aluminum and tin. *World Rev Nutr Diet* 1987; 54:255–285.

110. Pennington J. Aluminum content of foods and diets. *Food Addit Contam* 1988;5:161–232.

111. Greger J. Dietary and other sources of aluminum intake. In: Chadwick D, Whelan J, eds. *Aluminum in Biology and Medicine* Chichester, England: Wiley and Sons, Ltd; 1992.

112. Greger J. Aluminum in the diet and mineral metabolism. In: Sigel H, ed. *Metal Ions in Biological Systems.* New York, NY: Marcel Dekker; 1988.

113. Noel L, Leblanc J, Guerin T. Determination of several elements in duplicate meals from catering establishments using closed vessel microwave digestion with inductively coupled plasma mass spectrometry detection: estimation of daily dietary intake. *Food Addit Contam* 2003;20:44–56.

114. Lione A. Aluminum intake from non-prescription drugs and sucralfate. *Gen Pharmacol* 1985;16:223–228.

115. Greger J. Potential for trace mineral deficiencies and toxicities in the elderly. In: Bales C, ed. *Mineral Homeostasis in the Elderly* New York, NY: Alan R Liss, Inc;1989.

116. Wills M, Savory J. Aluminum toxicity and chronic renal failure. In: Sigel H, ed. *Metal Ions in Biological Systems* New York, NY: Marcel Dekker;1988.

117. Committee on Nutrition. Aluminum toxicity in infants and children. *Pediatrics* 1986;78:1150–1154.

118. Chadwick D, Whelan J, eds. *Aluminum in Biology and Medicine.* Chichester, England: Wiley and Sons, Ltd; 1992.

119. Flaten T. Aluminum as a risk factor in Alzheimer's disease, with emphasis on drinking water. *Brain Res Bull* 2001;55:187–196.

120. Flaten T, Alfrey A, Birchall J, et al. Status and future concerns of clinical and environmental aluminum toxicology. *J Toxicol Environ Healt* 1996;12:152–167.

121. Perl D. Aluminum and Alzheimer's disease, methodologic approaches. In: Sigel H, ed. *Metal Ions in Biological Systems.* New York, NY: Marcel Dekker; 1988.

122. Kruck R, McLachlan D. Mechanisms of aluminum neurotoxicity: relevance to human disease. In: Sigel H, ed. *Metal Ions in Biological Systems.* New York, NY: Marcel Dekker; 1988.

123. McDermott J, Smith I, Iqbal K, et al. Brain aluminum in aging and Alzheimer disease. *Neurology* 1979;29: 809–814.

124. Markesbery W, Ehmann W, Hosain T, et al. Instrumental neutron analysis of brain aluminum in Alzheimer's disease and aging. *Ann Neurol* 1981;10:511–516.

125. Epstein M. Effects of aging on the kidney. *Fed Proc* 1979;38:168–171.

126. Ganrot P. Metabolism and possible health effects of aluminum. *Environ Health Perspect* 1986;65:363–441.

127. Nielsen F. Ultratrace minerals. In: Shils M, Olson R, Shike M, Ross A, eds. *Modern Nutrition in Health and Disease.* Baltimore, MD: Williams and Wilkins; 1999.

128. Rajagopalan K. Molybdenum: an essential trace element in human nutrition. *Annu Rev Nutr* 1988;8:401–427.

129. Johnson J. Molybdenum. In: O'Dell B, Sunde R. eds. *Handbook of Nutritionally Essential Mineral Elements.* New York, NY: Marcel Dekker; 1997.

130. Abumrad N, Schneider A, Steel D, et al. Amino acid intolerance during prolonged total parenteral nutrition reversed by molybdate therapy. *Am J Clin Nutr* 1981;34: 2551–2559.

131. Pennington J, Jones J. Molybdenum, nickel, cobalt, vanadium, and strontium in total diets. *J Am Diet Assoc* 1987;87:1644–1650.

132. Tsongas T, Meglen R, Walravens P, et al. Molybdenum in the diet: an estimate of average daily intake in the United States. *Am J Clin Nutr* 1980;33:1103–1107.

133. Keen C, Zeidenberg-Cherr S. Manganese. In: Ziegler E, Filer L Jr, eds. *Present Knowledge in Nutrition,* 7th ed. Washington, DC: ILSI Press; 1996.

134. Doisy E. Micronutrient controls on biosynthesis of clotting proteins and cholesterol. In: Hemphill D, ed. *Trace Substances in Environmental Health.* Vol 6. Columbia, MO: University of Missouri Press; 1972.

135. Friedman B, Freeland-Graves J, Bales C, et al. Manganese balance and clinical observations in young men fed a manganese-deficient diet. *J Nutr* 1987;117:133–143.

136. Strause L, Saltman P, Smith K, et al. Spinal bone loss in postmenopausal women supplemented with calcium and trace minerals. *J Nutr* 1994;124:1060–1064.

137. Wedler F. Biochemical and nutritional roles of manganese: an overview. In: Klimis-Tavantis D, ed. *Manganese in Health and Disease.* Boca Raton, FL: CRC Press; 1994.

138. Leach R Jr. Biochemical role of manganese. In: Hoeckstra W, Suttie J, Ganther J, et al., eds. *Trace Element Metabolism in Animals-2.* Baltimore, MD: University Park Press; 1974.

139. Gibson R, MacDonald A, Martinez O. Dietary chromium and manganese intakes of a selected sample of Canadian elderly women. *Hum Nutr Appl Nutr* 1985; 39A:43–52.

140. Schwartz R, Apgar B, Wien D. Apparent absorption and retention of Ca, Cu, Mg, Mn, and Zn from a diet containing bran. *Am J Clin Nutr* 1986;43:444–455.

141. Bales C, Freeland-Graves J, Lin P-H, et al. Plasma uptake of manganese: response to dose and dietary factors. In: Kies C, ed. *Nutritional Bioavailability of Manganese.* Washington, DC: American Chemical Society; 1987.

142. Lin P-H, Freeland-Graves J. Effects of simultaneous ingestion of calcium and manganese in humans. In: Bales C, ed. *Mineral Homeostasis in the Elderly.* New York, NY: Alan R. Liss, Inc;1989.

143. Dougherty V, Freeland-Graves J, Behmardi F, et al. Interactions of iron (Fe) and manganese in males fed varying levels of dietary manganese. *Fed Proc* 1987; 46:914.

144. Halfrisch J, Powell A, Carafelli C, et al. Mineral balances of men and women consuming high fiber diets with complex or simple carbohydrates. *J Nutr* 1987; 117:48–55.

145. Greger J. Nutrition vs. toxicology of manganese in humans: evaluation of potential biomarkers. *Neurotoxicology* 1999;20:205–212.

146. Barceloux D. Manganese. *J Toxicol Clin Toxicol* 1999; 37:293–307.

147. Hauser R, Zesiewicz T, Rosemurgy A, et al. Manganese intoxication and chronic liver failure. *Ann Neurol* 1994; 36:871–875.

148. Nieboer E, Tom R, Sanford W. Nickel metabolism in man and animals. In: Sigel H, ed. *Metal Ions in Biological Systems.* New York, NY: Marcel Dekker; 1988.

149. Nielsen F. Nickel. In Mertz W, ed. *Trace Elements in Human and Animal Nutrition.* 5th ed. San Diego, CA: Academic Press; 1987.

150. Cronin E, Michiel A, Brown S. Oral challenge with nickel-sensitive women with hand eczema. In: Brown S, Sunderman F Jr, eds. *Nickel Toxicology* New York, NY: Academic Press; 1980.

CHAPTER 7

Smell, Taste, and Somatosensation in the Elderly

Valerie B. Duffy, PhD, RD and Audrey K. Chapo, MS, RD

Smell, taste and somatosensation (touch, pain, and temperature sensations) contribute to the sustenance of nutritional health and enjoyment of eating by receiving, processing, and reacting to information from the food world. The quality of this sensory information can influence whether or not we choose to ingest a food or beverage. The aroma of food may stimulate our appetite, even if we are not hungry. Once in the mouth, the taste, smell, and somatosensory sensations blend into a composite oral sensory experience. Foods and beverages that are appealing and diverse in oral sensations may stimulate us to eat more. Conversely, we may have less desire to eat if the quality of the oral sensory experience is less appealing, unpleasant, or void of diversity. Thus, our desire to eat, what we eat, and, ultimately, our nutritional status may be influenced by oral sensation. Understanding the physiological and psychological processes of oral sensation and how these processes may change with aging is important to promoting nutritional health and food enjoyment across aging.

First, there will be a review of oral sensory processes: the physiology of the sensory systems that respond to chemical stimuli and the psychology of our perceptual response. These processes will be reviewed within the context of normal taste, smell, and somatosensation, and within changes associated with aging and disease. There will then be a discussion of the potential impact of taste, smell, and oral somatosensory changes on nutrition in aged adults as well as methods to assess these changes.

ORAL SENSORY PROCESSING OF FOOD AND BEVERAGE FLAVORS

Taste, olfaction, and somatosensory systems respond to chemicals such as those that make up foods and beverages; thus, they are often referred to as chemosenses. The sense of smell allows detection, recognition, and exact identification of odors from the environment and from the oral cavity (Figure 7–1). For example, we use the sense of smell to detect the off-odors of souring milk, to recognize that cookies are flavored with rum extract, or to identify red Bordeaux from Pinot Noir. True taste (gustation) is the perception of saltiness, sweetness, sourness, and bitterness; support exists for umami, the meaty flavor of glutamate, as the fifth basic taste quality.[1] The somatosensory system is responsible for mouth feel/texture and chemesthetic qualities like irritation and astringency as well as temperature of foods and beverages.

Although functionally similar, taste, smell, and somatosensation are perceived through separate neurophysiologic systems that carry sensory information from the receptors to the brain. Mechanical stimuli (eg, fat) stimulate touch afferents in the oral cavity such as in fungiform

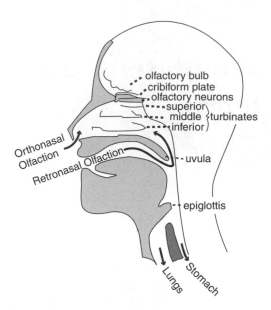

Figure 7–1 The Two Pathways For Olfactory Perception
Odors are perceived through the nostrils (ie, orthonasal olfaction) and through the oral cavity (ie, retronasal olfaction). Both pathways carry the odor to the olfactory neurons where the chemical signal (ie, odor) is transduced into a nervous signal.

papillae that may act as oral sensors to viscous substances that move across the tongue.[2] Chemical stimuli (tastants, odorants, and irritants) must reach and be adsorbed to a specific receptor cell. These receptor cells have long extensions (cilia or microvilli) that provide enough surface area for adsorption. The high level of specificity of the receptor cells makes it possible for the chemosensory system to detect and differentiate the slightest variances in chemical stimuli. Chemicals that only differ in chirality may generate radically different perceptions. For example, D- and L-isomers of carvone produce the distinctly different olfactory sensations of caraway and spearmint.[3] Although the human olfactory system has the potential to distinguish an unlimited number of chemicals, in reality the odorants that people differentiate number only in the hundreds.[4] Odorants must be volatile, hydrophobic, and have relatively low molecular weight. Similar chemical specificity also occurs

for taste; a number of compounds may produce a sweet taste, but the quality of each sweet taste may vary slightly. The receptor cells also transduce the chemical stimuli into electrical signals, transforming chemical signals into action potentials. Throughout life, receptor cells undergo a cycle of regulated neurogenesis, including birth, maturation, and programmed death throughout life. Most taste receptors live 10 days[5] and are continually replaced. Olfactory receptors live a varied life span based on regulation of neurogenesis by extrinsic (eg, exposure to microorganisms) and intrinsic (eg, growth factors) factors (see Mackay-Sim[6] for a review). There is great interest in understanding olfactory neurogenesis for possible tissue transplantation.

PHYSIOLOGY OF SMELL, TASTE, AND SOMATOSENSATION

Smell

Olfactory stimuli reach the olfactory system through two pathways: from the environment through the nostrils (orthonasal route) and from the mouth through the nasopharynx (retronasal route) (Figure 7–1). Both routes transport odorants to the olfactory epithelium, which is located on the dorsal aspect of the nasal cavity in the septum, extending from the superior turbinate to the anterior middle turbinate, a region larger than once believed.[7] The olfactory epithelial area varies across individuals and, with aging, appears to be replaced by respiratory epithelium.[8] Individuals with congenital anosmia (ie, without a sense of smell) have greatly reduced or absent olfactory epithelium.[9] Women consistently outperform men on olfactory tests,[10,11] in part because of female sex hormone influences on olfactory perception,[12–14] the anatomy of the nasal cavity,[15] and verbal processing skills in women applied to odor identification and memory tasks.[16]

The act of eating perfectly exemplifies the dual nature of olfactory perception. We perceive food odors passively through normal breathing (orthonasal olfaction). Sniffing increases the intensity of odors by causing turbulent airflow through the nasal cavity and increasing the concentration of odor molecules that reach the olfactory receptors.[17] We appreciate the full bouquet of a wine by holding the glass close to the nose and sniffing. Interestingly, nasal dilators amplify olfactory functioning by increasing the amount of inspired odorant that reaches the olfactory receptors.[18] In the mouth, foods and beverages present a complex mixture of smell, taste, and somatosensory sensations. Foods and beverages that are cold or have flavoring embedded may provide little olfactory stimulation until actually placed in the mouth. Chewing and mouth movements serve to volatilize odorants in the food via warming and mechanical action, and with the addition of swallowing, creates a pressure differential sufficient to pump these volatile odorants up through the oropharynx and nasopharynx to the olfactory epithelium (retronasal olfaction).[19] Analogous to the sniffing, the tongue, cheek, and throat movements must work in harmony to release and transport olfactory volatiles for full retronasal perception.

The olfactory epithelium should respond similarly to an odorant whether it is delivered through the nostrils or through the oral cavity. However, consider the anticipation that accompanies a brewing cup of coffee. The aroma permeates the kitchen and when brewing is finished, you pour yourself a cup. The retronasal flavor of the coffee does not elicit the same sensations as the orthonasal odor. Rozin[20] describes the qualitative differences between olfactory stimuli perceived from the nose and from the mouth. The volatile components of the coffee mix with the coffee bitterness, the hot temperature, and the feel of the coffee in your mouth. All of these factors modulate perception of the coffee odorants perceived in the mouth differently from those perceived through the nostrils. The perceptual localization of retronasal olfaction to the mouth has long been attributed to touch,[21] although evidence shows that taste also influences retronasal olfaction.[22] Patients report retronasal olfactory impairment with medically induced[23,24] or experimentally induced[25,26] loss of taste from the anterior tongue. Conversely, individuals who are genetic supertasters report greater retronasal olfactory intensity from model foods.[27]

The olfactory epithelium has olfactory receptor cells, supporting cells, and basal cells (Figure 7–2). The olfactory receptors are the olfactory neurons, which transmit the duration of exposure, identity, and concentration of thousands of

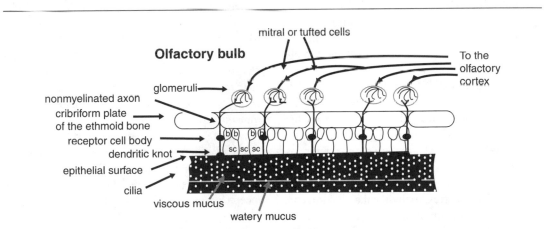

Figure 7–2 Peripheral Olfactory Pathways
The olfactory mucosa has olfactory receptor cells (receptor cell body, dendritic knob, and cilia noted), support cells (sc) and basal cells (b). The unmyelinated axons of the olfactory receptor cells project centrally through the cribriform plate of the ethmoid bone and terminate in the glomeruli of the olfactory bulb. The olfactory bulb neurons (mitral or tufted cells) project centrally to the olfactory tract. (Adapted from Greer[34]).

different odors through the primary olfactory center (the olfactory bulb) and to the secondary sensory centers in the central nervous system (the primary olfactory cortices). The supporting cells secrete mucus, and basal cells serve to generate new olfactory receptors. The size of the human olfactory epithelium is 1 to 2 cm², one-hundredth the size of that of the dog, an animal that possesses a much keener sense of smell. Nonetheless, a 2 cm² area of human olfactory tissue is estimated to contain 6 million ciliated olfactory cells.[28]

Odorants reach olfactory receptors on the cilia distributed throughout the olfactory epithelium by passing through a mucus layer (Figure 7–2), which may serve to concentrate and amplify the chemical message.[29] The odorants either pass through this mucus layer by diffusion[30] or by facilitated diffusion with a transport protein.[31] Odorant binding to the receptor proteins initiates the transduction cascade (ie, the conversion of the chemical signal to an electrical signal) by activating a GTP-binding protein (G protein)-linked receptor superfamily[32] to stimulate the adenylate cyclase enzyme cascade and the production of cAMP (cyclic adenosine 3′,5′-monophosphate) second messenger system (see Moon and Ronnett[32] for a review). cAMP mediates depolarization of the olfactory receptor cell and the action potential is carried by the nonmyelinated axon of the receptor cell (ie, olfactory nerve) through the cribriform plate to the olfactory bulb. The receptor cells synapse on the dendrites of the mitral or tufted cells in the glomeruli of the olfactory bulb (see Greer[34] for a review), which appears to fine-tune the odor message from the olfactory receptors via mapping the odor quality based on the chemical structure of the odorant as well as odor concentration.[35] The axons of the mitral and tufted cells transmit the sensory message to the olfactory cortex, including the piriform cortex where the incoming odor messages are compared with a template of past experiences ("This complex wine is a 25-year old Port."), to other broader cortical regions and limbic brain structures, including the orbitofrontal cortex ("The Port has a sweet taste and rich full texture."), hippocampus and amygdala for odor memory ("The flavor of this Port is similar to one I tasted last year."), and the hypothalamus as the feeding center ("I'll have another glass of this Port.").

Taste

True tastants (salt, sugar, sour, bitter) stimulate taste receptors located in special end organs (taste buds) on the tongue, soft palate, pharynx, larynx, and epiglottis. Taste buds on the tongue are held within gustatory papillae: the fungiform papillae on the anterior tongue, the foliate papillae on the posterior lateral sides of the tongue, and the circumvallate papillae, which extend in a rearward-facing chevron across the back of the tongue (Figure 7–3). Humans show large variation in both number of fungiform papillae and the taste buds on these papillae.[36] This variation appears to relate to sensory abilities. Genetic supertasters, who rate 6-*n*-propylthiouracil as extremely bitter, have the highest density of fungiform papillae and taste buds upon them.[37] Compared to nontasters, supertasters taste greater intensity from salt, sweet, sour, and bitter compounds as well as a number of somatosensory sensations.[2,38]

Taste buds contain between 50 and 150 cells that form into a discrete ovoid structure. These cells are divided into basal cells (from which new taste cells originate) and three types of elongated bipolar cells (dark, intermediate, and light), which have microvilli that extend through a taste pore into the oral environment. The microvilli appear to contain the taste receptors. To reach the microvilli, tastants become dissolved in saliva and a mucus layer for transport to taste receptors (individuals with diminished salivary production can show impaired taste perception).[39] Gustatory papillae contain taste receptor cells that respond to all basic taste qualities.[*] The gustatory stimuli interact with the taste receptor, which results in depolarization of the re-

---

[*]Humans can perceive salt, sweet, sour, and bitter on all parts of the oral cavity that contain taste receptors. As pointed out by Bartoshuk, the idea of a tongue map (the ability to perceive certain taste qualities on specialized areas of the tongue) is an "enduring scientific myth" that continues to show up in children's books and even some professional references.[40] By painting taste solutions on the areas of cranial nerve innervation, one can easily disprove the taste map.

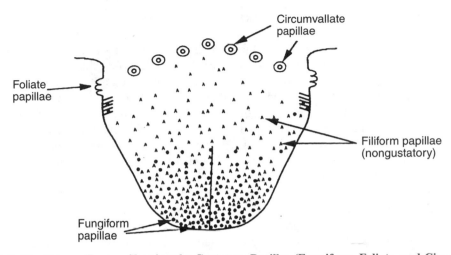

Figure 7–3 The Human Tongue Showing the Gustatory Papillae (Fungiform, Foliate, and Circumvallate Papillae) and the Nongustatory Filiform Papillae

ceptor and transmission of the electrical signal. The mechanism of taste transduction is specific for the type of gustatory stimuli.[41] Taste transduction involves sodium and potassium ion channels and two second-messenger systems (adenylate cyclase and phosphatidylinositol systems). Acids and sodium salts activate the ion channels directly to depolarize the receptor. Sweet compounds and bitters stimulate G protein-coupled receptors and then second-messenger signaling cascades to depolarize the receptor. As reviewed by McBurney and Gent,[42] taste is analytic, referring to the ability to tell that mixtures of tastant, equated for concentration, are perceived as separate qualities (sour and sweet in lemonade) versus formation of a new quality (ie, synthesis). Because of the analytic nature, taste quality is coded by fibers within the taste nerves that respond best to a particular taste quality (ie, labeled line).

Branches of three cranial nerves innervate the taste buds on each side of the tongue and transmit the electrical signal to the medulla:[43] the chorda tympani nerve (branch of cranial nerve VII) innervates taste buds in the fungiform papillae and in the anterior foliate papillae; the lingual branch of the glossopharyngeal nerve innervates the taste buds in the posterior foliate papillae and in the circumvallate papillae; the superficial petrosal branch of the cranial nerve VII innervates taste buds on the soft palate; and the superior branch of the vagus nerve (cranial nerve X) innervates taste buds in the epiglottis. These cranial nerves project to the nucleus of the solitary tract (NST). This region receives information from the somatosensory and the olfactory systems. From the NST, the axons travel to the vetrobasal thalamus and then to the gustatory cortex, orbitofrontal cortex, amygdala, and lateral hypothalamus.

Taste and oral somatosensations appear to be under the control of sex hormone variation. Taste varies across the menstrual cycle,[2] rises to its peak at the first trimester of pregnancy, falls to the lowest point in pregnancy by the third trimester, and then declines across menopause.[44] The bitter taste quality appears to be most affected. Pregnancy-associated taste changes may support a healthy pregnancy by modulating response to the food world (eg, upregulation of bitter taste helps the mother avoid ingesting bitter poisons). Young women are also statistically more likely than young men to be supertasters.[37]

Somatosensation

Cranial nerve V, the trigeminal nerve, transmits the largest amount of somatosensory sensations from the face. Branches of this cranial nerve innervate the mucous membranes of the nasal cavity, oral cavity, and eye (see, Silver and Finger[45] for a comprehensive review of the anatomy of the trigeminal system), which supports the perceptual integration of trigeminal sensations with odor and taste sensations. Foods and beverages stimulate three of the four classes of sensory fibers and receptors in the trigeminal nerve: (1) tactile sensations such as particle size, texture, and creaminess stimulate mechanoreceptors; (2) temperature of foods and beverages stimulate thermoreceptors; and (3) irritants and pungent foods stimulate nociceptors.

Somatosensory sensations are tightly integrated with, but separate from, smell and taste sensations. Odor compounds, if concentrated enough, cause intranasal stimulation of olfactory and trigeminal nerves.[46,47] Concentrated or noxious odors also irritate the eye and affect change in the respiratory and circulatory systems to warn the organism that a harmful substance is present. Individuals with olfactory dysfunction may still be able to distinguish the presence of concentrated odors through intranasal stimulation of trigeminal nerve.[47] Strong tastants (eg, the concentrated citric acid or sodium chloride) can also stimulate the nociceptors and produce irritation on the tongue.[48,49] On the anterior tongue, up to 75% of the innervation of the fungiform papillae arises from the lingual branch of the trigeminal nerve.[50,51] On the posterior tongue, the glossopharyngeal nerve carries sensory fibers for pain and temperature.[52]

INTEGRATION OF SMELL, TASTE, AND SOMATOSENSATION

Peripheral sensory messages from foods and beverages are integrated in central sensory systems to form a composite sensation that elicits a hedonic response to motivate dietary behaviors. As described by Green,[52] licking exemplifies the peripheral messages. While licking maple walnut ice cream, the trigeminal nerve senses the coolness, creaminess, and texture of the ice cream and added nuts, and the chorda tympani nerve senses the sweetness. As the ice cream is moved to the back of the tongue, the melting and mouth movements release and pump the maple and walnut flavor volatiles to cranial nerve I for olfactory perception and stimulating more taste and somatosensory receptors. Oral sensations support appropriate swallowing reflexes[53] and loss of full oral sensory stimulation may decrease the ability to relearn to swallow with neurological impairment.[54] Sensory inputs from taste, olfaction, somatosensation, and vision are integrated, for example, within the orbitofrontal cortex to respond to feelings of hunger (ie, intensified sensations or hedonic response) and satiety (ie, suppressed sensation or hedonic response).[55]

Sensory integration is observed perceptually in mixtures of taste, odors, and trigeminal stimuli through additivity and suppression. For additivity, taste and retronasal olfactory sensation work synergistically to enhance overall oral sensation. That is, adding sweet to banana olfactory flavoring increases the perceived intensity of banana flavor,[56] and adding vanilla olfactory flavoring to a sweetener enhanced the perceived intensity of sweetness.[57] This enhancement appears to be learned[58] (eg, sweet taste is congruent with fruity olfactory flavor but not with savory olfactory flavors). For suppression, adding too much of a viscous agent diminishes sweetness and retronasal olfactory intensity within a mixture.[56]

Sensory inputs carried from the periphery via the cranial nerves appear to inhibit one another via centrally mediated mechanisms to respond to a stimulus of multiple components such as an odor that stimulates olfactory and trigeminal systems, a concentrated taste that has taste and trigeminal components, or a food that stimulates taste, retronasal olfaction, and oral somatosensation. Loss of input from one or more of the sensory inputs changes the composite sensation of the mixture as well as changes sensory experiences in the absence of stimulation (eg, phantom sensation). For orthonasal olfaction, the odor component (cranial nerve I) inhibits the trigeminal component (cranial nerve V) of an odor such that loss of the odor component releases the inhibition to increase the perceived intensity of the trigeminal component as seen in individuals without a sense of smell.[59] Loss of taste functioning on individual areas of cranial nerve innervation (revealed by unilaterally applying taste solutions on areas of cranial nerve innervation)[60,61] influences taste from the other taste-specific cranial nerves, oral somatosensation from branches of cranial nerve V, and retronasal olfaction from cranial nerve I.

Loss of taste on the anterior tongue (chorda tympani nerve) releases the usual inhibition on taste from the other cranial nerves (cranial nerves IX, X) to maintain whole-mouth taste perception, even with extensive damage to the taste system. A dramatic example of the resilience of the taste system from an anecdote in *The Physiology of Taste*, written by Brillat-Savarin in the early 1800s, is explained by Bartoshuk.[40] In this case, a prisoner had the anterior portion of his tongue cut off as punishment. The prisoner did not complain of taste loss (reported being able to taste salt, sweet, sour, and bitter) but did have intense or painful sensations from very sour or bitter substances. The punishment removed chorda tympani taste projections to the central nervous system and released the inhibition of inputs from cranial nerves IX and X to maintain whole-mouth taste perception. Release of inhibition on taste has been shown in patients who had their chorda tympani nerve severed in surgery to remove acoustic neuromas[60] and those exposed to taste-related pathologies (eg, head trauma, upper respiratory tract infections, middle ear infections). Heightened sensations from the cranial nerves IX and X may also be the basis of dysgeusia, tastes that exist in the absence of apparent taste stimulation.[62,63]

Anesthesia studies provide an experimental model for studying interactions between taste and oral sensory nerves and provide insights to clinical observations. Unilateral anesthesia of CN VII abolishes taste on the ipsilateral anterior tongue while intensifying some qualities (especially bitterness) on the contralateral, posterior tongue (innervated by CN IX).[62,63] In 1965, Bull[24] described oral sensory changes in individuals who underwent unilateral chorda tympani damage during middle ear surgery. Approximately two of three complained of alterations in "taste," including inability to differentiate between coffee and tea, and the perception that foods, such as bread and chocolate, were "doughy" and "greasy," respectively. These complaints represent changes in true taste, oral somatosensation, and retronasal olfaction. Unilateral anesthesia of CN VII can result in contralateral intensification of an oral irritant mediated by CN V, particularly for genetic supertasters.[64] Release of inhibition on the trigeminal nerve in response to loss of taste from the chorda tympani nerve may also be why the subjects reported painful sensations from concentrated tastants. Burning mouth syndrome, an oral pain phantom, has been associated with damage to chorda tympani taste particularly in those who have the greatest number of fungiform papillae (ie, supertasters).[65] Spatial loss of taste may also decrease retronasal olfactory sensations[25,26] as shown in the clinical observations of Bull.[74] The oral sensory nerves are not connected in the periphery, and thus, the sensory changes must originate in the central nervous system.

Exposure to conditions that damage taste nerves with aging could change the interactions between the oral sensory nerves, modifying the oral sensation from foods/beverages and thereby affecting food preference and dietary behaviors. Loss of taste from the chorda tympani nerve may change the oral sensory quality of concentrated salt,[66] which has taste as well as chemesthetic qualities.[67] Preliminary studies from our laboratory suggest intensified oral sensations from concentrated salt in solution in elderly women, as compared with young women, may result from reduced chorda tympani taste function.[66,68] Elderly females also reported that chicken broth with high levels of sodium chloride were experienced as less pleasant in this study[66,68] and others,[69] suggesting the existence of a sensory hindrance to consuming sodium from foods/beverages with apparent saltiness (eg, some commercial soups, soy sauce, and tomato-based juices).[70] These findings disprove the popular belief that preference for salt increases with age due to taste loss. A further discussion on the potential impact of spatial taste loss in the elderly on oral sensations and dietary behaviors follows.

GENETIC VARIATION IN TASTE AND ORAL SENSATION

Taste and oral sensations seen in the elderly are a result of the interplay between genetically mediated influences and those associated with the environment (eg, exposure to pathogens) and maturation (eg, sex hormone changes). Taste and oral sensation vary genetically. The discovery of genetic variation in the ability to taste the bitterness of compounds possessing the $N - C = S$ was accidental.[71] Nontasters report that 6-n-propylthiouracil (PROP), one of these compounds, is tasteless while tasters report that the compounds are bitter or intensely bitter. Bartoshuk et al[37] classified nontasters, medium, and supertasters based on increases in perceived intensity with increasing concentrations of PROP and showed that the three groups differed in the density of fungiform papillae and their taste buds. On average, supertasters have greater numbers of fungiform papillae and taste buds than do nontasters. Some of the variability in the bitterness of PROP and phenylthiocarbamide (PTC) can be explained by gene polymorphisms on chromosome 7q[72] but not enough to explain supertasting. It appears that supertasters are homozygous for genes on this region of chromosome 7 and have a high number of fungiform papillae;[73] the genetic control of fungiform papillae is presently unclear.

In comparison with nontasters, supertasters perceive more intensity from a number of salty, sweet, sour, and bitter compounds as well as a variety of oral irritants, including chili peppers (ie, capsaicin), black pepper (ie, pipperine), ginger (ie, zigerone), carbonation, and alcohol.[2,74] Supertasters also report the greatest tactile sensations from high-fat milk products[38] and salad dressings.[75] Recent data also show that supertasters report greater retronasal intensities than do nontasters.[27] Oral sensory differences associated with genetic variation in taste translate to differences in dietary behaviors as well as risk of chronic disease. Studies on interactions between aging and genetic variation in taste and its effects on dietary behaviors have just begun. Risk of oral sensory problems may also be greater for supertasters than for nontasters. For example, supertasters may have the highest propensity to experience oral pain in response to conditions and therapies that impair oral health (eg, cancer therapies).[76]

MEASUREMENT OF PERCEIVED TASTE, SMELL, AND SOMATOSENSATIONS

Psychophysics, a branch of psychology, involves the study of how perception relates to physical stimulation. This includes how smell, taste, and somatosensory sensations vary with the quality, concentration, and duration of exposure to odorants, tastants, and a range of touch, temperature, and pain stimuli. Psychophysical investigation can characterize both the relationship between the physical and perceptual worlds and how this relationship changes across aging. Examples of two psychophysical procedures include the determination of the concentration required for detection or recognition of a chemical (threshold) and how perceived intensity varies with changing concentration (suprathreshold). In olfaction, odor identification tasks (ie, the ability to identify correctly a number of odorants) are a standard psychophysical procedure. Drawing heavily from psychophysical tradition, sensory evaluation includes hedonic responses to taste, smell, and oral somatosensory stimuli.

Valid psychophysical techniques are necessary to understand fully the effect of age-related physiological changes on sensory perception. Below is a description of the common psychophysical techniques.

Threshold

Threshold is sensitivity to a particular chemosensory stimulus and represents the lowest concentration needed to elicit a sensation (absolute sensitivity or detection threshold) or to recognize a sensation (recognition threshold). Thresholds are very simple to compare across individuals, whether within a cohort of elderly individuals or across age cohorts. A high threshold (or low sensitivity) indicates that an individual requires a high concentration to first perceive a stimulus.

For olfactory thresholds, the procedure must ensure delivery of a consistent concentration (ie, parts per billion) of odorant through devices such as porous paper dipped in odorant, sniff or squeeze bottles containing the odorant diluted in water or oil, or an olfactometer.[77] Historically, threshold methods were plagued by bias related to the arbitrary decision point of the subject; that is, one participant might say "Yes, I smell something" at the smallest hint while another participant may wait to be absolutely sure he/she smells something before saying, "Yes, I smell something," when in fact, the two subjects have the same threshold. As a result, methods that forced subjects to make a choice were developed. One such technique for assessing threshold is the two-alternative forced choice version of the ascending method of limits.[78] For example, in olfactory threshold testing, the subject is presented with two squeeze bottles, one with an odorant at the weakest concentration (nondetectable level) and the other only with the diluent (the order of presentation is random). The subject is asked to squeeze and sniff one bottle at a time and judge which bottle is stronger (forced choice). If correct, he or she is tested again with the same concentration. If the individual judges incorrectly, a stronger concentration is presented (ascending method of limits). Threshold is the concentration at which the subject makes four or five consecutive correct choices in a row.

The staircase procedure, a variant of the method of limits, is another threshold method used frequently in clinical and experimental procedures. In this procedure, the subject responds to stimuli that are above and below the threshold level. In taste thresholds, for example, the subject is presented with two solutions, one the stimuli (nondetectable level), the other diluents (usually water). If the subject makes one or two consecutive correct choices, the tester decreases the concentration and makes the task more diffi-

cult. If the subject judges incorrectly, the tester increases the concentration and makes the task easier. A reversal is the point at which the direction of the concentration given changes. The threshold value is calculated as the mean concentration of all reversals (generally six reversals, balanced with equal number of reversals at the highest and lowest concentrations with the first reversal not counted). (See Doty and Laing[77] and McBurney and Collins[79] for more information.)

When interpreting threshold elevations in aging, it is important to note that the process relies on both sensory and nonsensory data. Thresholds can show large variability, which makes repeat testing highly recommended to ensure the validity of the measurement.[78]

The utility of using thresholds to understand responses to more intense sensations needs to be examined especially in relation to dietary behaviors. For olfactory perception, it appears that threshold and suprathreshold performance are equivalent.[80] That is, a subject tested with an elevated threshold (low sensitivity) would also perceive lower intensities to more concentrated (suprathreshold) odors. This may be true for orthonasal olfaction if the trigeminal component of the odor is low, as is the case for phenyl ethyl alcohol (rose) where this may not hold for an odorant with a strong trigeminal component, like naphthalene (mothballs). For taste, threshold performance can dissociate with suprathreshold performance such that those with the lowest thresholds (ie, highest sensitivity) may not be those who taste higher concentrations as most intense.[81] As such, thresholds have little utility in predicting dietary behavior. For example, PROP suprathreshold bitterness was a better and significant predictor of alcohol intake than was PROP threshold.[82] The food and beverage world is one of suprathreshold sensation, rarely tapping sensations close to the threshold level. It is not surprising that studies employing only threshold measures have failed to find taste effects on food acceptance or intake.[83,84] Thus, suprathreshold measures are required to explore fully associations between variation in oral sensation and dietary behaviors.

Identification Tasks

Identification tasks are used most frequently in the measurement of olfactory perception. Subjects perceive and identify odorants, usually being prompted with a list of odors (tested odors and those that are distracters). Odor identification requires cognition, memory, and familiarity with the odorants. Correct odor identification requires sufficient sensory information to detect and recognize the odor as familiar, retrieve the odor name from long-term memory, and form the odor-word relationship.[85] Individuals without sensory impairment have difficulty linking an odor to a verbal description[4] in what has been called the "tip of the nose" phenomenon.[86] Experimental designs should control for the potential of cognitive difficulties exaggerating the degree of age-related olfactory impairment.[87] Because semantic coding and memory play a central role in odor identification,[88] it is critical that odor identification procedures can be constructed to measure primarily sensory functioning. In fact, observed age-related differences in odor recognition can disappear after controlling for odor naming ability.[89] Screening subjects for cognitive functioning may provide information as to whether or not an identification task is appropriate for the individual. Previous research shows that the elderly perform better on odor identification tasks that include odors from their childhood.[85] The odors in the test should be familiar to the age cohort, including consideration for cultural differences. The task should minimize difficulties with retrieving odor names by providing a list of odors to choose from. Allowing individuals to select the correct odor name from a list and retesting missed items after correct feedback can decrease the cognitive challenges of odor identification tasks.[90]

Scaling Sensory Intensity or Hedonics

The clinician or experimenter can measure how perceived intensity or level of liking or disliking varies with concentration of an odorant, tastant, or irritant, using concentrations that range from barely detectable levels to strong, very strong, and even strongest imaginable sensation. This is referred to as direct scaling or measuring the relationship between perceived intensity and concentration to produce a function. A steep function is when perceived intensity rises greatly with an increasing in concentration whereas a flat function is a small rise in perceived intensity with increasing concentration. The primary concern with this measurement is the comparison of intensity judgments between individuals with validity.[91] That is, how does one subject's judgment of "strong" compare to another's judgment? Are the two sensations equal? How can one be sure if people cannot share each other's sensory experiences?

The general techniques for measuring perceived intensity are reviewed below, including those with labeled scales or magnitude estimation, which either match the intensity of the stimulus to the length of the line, the adjective descriptor, or another sensation. The literature on taste and smell in aging includes a variety of scaling methods.[81] Understanding the use and limitation of each type of scaling method will support the appropriate interpretation of studies on sensory perception and aging. Correct use of scaling techniques has application beyond measuring sensory perception, including measuring hedonic feelings toward foods and even feelings of satisfaction with patient care services. It also has application for being able to detect changes in behavior and quality of life over time or in response to an intervention.[91]

Labeled Scales

In the food world, variants of the Natick 9-point category scale (1 = very weak, 5 = medium, 9 = very strong)[92] are often seen. The subjects assign a number between 1 and 9 to indicate the intensity of the stimulus. Figure 7–4 shows a nine-point scale applied to saltiness of a solution or sampled broth.[69] Category scales only order the intensity of stimuli from low to high,[93] and thus, when a person judges one stimulus as "3" and another "6," the only reasonable conclusion is that the second stimulus was stronger than the first. This

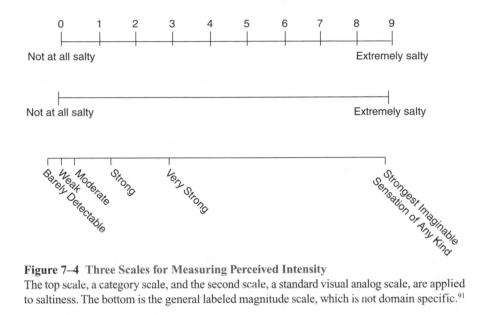

Figure 7–4 Three Scales for Measuring Perceived Intensity
The top scale, a category scale, and the second scale, a standard visual analog scale, are applied to saltiness. The bottom is the general labeled magnitude scale, which is not domain specific.[91]

method of scaling neither reflects how much stronger one stimulus is compared with another (ie, a measure of relative intensity) nor provides a measure of absolute intensity because the clinician or experimenter can never assume that the labels of the scale (eg, "strong") mean the same intensity to all individuals. These scales can be used to make within-subject comparisons (ratings of pain within a single person across a number of days) but not between two subjects.

The other problem with the category scale (as well as the visual analog scale) as shown in Figure 7–4 is that the adjectives are anchored to a particular sensation, in this case saltiness. This falsely assumes that the top saltiness intensity is equivalent to all. That is, let's assume that young and aged subjects rate the saltiness of increasing concentrations of broth as done in the experiment by Drewnowski et al,[69] who found that the young and aged rated them equally. Next, the same subjects rate the intensity of the saltiness on a scale anchored at the top to "strongest imaginable sensation of any kind" and the average rating for the aged exceeds the average rating for the young subjects. In reality the aged subjects could experience more intensity from salt in chicken broth because the salt stimulates

salty taste as well as irritation, the latter more intense. In fact, that is what was found.[90] Inappropriate use of scaling has been presented in greater depth elsewhere.[91]

Figure 7–4 shows two different labeled lines that vary in type and placement of adjectives: a standard visual analog scale and the general Labeled Magnitude Scale (gLMS),[91] which generalizes the Labeled Magnitude Scale[94,95] to apply to all sensations, not just to those in a particular domain (eg, oral sensation). The tape-pull method[96] (subjects pull a retractable metal tape with the length of the tape reflecting the intensity of stimuli) is a variant of the line length but without adjective labels. The visual analog scale can have the same inherent problems of a category scale if anchored to a particular domain of interest (Figure 7–4). The gLMS[91,94] produces relative intensity data (the visual analog scale also may provide this type of data) and has adjectives placed in a nearly logarithmic manner, a pattern that has been empirically proven to exist across a variety of sensory domains for intensity and hedonic measures.[91] The placement of the adjectives also limits ceiling effects or the inability of the subject to express the true increase in the perceived intensity of increasing concentrations. But most important, labeled lines used to scale perceived intensity or degree of liking/disliking can be used to make across-group comparisons (eg, young vs. aged) only if we can assume that the adjectives have the same meaning, on average, across the groups. Magnitude matching eliminates the need to make these assumptions.

Magnitude Estimation

Magnitude estimation requires a subject to assign a number to represent the intensity of a stimulus, according to the following instructions:

> "Please tell me how strong or weak a series of tastes and sounds is to you by providing a number to represent the intensity. The larger the number, the stronger the taste or sound. Conversely, the smaller the number, the weaker the taste or sound. You can use any numbers that you desire. However, I will ask you to judge the tastes and sounds relative to the first one you perceive. That is, if the second stimulus is three times stronger than the first, provide a number that is three times larger than the first number. If the second stimulus is a third as strong, then give a number that is a third as large."

With this scale the perceived intensities are relative: a judgment of "8" reflects an intensity twice that of a judgment of "4." Magnitude estimation can limit ceiling effects. For example, in line with the preceding instructions, the subject might feel that he or she would use a 1 to 10 scale to judge the intensity of salt solutions. Upon tasting the solutions, the subject gives a "4" to the first solution and an "8" to the second solution. The subject feels the third solution is twice as strong as the second solution. Magnitude estimation allows them the freedom to use "16" even though they might have originally thought they would use a 1 to 10 scale. Some line scales may not afford this freedom, and thus are subject to ceiling effects.

Magnitude estimation assumes that individuals can use numbers appropriately. The practice task of judging the distance between two points can quickly train the subject to assign numbers that represent magnitude with ratio properties. The following is a practice setting (the order of presentation can be varied):

> "Please assign a number to represent the distance between my two fingers (such as 5 inches in space), between my two hands (such as shoulder width apart), again between my two hands (such as full arm span), between my two fingers (such as 1 inch apart), and again between my two fingers (such as $^1/_2$ inch apart)."

Magnitude estimation does not allow comparison of perceived intensity across subjects unless the meaning and use of the number scale are standardized. One subject may have used a 1 to 50 number scale, another a 1 to 15. The clinician or experimenter cannot assume that "15" equaled the intensity of "50" because the numbers only have meaning to the subject. The problem may be addressed by asking the subject the meaning of his or her scale after the session is completed.[97] For this technique, subjects are asked, "If you did or had experienced something as 'very strong,' what number would you have provided?" The subject would then generate numbers for all the desired adjectives of intensity. The only limitation is the assumption that the adjectives mean the same thing to all of the subjects. Another way to standardize the number scale or magnitude estimate data is through the use of magnitude matching.

Magnitude Matching

This procedure matches the intensity judgments from one sensory continuum to another, or across qualities within a sensory continuum (also called cross-modality matching). One sensory stimulus serves as the standard and the assumption is that sensations from the standard and sensation of interest are not correlated. Marks and Stevens[98–100] developed this procedure to use with magnitude estimate data. For example, in measuring perceived odor intensity in young and older adults, the standard could be the intensity of sodium chloride (with the assumption that intensity of NaCl shows less risk of loss with aging and thus is perceived equally in both age groups). In the session, subjects would judge the intensity of a concentration series of odors and NaCl solutions, usually presented in a random order. The experimenter would instruct the subject to provide magnitude estimate data and to use the same number scale to judge the intensity of odors and tastes. For comparison within and between cohorts, the odor intensities would be standardized with the NaCl intensities.

The primary limitation of magnitude matching is the identification of an appropriate standard. If the perceived intensity of the standard shows an association with age, finding true differences between young and elderly in the perceived intensity of the sensation of interest is nearly impossible. Preliminary data have shown that NaCl may not be an appropriate standard for across-age comparisons;[66] remembered nonoral sensations (eg, loudness of a whisper, the dark-light transition of walking out of a movie theater into the sunshine, or the chill of an icy wind) appear to offer a more reasonable standard. By using the label "strongest imaginable sensation of any kind" on the gLMS, we can see psychophysical functions for taste that are equivalent to those produced by magnitude matching.[101] This suggests that the gLMS produces valid across-group comparisons for taste. Responses measured with scales like the gLMS may be checked with normalizing the data to a standard.[82,102] That is, the preceding example could be repeated using the gLMS and intensity of remembered nonoral sensations to examine perceived odor intensity in young and older adults.

Misuse of Standards in Psychophysical Testing

Some experimental designs have included the use of standards that inappropriately force subjects to assign similar ratings for very different perceptual experiences. A complete explanation of this error can be found in the literature.[81] Although a number of aging studies have used these inappropriate standards, here are the details of one study.[103] In this experiment, investigators were interested in determining the perceived saltiness of tomato juices that varied in NaCl and citric acid concentration. Before sampling the

tomato juices, the subjects (young and elderly) were given standards for the "least salty" as "tomato juice with no added salt" and "most salty" as "tomato juice with 1.5% NaCl." The subjects were told to make their intensity judgment on a 10 cm line relative to these two standards. This is a very different procedure than magnitude matching. In this procedure, subjects are forced to comply with these set standards. What if the standards were not perceived equally by all subjects? What if the 1.5% NaCl in the tomato juice was not the saltiest stimulus? Citric acid can add to the perceived intensity of saltiness and the highest concentration of citric acid in tomato juice might have been the most intense saltiness to some subjects. This paradigm could accommodate neither these possibilities nor the difference between young and elderly cohorts.

Additional Psychophysical Measures

A number of additional tests are available to measure smell, taste, and somatosensation. Individuals use odor memory to recognize and recall odors that are presented in testing. Odors evoke memories with a high level of emotional salience, and it is this emotionality that distinguishes odor memory from those evoked by other sensory systems.[104] Odor memory tests are used in research to understand changes associated with aging, central olfactory processing, such as why women outperform men on odor memory tests.[105] This review will not describe odor memory testing procedures because some research shows that information on olfactory functioning gleaned from odor memory tests is similar to that from detection thresholds, discrimination, and identification tasks.[106] Odor memory tasks related to diseases associated with aging are discussed below.

Summary of the Psychophysical Techniques for Aging Studies

Thresholds provide a measure of sensitivity but may or may not reflect the ability to perceive stimuli at concentrations relevant to eating.

Suprathreshold tasks measure perception of real-world stimuli. For perceived intensity measures, the scaling method must (1) allow subjects to express the range of their sensations (which will eliminate the ceiling effect); (2) avoid the use of a standard to assign a particular value or the limits of the scale; (3) use a labeled scale that allows comparison of relative intensities; and (4) provide a valid way to compare perceived intensity across subjects (eg, magnitude matching). In the performance of identification tasks (primarily for olfaction), the method must attempt to separate sensory influences from cognitive influences. Psychophysical tasks that utilize foods and beverages may have the most application in the exploration of the relationship between oral sensory functioning and nutritional outcomes.

FUNCTIONAL MEASURES OF SMELL, TASTE, AND SOMATOSENSATION

Researchers and clinicians use electrophysical measurement of olfactory function to extend the information gleaned from psychophysical evaluation.[107] This technology involves recording brain potentials, magnetic responses, and changes in blood flow in response to odors. Olfactory event-related potentials (OERP) can help determine structures involved in causing olfactory dysfunction and thus suggest the availability of treatments. OERP can be particularly helpful in diagnosing olfactory disturbances in dementia disorders where you want to minimize the cognitive demands of the olfactory testing.[108] Testing involves giving an odor stimulus and asking the participant to respond to the stimulus while minimizing visual, somatosensory, or auditory sensory inputs that could affect the OERP.[107] The OERP provides information on the length of time it takes to show a significant change in neural electrical response to the odor (ie, latency) and the magnitude of neural response (ie, amplitude).

Imaging neural responses to odors in noninvasive ways has been used to increase understanding of central olfactory processing, including positron emission tomography (PET) and functional magnetic resonance imaging (fMRI). As described in a review,[109] the PET and fMRI indirectly measure neural activity through changes in metabolic activity and blood flow to answer questions about what areas of the brain respond to odors and oral sensations and how behavioral response is formed (eg, "This ice cream is strawberry and I like it.").

SMELL, TASTE, AND SOMATOSENSORY CHANGES ASSOCIATED WITH AGING

Clinicians can assess normal sensory functioning (ie, normosmic, normogeusic) and reveal a range of disorders in smell, taste, and somatosensation. In olfaction, individuals can suffer from diminished (hyposmia) or absent (anosmia) ability to perceive one, a few, or all tested odorants.[110] Specific anosmia may be a genetic variation and not a disorder. For example, 6% of adults are estimated to have a specific anosmia to the musky compounds galoxide and andostenone.[111,112] Altered olfactory perception or dysosmia also exists. Dysosmia can be the distortion of odor quality (parosmia, for example, smelling burnt paper instead of baby powder) or a phantom olfactory sensation with no apparent olfactory stimulus (olfactory hallucinations, phantosmia).[110]

In taste, individuals can also show diminished (hypogeusia) or absent (ageusia) taste perception. Total ageusia is very rare;[113,114] of over 1100 individuals seeking help for taste disturbances, less than 1% had confirmed ageusia or severe hypogeusia (severe hyposmia/anosmia was more common in 32% of individuals). The ability to taste with the whole mouth is maintained despite major damage to the nerves that subserve taste. As with olfaction, individuals can suffer from altered taste perception (dysgeusia). Chronic dysgeusia or a persistent salt, sweet, sour, or bitter sensation can result from a stimulus in the mouth (eg, the taste of an oral infection) or something that leaks into the mouth from the blood stream (eg, bitter taste from medications). Dysgeusia can also be a phantom sensation generated by spontaneous activity in the nervous system in the absence of stimulation (analogous to phantom limb sensations). Individuals can experience metallic oral sensations in response to a food or beverage as well as a phantom sensation. The metallic quality may arise from taste, tactile, and/or retronasal sensations.[115]

Somatosensory perceptions can also be altered. Loss of sensitivity can occur to touch sensations (numbness) and to chemical irritants (desensitization). Chemical desensitization can occur through the application and removal of capsaicin (the burn of chili pepper).[116] This desensitization property can provide an effective means of analgesia for peripheral sources of oral pain.[76] Individuals can also perceive pain or hypersensitivity to somatosensory stimuli as well as oral pain phantoms (eg, burning mouth syndrome).

The following discussion is from studies on taste, smell, and somatosensory perception in aging that incorporates some caution in presenting some of the findings, reflecting the limitations of the psychophysical procedures outlined earlier. With this consideration, the data support that age-related olfactory dysfunction is more common than taste dysfunction. Somatosensory sensations also appear stable across age, although there are some age-related declines in trigeminal sensation via the nares but increases in oral trigeminal sensations in response to localized taste losses. It is important to mention that complaints of "taste loss," if sensory, are olfactory problems. Individuals usually are both unable to separate and distinguish taste from smell when a chemosensory stimulus is placed in the mouth. They are also unable to distinguish the contributions of taste and smell to the overall intensity of a chemical stimulant.[117,118] Individuals usually attribute the flavor of food as "taste" to resolve ambiguities between taste and retronasal olfaction.[118] Clinicians must carefully question older adults to understand their complaint, and if sensory, assess whether the complaint is taste or smell.

The Sense of Smell and Aging

Most studies support the thesis that olfaction shows age-related declines. It is hypothesized that aging alone produces a gradual loss of ol-

factory dysfunction that is often unrecognized. Olfactory loss associated with dementia disorders may also be gradual, in some cases paralleling the decline in cognitive functioning. A more precipitous loss of olfactory perception could indicate an overriding environmental insult such a nasal/sinus disease, head trauma, and upper respiratory tract infections. Older adults show a range of functioning from total loss (anosmia) to diminished ability (hyposmia) to a sense of smell equal to younger adults (normosmia). It is difficult to separate olfactory losses of aging from those caused by disease and environmental insults. Analysis of data from the Baltimore Longitudinal Study of Aging[119] shows age-related declines in olfactory perception in a group of aged males and females without overt disease.

Olfaction is more vulnerable than taste to loss with aging because of its anatomical structure and because aging associates with changes in peripheral and central components.[120] Olfactory information is carried by only cranial nerve I; taste is transmitted by branches of three different cranial nerves (VII, IX, X). The olfactory nerve must travel through the ethmoid bone and can be severed with a specifically located head trauma. The olfactory receptors are embedded in a relatively small region of the superior sinus region whereas taste has receptors (taste buds) on the tongue, palate, and in the throat. Because the olfactory neurons also serve as olfactory receptors, they are directly exposed to environmental insults such as toxins and infectious agents. Although olfactory neurons can regenerate, they must do so by reinnervating the olfactory bulb and there are age-related declines in the number of functional cells in the olfactory bulb.[121] These changes may arise from repeated exposure to environmental insults versus age per se. Neurogenesis may be impaired in disease and, across aging, results in less functioning olfactory receptors, according to data from animal models.[122,123] In taste, the neurons are protected because there are specialized taste receptors and epithelial cells.

A number of studies provide indications of age-related prevalence of olfactory impairment (ie, the total number of cases at a given point of time). Some include measured olfactory functioning across age cohorts with elderly recruited from long-term facilities,[124] from those who read *National Geographic* magazine,[10] and from a large population-based study.[11] Another is a statistical sampling of U.S. adults with self-reported olfactory impairment.[125]

The first of these studies included more than 1900 individuals from ages 5 to 99 years[124] and measured olfactory perception with the University of Pennsylvania Smell Identification Test (UPSIT).[126] The purpose of the study was to establish normative data for the UPSIT, and the elderly sample was selected from long-term care facilities. The UPSIT has 40 odors and a multiple-choice format. Subjects scratch and sniff the odor and try to identify the odor from three distracters. From the data, Doty and colleagues[124] concluded the following: peak olfactory performance occurred between the third and fourth decades; women had higher olfactory performance than men; and up to 50% of individuals over the age of 65 had major olfactory impairment. The National Geographic Smell Survey[10] included 1.2 million free-living individuals who responded to a six-odor, scratch-and-sniff-type test that was inserted in the *National Geographic* magazine. Age-related declines were seen in ability to detect and correctly identify each odor as well as average perceived intensity of the odorants. Elderly individuals from this sample who denied exposure to insults of the olfactory system had less olfactory dysfunction, according to across-cohort comparisons.[127] The final involved olfactory testing added to a follow-up examination of a population-based study of sensory loss and aging of more than 2400 residents from Beaver Dam, Wisconsin who ranged in age from 53 to 94 years.[11] Trained personnel administered the eight-item odor identification task; participants responded to illustrations of odors and distracters. The overall prevalence was 24.5%, with rates increasing with age (62% of those over age 80 were impaired) and greater in men and those reporting exposures to environmental insults that increase risk of olfactory dys-

function (eg, nasal/sinus disease, smoking, upper respiratory tract infections).[11]

A statistical sampling of U.S. adults for reported chronic smell disorders was completed in the 1994 Disability Supplement to the National Health Interview Survey of 107,469 individuals.[125] The overall prevalence was 1.4% of adults, with the highest in individuals over the age of 75 (46 per 1000) and the next highest group being those 65 to 74 years (26.5 per 1000). Of the total sample over the age of 65 years, 40% reported chronic problems with their sense of smell. Although this survey is a statistical sampling, it relies on reported smell disorders. There is a lack of awareness regarding disorders of the sense of smell,[128] and self-reported olfactory dysfunction becomes less accurate with age.[11]

A number of issues deserve attention related to olfactory functioning across aging; some of these were based on a critical review of the olfactory and aging literature by Cain and Stevens.[80]

1. Does the olfactory loss in aging influence the entire range of perceptual experience from an elevation of thresholds (ie, lower sensitivity) to reduced perception of more concentrated stimuli?
2. Is the age-related loss equal for all olfactory stimuli or are some qualities more vulnerable to losses with aging than others?
3. Important to geriatric nutrition, does aging influence the perception of odors and olfactory flavors equally? That is, are there factors that impair the ability to perceive the full flavor of food even if the older adult has a normal sense of smell?
4. Do functional measures of olfactory perception show age-related declines?

Threshold Vs. Suprathreshold Perception

The elderly, on average, require from twofold to 100-fold higher concentration to recognize the quality of an odorant (recognition threshold).[78,80] Using magnitude matching, Stevens and colleagues[129] were the first to report reduced odor intensities in elderly subjects. The testing was first conducted using an auditory standard and was repeated with sodium chloride as a standard.[130] This latter study showed greater age-related impairment to olfaction than to taste. In comparing perceived intensities of six odors that varied in quality, Stevens and Cain[131] found age-related olfactory losses for weak and strong odorants. Thus, a substantial elevation in threshold would reflect a reduced ability to perceive more concentrated olfactory stimuli. Thresholds, however, may be more sensitive than suprathreshold measures to losses in olfactory perception associated with dementia disorders.[132] Odor memory declines with aging similar to declines seen in odor sensitivity and odor identification.[105]

Age-related Olfactory Losses Do Not Appear Quality Specific

Other sensory systems show quality-specific changes associated with aging, including hearing and taste. This does not appear to be true for the sense of smell based on current thinking quality specific changes with aging. The olfactory epithelium has over 300 different types of receptors coded by olfactory genes.[133] Odors stimulate a pattern of these receptors and the individual template of the pattern stored in memory. Losses of olfactory perception with aging are more likely to affect the intensity of response to these odors versus the quality per se. The data from the National Geographic Smell Survey suggest that age-related losses are not uniform across odors;[10] sweet and fruity odors may be most vulnerable to the physiological changes that accompany aging, while musky and spicy odors are relatively stable.[134] The difference in age-related declines across these odor groups may be explained by stimulus intensity differences between the sweet odors and those that are musky/spicy as well as the presence of trigeminal components to the odors.

Retronasal Vs. Orthonasal Olfaction and Aging

The elderly show less ability than young to identify food based solely on olfactory cues, according to studies using blended foods as the stimulus[135,136] and readily available foods and condiments.[137] Perceived intensity ratings of an orally sampled odorant (ethyl butyrate) are also lower in the elderly versus young.[138] In this study, subjects perceived the odorant retronasally with and without the nose pinched. The younger subjects, with the nose open, consistently gave stronger ratings to the overall intensity of ethyl butyrate solutions. The elderly did not notice a difference between the overall intensity with the nose pinched or open. Declines in retronasal olfaction appear in middle-aged adults. Cain et al.[139] reported that middle-aged and older individuals were equally unable to discriminate the presence of an olfactory seasoning (marjoram) in a food item (soup). Middle-aged adults also show decreased retronasal intensity, according to a preliminary study.[140] In this study, women rated the intensity of chocolate and orange flavoring delivered both orthonasally in plastic squeeze bottles with a pop-up spout and retronasally in a sucrose-sweetened gelatin. The middle-aged females, on average, exhibited lower orthonasal and retronasal olfactory perception than the young females. In summary, these studies suggest that an age-related decline in olfactory perception decreases the ability to perceive the full flavor of food, and that these losses may occur in middle age.

Defects of the olfactory system could impair olfactory perception regardless of whether the odors were delivered through the nostrils or the oral cavity. However, clinical conditions show dissociation between retronasal and orthonasal olfaction. Full retronasal olfactory perception requires sufficient mastication to release volatiles from foods as well as adequate mouth and swallowing movements to create enough intraoral pressure to pump the volatiles from the mouth retronasally to the olfactory epithelium.[19] Burdach and Doty[19] hypothesize that the elderly are neither able to release food volatiles effectively nor to generate enough active turbulent airflow to transport these released volatiles to the olfactory cleft. Conditions that impair chewing and mouth and swallowing movements could diminish retronasal perception, even with an intact olfactory system. The elderly can show impairment in chewing, even with natural dentition.[141]

By testing orthonasal and retronasal olfactory perception in a group of reportedly healthy elderly women, we[142] found diminished retronasal sensitivity in women who wore complete maxillary dentures or with dentures that at least covered the palate of the mouth. The retronasal measure was a sweetened gelatin that varied in orange flavoring from subthreshold to threshold levels. Orthonasal olfaction was measured with a standard measure of olfactory dysfunction.[90] The denture effect on retronasal sensitivity was independent of the ability to perceive odors through the nostrils. That is, some older women had a normal sense of smell but needed high levels to first detect the orange flavoring. The limitation of this study was that the functional ability of the dentures was not directly measured. Factors such as the stability, retention, and occlusion of the dentures could be important to perceiving retronasal olfaction fully. Many other oral conditions and swallowing disorders could have the potential to diminish retronasal olfaction. A number of studies report diminished food enjoyment with oral health problems, such as oral pain and periodontal disease;[143] impaired retronasal olfaction could cause some of the diminished enjoyment.

Spatial taste losses also impair retronasal olfaction independently from orthonasal perception as suggested by clinical[23,24] and experimental data with temporary anesthesia of the chorda tympani nerve[25] alone or with the lingual nerve.[26] Preliminary data suggest that the elderly perceived less intensity from retronasal olfactory stimuli because of spatial taste losses from the chorda tympani nerve as well as orthonasal olfactory impairment.[27] That is, retronasal olfaction is vulnerable to losses because of impairments in the olfactory and gustatory systems.

Interestingly, individuals with laryngectomies can exhibit diminished ability to perceive odors through the nostrils but intact ability to perceive olfactory flavors retronasally.[144] The laryngectomy interrupts the normal path of air traveling from the nose or mouth to the lungs and allows the individual to breathe through a stoma in the throat. The patients complained that they could not smell odors but did not notice a diminished flavor of food. Orthonasal olfaction was impaired because the air carrying odors does not pass through the nostrils during breathing. Olfactory flavor perception remained intact because eating allows the olfactory volatiles to reach the olfactory epithelium retronasally. Retronasal olfactory perception also exceeds that of orthonasal perception in chronic rhinosinusitis with nasal polyposis and mechanical obstruction in the anterior portion of the olfactory cleft.[145]

Functional Measures of Olfactory Perception Show Age-related Declines

Olfactory event-related potentials show age-related declines in amplitude and latency of response to an odor.[146,147] Aging effects were also seen with fMRI imaging of odor identification.[148] Neuroimaging studies with fMRI in young vs. aged adults show that aged have decreased cerebral activities in response to odors in the piriform cortex, entorhinal cortex, and amygdala in response to orthonasally[148,149] and retronasally introduced odorants.[150]

The Sense of Taste and Aging

Total ageusia is rarely seen. Data from the University of Pennsylvania Smell and Taste Center serve as compelling evidence in support of this statement. In over 1000 individuals presenting to this Center with "taste loss," less than 1% had measurable taste impairment while 32% had severe olfactory dysfunction.[113,114]

Altered taste sensations are more common. According to data from the 1994 Disability Supplement to the National Health Interview Survey of 107,469 individuals,[125] participants reported on chronic taste problems, including inability to taste salt and sweet as well as the presence of "inappropriate" tastes in the mouth. Age-related increases were seen primarily in the presence of inappropriate tastes (the smallest age-related increases were seen with inability to taste salt or sweet) with up to 41% of those older than 65 years of age reporting a chronic taste problem.

Researchers appear to agree that aging is associated with elevated taste thresholds with some differences across qualities and within bitter qualities. Taste threshold does not reflect the ability to perceive concentrated tastes, such as those you would experience during eating.[81] Some of the studies that hypothesize taste impairment in elderly adults incorporate elements that retain the psychophysical scaling problems mentioned earlier. Aging can be associated with loss of taste perception in individual areas of cranial nerve innervation that do not produce whole-mouth taste loss but can alter oral somatosensory, retronasal, and even dietary-related behaviors. Taste can be damaged without showing changes in numbers of fungiform papillae. These papillae are formed early in gestation[151] and remain intact unless the trigeminal nerve is damaged.[2,152] Thus, an individual with taste-related pathology may present elevated thresholds or depressed bitter intensity[153] relative to the number of fungiform papillae. The number of taste receptors (ie, taste buds) does not appear to change with aging.[154] Even within animal models, there is not support for changes in the peripheral taste system with aging.[155,156] Nonetheless, a recent study has shown decreases in laryngeal taste bud number as well as secretory/motor neurons in elderly versus young rats.[157]

It is important to also discuss (1) age-related elevations in taste thresholds; (2) suprathreshold taste perception and aging; and (3) cranial nerve interactions to affect oral sensation.

Elevated Taste Threshold in Aging

Aging associates with elevations across all taste qualities,[158,159] even when including only those elderly adults who are healthy, without dentures, and not taking prescription medication. The latter finding strengthens the argument that the effects are due to aging versus disease. Across qualities, NaCl shows the greatest age-related elevation, sucrose the least. There are also compound-specific elevations in bitter threshold associated with aging.[160] The elderly also show elevated thresholds for taste within taste mixtures (eg, elevated NaCl threshold in a mixture of cit-

ric acid or tomato soup).[161] It is important to note, however, that subjects confuse the qualities of saltiness (NaCl) and sourness (citric acid).

Suprathreshold Taste Perception and Aging

Because performance on a taste threshold may not indicate how intensely one perceives concentrated tastants,[81] attention to suprathreshold taste function should provide the most information about the taste world of older adults. The scientific literature reflects that the primary method used to assess suprathreshold function in the aging is perceived intensity (identification tasks are less interesting because there are a limited number of taste qualities). Many of the studies examining taste and aging have methodological issues that make interpreting the findings difficult.[81]

A number of studies with magnitude matching as the psychophysical method do not find age-related reductions in perceived intensity for tastants except for reductions in intensity of bitter compounds. There is also support for concentrated tastants that elicit trigeminal sensations to be perceived as more intense in elderly. The validity of magnitude matching, the gold standard psychophysical method, hinges on the ability to find a standard that does not show changes with aging.[91] Using a valid standard allows comparison of taste intensity between young and elderly subjects. A number of studies have been conducted using an auditory standard.[130,162–164] The auditory standard was low frequency and relatively high intensity (aging associates with largest losses to the perception of high-frequency, low-intensity sounds). Two of the three studies[130,162] reported that the perceived intensity judgments of young and elderly subjects overlapped. The other[163] found small age-related reductions in perceived intensity of tastes in solution in the elderly, most notably for bitter compounds and umami. We have also observed age-related reductions in bitter taste perception in females, this decline appears to occur with menopause.[165] Age-related differences in taste intensity appear to be less pronounced during eating when interactions between taste, smell, and oral somatosensations influence overall flavor intensity.[163]

By using magnitude matching with remembered nonoral sensations as the standard, elderly females compared to young females produced the highest ratings for concentrated salt in solution and in broth as well as the greatest aversion to the most concentrated stimuli.[66] Mojet et al.[163] also showed that elderly women gave the highest intensity ratings to concentrated salt. At high concentrations, salts elicit taste and irritation sensations.[67] The irritation qualities could be heightened with aging because exposure to environmental insults (eg, head injury, ear infections) produce quality- and area-specific taste losses and not losses in oral irritation. Age-related loss of bitter may release the usual inhibition on oral irritation, as suggested in models for burning mouth syndrome as discussed earlier.

Elderly adults can show discrete losses of taste to areas of cranial nerve innervation.[166] It is uncertain if these losses occur with aging or because of conditions that damage individual cranial nerves. Because of the redundancy in innervation, the discrete losses of taste go unnoticed. If the damage to one cranial nerve is substantial, the elderly could have a dysgeusia that could add to the intensity of taste stimuli via release of inhibition. This was described by Bartoshuk;[166] elderly subjects perceived weak taste solutions as more intense than did young subjects. Elderly subjects may also complain of dysgeusia.

Somatosensation and Aging

Although older adults show lower touch sensitivity than younger adults on various body loci including the tongue,[167] aging does not associate with diminished intensity of oral somatosensory sensations. Weiffenbach et al.[168] reported that age did not associate with a difference in perceived intensity of thickened liquids (thickened with methylcellulose). Perception of temperature in the mouth also does not appear to show age-related changes.[168,169]

Data from our laboratory suggest that spatial losses of taste can actually increase the intensity of oral somatosensory experiences similar to the intensification of irritation qualities from concentrated NaCl. Bartoshuk and colleagues[170] report that older women ($\geq$53 years) rated greater burn from oral capsaicin than young females and men. The rated capsaicin burn was especially high in those older women who were genetic supertasters. With menopause, there may be some loss of bitter perception, especially to the anterior tongue. The loss of taste on the anterior tongue (cranial nerve VII) could make the response to irritation (cranial nerve V) on the anterior tongue even more pronounced. This may have clinical relevance. Age is associated with a dramatic increase in the incidence of neuropathic pain conditions, including postherpetic neuralgia and trigeminal neuralgia.[171] Also, burning mouth syndrome, a syndrome characterized by an excruciating oral pain phantom sensation, afflicts primarily postmenopausal women. It may be that taste and pain interactions play a role in the etiology of burning mouth syndrome.[65] Individuals with this oral pain phantom were more likely than age-matched controls to have taste damage from the chorda tympani and the highest number of fungiform papillae (ie, genetic supertasters). Interactions between taste and somatosensory sensations can also affect the oral sensation from fat. Creaminess/textural sensations are the primary oral cue for fat in the mouth. In our laboratory, we found that aged women were more likely to report greater creamy sensations from a range of sampled high-fat foods than did younger adults.[68] They also reported greater preference for high-fat foods on a survey and in response to sampled high-fat foods. The aged women also showed significant depression in chorda tympani taste, especially for bitterness. Thus, loss of taste on the anterior tongue could enhance somatosensory input from high-fat foods and make them more pleasurable.

Perception of nasal trigeminal sensations also shows some age-related declines. Individuals over the age of 60 were less able than young adults to tell which side an odor was presented as a test of nasal trigeminal sensitivity.[172] Perception of irritation through the nasal cavity shows age-related declines. In comparison with younger adults, older individuals report less pungency in carbon dioxide inhaled through the nostrils.[129] Despite these apparent losses of nasal trigeminal perception, the elderly are still able to use trigeminal sensations for the perception and discrimination of odorants.[173]

CAUSES OF SMELL, TASTE, AND ORAL SOMATOSENSORY DISORDERS

Interest in the causes of chemosensory dysfunction was stimulated in the 1970s when the National Advisory Neurological and Communicative Disorders and Stroke Council estimated that 2 million adults suffered from taste or smell disorders, a figure that probably does not include the level of dysfunction seen in elderly adults.[174] Nationally, over 200,000 visits per year are made to physician's offices with the complaint of partial or complete loss of smell or taste.[175] The following section reviews the causes of smell, taste, and oral somatosensory disturbances, including changes specifically associated with aging.

The most common causes of olfactory dysfunction in patients without major systemic diseases are upper respiratory tract infections, head trauma, inflammatory diseases (eg, chronic nasal/sinus disease, allergic rhinitis), and neurodegenerative diseases.[110,114] These diseases diminish olfactory perception through one or a combination of these factors: (1) reduced ability to transport odorants to the olfactory receptors; (2) damage to the sensory receptors that receive and transduce the olfactory message; and (3) damage to the peripheral or central neurophysiological systems. More common in the aged are neurodegenerative diseases of the central nervous system (eg, Alzheimer's disease and Parkinson's disease), which have a comorbidity of olfactory dysfunction. Less common causes of olfactory dysfunction are congenital disorders, toxic exposures, and medications. Individuals with chronic systemic disease can also show olfactory disorders.

Taste disorders can also result from conditions that disrupt the transport of stimuli to the receptors and those that disrupt the neural pathways necessary for taste perception.[176,177] Taste loss can occur at specific areas of cranial nerve innervation, but these usually go unnoticed. Individuals are most troubled by dysgeusia (persistent salty, sweet, sour, or bitter sensation), especially if chronic.[178] If the patient cannot describe the sensation as salty, sweet, sour, or bitter, then it is a dysosmia or parosmia. Most troubling is the fact that these disorders may not be evaluated correctly and instead may be treated as psychiatric problems.

The primary causes of smell, taste, and oral somatosensory disorders are discussed below. More extensive descriptions of olfactory disorders are in the cited literature.[110,177]

Upper Respiratory Tract Infections (URI)

URIs diminish olfactory perception through nasal obstruction and viral damage to the olfactory receptors. Olfactory dysfunction may occur after repeated bouts of URI. Some individuals may be more susceptible to olfactory dysfunction than others.[11] The effect of the common cold on olfactory abilities has been shown through direct experimental investigation.[179] After inoculation with a common cold virus, volunteers showed elevated odor thresholds, the level of elevation predicted by the degree of nasal obstruction. The URI virus primarily affects the peripheral olfactory processes, although viruses can invade the central nervous system via the olfactory receptor cells, especially with age-related degradation of the olfactory epithelium.[180] Through electron-microscopic observations,[9] individuals with post-URI olfactory dysfunction had reduced numbers of olfactory receptor cells with cilia. There is no known treatment of URI-related olfactory dysfunction, although it is important to rule out nasal/sinus disease involvement.[181] There have been suggestions that alpha lipoic acid treatment supports regeneration of olfactory nerves to restore olfactory perception after URI-related olfactory dysfunction.[182] However, the effects of the treatment cannot be separated from spontaneous recovery of olfactory functioning and the treatment has neither stood the challenge of double-blinded placebo control trial nor shown a dose-related response to improve olfactory functioning. Most patients with URI-related olfactory loss show olfactory improvement, although noticeable improvement may take years.[183] Patients with URI-related olfactory loss (and head trauma) may exhibit dysosmia (the distortion of an odor when an odor is present), which subsides over time. Prevention of upper respiratory tract infections (or the flu) may be the best way to avoid the risk of olfactory dysfunction. Individuals with infection from the human immunodeficiency virus early in the disease process show elevated olfactory thresholds that may be related to respiratory tract infections[184,185] and declines in olfactory identification that parallels disorders that are associated with the development of Acquired Immunodeficiency Syndrome.[184,186]

The viruses that cause URI can also damage taste from individual areas of cranial nerve innervation (eg, loss of taste on the anterior tongue). The individual would not report a loss of ability to taste salt, sweet, sour, or bitter, but as stated previously, the spatial loss, if severe enough, could alter the balance in taste, oral somatosensory, and retronasal sensation. In fact, some taste qualities could be diminished yet whole-mouth oral sensations could remain intact due to interactions between cranial nerves innervating the oral cavity for taste.[187]

Pathologies of the Middle Ear

A number of pathologies damage the chorda tympani nerve as it passes through the middle ear (eg, otitis media). Some surgeries also damage the chorda tympani nerve (eg, acoustic neuroma surgery). Patients with pathological or surgical damage of the chorda tympani nerve show unilateral or bilateral taste impairment to the anterior tongue for one or all taste qualities, depending on the extent of the nerve damage.[60,188] However, patients rarely report a change in taste perception even when the chorda tympani nerve is cut. Whole-mouth taste perception is maintained because the remaining taste nerves apparently compensate for the loss of taste in one area of the mouth. In fact, surgical or experimental manipulation of the chorda tympani nerve can result in increased taste sensations from the area innervated by cranial nerve IX; this may be the basis of dysgeusia that results from nerve stimulation and not from a substance present in the mouth.

Head Trauma

Head trauma can cause more severe chemosensory losses than either URIs or nasal sinus disease.[114] In aged individuals, head trauma often results from falls. The incidence of anosmia in those with head trauma range from as low as 5% to 60%.[189] A direct relationship exists between severity of brain injury and the degree of olfactory dysfunction in closed head injuries.[190] More severe head trauma results in a higher frequency of anosmia, especially in those injuries involving frontal and occipital blows.[191] The mechanisms for head injury–related olfactory loss involve peripheral damage to the olfactory nerves and the nose and central damage to the olfactory centers in the brain.[191] The most common cause of olfactory loss is thought to be the severing of the olfactory nerves where they pass through the cribriform plate of the ethmoid bone as the result of the coup-contra-coup forces (impact causes the brain to bump the opposite side of the skull).[192] Patients with head trauma–related olfactory dysfunction can show disorganization of cells in the olfactory epithelium and few olfactory cilia that reach the epithelial surface[9] and damage to the olfactory bulb and tracts and the inferior frontal lobes.[193] Only a few patients (up to 35%) show slight improvements in olfactory perception over time.[183,193]

Head trauma can also cause complete taste loss, but the incidence is very low (0.4% to 0.5%).[192] More common is spatial taste loss.[194] Head trauma may damage the chorda tympani nerve more frequently than the glossopharyngeal nerve because the former is more vulnerable to injury where it passes through the temporal bone.[192] Because of the compensating interactions between the taste nerves, patients do not usually complain of taste loss with head trauma unless the loss is extensive.

Chronic Nasal and Sinus Diseases

Chronic nasal and sinus diseases are associated with swollen tissues, polyps, tumors, and deformities, all of which can obstruct the odorant from traveling through the nasal passages to the olfactory epithelium.[145] Olfactory impairment from chronic nasal and sinus disease involves conduction loss (ie, inflammation inhibiting odorant binding to receptors) and changes to the olfactory receptors and epithelium because olfactory functioning is rarely fully recovered with pharmacological and surgical treatment of the underlying nasal and sinus disease.[110] Conductive causes of olfactory dysfunction are treatable and differentiated from nonconductive causes with oral steroids.[181] According to the National Health Interview Survey of 1994, 15% of older adults report chronic sinusitis.[195] Age is also associated with increased nasal resistance (decreased nasal airflow), physical changes in the nasopharynx, and the relationship between nasal and pulmonary airflow.[196] Allergic rhinitis can elevate olfactory thresholds via modifying the amount and chemical composition of the mucus secretion;[197] the allergic response;[198] and the level of inflammation in the sinus tissues.[199] Individuals with allergic rhinitis may also have greater risk of viral infections as a cause of olfactory dysfunction.[200] Up to 23% of individuals who suffer from allergic rhinitis suffer from elevated olfactory thresholds,[199] and according to the National Health Interview Survey of 1994, 8% of older adults report allergic rhinitis without asthma.[195]

Nasal/sinus disease may be the only treatable form of olfactory dysfunction. Diagnosis of this condition must be done by an otolaryngologist and usually includes the patient history, physical examination, and CT scans.[201] There is a good correspondence between self-reported olfactory dysfunction and measured dysfunction in individuals with olfactory dysfunction associated with chronic nasal/sinus disease.[110] If patients notice fluctuations in their sense of smell with exacerbation of nasal/sinus conditions, they may benefit from aggressive therapy to prevent the olfactory disturbances associated with more chronic conditions. Medical management of nasal/sinus disease includes controlling the causes of the inflammation (eg, allergens causing allergic rhinitis, nasal infections) and level of the inflammation (eg, systemic or topical corticosteroids).[110] Some nasal/sinus diseases require surgical interventions (eg, severe sinusitis and nasal polyposis). Just over half of the individuals with progressive sinusitis had olfactory improvements with endoscopic sinus surgery.[202]

Menopause

Diminished estrogen may influence taste and olfactory functioning and the normal balance of oral sensation. A synthesis of cross-sectional data suggests that taste is upregulated in women during childbearing age and then declines across menopause.[2] There are significantly fewer supertasters among elderly than young women.[38] Although hormone replacement has been hypothesized to aid in the preservation of olfactory functioning with aging, it has not been shown to produce improved performance on a variety of olfactory tests.[203]

Neurodegenerative Disorders

Olfactory dysfunction is reported in a wide range of neurodegenerative disorders, including Alzheimer's disease (AD), Parkinson's disease (PD) (and variants), Huntington's disease, and Down's syndrome,[132] as shown through a meta-analysis of 43 studies.[204] Olfactory dysfunction appears to be an early marker in those at risk for developing AD,[205] and most patients with AD have but are unaware of olfactory dysfunction.[128] Performance on odor identification corresponds closely with brain areas involved in the neuropathology of AD, and thus these olfactory tests should be added to the battery of tests to diagnoses probable AD.[206] Olfactory testing can assist in the differential diagnosis of AD versus depression and affective disorders.[207] The cause appears to be more than just a central nervous system disruption. Olfactory dysfunction provides an early marker for AD and PD, before there is marked brain disorganization and the level of dysfunction may be related to the disease progression in AD but not to that in PD. There appears to be a genetic vulnerability to olfactory dysfunction in AD related to the presence of a particular variant of the apolipoprotein E allele.[208]

Olfactory dysfunction is seen in 9 of 10 individuals with PD (a rate that exceeds the presence of tremors, a hallmark sign of PD), and they are unaware of the dysfunction.[209] The severity of PD does not correspond with the degree of olfactory dysfunction. Medications used to treat PD do not improve olfactory functioning.[132] Olfactory dysfunction may precede loss of motor function in individuals with a high-risk of developing PD.[210]

Systemic Diseases

A number of diseases have been associated with smell, taste, and oral somatosensory disorders. However, this association is often drawn from patient reports and is without valid measures of functioning. The level of impairment associated with these chronic diseases may relate to the severity of the disease, how the disease complications impair the sensory processes, and the side effects of the medications. Also, these chronic diseases impair nutritional health, which can also affect sensory functioning. The following is a review of some of the systemic diseases and the associated smell, taste, and oral somatosensory alterations.

Individuals with liver disease show elevated detection and recognition thresholds for both odorants[211] and tastes.[211,212] Recovery from the illness or correcting the nutrient deficiency (eg, vitamin A)[211] may improve functioning.[178] One study reported increases in taste and smell sensitivity for some compounds from pre to post liver transplantation for end-stage liver disease; the changes may relate to improvements in health and nutritional status and medications.[213]

Individuals on hemodialysis or peritoneal dialysis had significantly higher olfactory thresholds than matched controls; the level of olfactory impairment correlated with the severity of disease.[214] The renal transplantation patients did not show threshold elevations. Dialysis patients have a high frequency of complaints about food "taste" and enjoyment. The response may be hedonic[178] or sensory. Patients with chronic renal failure had fewer taste buds per fungiform papilla than healthy controls[215] (although it is not clear if the two groups differed in density of fungiform papillae, which varies genetically). Taste thresholds of individuals on continuous ambulatory peritoneal dialysis were higher for NaCl and bitter than age- and sex-matched controls.

Patients with cancer frequently report changes in the taste of food and changes in appetite. The cancer itself does not appear to cause a reduction in taste or olfactory perception unless it directly interrupts receptor sites or neural transmission.[76] Cancer therapies can alter smell, taste, and oral somatosensation. More research is needed on the influence of cancer (and its therapies) on olfactory perception. Ophir et al.[216] did report olfactory impairment extending beyond 6 months after radiation therapy. Chemotherapy, through eliciting nausea and vomiting, can cause conditioned food aversions. Because of the psychophysical errors in the study procedures, taste changes with chemotherapy are difficult to determine. Olfactory changes with chemotherapy have not really been investigated. Radiation therapy, especially if localized to the head and neck region, can result in "blindness of the mouth"[23] although the loss is not seen in all individuals; some may actually show intensified taste sensations.[76]

The effects of the neuropathic and vascular complications of diabetes appear to influence the level of chemosensory dysfunction. For example, individuals with diabetes mellitus complicated by macrovascular disease show higher risk of olfactory impairment, as measured with an odor identification task.[217] Individuals with type I diabetes with neuropathy have higher reported xerostomia and decreased salivary flow rates than matched controls;[218] these changes to oral health could diminish taste and retronasal olfaction. In type 2 diabetes, hedonic response to sweet beverages may be a function of dietary intake[219] as well as level of blood sugar control.[220] Higher preference was seen in those with greater intake of sweet foods and higher serum glucose. There also may be a genetic taste link to diabetes and resultant patterns of food preferences. In comparison with PROP supertasters, nontasters report less intensity from sucrose, greater preference for and intake of sweet foods,[221] and are more likely to be obese.[38]

An extensive list of diseases and conditions associated with olfactory disorders is provided by Murphy and colleagues.[110] For example, olfactory disorders are also reported with a number of psychiatric disorders, including schizophrenia.[132] Some diseases decrease olfactory perception by changing the quantity and quality of the mucus secretion and, thus, physically or chemically modifying olfactory perception.[222] For example, patients with cystic fibrosis exhibit olfactory dysfunction. This disease changes the chemical make-up and viscosity of mucus secretions, which impedes the odorant from reaching the olfactory receptors. Individuals with Sjögren's syndrome can complain of taste and olfactory problems[39] because the disease impairs salivary gland and mucus production. Sjögren's syndrome can elevate taste thresholds but leave the ability to perceive real-world taste concentrations (ie, suprathreshold concentrations) unimpaired.[39] Although orthonasal olfaction does not appear abnormal in Sjögren's syndrome as measured by an olfactometer,[223] retronasal olfaction could be blunted if the impaired oral secretions limit the release and active transport of food volatiles to the olfactory receptors.

Exposures

A number of airborne compounds, toxic metals, irritant gases, and solvents are toxic to the olfactory system and impair olfactory perception indirectly (impeding the flow of odorants to the olfactory receptors) or directly (damaging the olfactory epithelium and/or central olfactory processing).[224]

Medications

The elderly are at risk for drug-nutrient interactions because they often take multiple medications to control chronic diseases. It is important to determine whether or not medications influence food intake in older adults through the alteration of chemosensory perception. Medications that alter taste and olfactory perception have been reviewed,[225] including those used to treat hypertension and hyperlipidemia.[226] Following is a description and summary of some of the effects of medication on taste, smell, and oral somatosensation.

Medications could have a direct effect on these sensory processes by impairing the transport of stimulus to the receptor and changing the peripheral structures and sensory transduction mechanisms. For example, medications with the side effect of xerostomia and/or drying of the nasal mucous membranes could hinder the tastant or odorant from reaching the receptors. This could result in diminished olfactory or taste perception, although this has not been shown clinically. Xerostomia can increase the risk of oral infections and periodontal disease and produce altered taste (ie, dysgeusia) and oral pain.[143] Medications can enter the mouth through the saliva[227] and gingival fluid[228] to produce a dysgeusia (the quality of which may be bitter to match the usual taste of medications), an olfactory sensation,[229] and even other sensations (eg, metallic). Medications that are not introduced to or through the mouth but rather in the blood may also stimulate taste (venous taste phenomenon)[230] or olfactory sensations.[229]

Medications can influence our preference for foods through conditioned aversions. Conditioned food aversions can occur with medications that induce nausea and vomiting:[231] the individual associates the discomfort of the nausea and vomiting with the food eaten directly before the illness, even if the cause of the illness was not the food. These aversions are reported frequently in the literature as one mechanism for the loss of appetite and the change in preference for foods as the result of cancer and its therapies.

The clinician should take caution in interpreting the reports of chemosensory changes with medications.[226] Patient reports may represent a combination of sensory and nonsensory issues, as well as confusions between taste, olfaction, and somatosensory changes. Thorough investigations on the effect of medications on chemosensory mechanisms, including studies with valid psychophysical measurements to characterize the threshold and suprathreshold influences of medications, are yet to be completed. Each patient should receive an individual assessment of sensory-related complaints. Careful interviewing of the patient will help the clinician determine if the change is sensory or nonsensory. Working with the health care team and changing medications might alleviate some of the complaints and lower the risk of drug-nutrition interactions.

Oral Health

Oral health is necessary for adequate oral sensations. Ship[143] provides a review of some of the oral conditions that can alter oral taste and smell, including infections, oral lesions, xerostomia, poorly fitting dental prostheses, and oral problems associated with systemic disease. Changes to oral health in the elderly are primarily due to diseases/conditions and accompanying treatments rather than changes due to old age.[143] Tobacco and alcohol addiction also diminish taste and olfactory perception through decreases in oral health. These conditions can cause dysosmia (smelling the infection in the mouth), dysgeusia (tasting the by-products of the oral infection), and diminished retronasal olfactory sensations.

IMPACT OF NUTRITIONAL STATUS ON CHEMOSENSORY FUNCTION IN AGING

Nutritional deficiencies or toxicities could influence any of the neurological or biochemical processes in smell, taste, and oral somatosensation. However, as reviewed,[232] chemosensory disturbances are not consistently seen with minimal malnutrition and instead are associated with marked nutritional deficiencies or toxicities. Indeed an intervention to improve nutrient intake and lean body mass in frail elderly resulted in improved lean body mass and improvement of nutritional status without any change in measured or perceived olfactory perception.[233]

However, a special note on zinc is required. Zinc deficiency has been associated with taste loss; zinc supplementation may improve taste perception in individuals with zinc deficiency related to chronic diseases[234,235] and in head and neck cancer treated with irradiation.[236] It may be that the disease[237] or other nutrient deficiencies (eg, magnesium[235] and/or protein status)[238] may be more important than zinc nutrition to maintain taste functioning. However, most of the studies on taste and nutritional status are conducted with threshold measures that may not indicate ability to perceive tastes usual to foods and beverages. Thus, the documented taste disorders may have little association with food behaviors.[212]

Individuals show taste and olfactory disorders without dietary inadequacies or obvious nutritional risk.[239,240] Thus, does the zinc deficiency cause taste and olfactory disturbances in the elderly? Zinc supplementation for otherwise healthy individuals with chemosensory disorders appears to be of no benefit. Most individuals who have taken zinc for chemosensory disorders report no improvement in their condition[241] and show no difference in sensory function than those not taking zinc.[114] The ineffectiveness of zinc supplementation for chemosensory functioning was also demonstrated in two, double-blinded studies.[242,243] Lower zinc status also was not associated with taste acuity in elderly subjects.[244] However, elderly individuals with biochemically measured zinc deficiency may show improved taste acuity with zinc supplementation.[245] In summary, the benefit of zinc supplementation to improve food flavor perception in the elderly is still not substantiated. Olfactory perception shows the greatest age-related dysfunction, yet the benefit of zinc supplementation to olfactory functioning is questionable. It remains unclear whether aged individuals would notice improved oral sensory functioning in response to the zinc supplementation and if this improvement would have a positive impact on their dietary behaviors.

IMPACT OF SMELL, TASTE, AND ORAL SOMATOSENSATION ON NUTRITION IN AGING

The sensory qualities of food play an important role in influencing what we choose to eat. Olfactory information may be critical in shaping what we like to eat because it allows the exact identification of foods and beverages. Orthonasal olfaction can stimulate appetite through perceiving food odors in the environment. Once food is in the mouth, taste, retronasal olfaction, and somatosensory sensations combine to provide the composite sensation of flavor. Our preference for foods and beverages smelled through the nostril may be very different than our preference for foods and beverages experienced as the composite sensation of flavor.[20] For example, the Jamaican fruit "stinking toe" has a very unpleasant aroma but, when placed in the mouth, produces a wonderful sensation.

Very little of food preference is innate. Human beings are born liking sweet and disliking bitter.[246] The rest of our food likes and dislikes are learned[247] using sensory experiences from the food world. We couple the flavor of food with a positive learning experience.[248,249] An olfactory flavor of a food is liked because it is paired with sweetness, a quality we are predisposed to liking. Basic to life is learning to like foods and beverages that provide a source of energy. Negative learning also occurs and produces food dislikes. We couple the specific olfactory flavor of a food with the negative experience of nausea and vomiting;[250] these learned food aversions can be very powerful and last years. It is important to note that sociocultural factors can modulate the biological factors that drive food likes and dislikes, and, thus, what is actually consumed.[251]

The question of interest is whether or not the oral sensory profile of the food and beverage world changes enough with aging to change food preferences and the patterns of food selection that have developed over a lifetime. Theoretically, oral sensations from foods and beverages change across aging because of repeated exposures to the aforementioned diseases/conditions or the aging process itself. Older adults may have different patterns of food preferences than young adults in part because of oral sensory changes. If the changes to oral sensation are extreme enough to be noticed, an older adult may report changes in the desire to eat as well as the satiety responses to the food and beverage sensations (sensory-specific satiety). A change in food preference, appetite, cravings, and satiety response could ultimately influence food selection and nutritional status parameters, such as body weight and the ability to manage diet-related chronic diseases. The hypothesized association between changes in smell, taste, and oral somatosensation; dietary behaviors; and nutritional status is shown in Figure 7–5.[252]

Some of the research on the impact of age-related changes in oral sensation and dietary behaviors comes from individuals who sought help for taste, smell, or oral sensory complaints from the few National Institutes of Health–funded clinical research centers that specialized in taste and smell disorders. These individuals were troubled enough by their disorders to seek out one of a few of these centers, even if there was little hope for a cure. Most reported changing their eating habits because of the disorder, although the specific response varied. Applying the nutrition findings from this group of health-seeking individuals to the elderly is not appropriate. The elderly may neither notice nor seek medical treatment for olfactory and oral sensory changes. They also may merely maintain food habits that were established over their lifetime. Other research on the impact of age-related changes in oral sensation and dietary behaviors comes from studies on healthy, free-living older adults compared to younger cohorts.

Older adults could consciously or unconsciously modify well-established food preferences

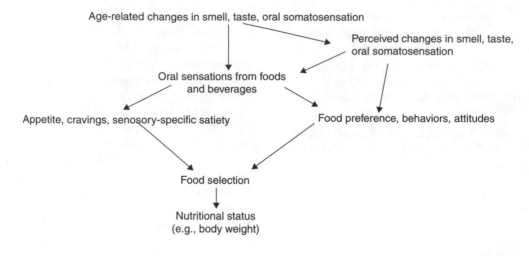

Figure 7–5 Hypothesized Association Between Age-related Changes in Smell, Taste, and Oral Somatosensation; Dietary Behaviors; and Nutritional Status

and behaviors in response to changes in oral sensation. The modification could fit two extreme patterns as seen in patients who seek treatment for taste, smell, and somatosensory disorders: "indiscriminate eating" and "compensation eating."[253] These patterns serve only as a description of the potential nutritional response to age-related changes.

Indiscriminate Eating

Older adults with changes in oral sensation eat less for pleasure. They experience less olfactory cues to stimulate appetite. The flavor of food is diminished and everything has a "blah" flavor. This decreases enjoyment of eating and may decrease the drive for flavor diversity (ie, decreased sensory-specific satiety).[254] Nutritional risk could result if the diet becomes monotonous, decreasing the ability to meet nutritional requirements and, in the extreme, causing weight loss.

Compensation Eating

The older adult with changes in oral sensation uses sensory and nonsensory strategies to maintain enjoyment of eating. This may include relying on the taste (eg, sweet foods) and creamy components of food for enjoyment. Nutritional risk could occur with excessive intake of sweet and high-fat foods, causing an energy imbalance and increasing the risk of obesity. In the nonsensory domain, the individual may select food more for its ability to maintain health and manage chronic disease than for sensory qualities.

The following questions related to this conceptual model and general nutrition patterns need to be addressed:

1. Do the elderly notice changes in olfactory perception and oral sensation with aging and how does the awareness influence nutritional outcomes?
2. Do olfactory dysfunction and resultant changes in oral sensation influence food preference and food intake in elderly individuals?
3. Do these changes increase nutritional risk in elderly individuals?

Self-rated Olfactory and Oral Sensory Changes with Aging

One's perception of health and changes with aging can provide a useful proxy for measured health status, an understanding of the processes through which an individual evaluates and acts on symptoms, and a historical complement to a single measure of functioning. Study of these perceptions will ultimately enhance the understanding of how olfactory and oral sensory changes affect nutritional health and eating enjoyment. Indeed, questions about oral sensation to detect nutrition problems appear in the Minimum Data Set (Version 2.0) resident assessment instrument for long-term care facilities,[255] section K on oral/nutritional status, such as the following:

> Complaints about the taste of many foods— The sense of taste can change as a result of health conditions or medications. Also, complaints can be culturally based—eg someone used to eating spicy foods may find nursing facility meals bland.

Data from the National Geographic Survey (1.2 million responses, 20% over the age of 60 years) show a decline in self-reported smell perception with increasing age.[10] Males rated smell perception lower at each age from teens to the ninth decade, whereas with females, mean rating increased to a peak rating in the fourth decade and then declined at a slope equal to that of males. Although ratings of olfactory perception show age-associated declines, many of the elderly do not notice major olfactory impairments.[128] Ship and Weiffenbach[119] examined the sensitivity and specificity of self-rated olfactory functioning and found that impaired individuals were less likely to report a dysfunction and that normosmic individuals were unlikely to complain of an olfactory dysfunction. However, Murphy et al[11] contend that self-rated olfactory abilities underestimate the prevalence of olfactory dysfunction.

Most individuals who seek treatment for olfactory dysfunction report that food is less flavorful and less enjoyable.[239,256] Foods and beverages present a complex mixture of stimuli. "Normal" taste, smell, and somatosensory sensations blend into a composite perceptual experience. With a change in ability to perceive some

or all of the olfactory components, the taste and somatosensory components may become more apparent. For example, dark chocolate may have a subtle blending of rich chocolately notes, plus the correct balance of the bitter cocoa with sweetness. Removing the retronasal chocolate input may only exaggerate the bitterness of the chocolate, even in the presence of sweetness. The reports of olfactory flavor changes with aging vary. Stevens[257] reports the responses of younger and older participants ($n = 276$) to the following "yes/no" questions:

1. Do you have a problem tasting?
2. Do you have a problem smelling?
3. Have you noticed changes in tastes of foods?
4. Do you enjoy food?

The food complaints appear low considering the large olfactory loss displayed with aging: only 17% of the elderly subjects answered "yes" to one or more of questions 1–3 and/or "no" to question 4; only 5.8% of the total complained of weakened food enjoyment all or some of the time. In contrast, nearly the entire younger group stated that eating is a great pleasure. The elderly individuals who reported "yes" to the preceeding questions attributed the problem to a lifelong lack of interest in food, restricted diets, the expense of foods, and denture problems.

A study of reportedly healthy elderly females ($n = 101$) included self-ratings of smell, taste, ability to sense the flavor of food, vision, and hearing at the time of the interview compared to when they were 30 to 35 years of age.[258] Although a seven-point categorical scale was used to solicit responses (extremely weaker–the same–extremely stronger), responses were folded into "loss," "no change," and "improved" categories (Figure 7–6). Ratings of loss of taste, smell, and flavor were much less than that for vision and hearing. One interpretation of these findings is that the chemical senses are more robust across aging, although the loss of olfactory functioning is thought to parallel that of vision and hearing.[259] A more likely interpretation

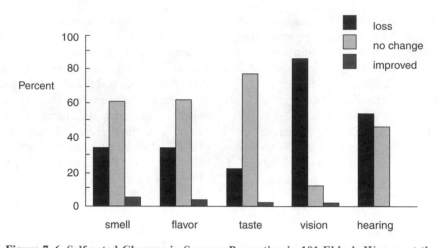

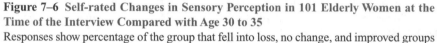

Figure 7–6 Self-rated Changes in Sensory Perception in 101 Elderly Women at the Time of the Interview Compared with Age 30 to 35
Responses show percentage of the group that fell into loss, no change, and improved groups

is olfactory functioning is not part of usual screening for older adults and they are unaware of the losses. Nonetheless, one of two elderly women reported a loss of ability to perceive odors and/or food flavors with aging. The same group had olfactory testing after rating their sensory abilities. Nearly half had olfactory dysfunction measured orthonasally (butanol threshold, odor identification task)[90] and/or retronasally[142] as reported.[260] At least 1 in 2 women were correct in rating their measured functioning as normal or dysfunctional, although approximately 1 in 6 women were in each of the discordant groups (reported loss with no measured dysfunction, reported no change with measured dysfunction).

The self-rating of sensory function requires individuals to evaluate their own sense of well-being, rate a perceptual experience, and, in relation to aging, compare current function to that of an earlier age. White and Kurtz.[261] contend that young and elderly are equally unable to assess their olfactory abilities correctly, but that each age group makes a different type of error in self-assessment. In patients who reported chemosensory disturbances, young patients underestimated their abilities while elderly patients seemed unaware of the deficit. Because this entails private and subjective responses, the quality

of the result ultimately relies on individuals being able to accurately rate their impression. Discordance between rated and measured perception could stem from an unwillingness to disclose the sensory loss, or the rate and magnitude of the loss. The individuals' attention to their sensory function or to their own health could also affect the discrepancy between rated and measured sensory function. Some elderly may not want to admit a loss of smell perception or may assume their smell function is good considering their age. Individuals may notice a sudden loss (as with an insult such as head trauma) or a problem temporarily related to the sense of smell more than the gradual loss of smell associated with aging. Indeed, those with sinusitis and diminished olfactory sensitivity do report impairments.[128] In aging, if the amount of loss exceeds a certain theoretical point, a person would notice it even if the decline occurred gradually. Finally, some people may not assign value to their sense of smell or may not exhibit overall health-seeking tendencies. Therefore, they may just assume that their sense of smell is adequate without really giving it any thought.

Having individuals rate their perception of physical difficulty may help determine the impact this difficulty has on health outcomes. For example, the perception of difficulty in chewing a food with any type of prosthesis was a larger determinant of food acceptance than actual mastication abilities.[262] An individual's perception of a chemosensory disorder potentates the negative effects on nutrition;[263] in a group of individuals who sought treatment for a chemosensory disorder, greater nutritional risk (eg, weight changes) was seen in individuals who reported that the disorder changed their interest in eating or felt that eating exacerbated the disorder. Comparison of self-rated and measured olfactory abilities related to food intake and body weight is discussed in the following section.

Food Preference and Age-related Changes to Smell and Oral Sensation

Most odors that we experience are complex mixtures of odorants. A change in the ability to perceive one or some of the odor molecules could change the hedonic response to the stimulus. For example, the elderly may rate characteristically unpleasant odors (eg, the smell of sulfur) as pleasant[10] because they are unable to perceive some of the odor compounds in the mercaptans that give it an unpleasant odor quality.

Most individuals who seek treatment for olfactory dysfunction report using food and non food related strategies to maintain food appreciation.[239] The most common strategies involved the use of primary taste qualities, spices, and trigeminal stimulants,[239] especially increased used of salt and/or sugar.[263] The taste or somatosensory properties of food may carry more importance in determining food preference and intake in individuals with olfactory impairment. We reported that elderly females with poorer olfactory functioning reported less preference for and intake of foods with strong sour (eg, citrus fruits) and bitter (eg, Brasicca vegetables) tastes.[260] With olfactory dysfunction, the sour or bitter taste may become more apparent and make the food less appealing. Texture is also an important component of food acceptance, being rated as the most important component of food identification and food enjoyment in individuals with congenital anosmia.[264]

An older person with olfactory dysfunction or oral sensory changes may compensate for changes in smell and oral sensation by preferring foods with a pleasant primary taste, those with a stronger olfactory component, or even those with a pungent sensation. Some of these preference patterns have been shown experimentally. Relating to compensating with pleasant tastes, elderly subjects report higher concentrations of salt and sweet as more preferable than do younger subjects.[265] However, in a preliminary study comparing NaCl sensory and hedonic responses to solution and chicken broth varying in levels of NaCl, aged females reported greater saltiness from and greater aversion to concentrated samples than the young did,[66] possibly due to age-related increases in irritation from release of inhibition on the trigeminal nerve.[68] Hedonic ratings converged with measures of intake; from 3-day diet records, aged females consumed less Na adjusted for body composition and reported less frequent use of added NaCl compared to young females.[70] In agreement, salt preferences have been shown to decrease with advancing age[266] and intake of salty snacks fell with age.[267] Another study showed that the aged gave lower hedonic ratings for 0.64 M NaCl in broth than the young; however, differences in intensity of concentrated NaCl across age groups were not shown.[69] The latter study employed a categorical scale and must be interpreted cautiously given the scaling issues addressed earlier.

Elderly adults may compensate for olfactory loss by preferring and consuming more sweets. In a sample of free-living elderly women, those with the poorest sense of smell reported the most frequent intake of sweet and high-fat foods.[260] Interestingly, elderly people with probable AD also show higher preference for sweets than do those without this dementia.[268] Although the researchers suggested a neurochemical basis for this pattern of food preference, olfactory dysfunction, an early marker for AD, may also contribute to this sweet preference. The combination of sweet and fat is pleasurable for many but may be especially so in those with olfactory impairment.[260] However, preference ratings for sweet foods in the elderly may not always predict intake of foods that are high in added sugar. De Jong et al.[269] found that although elderly subjects had greater preference for higher sucrose concentrations than young in a laboratory setting, this did not translate to greater sweet intake by elderly subjects in a naturalistic setting. We also observed that elderly females reported greater preference for high-fat sweets than young females yet reported consuming these foods least frequently.[270] A high level of cognitive restraint may cause discordance between preference and intake patterns, especially among health-seeking older adults.[271]

Older adults may have a greater preference for high-fat foods related to greater oral tactile sensations than do young adults, according to preliminary findings from our laboratory. In comparison with young females, elderly females showed chorda tympani taste losses but increased creamy sensations from high-fat foods.[68] The increased creamy sensations could arise from a release of inhibition on the trigeminal nerve. Because heightened creaminess is associated with increased preference (except for genetic supertasters),[38] older adults reported highest preference for high-fat foods. Preferences appeared to influence intake of dietary fat; older women consume more energy from fat and consumed high-fat meats and breakfast foods most frequently compared with young women.[68] Other studies support that aging combined with exposure to taste-related pathology increases preference for fat. Men over 30 years of age and with a history of severe otitis media report higher preferences for high-fat foods and have greater adiposity than those without this history.[272] Those reporting exposure to pathology that damages taste from cranial nerves VII and IX reported greatest preference for high-fat foods and had highest adiposity.[273]

Despite suggestions that individuals with olfactory dysfunction may find food less appealing due to more apparent bitter/sour qualities in the absence of olfactory components,[260] experimental findings and preliminary findings from our laboratory show that the elderly may have a greater range of food preferences because of

changes in olfactory perception. Experimentally, Pelchat[274] showed that older adults with measured olfactory dysfunction are less finicky and more willing to try novel food items. In a later study, this author[275] provided evidence for poorer olfactory perception in the willingness of the elderly to try novel food. Elderly with diminished ability to smell were more willing to try novel foods with unpleasant smells.

Being less finicky could present risks and benefits to the elderly. As a risk, older adults may be less able to use olfactory cues to tell that foods are spoiled and be more willing to eat these foods. As a benefit, older adults may be more willing to make their diets more healthful. Warwick and Schiffman[276] found that elderly people were less aware of changes in level of fat in milk products. In their study, both elderly and young rated liking for sweet/fat and salt/fat mixtures that varied in the level of fat. The level of fat did not influence preference for these mixtures in the elderly; the younger subjects showed differing preference with variation in level of fat in these mixtures. These findings suggest that decreasing the level of fat in diets of older adults does not have to disrupt food enjoyment.

Preliminary data from our laboratory supports that older adults may be more willing to consume vegetables that may have odor notes that are less pleasant (eg, sulfur notes in Brassica vegetables) or bitter taste qualities. Aged females reported greater liking and consumption of bitter foods (beverages, fruits, and vegetables) compared to young females.[270] The aged females in this study perceived less bitterness and/or sourness from quinine hydrochloride solutions, espresso, and grapefruit juice;[270] age-related decreases in bitter sensation are well accepted.[160,162,277] Because bitter sensations are known to decrease with age, loss of olfactory function may not always be a deterrence to consuming bitter foods/beverages, as suggested,[260] if the olfactory loss makes only very dim sensations of bitterness more apparent. Evidence exists supporting the idea that age-related losses of bitter sensation influence increased preference and intake of bitters in the aged.[266] PROP tasting also influences bitter acceptance and intake and these effects appear to be separate from aging, yet PROP effects persist across age cohorts.[278] Whereas acceptance and intake of bitters increases with age, both decrease with PROP bitterness. Age-by-PROP interactions could have implications for cancer as suggested by associations between colon polyps, PROP bitterness, and vegetable intake in older men.[279]

Appetite, Craving, and Satiety in Olfactory Dysfunction

Olfactory dysfunction can disrupt dietary behaviors[280] and cause loss of appetite and weight[281] in animals. In humans, the relationship between appetite and olfactory dysfunction is not consistent. Up to 48% of individuals seen for a chemosensory disturbance report a decreased appetite with the onset of the disorder.[256] In this same sample, food aversions were highest in those with multiple chemosensory disorders and altered taste or olfactory sensations, such as dysgeusia and paromsia.[256] Some researchers claim that chemosensory losses play a major role in the anorexia often observed in elderly people.[282] However, in a sample of free-living elderly women, even those with poorest olfactory function did not report less enjoyment of food or a poor appetite.[260]

Appetite or the desire to eat a food can be separate from ratings of preference, according to recent investigation.[283] Free-living elderly individuals and those from a long-term care facility reported the preference for liquid meal supplements. Both groups gave preference ratings for the supplement close to that of regular foods. Consumption of the supplements was better when the elderly were in groups instead of being alone. Preference did not necessarily match willingness to consume the supplement.

The elderly appear to report less food cravings, as defined by an intense desire to eat a particular food.[284] In an experimental study with young and elderly men and women, Pelchat and Schaefer[284] looked at number of cravings in response to sensory deprivation with a monotonous diet (complete liquid supplement). Young females and males had an increased number of cravings in response to the monotonous diet; elderly females did not. Interestingly, the elderly subjects had lower olfactory sensitivity (threshold measure) and olfactory sensitivity correlated with the craving response to the monotonous diet. That is, the greater the olfactory sensitivity, the more cravings. More research in this area is needed, yet these data do suggest the olfactory declines could increase the risk of monotonous, less diverse diets.

Food flavor could influence both the kinds of foods selected and the total food intake, possibly through "sensory-specific satiety."[254] According to this theory, as a person eats a food, the pleasantness of its flavor decreases while the pleasantness of other foods not consumed decreases much less or remains constant. Sensory-specific satiety has an effect on the quantity of food eaten at a meal[285] and may promote diversity of dietary intake. Therefore, olfactory dysfunction and a large change in flavor perception could modify the physiologic response to food, decrease the drive for flavor diversity, and increase the likelihood of consuming a monotonous diet.[286]

The association between olfactory perception and sensory-specific satiety in young and older subjects was tested by Rolls and McDermott.[287] In this study, subjects from four age cohorts (adolescent, young adult, middle-aged, and elderly) participated in sensory-specific satiety measures and in a standard measure of orthonasal olfaction (UPSIT-Scratch and Sniff Odor Identification Test).[126] For the sensory-specific satiety measures, subjects sampled and rated the pleasantness of the taste, odor, appearance, and texture of a number of foods (including the first serving of low-fat strawberry yogurt). They then consumed a second serving of low-fat strawberry yogurt and provided pleasantness ratings of eaten (yogurt) and uneaten foods (other sampled foods). Elderly subjects did not show sensory-specific satiety; they rated as much pleasantness and desire to eat the second serving of the strawberry yogurt as they did the first serving. Interestingly, there was no significant relationship between measured orthonasal olfaction and the sensory-specific response in the elderly (even though elderly subjects had lower olfactory functioning than was tested in the other age cohorts). However, the lack of association might relate to a combination of orthonasal and retronasal difficulties. Some of the middle-aged and elderly subjects wore dentures and these subjects did not appear to report as great a change in the "taste" of yogurt from first to second exposures. The presence of dentures could diminish retronasal olfaction (even more than that observed for orthonasal olfaction) and blunt the sensory-specific satiety response in the elderly subjects.

Intake and Body Weight and Age-related Changes in Olfaction and Oral Sensation

Most individuals who seek evaluation for a chemosensory disorder report that they change their eating habits in response to the chemosensory disorder,[239,256,263] yet report consuming an adequate nutrient intake (intakes >66% of the RDA).[239] Free-living elderly women with lower olfactory perception had higher intakes of nutrients that increase risk of heart disease (high intake of energy from saturated fat, lower polyunsaturated to saturated fat intake, higher total fat intake).[260] Those with olfactory dysfunction may also be less willing to cook for themselves or to eat a variety of foods.[260] The latter findings may emphasize the importance of senior meal opportunities that aim to provide older adults with at least one nourishing meal each day. Chemosensory changes with aging may be advantageous to some older adults. These changes may make it easier for the older adult to base food selection on the nutritional value of foods instead of only the sensory qualities.

Studies on the relationship between changes in smell and oral sensation come from those who seek medical attention for chemosensory disorders and free-living older adults. In clinical patients, Ferris and Duffy[239] found a strong relationship between a reported increased food intake, obesity, and smell dysfunction, especially in elderly females. Individuals with olfactory dysfunction and increased food intake often reported "not feeling satisfied with eating". "I eat more because I hope that the next bite will taste better." The association between olfactory dysfunction and weight gain was also uncovered by Mattes and Cowart.[256] Males may show a different association between weight and olfactory dysfunction. Ferris and Duffy[239] reported that of those males who were underweight, most were anosmic. A higher risk of weight loss was also observed in individuals who suffer from multiple chemosensory disorders[256] and burning mouth syndrome.[114]

The impact of measured olfactory dysfunction and interactions between measured and self-rated olfactory perception on food intake and adiposity were examined in a study of 80 free-living elderly women who reported good health.[258,260,288] Before olfactory testing, the women rated their sense of smell at the present time and changes in smell and food flavor since an earlier age. Retronasal olfaction was measured via a model food[142] and orthonasal functioning with a standard clinical measure.[90] Those with a poorer sense of smell (either orthonasal or retronasal) had less interest in food-related activities, more frequent intake of sweet foods, and greater intake of a diet that increases risk of cardiovascular disease (eg, higher energy from saturated fat) in an interviewed food frequency and dietary analysis of five, nonconsecutive food records.[260] The women were categorized into concordant and discordant groups based on the correspondence between measured and self-rated olfactory perception.[258,288] Those who had good retronasal sensitivity and rated a good sense of smell presented with the least nutritional risk, consuming the highest intakes of fruits and vegetables as well as high-fiber grains and seeds and having a normal body mass index. Women who perceived an olfactory dysfunction despite a normal measured function were significantly more likely to be obese and have more frequent intake of high-fat, salty meats and lower dietary diversity than those who had measured dysfunction or those who did not believe that they had an olfactory problem. These data suggest that perceiving the problem may be as much of a risk to good nutrition as having measured olfactory dysfunction, an effect seen previously as applied to dietary behaviors in measured and perceived chewing difficulty.[262]

ASSESSING CHEMOSENSORY COMPLAINTS IN OLDER ADULTS

An older person may complain food just does not "taste" good anymore. He or she may also report not enjoying eating. There are questions and psychophysical tools that dietetics practitioners can use to assess the chemosensory complaint or whether a chemosensory disorder contributes to the lack of enjoyment from eating. If a chemosensory dysfunction is suspected, additional physical examinations, including otolaryngological, neurological, and dental evaluations, can assess the probable cause of the disorder.

Determining If the Complaint Is Sensory or Nonsensory

Individuals may complain about the "taste" of foods for a number of reasons other than problems with chemosensory perception. Pleasure from eating and appetite can act separately from the sensory input of foods and beverages. Simple questions may help the clinician start to distinguish a sensory from a nonsensory problem.

Questions About the Complaint

- "What does the food 'taste' like to you? Can you taste salt, sweet, sour (for example, lemon or vinegar), and bitter (for example, strong coffee or even a medication)?" Answers to these questions help determine if the complaint is sensory and help rule out a taste problem.
- "How long have you had the problem? Was the change gradual or sudden?" Answers to these questions help determine if the complaint is a chronic versus an acute problem.
- "Do you associate the complaint with any specific problem?" Answers to this and the proceeding question may help determine if the condition is associated with one of the pathologies that cause chemosensory disorders. The question could then be expanded to request a history of specific chemosensory-related conditions.
- "Does the problem change . . . is the problem better on some days than others?" Individuals with olfactory dysfunction associated with nasal/sinus disease may report fluctuations in the ability to smell. Individuals may benefit from a complete evaluation by an otolaryngologist to rule out nasal/sinus disease, which is the only treatable cause of olfactory disorders.
- "Do odors smell as they should? Does, for example, peanut butter smell like peanut butter? Do you think you could tell what you were eating if your eyes were closed?" These questions address the sense of smell, not only diminished orthonasal olfaction, but also odor distortions and retronasal perception.
- "Do you have a persistent taste in your mouth, such as a persistent salt, sweet, sour, or bitter taste?" This question should help determine if the individual has a dysgeusia. The individual may not be able to describe the quality as salt, sweet, sour, or bitter and may instead describe the quality as something vague (eg, "yuck" or foul). This may be an olfactory sensation related to the smell of an infection.
- "Are you suffering from oral pain, burning, prickling, or numbness on your tongue or in your mouth?" These questions are designed to reveal a somatosensory disturbance associated with the "taste complaint." Individuals who respond positively to this question may benefit from further dental or medical evaluation.

Nutritional Consequences of the "Taste Complaint"

- "Have you changed your eating habits in response to the change in the way food 'tastes?' Are you avoiding any foods because of the problem? Have you changed the types of foods you eat since the problem started? Are you adding anything to your foods to make the 'taste' of the food any better?" A chemosensory disorder may have a negative impact on nutritional health if the individual complains of a chemosensory problem and/or complains that the problem has influenced his or her eating habits.[256]

- "Are you taking any vitamin, mineral, dietary supplements or using alternative therapies because of your disorder?" Individuals who present to clinical research centers with chemosensory disorders have reported frequent use of supplements.[239] Because these conditions are usually untreatable, individuals may turn to alternative therapies.
- "How is your appetite? Has your appetite changed since the problem started?"
- "Do you enjoy eating? Has your enjoyment of eating or activities related to food and eating changed since the problem started?"
- "Has your weight changed in response to the problem?"

The client may need to answer additional questions about the disorder and the nutritional outcomes to determine if the problem is sensory or nonsensory. These may include specific questions about feelings of health and happiness. Individuals may feel depressed because the disorder has disrupted their eating and food behaviors. With olfactory dysfunction, the older person may not feel as confident cooking or may stop entertaining friends and family because of decreased enjoyment in cooking. If the chemosensory dysfunction is disruptive enough to their feelings of well-being, they may need to seek assistance in coping with the disorder.[289]

Screening for Taste and Olfactory Functioning

The sense of taste is the easiest to test with stimuli readily available (table salt, sugar, sour—lemon or vinegar, and bitter—instant coffee crystals). Ask the individual to identify the taste of the four stimuli. Clinicians can also test taste spatially in a screening procedure,[76] especially to the anterior tongue (taste, chorda tympani nerve), using a salt (1 tsp salt in $\frac{1}{2}$ cup of water) and bitter (1 tsp instant coffee in 1 medicine cup of water) and having patients report the intensity on the gLMS (Figure 7–4), where the top of the scale is anchored to any sensation, not just oral sensations. Patients that report these stimuli as less than "weak" have probable taste damage.

A number of odor identification tasks are available to use in a clinical setting. The odor identification task from the Connecticut Chemosensory Clinical Research Center Test[90] can provide a low-cost olfactory screen. The odors are baby powder, chocolate, cinnamon, coffee, mothballs, peanut butter, Ivory® soap, and a trigeminal probe (Vicks Vapo-Steam®). Place the odor in a covered jar and conceal the stimulus to reduce nonolfactory cues. Have the subjects identify the odors from a list of odors and distracters.[90] Provide correct feedback and present misidentified items a second time. If subjects miss four out of the seven nontrigeminal odors (even after giving correct feedback and presenting missed items a second time), they have probable hyposmia and should have more in-depth olfactory evaluation by an otolaryngologist. Failure to identify Vicks (especially after feedback) suggests malingering rather than true olfactory loss.

The University of Pennsylvania Smell Identification Test (UPSIT)[126] is a commercially available test of olfactory functioning (Sensonics, Inc., Haddonfield, NJ) and includes 40 "scratch-and-sniff" odorants and a multiple-choice format. Normative data on a large number of subjects according to age and sex allows the determination of the level of olfactory functioning (ie, anosmia, hyposmia) and what the level is relative to age and sex. Individuals with olfactory dysfunction should be evaluated by an otolaryngologist.[290]

Olfactory tests that include measuring the perception of retronasal olfaction might more fully capture the sensory experience of eating. Clinicians can use jelly beans as a way to test retronasal olfaction (gourmet jelly beans may provide the best stimuli because olfactory components are distinctive). The first task is to distinguish taste from olfactory flavor. Have the clients sample the jelly bean with their noses plugged (avoid visual cues as to the flavor of the jelly bean). Then have the client unplug the nose and ask if the jelly bean "tastes" any differently. With the nose plugged, one should only be able to sense the taste and somatosensory cues from foods and beverages. However, opening the nostrils allows retronasal transport of the odorants to the olfactory epithelium. If clients do not notice a difference between the nose plugged and unplugged, they have impaired retronasal olfaction. Some individuals cannot fully plug their nostrils to inhibit retronasal olfactory sensation, thus, the jelly beans can also be used in an identification task. Select the jelly bean flavors that might be most familiar to your clients and set up a selection list that includes the correct labels and distracters. Be sure to give feedback and retest missed items to increase the chance of testing only olfactory perception. Misidentification of more than half of the jelly beans probably would constitute olfactory impairment in older adults. Heilmann and colleagues[137] developed a retronasal test kit of 20 foods in powder form (eg, spices, instant soups) that produced good test-retest reliability in healthy subjects; the test proved able to detect age-related losses in retronasal olfaction and thus may be a reasonable tool for retronasal olfactory assessment in a clinical setting.

The Complaint of Dysgeusia

Dysgeusias are very disturbing disorders to the individual and are difficult to diagnosis. They often do not have a treatment. In practice, clinicians can use a combination of questions and topical anesthesia as tools for diagnosing the origins of dysgeusia.[151] First, determine that the patient has a persistent taste. If the topical anesthetic abolishes the taste, then it may be that the dysgeusia results from something present in the mouth (eg, tasting an oral infection) or from a taste seeping into the mouth from the blood (as with a medication). Addressing the cause may alleviate the dysgeusia. If the taste is not changed

or is intensified by the topical anesthetic, it may be a centrally mediated phantom sensation. The clinician must take care in administering and assessing the results of the topical anesthetic.[151] If the effect of the anesthetic is not complete, an inappropriate conclusion may be drawn. To avoid this, test the thoroughness of the anesthesia by applying a taste stimulus. Care should be taken as well to avoid any adverse reactions, such as aspiration, from the topical anesthetic. There is some evidence that dysgeusias and phantom oral pains may respond to benzodiazepines.[65] The rationale for this treatment is that the oral pain is centrally mediated and possibly controlled through the trigeminal nucleus of the medulla. Taste appears to inhibit oral pain through gamma-amino butyric acid (GABA). Clonazepam, a GABA receptor agonist, intensifies the inhibition produced by GABA, and thus can suppress the oral pain and taste phantoms. An individual who has intensification of a dysgeusia from a topical anesthetic should have further medical and dental evaluation.

NUTRITIONAL INTERVENTIONS FOR CHEMOSENSORY DISORDERS IN THE ELDERLY

From the nutritional and chemosensory assessment, clinicians can create individualized nutritional care plans to help clients maintain their nutritional health and enjoyment of eating despite the olfactory impairment and changes in oral sensation. Individuals can utilize a number of strategies to compensate for loss. Because the ability to taste is stable with aging, the primary taste qualities of foods and beverages can be important predictors of food enjoyment. Sweet or salty foods, especially those that are also high in fat, may be particularly enjoyable to individuals with olfactory dysfunction. Changes in oral sensation may actually blunt the less pleasant flavors of some vegetables and fruits and increase their acceptance and intake in the elderly. Acceptance of fruits and vegetables can also be enhanced in the older adult with olfactory dysfunction by masking the bitterness with either salt[291] or sweet compounds.[277] Somatosensory sensations can also provide another dimension to a meal. Variation in the texture, the pungency, and the temperature of foods may help maintain interest in eating with diminished or absent olfactory cues. The color and presentation of food, or "eating with the eyes," may help stimulate appetite and food enjoyment, especially for those with olfactory dysfunction.

Using stronger olfactory flavorings in foods/beverages may provide a means to compensate for age-related decreases in olfactory oral sensations. de Graaf and colleagues[292] showed that elderly subjects, in comparison with young subjects, reported greater preference for many olfactory flavorings in common food products. A number of research studies have examined the impact of enhancing the flavor of foods on food intake and nutritional parameters in free-living older adults[293] and elderly long-term care residents.[294–296] Flavor intensification differs from the addition of spices, herbs, and salt, as reviewed by Schiffman,[297] to include adding odorants extracted from foods (natural) or synthesized or nonvolatile compounds that intensify existing odorants (eg, salt, sweet, MSG—the sodium salt of glutamic acid). In a cross-over controlled intervention study, Schiffman[298] found that seniors who participated in meals at a retirement center reported increases in aroma, overall liking, and overall satisfaction during a 4-week period of flavor- and MSG-enhanced foods (entrees, soups, sauces, vegetables, pastas) as compared with the unenhanced period. In an intervention study comparing young and elderly responses, free-living elderly were unaffected in pleasantness ratings of flavor-enhanced oat bran product (even though they had measured olfactory impairment) and the flavor enhancement did not result in the elderly consuming more of the product.[293] The young reported lowest preference ratings for and lowest intake of the product.

The strategies to compensate for the olfactory dysfunction may be critical to maintain nutritional health and food enjoyment in long-term care residents. The resident may be on a restricted diet, which could limit use of sweet and salty foods to compensate for sensory changes. Chewing and swallowing difficulties also limit the ability to use texture as a way to vary the sensory qualities of foods. Pureed food also may not have the vibrant colors of fresh foods. Long-term care residents, especially those with olfactory impairments, may benefit from liberalizing the diet restrictions in order to stimulate appetite and maintain food enjoyment and the quality of life.[299]

Many initiatives in long-term care facilities continue to combat the effects of olfactory dysfunction and changes in oral sensation on nutritional risk of the older adult. Applying culinary arts techniques will enhance the overall sensory appeal of foods and beverages, including visual presentation and oral sensory appeal, especially for salt, sugar, and texture-modified diet. Increasing the socialization during mealtime results in improved intake, even in residents who do not report changes in food preference.[283] Flavor-enhanced foods show positive effects in elderly residents who live in long-term care facilities, including increases in intake and body weight[295,296] and some measures of nutritional status.[294,297]

SUMMARY

Nutrition plays a vital role in the health and well-being of older adults. Taste, smell, and oral somatosensation contribute to food enjoyment and nutritional health, receiving sensory input from the food world. Through the process of aging and the continual exposure to environmental insults, the elderly are at risk for loss of olfactory perception and changes to oral sensation. Poorly fitting dentures may further increase the risk of olfactory dysfunction by reducing retronasal processing of olfactory food flavor. Loss of true taste as perceived with the whole mouth is rare because of the tremendous redundancy in cranial nerves that carry taste sensations from the environment to the brain. However, recent evidence shows that localized loss of taste from an individual area of cranial nerves can alter oral sensations from foods and beverages and change food preferences and patterns of food intake. Localized losses of taste, if extreme enough and/or coupled with genetic supertasting, can result in dysgeusias (ie, persistent tastes with or without oral stimulation) and oral pain syndromes that impair the quality of life and the ability to obtain oral nourishment.

Older adults who complain of olfactory loss, of oral sensory disturbances, or that eating is not enjoyable deserve a thorough assessment. There are a limited number of treatments for chemosensory disturbances if the sensory system is damaged. Chemosensory disorders can improve if the underlying cause is treatable, such as through the modification of medications or alleviation of the underlying condition. Treatable or not, olfactory and oral sensory disorders can influence nutritional health. Practitioners should assess the nutritional impact of measured or perceived disorders on the quality of the eating experience and nutritional health in older adults. The nutritional response to the olfactory loss is not uniform. Dietetics practitioners should develop individualized nutritional care plans for older adults with reported or suspected taste, smell, and oral somatosensory disturbances.

ACKNOWLEDGMENTS

Manuscript preparation was supported by NIA RO3AG1861, NIDCD 00283, and NRICGP/USDA 2002-00788. Thank you to John Hayes, MS, for helpful review and editing of this manuscript.

REFERENCES

1. de Araujo IE, Kringelbach ML, Rolls ET, Hobden P. Representation of umami taste in the human brain. *J Neurophysiol* Jul 2003;90(1):313–319.

2. Prutkin JM, Duffy VB, Etter L, et al. Genetic variation and inferences about perceived taste intensity in mice and men. *Physiol Behav* 2000;61(1):161–173.

3. Pickenhagan W. Enantioselectivity in odor perception. In: Teranishi R, Buttery R, Shahidi F, eds. *Flavor Chemistry: Trends and Development* Washington, DC: American Chemical Society; 1989:151–157.

4. Engen T. Remembering odors and their names. *American Scientist* 1987;75:497–503.

5. Beidler L, Smith J. Effects of radiation therapy and drugs on cell turnover and taste. In: Getchell T, Doty R, Bartoshuk L, Snow J, eds. *Smell and Taste in Health and Disease*. New York, NY: Raven Press; 1991:753–763.

6. MacKay-Sim A. Neurogenesis in the adult olfactory neuroepithelium. In: Doty R, ed. *Handbook of Olfaction and Gustation*. New York, NY: Marcel Dekker; 2003:93–113.

7. Leopold DA, Hummel T, Schwob JE, Hong SC, Knecht M, Kobal G. Anterior distribution of human olfactory epithelium. *Laryngoscope* Mar 2000;110(3 Pt 1):417–421.

8. Paik SI, Lehman MN, Seiden AM, Duncan HJ, Smith DV. Human olfactory biopsy. The influence of age and receptor distribution. *Arch Otolaryngol Head Neck Surg* Jul 1992;118(7):731–738.

9. Moran D, Jafek B, Eller P, Rowley JD. Ultrastructural histopathology of human olfactory dysfunction. *Microsc Res Tech* 1992;23(2):103–110.

10. Wysocki CJ, Gilbert AN. The National Geographic smell survey: effects of age are heterogeneous. Nutrition and the chemical senses in aging: recent advances and current research needs. *NY Acad Sci* 1989;561:12–28.

11. Murphy C, Schubert C, Cruickshanks K, Klein B, Klein R, Nondahl D. Prevalence of olfactory impairment in older adults. *JAMA* 2002;288(18):2307–2312.

12. Doty R, Snyder P, Huggins G, Lowry L. Endocrine, cardiovascular, and psychological correlates of olfactory sensitivity changes during the human menstrual cycle. *J Comp Physiol Psychol* 1981;95:45–60.

13. Gilbert A, Wysocki C. Quantitative assessment of olfactory experience during pregnancy. *Psychosomatic Med* 1991;53:693–700.

14. Navarrete-Palacios E, Hudson R, Reyes-Guerrero G, Guevara-Guzman R. Lower olfactory threshold during the ovulatory phase of the menstrual cycle. *Biol Psychol* 2003;63(3):269–279.

15. Hornung D, Leopold DA. Relationship between uninasal anatomy and uninasal olfactory ability. *Arch Otolaryngol Head Neck Surg* 1999;125(1):53–58.

16. Oberg C, Larsson M, Backman L. Differential sex effects in olfactory functioning: the role of verbal processing. *J Int Neuropsychol Soc* 2000;8(5):691–698.

17. Laing D. Optimum perception of odor intensity by humans. *Physiol Behav* 1985;34:569–574.

18. Hornung D, Smith D, Kurtz D, White T, Leopold D. Effect of nasal dilators on nasal structures, sniffing strategies, and olfactory ability. *Rhinology* 2001;39(2):84–87.

19. Burdach K, Doty R. The effects of mouth movements, swallowing and spitting on retronasal odor perception. *Physiol Behav* 1987;41(4):353–356.

20. Rozin P. "Taste-smell confusions" and the duality of the olfactory sense. *Percept Psychophys* 1982;31(4):397–401.

21. Hollingworth H, Poffenberger A. *The Sense of Taste.* New York, NY: Moffat, Yard and Company; 1917.

22. Bartoshuk L, Duffy V, Fast K, Snyder D. Genetic differences in human oral perception: advanced methods reveal basic problems in intensity scaling. In: Prescott J, Tepper B, eds. *Genetic Variation in Taste Sensitivity.* New York, NY: Marcel Dekker Inc; 2004:5–20.

23. MacCarthy-Leventhal E. Post radiation mouth blindness. *Lancet* 1959;19:1138–1139.

24. Bull T. Taste and the chorda tympani. *J Laryngol Otol* 1965;79:479–493.

25. Fast K, Bartoshuk L, Kveton J, Duffy V. Unilateral anesthesia of the chorda tympani nerve suggests taste may localize retronasal olfaction [abstract]. *Chem Senses* 2000;25:614–615.

26. Snyder D, Dwivedi N, Mramor A, Bartoshuk L, Duffy V. Taste and touch may contribute to the localization of retronasal olfaction: unilateral and bilateral anesthesia of cranial nerves V/VII. *Soc Neurosci Abstr* 2001;27: 711–727.

27. Duffy V, Chapo A, Hutchins H, Snyder D, Bartoshuk L. Retronasal olfactory intensity: associations with taste. *Chem Senses* 2003;28:A-33.

28. Moran D, Rowley J, Jafek B. Electron microscopy of human olfactory epithelium reveals a new cell type: the microvillar cell. *Brain Res* 1982;253:39–46.

29. Lancet D. Vertebrate olfactory reception. *Ann Rev Neurosc* 1986;9:329–356.

30. Getchell T, Getchell M. Regulatory factors in the vertebrate olfactory mucosa. *Chem Senses* 1990;15:223–231.

31. Pevsner J, Snyder S. Odorant-binding protein: odorant transport function in the vertebrate nasal epithelium. *Chem Senses* 1990;15:217–222.

32. Buck L. Information coding in the vertebrate olfactory system. *Annu Rev Neurosci* 1996;19:517–544.

33. Moon C, Ronnett G. Molecular neurobiology of olfactory transduction. In: Doty R, ed. *Handbook of Olfaction and Gustation.* New York, NY: Marcel Dekker, Inc.; 2003: 75–91.

34. Greer C. Structural organization of the olfactory system. In: Getchel T, Doty R, Bartoshuk L, Snow J, eds. *Smell and Taste in Health and Disease.* New York, NY: Raven Press; 1991:65–81.

35. Xu P, Greer C, Shepherd G. Odor maps in the olfactory bulb. *Comp Neurol* 2000;422:489–495.

36. Miller I, Reedy F. Variation in human taste bud density and taste intensity perception. *Physiol Behav* 1990;47: 1213–1219.

37. Bartoshuk L, Duffy V, Miller I. PTC/PROP tasting: anatomy, psychophysics, and sex effects. *Physiol Behav* 1994;56(6):1165–1171.

38. Duffy VB, Lucchina LA, Bartoshuk LM. Genetic variation in taste: potential biomarker for cardiovascular disease risk? In: Prescott J, Tepper B, eds. *Genetic Variation in Taste Sensitivity.* New York, NY: Marcel Dekker Inc, 2003:197–229.

39. Weiffenbach J, Schwartz L, Atkinson J, Fox P. Taste performance in Sjögren's syndrome. *Physiol Behav* 1995; 57(1):89–96.

40. Bartoshuk L. The biological basis of food perception. *Food Qual Pref* 1993;4:21–32.

41. Kinnamon S, Margolskee R. Mechanisms of taste transduction. *Curr Opin Neurobiology* 1996;6:506–513.

42. McBurney D, Gent J. On the nature of taste qualities. *Psychological Bulletin* 1979;86(1):151–167.

43. Pritchard T. The primate gustatory system. In: Getchell T, Doty R, Bartoshuk L, Snow JJ, eds. *Smell and Taste in Health and Disease.* New York, NY: Raven Press; 1991:109–125.

44. Duffy V, Bartoshuk L, Striegel-Moore R, Rodin J. Taste changes across pregnancy. *NY Acad Sci* 1998;855:805–9.

45. Silver W, Finger T. The trigeminal system. In: Getchell T, Doty R, Bartoshuk L, Snow JJ, eds. *Smell and Taste in Health and Disease.* New York, NY: Raven Press; 1991: 97–108.

46. Cometto-Muniz JE, Cain WS, Abraham MH, Gola JM. Ocular and nasal trigeminal detection of butyl acetate and toluene presented singly and in mixtures. *Toxicol Sci* Oct 2001;63(2):233–244.

47. Doty R, Brugger W, Jurs P, Orndorff M, Snyder P, Lowry L. Intranasal trigeminal stimulation from odorous volatiles: psychometric responses from anosmic and normal humans. *Physiol Behav* 1978;20:175–185.

48. Green BG, Gelhard B. Salt as an oral irritant. *Chem Senses* 1989;14(2):259–271.

49. Green B, Hayes J. Capsaicin as a probe of the relationship between bitter taste and chemesthesis. *Physiol Behav* 2003;79(4–5):811–821.

50. Whitehead M, Beeman C, Kinsella B. Distribution of taste and general sensory nerve endings in fungiform papillae of hamsters. *Am J Anat* 1985;173:185–201.

51. Whitehead MC, Kachele DL. Development of fungiform papillae, taste buds, and their innervation in the hamster. *J Comp Neurol* 1994;340:515–530.

52. Green B. Thermal perception on lingual and labial skin. *Perception Psychophysics* 1984;36(3):209–220.

53. Pelletier C, Lawless H. Effect of citric acid and citric acid-sucrose mixtures on swallowing in neurogenic oropharyngeal dysphagia. *Dysphagia* 2003;18(4): 231–241.

54. Bartoshuk L, Duffy V, Leder S, Snyder D. Oral sensation: genetic and pathological sources of variation. *Dysphagia* 2003;14(2):3–9.

55. Rolls ET, Scott T. Central taste anatomy and neurophysiology. In: Doty R, ed. *Handbook of Olfaction and Gustation*. New York, NY: Marcel Dekker Inc.; 2003: 679–705.

56. Hollowood T, Linforth R, Taylor A. The effect of viscosity on the perception of flavour. *Chem Sense* 2002; 27:583–591.

57. Sakai N, Kobayakaw T, Gotow N, Satio S, Imada S. Enhancement of sweetness ratings of aspartame by a vanilla odor presented either by orthonasal or retronasal routes. *Percept Psychophys* 2001;92:1002–1008.

58. Noble A. Taste-aroma interactions. *Trends Food Sci Technol* 1996;7:439–444.

59. Cain WS. Olfaction and the common chemical senses: some psychophysical contrasts. *Sensory Proc* 1976;1: 57–67.

60. Kveton J, Bartoshuk L. The effect of unilateral chorda tympani damage on taste. *Laryngoscope* 1994;104(1): 25–29.

61. Sipiora M, Murtaugh M, Gregoire M, Duffy V. Bitter taste perception and severe vomiting during pregnancy. *Physiol Behav* 2000;69(3):259–267.

62. Lehman CD, Bartoshuk LM, Catalanotto FC, Kveton JF, Lowlicht RA. Effect of anesthesia of the chorda tympani nerve of taste perception in humans. *Physiol Behav* 1995;57:943–951.

63. Yanaglsawa K, Bartoshuk LM, Catalanotto FA, Karrer TA, Kveton JF. Anesthesia of the chorda tympani nerve and taste phantoms. *Physiol Behav* 1997;63(3):329–335.

64. Tie K, Fast K, Kveton J, et al. Anesthesia of chorda tympani nerve and effect on oral pain [abstract]. *Chem Senses* 1999;24(5):609.

65. Grushka M, Bartoshuk L. Burning mouth syndrome and oral dysesthesias. *Can J Diag* June 2000:99–109.

66. Chapo A, Phillips M, Ilich J, Duffy VB. Sodium chloride (NaCl) saltiness: are older females more responsive? *Gerontologist* 2001;41(special issue 1):83.

67. Green B, Gelhard B. Salt as an oral irritant. *Chem Senses* 1989;14(2):259–271.

68. Chapo A, Bartoshuk L, Ilich J, Duffy V. Age-related differences in fat perception and dietary behaviors. *Chem Senses* 2002;27:A19–A20.

69. Drewnowski A, Henderson S, Driscoll A, Rolls B. Salt taste perceptions and preferences are unrelated to sodium consumption in healthy older adults. *J Amer Diet Assoc* 1996;96:471–474.

70. Chapo A. *Age-related changes in oral sensation: associations with preference for and intake of dietary salt and fat* [master's thesis]. Storrs, CT: School of Allied Health, University of Connecticut; 2002.

71. Fox AL. Six in ten "tasteblind" to bitter chemical. *Science News Letter* 1931;9:249.

72. Kim UK, Jorgenson E, Coon H, Leppert M, Risch N, Drayna D. Positional cloning of the human quantitative trait locus underlying taste sensitivity to phenylthiocarbamide. *Science* February 21, 2003;299(5610): 1221–1225.

73. Bartoshuk L, Duffy V, Fast K, et al. What makes a supertaster? [abstract] *Chem Senses* 2001;26(8):1074.

74. Prescott J, Swain-Campbell N. Responses to repeated oral irritation by capsaicin, cinnamaldehyde and ethanol in PROP tasters and nontasters. *Chem Senses* 2000;25: 239–246.

75. Tepper B, Nurse R. Fat perception is related to PROP Taster Status. *Physiol Behav* 1997;61(6):949–954.

76. Duffy V, Lucchina L, Fast K, Bartoshuk L. Oral sensation and cancer. In: Berger A, Portnoy R, Weissman D, eds. *Principles and Practice of Palliative Care and Supportive Oncology*. 2nd ed. Philadelphia, PA: JB Lippincott Company; 2002:178–193.

77. Doty R, Laing D. Psychophysical measurement of human olfactory function, including odorant mixture assessment. In: Doty R, ed. *Handbook of Olfaction and Gustation*. New York, NY: Marcel Dekker Inc.; 2003: 203–228.

78. Stevens J, Dadarwala A. Variability of olfactory thresholds. *Chem Senses* 1993;13:643–653.

79. McBurney DH, Collings VB. *Introduction to Sensation/ Perception*. 2nd ed. Englewood Cliffs, NJ: Prentice Hall; 1984.

80. Cain WS, Stevens J. Uniformity of olfactory loss in aging. Presented at Nutrition and the Chemical Senses in Aging: Recent Advances and Current Research Needs; 1989; New York, NY.

81. Bartoshuk L, Duffy V. Taste and smell. In: Masoro E, ed. *Aging*. Vol Section 11. New York, NY: Oxford University Press; 1995;363–375.

82. Duffy V, Peterson J, Bartoshuk L. Bitterness of 6-n-propylthiouracil (PROP) associates with alcohol sensation and intake. *Physiol Behav* Under review.

83. Jerzsa-Latta M, Krondl M, Coleman P. Use and perceived attributes of cruciferous vegetables in terms of genetically-mediated taste sensitivity. *Appetite* 1990;15: 127–134.

84. Kranzler H, Moore P, Hesselbrock V. No association of PROP taster status and parental history of alcohol dependence. *Alcoholism: Clin Exper Res* 1996;20(8): 1495–1500.

85. Wood JB, Harkins SW. Effects of age, stimulus selection, and retrieval environment on odor identification. *J Gerontol* 1987;42(6):584–588.

86. Lawless H, Engen T. Association to odors: interference, memories, and verbal labeling. *J Exper Pysch* 1977;3: 52–59.

87. Corwin J. Assessing olfaction: cognitive and measurement issues. In: Serby M, Chobor K, eds. *Science of Olfaction*. Berlin: Springer-Verlag; 1992:335–354.

88. Lehrner J, Gluck J, Laska M. Odor identification, consistency of label use, olfactory threshold and their relationship to odor memory over the human lifespan. *Chem Senses* 1999;24:337–346.

89. Larsson M, Backman L. Age-related differences in episodic odour recognition: the role of access to specific odour names. *Memory* 1997;5(3):361–378.

90. Cain WS, Gent JF, Goodspeed RB, Leonard G. Evaluation of olfactory dysfunction in the Connecticut Chemosensory Clinical Research Center. *Laryngoscope* 1988;98:83–88.

91. Bartoshuk L, Duffy V, Fast K, Green B, Snyder D. Labeled scales (eg, category, Likert, VAS) and invalid across-group comparisons: what we have learned from genetic variation in taste. *J Food Qual Pref* 2002; 14:125–138.

92. Kamen J, Pilgrim F, Gutman N, Kroll B. Interactions of suprathreshold taste stimuli. *J Exp Psychol* 1961;62: 348–356.

93. Stevens S. The psychophysics of sensory function. In: Rosenblith W, ed. *Sensory Communication*. Cambridge, MA: MIT Press; 1961:1–33.

94. Green B, Shaffer G, Gilmore M. A semantically-labeled scale of oral sensation with apparent ratio properties. *Chem Senses* 1993;18:683–702.

95. Green B, Dalton P, Cowart B, Rankin K, Higgins J. Evaluation of the labeled magnitude scale for measuring sensations of taste and smell. *Chem Senses* 1996;21: 323–334.

96. Weiffenbach J, Cowart B, Baum B. Taste intensity perception in aging. *J Gerontol* 1986;41:460–468.

97. Moskowitz H. Magnitude estimation: notes on what, how, when, and why to use it. *J Food Qual* 1977;1: 195–228.

98. Marks L, Stevens J, Bartoshuk L, Gent J, Rifkin B, Stone V. Magnitude matching: the measurement of taste and smell. *Chem Senses* 1988;13:63–87.

99. Stevens J, Marks L. Cross-modality matching functions generated by magnitude estimation. *Percept Psychophys* 1980;27:379–389.

100. Marks L, Stevens J. Measuring sensation in the aged. In: Poon L, ed. *Aging in the 1980's: Psychological Issues*. Washington, DC: American Psychological Association; 1980:592–598.

101. Bartoshuk L, Duffy VB, Green B, Hoffman H, et al. Valid across-group comparisons with labeled scales: the gLMS vs. magnitude matching. *Physiol Behav* 2004; Aug 82(1):109–114.

102. Snyder D, Lucchina L, Duffy V, Bartoshuk L. Magnitude matching adds power to the labeled magnitude scale [abstract]. *Chem Senses* 1996;21(5):673.

103. Little A, Brinner L. Taste responses to saltiness of experimentally prepared tomato juice samples. *J Am Diet Assoc* 1984;84:1022–1027.

104. Herz RS. Are odors the best cues to memory? A cross-modal comparison of associative memory stimuli. *Ann N Y Acad Sci* November 30, 1998;855:670–674.

105. Choudhury E, Moberg P, Doty R. Influences of age and sex on a microencapsulated odor memory test. *Chem Senses* 2003;28(9):799–805.

106. Doty RL, Smith R, McKeown DA, Raj J. Tests of human olfactory function: principal components analysis suggests that most measure a common source of variance. *Percept Psychophys* 1994;56:701–707.

107. Kobal G. Electrophysical measurement of olfactory function. In: Doty R, ed. *Handbook of Olfaction and Gustation*. New York, NY: Marcel Dekker Inc.; 2003: 229–249.

108. Wetter S, Murphy C. A paradigm for measuring the olfactory event-related potential in the clinic. *Int J Psychophysiol* July 2003;49(1):57–65.

109. Sobel N, Johnson B, Mainland J, Yousem D. Functional neuroimaging of human olfaction. In: Doty R, ed. *Handbook of Olfaction and Gustation*. New York, NY: Marcel Dekker Inc.; 2003:251–273.

110. Murphy C, Doty R, Duncan HJ. Clinical disorders of olfaction. In: Doty R, ed. *Handbook of Olfaction and Gustation*. 2nd ed. New York, NY: Marcel Dekker Inc.; 2003:461–478.

111. Bremner EA, Mainland JD, Khan RM, Sobel N. The prevalence of androstenone anosmia. *Chem Senses* 2003;28(5):423–432.

112. Amoore J. Specific anosmia and the concept of primary odors. *Chem Senses Flavor* 1977;2:267–281.

113. Pribitkin E, Rosenthal MD, Cowart BJ. Prevalence and causes of severe taste loss in a chemosensory clinic population. *Ann Otol Rhinol Laryngol* November 2003; 112(11):971–978.

114. Deems D, Doty R, Settle R, et al. Smell and taste disorders: an analysis of 750 patients from the University of Pennsylvania Smell and Taste Center. *Arch Otolaryng Head Neck Surg* 1991;117(5):519–528.

115. Lawless H, Schlake S, Smythe J, et al. Metallic taste and retronasal smell. *Chem Senses* 2004;29:25–33.

116. Green B. Capsaicin sensitization and desensitization on the tongue produced by brief exposures to a low concentration. *Neurosci Lett* 1989;107:173.

117. Mozell M, Smith B, Smith P, Sullivan L, Swender P. Nasal chemoreception in flavor identification. *Arch Otolaryngol* 1969;90:367–373.

118. Murphy C, Cain WS, Bartoshuk LM. Mutual action of taste and olfaction. *Sensory Processes* 1977;1:204–211.

119. Ship J, Weiffenbach J. Age, gender, medical treatment and medication effects on smell identification. *J Gerontol* 1993;48:M26–M32.

120. Cowart B, Young I, Feldman R, Lowry L. Clinical disorders of smell and taste. *Occ Med* 1997;12(3): 465–483.

121. Meisami E, Mikhail L, Baim D, Bhatnagar K. Human olfactory bulb: aging of glomeruli and mitral cells and a search for the accessory olfactory bulb. *Ann NY Acad Sci* 1998;30(855):708–715.

122. Kern RC, Conley DB, Haines GK 3rd, Robinson AM. Pathology of the olfactory mucosa: implications for the treatment of olfactory dysfunction. *Laryngoscope* 2004;114(2):279–285.

123. Conley DB, Robinson AM, Shinners MJ, Kern RC. Age-related olfactory dysfunction: cellular and molecular characterization in the rat. *Am J Rhinol* 2003; 17(3):169–175.

124. Doty RL, Shaman P, Applebaum SL, Giberson R, Siksorski L, Rosenberg L. Smell identification ability: changes with age. *Science* 1984;226(4681):1441–1442.

125. Hoffman H, Ishii E, MacTurk R. Age-related changes in the prevalence of smell/taste problems among the United States adult population. Results of the 1994 disability supplement to the National Health Interview Survey (NHIS). *Ann NY Acad Sci* 1998;855:716–722.

126. Doty R, Shaman P, Dann M. Development of the University of Pennsylvania smell identification test: a standardized microencapsulated test of olfactory function. *Physiol Behav* 1984;34:489–502.

127. Barber C. Olfactory acuity as a function of age and gender: a comparison of African and American samples. *Int J Aging Hum Devel* 1997;44(3):317–334.

128. Nordin S, Monsch A, Murphy C. Unawareness of smell loss in normal aging and Alzheimer's disease: discrepancy between self-reported and diagnosed smell sensitivity. *J Gerontol B Psychol Sci Soc Sci* 1995;50: P187–192.

129. Stevens J, Plantinga A, Cain W. Reduction of odor and nasal pungency associated with aging. *Neurobiol Aging* 1982;3:125–132.

130. Stevens JC, Bartoshuk LM, Cain WS. Chemical senses and aging: taste versus smell. *Chem Senses* 1984;9(2): 167–178.

131. Stevens JC, Cain WS. Age-related deficiency in the perceived strength of six odorants. *Chem Senses* 1985; 10(4):515–529.

132. Doty RL. Odor perception in neurodegenerative diseases. In: Doty R, ed. *Handbook of Olfaction and Gustation*. New York, NY: Marcel Dekker Inc.; 2003: 479–501.

133. Matsunami H. A multigene family encoding a diverse array of putative pheromone receptors in mammals. *Cell* 1997;(90)4:775–8422.

134. Russel M, Cummings B, Profitt B, Wysocki C, Gilbert A, Cotman C. Life span changes in the verbal categorization of odors. *J Gerontol: Psych Sci* 1993;48(2): P49–P53.

135. Schiffman SS. Food recognition by the elderly. *J Gerontol* 1977;32:586–592.

136. Murphy C. Cognitive and chemosensory influences on age-related changes in the ability to identify blender foods. *J Gerontol* 1985;41(1):47–52.

137. Heilmann S, Strehle G, Rosenheim K, Damm M, Hummel T. Clinical assessment of retronasal olfactory function. *Arch Otolaryngol Head Neck Surg* 2002;128: 414–418.

138. Stevens J, Cain W. Smelling via mouth: Effect of aging. *Percep Psychophys* 1986;40(3):142–146.

139. Cain W, Reid F, Stevens J. Missing ingredients: aging and the discrimination of flavor. *J Nutr Elder* 1990; 9(3):3–15.

140. Dabrila G, Duffy V. Middle-aged females exhibit lower orthonasal and retronasal olfactory perception than young females. *Chem Senses* 1996;21(5):591–592.

141. Feldman R, Kapus K, Alman J, Chauncey H. Aging and mastication: changes in performance and in the swallowing threshold with natural dentition. *J Am Geriatr Soc* 1980;28:97–103.

142. Duffy V, Cain W, Ferris A. Measurement of sensitivity to olfactory flavor: application in a study of aging and dentures. *Chem Senses* 1999;24(6):671–677.

143. Ship J. The influence of aging on oral health and consequences for taste and smell. *Physiol Behav* 1999; 66(2):209–215.

144. Ritter F. Fate of olfaction after laryngectomy. *Arch Otolaryngol* 1964;79:169–171.

145. Landis BN, Giger R, Ricchetti A, et al. Retronasal olfactory function in nasal polyposis. *Laryngoscope* 2003;113(11):1993–1997.

146. Murphy C, Morgan CD, Geisler MW, et al. Olfactory event-related potentials and aging: normative data. *Int J Psychophysiol* 2000;36(2):133–145.

147. Covington J, Geisler M, Polich J, Murphy C. Normal aging and odor intensity effects on the olfactory event-related potential. *Int J Psychophysiol* 1999;32(3): 205–214.

148. Suzuki Y, Critchley H, Suckling J, et al. Functional magnetic resonance imaging of odor identification: the effect of aging. *J Gerontol A Biol Sci Med Sci* 2001; 56(12):M56–60.

149. Ferdon S, Murphy C. The cerebellum and olfaction in the aging brain: a functional magnetic resonance imaging study. *Neuroimage* 2003;20(1):12–21.

150. Cerf-Ducastel B, Murphy C. FMRI brain activation in response to odors is reduced in primary olfactory areas of elderly subjects. *Brain Res* 2003;986(1–2):39–53.

151. Miller IJ, Bartoshuk L. Taste perception, taste bud distribution, and spatial relationships. In: Getchel T, Doty R, Bartoshuk L, Snow J, eds. *Smell and Taste in Health and Disease*. New York, NY: Raven Press; 1991:205–233.

152. Zuniga J, Miller I. Effects of chorda-lingual nerve injury and repair on human taste. *Chem Senses* 1994; 19:657–665.

153. Fast K, Duffy V, Bartoshuk LM. New psychophysical insights in evaluating genetic variation in taste. In: Rouby C, Schaal B, Dubios D, Gervais R, Holley A, eds. *Olfaction, Taste and Cognition*. Cambridge, England: Cambridge University Press; 2002.

154. Miller IJ. Human taste bud density across adult age groups. *J Gerontol* 1988;43:B26–B30.

155. Mistretta C. Anatomy and neurophysiology of the taste system in aged animals. Presented at: Nutrition and the Chemical Senses in Aging: Recent Advances and Current Research Needs; 1989; Sarasota, FL.

156. Mistretta C. Developmental neurobiology of the taste system. In: Getchel T, Doty R, Bartoshuk L, Snow J, eds. *Smell and Taste in Health and Disease*. New York, NY: Raven Press; 1991:35–64.

157. Yamamoto Y, Tanaka S, Tsubone H, Atoji Y, Suzuki Y. Age-related changes in sensory and secretomotor nerve endings in the larynx of F344/N rat. *Arch Gerontol Geriatr* 2003;36(2):173–183.

158. Murphy C. Taste and smell in the elderly. In: Meiselman HL, Rivlin RS, eds. *Clinical Measurement of Taste and Smell*. Vol 1. Lexington, MA: Collamore Press; 1986: 343–367.

159. Mojet J, Christ-Hazelhof E, Heidema J. Taste perception with age: generic or specific losses in threshold sensitivity to the five basic tastes? *Chem Senses* 2001;26(7):845–860.

160. Cowart B, Yokomukai Y, Beauchamp G. Bitter taste in aging: compound-specific decline in sensitivity. *Physiol Behav* 1994;56(6):1237–1241.

161. Stevens J, Cain W. Changes in taste and flavor in aging. *Crit Rev Food Sci and Nutr* 1993;33(1):27–37.

162. Bartoshuk LM, Rifkin B, Marks LE, Bars P. Taste and aging. *J Gerontol* 1986;41(1):51–57.

163. Mojet J, Heidema J, Christ–Hazelhof E. Taste perception with age: generic or specific losses in supra-threshold intensities of five taste qualities? *Chem Senses* 2003;28(5):397–413.

164. Lucchina L, Bartoshuk L, Duffy V, Ferri SA, Mark SL. Preliminary examination of suprathreshold olfactory and taste perception: free-living elderly females exhibit greater olfactory than taste impairment [abstract]. *Chem Senses* 1994;19.

165. Weiffenbach J, Duffy V, Fast K, Cohen Z, Bartoshuk L. Bitter-sweet age, sex and PROP (6-n-propylthiouracil) effects: a role for menopause? [abstract]. *Chem Senses* 2000;25:639.

166. Bartoshuk L. Taste: robust across the age span? Presented at: Nutrition and the Chemical Sense in Aging: Recent Advances and Current Research Needs; 1989; Sarasota, FL.

167. Stevens J, Choo K. Spatial acuity of the body surface over the life span. *Somatosens Mot Res* 1996;13(2): 153–166.

168. Weiffenbach J, Tylenda C, Baum B. Oral sensory changes in aging. *J Gerontol* 1990;45(4):M121–M125.

169. Calhoun K, Gibson B, Hartley L, Minton J, Hokanson J. Age-related changes in oral sensation. *Laryngoscope* 1992;102:109–116.

170. Bartoshuk L, Caseria D, Catalanotto F, et al. Do taste-trigeminal interactions play a role in oral pain? [abstract]. *Chem Senses* 1996;21:578.

171. Heft M. Orofacial pain. *Clin Geriatr Med* 1992;8: 557–568.

172. Wysocki C, Cowart B, Radil T. Nasal trigeminal chemosensitivity across the adult life span. *Percept Psychophys* 2003;65(1):115–122.

173. Laska M. Perception of trigeminal chemosensory qualities in the elderly. *Chem Senses* 2001;26(6):681–689.

174. US Department of Health and Human Services, National Institute of Neurological and Communicative Disorders and Stroke. *Report of the Panel on Communicative Disorders to the National Advisory Neurological and Communicative Disorders and Stroke Council*. National Institutes of Health; 1979:79–1914.

175. Disorders NIoDaOC. *National Strategic Research Plan. Smell, Taste and Touch and Chemosensory Disorders*. Bethesda, MD: US Department of Health and Human Services, Public Health Service, National Institutes of Health; 1995. No. 95-3711.

176. Snow JJ, Doty R, Bartoshuk L, Getchell T. Categorization of chemosensory disorders. In: Getchell T, Doty R, Bartoshuk L, Snow JJ, eds. *Smell and Taste in Health and Disease*. New York, NY: Raven; 1991:445–447.

177. Bromley S, Doty R. Clinical disorders affecting taste: evaluation and management. In: Doty R, ed *Handbook of Olfaction and Gustation*. 2nd ed. New York, NY: Marcel Dekker Inc.; 2003:935–957.

178. Deems R, Friedman M, Friedman L, Maddrey WC. Clinical manifestations of olfactory and gustatory disorders associated with hepatic and renal disease. In: Getchel T, Doty R, Bartoshuk L, Snow J, eds. *Smell and Taste in Health and Disease*. New York, NY: Raven Press; 1991:805–816.

179. Akerlund A, Bende M, Murphy C. Olfactory threshold and nasal mucosal changes in experimentally induced common cold. *Acta Otolaryngol (Stockh)* 1995;115(1): 88–92.

180. Baker H, Genter M. The olfactory system and nasal mucosa as portals of entry of viruses, drugs, and other exogenous agents into the brain. In: Doty R, ed. *Handbook of Olfaction and Gustation*. New York, NY: Marcel Dekker Inc.; 2003:549–573.

181. Seiden A, Duncan H. The diagnosis of a conductive olfactory loss. *Laryngoscope* 2001;111(1):9–14.

182. Hummel T, Heilmann S, Huttenbriuk K. Lipoic acid in the treatment of smell dysfunction following viral infection of the upper respiratory tract. *Laryngoscope* 2002;112(11):2076–2080.

183. Duncan H, Seiden A. Long-term follow-up of olfactory loss secondary to head trauma and upper respiratory tract infection. *Arch Otolaryngol Head Neck Surg* 1995;121(10):1183–1187.

184. Mueller C, Temmel A, Quint C, Rieger A, Hummel T. Olfactory function in HIV-positive subjects. *Acta Otolaryngol* 2002;122:67–71.

185. Murphy C, Davidson T, Jellison W, et al. Sinonasal disease and olfactory impairment in HIV disease: endoscopic sinus surgery and outcome measures. *Laryngoscope* 2000;110:1707–1710.

186. Westervelt H, McCaffrey R, Cousins J, Wagle W, Haase R. Longitudinal analysis of olfactory deficits in HIV infection. *Arch Clin Neuropsychol* 1997;21(6):557–565.

187. Bartoshuk L, Duffy V, Reed D, Williams A. Supertasting, earaches and head trauma: genetics and pathology alter our taste worlds. *Neurosci Biobehav Rev* 1995,20(1):79–87.

188. Bartoshuk L, Duffy V, Reed D, Williams A. Supertasting, earaches and head injury: genetics and pathology alter our taste worlds. *Neurosci Biobehav Rev* 1996;20(1):79–87.

189. Costanzo R, DiNardo L, Reiter E. Head injury and olfaction. In: Doty R, ed. *Handbook of Olfaction and Gustation.* New York, NY: Marcel Dekker Inc.; 2003: 629–638.

190. Green P, Rohling M, Iverson G, Gervais R. Relationships between olfactory discrimination and head injury severity. *Brain Inj* 2003;17(6):479–496.

191. Sumner D. Post-traumatic anosmia. *Brain* 1964;87: 107–120.

192. Costanzo R, Zasler N. Head trauma. In: Getchell T, Doty R, Bartoshuk L, Snow JJ, eds. *Smell and Taste in Health and Disease.* New York, NY: Raven Press; 1991: 711–730.

193. Yousem D, Geckle R, Bilker W, McKeown D, Doty R. Posttraumatic olfactory dysfunction: MR and clinical evaluation. *Am J Neuroradiol* 1996;17(6):1171–1179.

194. Solomon G. *Patterns of Taste Loss in Clinic Patients with Histories of Head Trauma, Nasal Symptoms, or Upper Respiratory Infections* [thesis]. Yale University School of Medicine; 1991.

195. Adams P, Marano M. Current estimates from the National Health Interview Survey, 1994. National Center for Health Statistics. *Vit Health Stat* 1995; 10(193):81–82.

196. Edelstein D. Aging of the normal nose in adults. *Laryngoscope* 1996;106:1–25.

197. Hinriksdottir I, Murphy C, Bende M. Olfactory threshold after nasal allergen challenge. *J Otorhinolaryngol Relat Spec* 1997;59(1):36–38.

198. Apter A, Mott A, Frank M, Clive JM. Allergic rhinitis and olfactory loss. *Ann Allergy Asthma Immunol* 1995; 75(4):311–316.

199. Cowart B, Flynn-Rodden K, McGeady S, Lowry L. Hyposmia in allergic rhinitis. *J Allergy Clin Immunol* 1993;91(3):747–751.

200. Apter A, Gent J, Frank M. Fluctuating olfactory sensitivity and distorted odor perception in allergic rhinitis. *Arch Otolaryngol Head Neck Surg* 1999;125(9): 1005–1010.

201. Leopold D, Bartels S. Evaluation of olfaction. *J Otolaryngol* 2002;31(1):S18–23.

202. Downey L, Jacobs J, Lebowitz R. Anosmia and chronic sinus disease. *Otolaryngol Head Neck Surg* 1996; 115(1):24–48.

203. Hughes L, McAsey M, Donathan C, Smith T, Coney P, Struble R. Effects of hormone replacement therapy on olfactory sensitivity: cross-sectional and longitudinal studies. *Climacteric* 2002;5(2):140–150.

204. Mesholam R, Moberg P, Mahr R, Doty R. Olfaction in neurodegenerative disease: a meta-analysis of olfactory functioning in Alzheimer's and Parkinson's diseases. *Arch Neurol* 1998;55:84–90.

205. Bacon Moore A, Paulsen J, Murphy C. A test of odor fluency in patients with Alzheimer's and Huntington's disease. *J Clin Exp Neuropsychol* 1999;21:341–351.

206. Murphy C, Jernigan T, Fennema-Notestine C. Left hippocampal volume loss in Alzheimer's disease is reflected in performance on odor identification: a structural MRI study. *J Int Neuropsychol Soc* 2003;9(3):459–471.

207. McCaffrey R, Duff K, Solomon G. Olfactory dysfunction discriminates probably Alzheimer's dementia from major depression: a cross-validation and extension. *J Neuropsychiatr Clin Neurosci* 2000;12:29–33.

208. Wetter S, Murphy C. Apollpoprotein E 4 positive individuals demonstrate delayed olfactory event-related potentials. *Neurobiol Aging* 2001;22:439–447.

209. Doty RL, Deems D, Setellar S. Olfactory dysfunction in parkinsonism: a general deficit unrelated to neurologic signs, disease stage, or disease duration. *Neurology* 1988;38:1237–1244.

210. Berendse H. Subclinical dopaminergic dysfunction in asymptomatic Parkinson's disease patients' relatives with a decreased sense of smell. *Ann Neurol* 2001;50: 34–41.

211. Garrett-Laster M, Russell R, Jacques P. Impairment of taste and olfaction in patients with cirrhosis: the role of vitamin A. *Human Nutr Clin Nutr* 1984;38C:203–214.

212. Madden A, Bradbury W, Morgan M. Taste perception in cirrhosis: its relationship to circulating micronutrients and food preferences. *Hepatology* 1997;26(1):40–48.

213. Bloomfeld R, Graham B, Schiffman S, Killenberg P. Alterations of chemosensory function in end-stage liver disease. *Physiol Behav* 1999;66(2):203–207.

214. Griep M, Van der Niepen P, Sennesael J, Mets T, Massart D, Verbeelen D. Odour perception in chronic renal disease. *Nephrol Dial Transplant* 1997;12: 2093–2098.

215. Astback J, Fernstrom A, Hylander B, Arvidson K, Johansson O. Taste buds and neuronal markers in patients with chronic renal failure. *Perit Dial Int* 1999;19 (suppl):S215–223.

216. Ophir D, Guterman A, Gross-Isseroff R. Changes in smell acuity induced by radiation exposure of the olfactory mucosa. *Arch Otolaryngol Head Neck Surg* 1988;114:853–855.

217. Weinstock R, Wright H, Smith D. Olfactory dysfunction in diabetes mellitus. *Physiol Behav* 1993;53:17–21.

218. Moore P, Guggenheimer J, Etzel K, Weyant R, Orchard T. Type 1 diabetes mellitus, xerostomia, and salivary flow rates. *Oral Surg Oral Med Oral Pathol Oral Radiol Endod* 2001;92(3):281–291.

219. Tepper B, Hartfiel L, Schneider S. Sweet taste and diet in type II diabetes. *Physiol Behav* 1996;60:13–18.

220. Tepper B, Seldner A. Sweet taste and intake of sweet foods in normal pregnancy and pregnancy complicated by gestational diabetes mellitus. *Am J Clin Nutr* 1999; 70(2):277–284.

221. Duffy V, Peterson J, Dinehart M, Bartoshuk L. Genetic and environmental variation in taste: associations with sweet intensity, preference, and intake. *Topics Clin Nutr* 2003;18:209–220.

222. Getchell M, Mellert T. Olfactory mucus secretion. In: Getchell T, Doty R, Bartoshuk L, Snow JJ, eds. *Smell and Taste in Health and Disease*. New York, NY: Raven Press; 1991:83–95.

223. Rasmussen N, Brofeldt S, Manthorpe R. Smell and nasal findings in patients with primary Sjögren's syndrome. *Scand J Rheumatol Suppl* 1986;61:142–145.

224. Hastings L, Miller M. Influence of environmental toxicants on olfactory function. In: Doty R, ed. *Handbook of Olfaction and Gustation*. New York, NY: Marcel Dekker Inc.; 2003:575–591.

225. Schiffman S. Taste and smell losses in normal aging and disease. *JAMA* 1997;278:1357–1362.

226. Doty RL, Philip S, Reddy K, Kerr K. Influences of antihypertensive and antihyperlipidemic drugs on the senses of taste and smell: a review. *J Hypertension* 2003;21:1805–1813.

227. Steele W, Stuart J, Whiting B. Serum, tear, and salivary concentrations of methotrexate in man. *Br J Clin Pharmacol* 1979;7:207–211.

228. Alfano M. The origin of gingival fluid. *J Theor Biol* 1974;47:127–136.

229. Maruniak J, Silver W, Moulton D. Olfactory receptors response to blood-borne odorants. *Brain Res* 1983; 265:312–316.

230. Matsuyama H, Tomita H. Clinical applications and mechanisms of intravenous taste tests. *Auris Nasus Larynx* 1986;13:S43–S50.

231. Garb J, Stunkard A. Taste aversions in man. *Am J Psych* 1974;131:1204–1207.

232. Friedman M, Mattes R. Chemical senses and nutrition. In: Getchell T, Doty R, Bartoshuk L, Snow JJ, eds. *Smell and Taste in Health and Disease*. New York, NY: Raven Press; 1991:391–404.

233. de Jong N, Chin A, Paw M, de Graaf C, van Staveren W. Effect of dietary supplements and physical exercise on sensory perception, appetite, dietary intake and body weight in frail elderly subjects. *Br J Nutr* 2000;83(6): 605–613.

234. Weisman K, Christensen E, Dreyer V. Zinc supplementation in alcoholic cirrhosis: a double-blind clinical trial. *Acta Med Scand* 1979;205:361–366.

235. Mahajan S, Prasad A, Lambujon J, Abbasi A, Briggs W. Improvement of uremic hypogeusia by zinc: a double-blinded study. *Am J Clin Nutr* 1980;33:1517–1521.

236. Ripamonti C, Zecca E, Brunelli C, et al. A randomized, controlled clinical trial to evaluate the effects of zinc sulfate on cancer patients with taste alterations caused by head and neck irradiation. *Cancer* 1998;82(10): 1938–1945.

237. Sturniolo G, D'Inca R, Parisi G, et al. Taste alterations in liver cirrhosis: are they related to zinc deficiency. *J Trace Elem Electrolytes Health Dis* 1992;6(1):15–19.

238. Tabuchi R, Econ M, Ohara I, Agr D. Influence of zinc supplementation to diets at graded levels of protein on taste sensitivity, morphological changes of tongue epithelia and serum zinc concentration in growing rats. *J Am Coll Nutr* 1996;15(3):303–308.

239. Ferris AM, Duffy VB. The effect of olfactory deficits on nutritional status: does age predict individuals at risk? Nutrition and the chemical senses in aging: recent advances and current research needs. *NY Acad Sci* 1989; 561:113–123

240. Ferris AM, Schlitzer JL, Schierberl MJ, et al. Anosmia and nutritional status. *Nutr Res* 1985;5:149–156.

241. Price S. The role of zinc in taste and smell. In: Meiselman H, Rivlin R, eds. *Clinical Measurement of Taste and Smell*. New York, NY: Macmillan; 1986:443–445.

242. Henkin R, Schechter P, Friedwald W, Demets D, Raff M. A double blind study of the effects of zinc sulfate on taste and smell dysfunction. *Am J Med Sci* 1976; 272:285–299.

243. Greger J, Geissler A. Effects of zinc supplementation on taste acuity of the aged. *Am J Clin Nutr* 1978;31: 633–637.

244. Bales C, Stenman L, Freeland-Graves J, Stone J, Young R. The effect of age on plasma zinc uptake and taste acuity. *Am J Clin Nutr* 1986;44:664–669.

245. Prasad A, Fitzgerald J, Hess J, Kaplan J, Pelen F, Dardenne M. Zinc deficiency in elderly patients. *Nutrition* 1993;9(3):218–224.

246. Mennella J, Beauchamp G. The early development of human flavor preferences. In: Capaldi E, ed. *Why We Eat What We Eat*. Washington, DC: American Psychological Association; 1996:83–112.

247. *Why We Eat What We Eat*. Washington, DC: American Psychological Association; 1996.

248. Capaldi E. Conditioned food preferences. In: Capaldi E, ed. *Why We Eat What We Eat*. Washington, DC: American Psychological Association; 1996:53–80.

249. Birch L, Fisher J. Development of eating behaviors among children and adolescents. *Pediatr* 1998;101: 539–549.

250. Schafe G, Bernstein I. Taste aversion learning. In: Capaldi E, ed. *Why We Eat What We Eat*. Washington, DC: American Psychological Association; 1996:31–51.

251. Rozin P. Sociocultural influences on food selection. In: Capalid E, ed. *Why We Eat What We Eat*. Washington, DC: American Psychological Association; 1996: 233–263.

252. Shepherd R. Sensory influences on salt, sugar and fat intake. *Nutr Res Rev* 1988;1:125–144.

253. Ship J, Duffy V, Jones J, Langmore S. Geriatric oral health and its impact on eating. *J Am Geriatr Soc* 1996; 44:456–464.

254. Rolls B. Sensory-specific satiety. *Nutr Rev* 1986;44(3): 93–101.

255. Centers for Medicaid and Medicare Services. MDS 2.0 Information Site. Accessed March 4, 2004.

256. Mattes R, Cowart B. Dietary assessment of patients with chemosensory disorders. *J Am Diet Assoc* 1994; 94(1):50–56.

257. Stevens J. Food quality reports from noninstitutionalized aged. Presented at: Nutrition and the Chemical Senses in Aging: Recent Advances and Current Research Needs; 1989; Sarasota, FL.

258. Duffy V. *Olfactory Dysfunction, Food Behaviors, Dietary Intake, and Anthropometric Measures in Single-living, Elderly Women* [doctoral dissertation]. University of Connecticut; 1992.

259. Doty R. Influence of age and age-related diseases on olfactory function. *Ann NY Acad Sci* 1989;561:76–86.

260. Duffy V, Backstrand J, Ferris A. Olfactory dysfunction and related nutritional risk in free-living, elderly women. *J Amer Dietet Assoc* 1995;95(8):879–884.

261. White T, Kurtz D. The relationship between metacognitive awareness of olfactory ability and age in people reporting chemosensory disturbances. *Am J Psychol* 2003;116(1):99–110.

262. Wayler AH, Muench ME, Kapur KK, Chauncy HH. Masticatory performance and food acceptability in persons with removable partial dentures, full dentures, and intact natural dentition. *J Gerontol* 1984;39(3):284–289.

263. Mattes R, Cowart B, Schiavo M, et al. Dietary evaluation of patients with smell and/or taste disorders. *Am J Clin Nutr* 1990;51:233–240.

264. Doty R. Food preference ratings of congenitally anosmic humans. In: Kare M, Maller O, eds. *Chemical Senses and Nutrition*. Vol II. New York, NY: Academic Press; 1977:315–325.

265. Murphy C, Withee J. Age-related differences in the pleasantness of chemosensory stimuli. *Psychol Aging* 1986;1(4):312–318.

266. Snyder D, Duffy V, Fast K, et al. Food preferences vary with age and sex: a new analysis using the general Labeled Magnitude Scale. *Chem Senses* 2001;26(8): 1050.

267. Snyder D, Duffy V, Hoffman H, Ko C, Bartoshuk L. Relationships between food preference and intake across the lifespan: new findings from NHANES III and USDA surveys. *Chem Senses* 2002;27:A19.

268. Mungas D, Cooper J, Weiler P, Gietzen D, Franzi C, Bernick C. Dietary preference for sweet foods in patients with dementia. *J Amer Geriatr Soc* 1990;38: 999–1007.

269. de Jong N, de Graaf C, van Staveren W. Effect of sucrose in breakfast items on pleasantness and food intake in the elderly. *Physiol Behav* 1996;60(6):1453–1462.

270. Chapo A, Bartoshuk L, Duffy V. Age-related changes in bitter and sweet sensations may influence dietary behaviors. *Chem Senses* 2003;28:A-41.

271. Lähteenmäki L, Tuorila H. Three-factor eating questionnaire and the use and liking of sweet and fat among dieters. *Physiol Behav* 1995;57(1):81–88.

272. Snyder D, Duffy V, Chapo A, Bartoshuk L. Food preferences mediate relationships between otitis media and body mass index. *Appetite* 2003;40:360

273. Chapo A, Alex J, Coelho D, Duffy V, Snyder D, Bartoshuk L. The influence of head trauma (HT), otitis media (OM), and tonsillectomy on oral sensation, fat acceptance and body mass index (BMI). *Chem Senses* In press.

274. Pelchat M, LaChaussee J. Food cravings and taste aversions in the elderly. *Appetite* 1994;23:193.

275. Pelchat M. You can teach an old dog new tricks: olfaction and responses to novel foods by the elderly. *Appetite* 2000;35:153–160.

276. Warwick Z, Schiffman S. Sensory evaluation of fat-sucrose and fat-salt mixtures: relationship to age and weight status. *Physiol Behav* 1990;48:633–636.

277. Schiffman S, Gatlin L, Satttely-Miller E, et al. The effect of sweeteners on bitter taste in young and elderly subjects. *Brain Res Bull* 1994;35(3):189–204.

278. Chapo A, Bartoshuk L, Brownbill R, Hutchins H, Ilich J, Duffy V. Age and genetic influences bitterness perception and dietary behaviors for bitter liquids and vegetables. Presented at: International Congress of Dietetics Meeting; 2004; Chicago, IL.

279. Basson M, Bartoshuk L, DiChello S, Weiffenbach J, Duffy V. Colon cancer and genetic variation in taste. *Chem Senses* 2003;28:A-123.

280. Tews J, Repa J, Nguyen H, Harper A. Protein selection by olfactory bulbectomized rats. *Nutr Rep Intl* 1985;31: 797–803.

281. May K. Association between anosmia and anorexia in cats. Presented at: Ninth International Symposium on Olfaction and Taste. *NY Acad Sci* 1986; 510: 480–82.

282. Schiffman S, Warwick Z. Use of flavor-amplified foods to improve nutritional status in elderly persons. Presented at: Nutrition and the Chemical Sense in Aging: Recent Advances and Current Research Needs. *NY Acad Sci* 1989; 561:267–276.

283. McAlpine S, Harper J, McMurdo M, Bolton-Smith C, Hetherington M. Nutritional supplementation in older adults: pleasantness, preference and selection of sip-feeds. *Br J Health Psychol* 2003;8(Pt 1):57–66.

284. Pelchat M, Schaefer S. Dietary monotony and food cravings in young and elderly adults. *Physiol Behav* 2002;68:353–359.

285. Rolls BJ, Rolls ET, Rowe EA, Kingston B, Megson A, Gunary R. Variety in a meal enhances food intake in man. *Physiol Behav* 1981;26:215–221.

286. Rolls B. Aging and appetite. *Nutr Rev* 1992;50(12): 422–426.

287. Rolls B, McDermott T. Effects of age on sensory-specific satiety. *Am J Clin Nutr* 1991;54:988–996.

288. Duffy V, Ferris A. Measured and self-rated olfactory dysfunction, dietary intake, and body mass index (BMI) in free-living elderly women. *FASEB J* 1993;7:A82.

289. Tennen H, Affleck G, Mendola R. Coping with smell and taste disorders. In: Getchell T, Doty R, Bartoshuk L, Snow JJ, eds. *Smell and Taste in Health and Disease.* New York, NY: Raven Press; 1991:787–802.

290. Holbrook E, Leopold D. Anosmia: diagnosis and management. *Curr Opin Otolaryngol Head Neck Surg* 2003;11(1):54–60.

291. Breslin P, Beauchamp G. Suppression of bitterness by sodium. *Chem Senses* 1995;20:609–623.

292. de Graaf C, Polet P, van Staveren W. Sensory perception and pleasantness of food flavors in elderly subjects. *J Gerontol Psychol Sci* 1994;49:P93–P99.

293. Koskinen S, Kalviainen N, Tuorila H. Flavor enhancement as a tool for increasing pleasantness and intake of a snack product among the elderly. *Appetite* 2003; 41(1):87–96.

294. Schiffman S, Warwick Z. Effect of flavor enhancement of foods for the elderly on nutritional status: food intake, biochemical indices, and anthropometric measures. *Physiol Behav* 1993;53(2):395–402.

295. Mathey M, Siebelink E, de Graaf C, Van Staveren W. Flavor enhancement of food improves dietary intake and nutritional status of elderly nursing home residents. *Gerontol A Biol Sci Med Sci* 2001;56(4):M200–205.

296. Henry C, Woo J, Lightowler H, et al. Use of natural food flavours to increase food and nutrient intakes in hospitalized elderly in Hong Kong. *Int J Food Sci Nutr* 2003;54(4):321–327.

297. Schiffman S. Intensification of sensory properties of foods for the elderly. *J Nutr* 2000;130:927–930.

298. Schiffman S. Sensory enhancement of foods for the elderly with monosodium glutamate and flavors. *Food Rev Int* 1998;14:321–333.

299. Position of the American Dietetic Association: Liberalized diets for older adults in long-term care. *J Am Diet Assoc* 2002;102:1316–1323.

CHAPTER 8

Oral Health in the Elderly

*Wendy E. Martin, DDS, Michèle Saunders, DDS, MS, MPH,
and Susan P. Stattmiller*

As the first segment of the gastrointestinal system, the oral cavity provides the point of entry for nutrients. The condition of the oral cavity, therefore, can facilitate or undermine nutritional status. If dietary habits are unfavorably influenced by poor oral health, then nutritional status may be compromised. However, nutritional status can also contribute to or exacerbate oral disease. General well-being is related to health and disease states of the oral cavity as well as the rest of the body. An awareness of this interrelationship is essential when the clinician is working with the older patient, since the incidence of major dental problems and the frequency of chronic illness and pharmacotherapy increase dramatically in older people.

REVIEW OF ANATOMY AND FUNCTIONS OF THE ORAL CAVITY

Anatomy of the Oral Cavity

The major parts of the oral cavity (Figure 8–1) are lips; vestibules; teeth; maxilla and mandible (upper and lower jaws, respectively); alveolar bone (termed *residual bone* if there are no teeth); gingivae (gums); hard and soft palates (roof of the mouth); tongue and mucous membranes (floor of the mouth); temporomandibular joint (TMJ); buccal mucosa (lining of the cheeks); salivary glands; and muscles of mastication and facial expression (orofacial musculature). Throughout the mouth, there are blood vessels, lymphatics, and nerves to ensure rapid communication between the oral cavity and other major organ systems.

At the lips, the skin of the face is continuous with the mucous membranes of the oral cavity. The bulk of the lips is formed by skeletal muscles and a variety of sensory receptors that judge the taste and temperature of foods. Their reddish color is due to an abundance of blood vessels near their surface.

The vestibule is the cleft that separates the lips and cheeks from the teeth and gingivae. When the mouth is closed, the vestibule communicates with the rest of the mouth through the space between the last molar teeth and the rami of the mandible.

Thirty-two teeth normally are present in the adult mouth: two incisors, one canine, two premolars, and three molars in each half of the upper and lower jaws. The teeth in the upper jaw are termed maxillary, and the teeth in the lower jaw are termed *mandibular.* The mandible is the movable member of the two jaws, whereas the maxilla is stationary. The components of an individual tooth provide a framework within which to appreciate changes that occur with age (Figure 8–2). Teeth are highly calcified structures composed of four parts: (1) enamel, the hard and brittle substance covering the outer surface of the crown of the tooth; (2) dentin, a bonelike substance forming the main body of the tooth, surrounding the pulp cavity, and covered by enamel on the crown and cementum on the root; (3) cementum, a

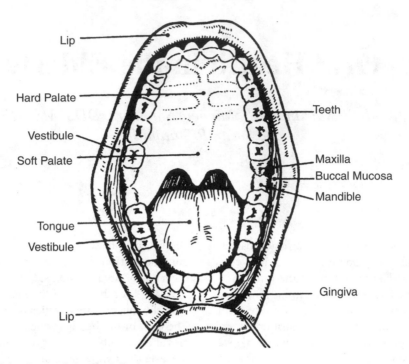

Figure 8–1 Major Parts of the Oral Cavity

bonelike substance that covers the tooth root; and (4) pulp chamber and canal(s), the soft central parts of the tooth that contain the blood vessels, nerves, and lymphatics. Each tooth in the mouth is surrounded and supported by alveolar bone. The visible portion of the tooth is termed the crown. The portion submerged below the gum line is the root. The region where these portions meet is called the *neck* of the tooth. The gingiva surrounds the necks of the teeth and covers the alveolar bone. It is composed of dense, fibrous tissue covered by a smooth vascular mucosa. The tooth roots are joined to the alveolar bone by periodontal ligaments.

The hard palate forms the roof of the mouth in the chewing area, and the soft palate lies just posterior to it. The floor of the mouth is formed by the tongue, which nearly fills the oral cavity when the mouth is closed, and mucous membranes. The tongue is a mobile mass of mostly skeletal muscle covered by a mucous membrane with numerous papillae on the surface.

The TMJ, located just anterior to the earlobe, is the only joint needed for chewing. A hinge-like movement occurs bilaterally in the TMJ during mouth opening and closing. During chewing, the mandible also exhibits protrusive and lateral movements.

The buccal mucosa forms the side walls of the oral cavity and contains numerous mucous glands. The secretions from these glands mix with food in the mouth to aid in both chewing and swallowing.

There are *three major* (bilateral) salivary glands, which secrete saliva into the mouth: parotid, submaxillary, and sublingual. The parotid glands are the largest, and their ducts open into the vestibules opposite the upper second molar teeth. The submaxillary (or submandibular) gland ducts open into the floor of the mouth under the tongue from their location in the angles of the mandible. The sublingual glands, the smallest of the major salivary glands, are embedded in the mucous membranes of the

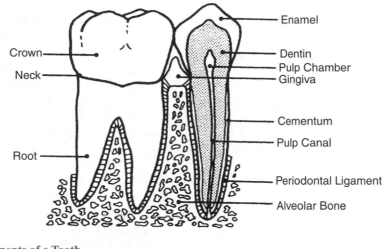

Figure 8–2 Components of a Tooth

floor of the mouth. Their ducts open under the tongue as well. The major salivary glands contribute about 95% of the total daily volume of saliva; the remaining 5% comes from numerous minor salivary glands in the mucous membranes of the lips, tongue, palates, and cheeks.[1] The primary role of saliva is to protect and maintain oral health.[2] In that regard, human saliva contains lubricatory factors (mucins) to keep oral tissues hydrated, pliable, and insulated; contains many antibacterial proteins that regulate colonization of oral bacteria; buffers the acid produced by oral bacteria to maintain tooth integrity; aids in carbohydrate digestion; mediates taste acuity; and is necessary for mastication and preparation of food for swallowing.[3–5]

The orofacial musculature consists of 4 muscles of mastication—the masseter, the lateral pterygoid, the medial pterygoid, and the temporalis muscles—and almost 20 muscles of facial expression. One of these facial muscles, the *buccinator,* acts as an accessory muscle of mastication by eliminating the space of the vestibule between the cheek and the jaws during chewing.

Functions of the Oral Cavity

The oral cavity serves in the masticating, tasting, and swallowing of food; as a phonetic box for speech; and as a secondary pathway for breathing. The major and minor salivary glands provide moisture to soften foods as well as supply carbohydrate-digesting enzymes.

Mastication (Chewing)

The teeth are designed for chewing; the anterior teeth provide a strong cutting action, and the posterior teeth provide a grinding action. The names of the teeth demarcate their four basic functions. The *incisors* cut or slice food, the *canines* tear food, the *premolars* shred food, and the *molars* grind food in preparation for swallowing.

Proper chewing is important in the digestion of all foods, especially most fruits and raw vegetables, which contain indigestible cellulose membranes that must be broken down before the food can be used by the body. Also, since digestive enzymes act only on the surfaces of food particles, the rate of digestion is highly dependent on the total surface area of the chewed food that is exposed to intestinal secretions.

The act of chewing has more significance than the mere preparation of food for swallowing. The food is moved around the mouth so that the taste buds are stimulated, and odors are released that stimulate the olfactory receptors. Much of the satisfaction and pleasure of eating depends on these stimuli.

Digestion in the Mouth

Saliva contains the digestive enzyme ptyalin (amylase), which functions to hydrolyze starches into two disaccharides, maltose and isomaltose. This is the first step in the digestion of carbohydrates. However, since food stays in the mouth for such a limited amount of time, only 3% to 5% of the starches that are eaten are hydrolyzed by the time the food is swallowed.[2] Most naturally occurring starches are digested poorly by ptyalin because they are protected by a thin cellulose cover. Cooking destroys these cellulose membranes and facilitates digestion in the mouth.

In general, swallowing can be divided into three stages: (1) the *voluntary stage,* which initiates the swallowing process; (2) the *pharyngeal stage,* which is involuntary and involves the muscular contractions for the passage of food through the pharynx to the esophagus; and (3) the *esophageal stage,* which is another involuntary phase that promotes the passage of food from the pharynx to the stomach. The oral cavity is involved with only the first (voluntary) stage of swallowing, which takes about 1 second.[6] When the food is ready to be swallowed, pressure from the tongue upward and backward against the palate forces the bolus of food posteriorly into the pharynx. From here on, the process of swallowing becomes automatic and usually cannot be stopped.

Speech

Speech is a complex behavior that integrates the processes of respiration, phonation, oral sensation, resonation, and articulation.[6] The mouth is one of the resonators for speech and other vocalizations. Speech relies heavily on the anatomic structures of the oral cavity, the three major organs of articulation are the lips, tongue, and soft palate.

ORAL HEALTH STATUS AND NEEDS IN THE ELDERLY

Oral Health Status

Oral health implies a state that is stable, relatively disease free, comfortable, and that permits adequate functioning for mastication, swallowing, and speech. Poor oral health may be viewed as a state of inadequate functioning resulting from decayed teeth; periodontal disease; ill-fitting dentures or lack of dentures; neglect of oral hygiene; and the presence of pain, inflammation, or infection in the oral cavity. Although few of these conditions pose mortality risks, they may lead to physical dysfunction, pain, and psychological anguish in the older patient.

A major criterion of successful aging is how well the individual maintains oral health, the ability to chew, the ability to talk, and personal satisfaction with appearance.[7] Unfortunately, the mouth often becomes one of the first areas of the body to be neglected by people who have chronic diseases and infirmities in old age.

There have been five national surveys indicating the oral status of the elderly. The older aged were excluded in two of the studies: the National Health Examination Survey of 1960–1962 excluded participants older than 79 years,[8] and the National Health and Nutrition Examination Survey (HANES I) of 1971–1974 included no subjects older than 74 years.[9]

In 1978, the National Institutes of Health (NIH) introduced an oral physiology and aging component to the Baltimore Longitudinal Study of Aging.[10] In Iowa, a longitudinal survey was initiated in 1981 to determine the prevalence and incidence of oral conditions in noninstitutionalized rural elderly Iowans. In 1987, the National Institute of Dental Research (NIDR) published national and regional data on the prevalence of oral conditions in 15,000 working adults and 5600 elderly people who attended multipurpose senior centers.[11] Useful data were obtained from this survey of adult oral health, even though the older participants were not entirely representative of the nation's elderly population. The findings disclosed that Americans are keeping their teeth longer, are going to the dentist more often for preventive checkups, are reducing the number of cavities in their mouths, and have practically eliminated edentulousness in middle age. However, serious dental problems still exist among elderly people (Table 8–1).

Table 8–1 Comparison of Oral Health Status of Employed Adults and Older Adults

Oral Status/Treatment Need	% of Employed Adults	% of Older Adults
Calculus deposits	83.9	88.9
Edentulousness	4.2	41.1
Gingival bleeding (after probing)	43.6	46.9
Gingival recession (1+ mm)	51.1	88.3
Periodontal attachment loss (1+ sites)	76.7	95.1
Retention of all teeth	36.7	2.1
Root caries	21.1	56.9
Visited dentist in past 2 years	79.6	56.4
Perceived need for dental care	50.4	36.0

Source: Reprinted from National Survey of Adult Dental Health, *Oral Health of United States Adults: National Findings*, 1987, National Institute of Dental Research.

Oral Health Needs

In general, studies reveal that many unmet treatment needs are affecting a large portion of the noninstitutionalized elderly population. This is true whether the study has been conducted by direct examination of patients or by survey. Data from HANES I indicated that 60% of elderly subjects had at least one dental treatment need.[9] The survey of rural elderly Iowans also found a high level of treatment needed: 40% required at least one restoration, 16% required at least one extraction, and 27% required some prosthodontic treatment; more than 60% of the dentate subjects needed some periodontal treatment.[12–14]

Many local studies and one statewide survey have documented the large need for dental care among institutionalized residents.[15–17] The results have ranged from 2.3 dental services needed per person with 3.2 services required for those having remaining natural dentition,[15] to 82.5% of 3247 patients screened in Vermont nursing homes in 1982.[16] In the latter study, examiners found that 37.2% of the residents required immediate attention to eliminate pain, infection, concern of malignancy, or a combination of these symptoms.

CHANGES IN ORAL AND CIRCUMORAL STRUCTURES WITH AGING

Overview

Differentiation of normal aging changes from disease processes in old age is of paramount importance. Not knowing the changes that occur with age might lead to excessive or unnecessary treatment. Erroneously evaluating a disease process as normal aging might have equally serious consequences. Unfortunately, lack of research on the aging oral cavity has resulted in a number of stereotypes and generalizations.[18] Standard graphs, tables, and information in many geriatric medical and dental textbooks show inevitable decrements with age. However, these studies included subjects who, although superficially healthy, in fact had some disease or were taking medication that affected oral function.[19] Therefore, most of this early information probably reflects oral changes due to disease or its treatment rather than dysfunctions related directly to increased age.

Hard Tissues

Bone

In the developmental years, bone resorption and deposition occur synchronously in the process of growth and remodeling. Alveolar bone, however, has a remodeling rate greater than that of the other bones of the body.[20] Bone is notably less active with maturity, although there is still some degree of continuing resorption and deposition. After age 35 to 40 years, approximately 1% of bone mass is lost per year in both men and women.[20]

As physical activity diminishes in the later years, so too does the demand for new bone formation. Resorption exceeds deposition, resulting in a net loss of bone. By the time old age is reached, atrophy has resulted from slow resorption with very little remodeling. Not only is there a generalized decline in bone volume,[21] but the composition of bone gradually alters, resulting in reduced resilience and increased brittleness and fragility (Chapter 12).[22]

Alveolar bone is one of the first bones to be affected by loss of mass. The periosteal and periodontal surfaces of alveolar bone become less resistant to harmful local oral trauma, inflammation, or disease.[23] This is a major factor contributing to periodontal disease, loss of teeth, and in the edentulous patient, inability to obtain adequate support and stability for dentures.[18,24] In both the maxilla and the mandible, the amount, extent, and uniformity of the bone loss differ with varying etiologies and health status.[25] It is now recognized that alveolar bone or residual ridge resorption is confounded by such factors as age, sex, race, and health status of the patient when the teeth are extracted; the tooth extraction technique; the diet of the patient; the presence of local factors; and the frequency of denture use.[25]

Teeth

It is frequently reported that the teeth themselves undergo changes with age (Table 8–2). Teeth differ from most other parts of the body in that the reparative or regenerative capacity of their constituent tissues is extremely limited. Also, the blood vessels and nerves become less active with age; as a result, the vitality of the average human tooth pulp lasts approximately 70 years.[2]

Attrition. The remaining natural teeth are likely to exhibit some flattening of the chewing surfaces induced by repeated contact with opposing teeth during masticatory movements. To compensate for the natural wear of these surfaces, human teeth erupt with their supporting structures throughout adult life.[26]

The patterns of tooth wear vary with each patient and are cumulative, since the enamel is incapable of repair or regeneration. The wear can range from minimal faceting to extreme loss of tooth substance, sometimes extending to the gin-

---

Table 8–2 Anatomic Changes in the Teeth with Age

Enamel
  Regeneration/repair-incapable
  Permeability-decreased

Dentin
  Permeability-decreased
  Sensitivity-decreased
  Calcification-increased
  Pain conduction-decreased
  Repair-capable with vital tooth pulp

Pulp chamber and canals
  Cellularity-decreased
  Innervation-decreased
  Tooth drainage-decreased
  Vascularity-decreased
  Volume-decreased (due to deposition of reparative dentin)

Apical foramen
  Size-decreased (may cause decreased pulp vascularity and innervation)

Cementum
  Deposition-continuous (major cause of decreased apical foramen size)
  Repair-capable with vital tooth pulp
  Resorption-increased susceptibility

Entire tooth
  Brittleness-increased (predisposing tooth to cracks, fractures, shearing)
  Darkening-increased
  Pain sensitivity-decreased
  Thermal sensitivity-decreased
  Translucency-decreased

giva. However, there is no agreement on the point at which physiologic attrition becomes pathologic or contributes to pathologic conditions.[27] In areas of excessive wear, reparative (or secondary) dentin is deposited on the walls of the pulp chamber and canals for protection. This, as well as reduced enervation, helps to explain the reduced tooth pain sensitivity and higher pain threshold in elderly people.

Temporomandibular Joint

The TMJ is a complex, diarthrodial joint capable of both swinging (hinge-like) and sliding motions on many axes. It undergoes functional remodeling throughout life, usually in response to changes in articulation of the teeth or alterations in the space between the maxilla and mandible. The functional changes in the TMJ are by no means confined to elderly individuals.

Signs of TMJ change include joint clicking, limitation of jaw opening, and deviation of the mandible during function, with the major symptom being pain. Researchers with the Baltimore Longitudinal Study of Aging assessed all of these for arteriosclerosis or obliteration of the capillaries.[28] More research into the aging TMJ is needed since these age-related changes may explain some of the masticatory problems in this age group.

Soft Tissues

Mucous Membranes

The stereotypic effect of aging on the oral mucosa is that atrophic changes occur. Clinically, these changes involve the surface epithelium's becoming thinner, drier, less elastic, less vascular, less firmly attached to the underlying connective tissue and bone, and more susceptible to injury from mild stresses.[22,29] Other changes occur as well with reduction in connective tissue and subcutaneous fat and increased linkage of collagen molecules. Some symptoms have been associated with these alterations, including xerostomia (mouth dryness) and sensations of pain or burning on the tongue, palate, or oral mucosa.[18] These changes, however, must be interpreted with caution. In critical reviews of the literature, Baum[18] and Hill[30] suggested that no conclusions could be drawn about whether atrophy of the oral mucosa is associated with aging. Other researchers have concluded that specific alterations of the oral tissues may instead be induced by a host of environmental factors, such as tobacco smoking or chronic systemic disease.[31]

Periodontium

Gingiva. The gum tissue of the elderly individual gradually recedes from the tooth, with subsequent exposure of more of the tooth surface and root. The degree that gingival recession progresses is related to age, tooth movement, inflammatory changes due to disease, oral care habits, and heredity.

Periodontal Ligament. The periodontal ligament is not one ligament, but a series of short, dense ligaments connecting the cementum of the tooth root to alveolar bone. Since the ligament is made up of connective tissues, aging affects it in the same way as it does other connective tissues in the body.[32] The result is a progressive loss of soft tissue attachment, leading to exposure of the root and loosening of the teeth within their bony sockets.

Tongue

The status of the tongue in aging, independent of diseased states and taste acuity, has not been studied in detail. Tongue vascularity changes very little compared with that of other organs because there is little tendency in this tissue for atherosclerosis or obliteration of the capillaries.[31] There is much controversy about whether aging is associated with atrophy of the papillae, increased formation of fissures, and decreasing sensitivity to gustatory stimuli in the tongue.[31,33–35]

Circumoral Tissues

Oral Musculature

Changes in aging oral musculature are consistent with those in aging muscle tissue in the body as a whole.[36] In general, there are reductions in muscle tone,[6] muscle performance,[37] number and activity of muscle cells, and number and size of the muscle fibers. Replacement of the muscle mass by fat or fibrous connective tissue results in generalized atrophy of the musculature attached to the bones in the oral cavity.[38]

Mastication. The muscles of mastication atrophy with age; this decreases the biting force and slows chewing performance.[39] The atrophy is probably due in part to disuse, since less muscular effort is required for chewing as a result of failing dentition or a progressively softer diet or both. In either case, the generalized loss of muscle mass decreases the biting force and can make chewing difficult.

Deglutition. Aging does not significantly affect the transit of the prepared food bolus through the mouth and pharynx.[40] However, the impact of decreased muscle mass and tone can make swallowing difficult and can alter the ability to form and prepare a bolus in the oral stage of swallowing.[6] Several studies[39–41] have demonstrated that as people age, they take longer and expend more effort to prepare a food bolus before swallowing.

Other Changes

Salivary Glands

In early reports, decreased salivary flow was generally considered to be concomitant with increased age.[18,42] Recent evidence indicates that the diminished salivary flow often noted in studies of elderly subjects is due to pathologic conditions or pharmacologic effects of medications, rather than aging.[2,5–7,42,43] Since diminished salivary flow does not occur in healthy, nonmedicated individuals,[44] these findings emphasize that the elderly person may be susceptible to situations and therapies that result in a reduction of saliva availability.

Sense of Taste

The sense of taste is a function of the taste buds in the mouth. Its importance in nutrition lies in the fact that it allows a person to select food in accord with personal desires and needs of the tissues for specific nutritive substances.

Taste Buds. The taste buds are found predominantly on three of the four different types of the tongue papillae (circumvallate, fungiform, and foliate), although they are also located in the epithelium of the palate, tonsillar pillars, and other points around the nasopharynx.[45] In early anatomic studies, marked decreases in the numbers and atrophy of the taste buds with aging were reported.[46] However, more recent investigations indicate there is no significant loss of taste buds in old age.[47]

Taste Sensitivity. Elderly people often complain of altered taste sensations (dysgeusia), decreased ability to perceive taste (hypogeusia), or complete loss of taste (ageusia). Few studies have been able to determine the reasons for these decrements in taste sensitivity.[45,48] One explanation is decreased salivary flow, since taste buds react only to dissolved compounds.

Although there is some agreement that taste sensitivity begins to decline after age 55 years, differences in research methods have produced different results.[49] Some studies have indicated that older adults need higher concentrations of the four primary sensations of taste (salty, sour, sweet, bitter) for identification than do children and younger adults.[50] Others have found that the taste buds detecting saltiness and sweetness are the first to deteriorate and that sensitivity to sour and bitter tastes declines later.[51,52] The use of psychophysical procedures found only minimal changes in taste sensitivity,[34] even though a steady decline in taste sensitivity with increasing age is still being found (Chapter 7).[34,35]

Sense of Smell

Smell is the least researched and understood sense. This is due in part to the location of the olfactory sensory receptors in specialized epithelial tissue of the nasal cavity and in part to the fact that the sense of smell is a subjective phenomenon that is not easily measured. In fact, much of what we call taste is actually smell, which largely determines the flavor and palatability of foods and beverages.[53]

Evidence of a decline in olfactory sensitivity with age is still very limited, and the cause of any decrement remains speculative.[54] Some investigators have found reduced smell sensitivity, with the greatest problems in recognition and identification of odors among persons older than 80 years.[55] Others have reported age-related losses with significant individual differences.[56] It has also been suggested that poor health and smoking may cause an even greater decline in smell sensitivity than does age alone.[56]

CHANGES IN ORAL AND CIRCUMORAL STRUCTURES WITH DISEASE

Overview

There are three major characteristics of dental diseases: universality, irreversibility, and cumulativeness (Table 8–3). Although these diseases are rarely debilitating or life threatening, there are indications that they have a significant impact on social, economic, and psychological areas of life, including the quality of life.[57] Older adults tend to place minimal importance on their oral health and accept functionally inadequate dentition as an unavoidable consequence of the aging process.

Many of the oral diseases that afflict the elderly are diseases of all age groups. Therefore, preventive dentistry remains an important aspect of their oral health care and should involve all three levels of prevention: (1) preventing initiation of disease, (2) preventing the progression and recurrence of disease, and (3) preventing the loss of function and loss of life.[58]

The prevention of dental disease requires that all individuals see a dentist at least yearly, whether they have natural teeth, no teeth, complete dentures, or a combination of teeth and dentures. First, this allows primary prevention procedures to be evaluated and reinforced regularly. Detrimental habits, environmental factors, and nutritional status all affect the likelihood that oral pathology will occur. As an example, poor oral hygiene significantly contributes to the diseases caused or aggravated by bacterial plaque infection,[59] and it is well known that the level of oral hygiene deteriorates with age.[60] Second, regular dental care can lead to early diagnosis and treatment of the pathologic conditions described below.

Hard Tissues

Bone

Resorption. Bone resorption is associated with loss of mineral content, increase in porosity, and generalized atrophy. Clinical observation of alveolar bone resorption has so far failed to provide a clear understanding of the mechanisms responsible. There is a portion of the population that shows bone loss without the other findings usually associated with active periodontal disease. This loss is also seen in the absence of dentition.[61]

Resorption of alveolar bone occurs in two dimensions. The mandible resorbs primarily in a vertical direction, resulting in loss of bone height. The maxilla resorbs primarily in a horizontal direction away from the covering lips and cheeks. This means that the chin will appear to protrude because the maxilla has receded horizontally and this leads to the characteristic "toothless look," which is a shortening of the distance between the chin and nose and a pulling inward of the lips.

Table 8–3 The Major Characteristics of Dental Diseases

1. *Universality*—Diseases of the oral cavity are the most prevalent of all diseases; dental caries and periodontal disease usually affect most people throughout life.
2. *Irreversibility*—The damage derived from the common oral diseases, such as dental decay or bone loss, is irreversible, although treatment can usually intercept its spread.
3. *Cumulativeness*—The structural losses induced in the teeth and their supporting alveolar bone by oral diseases are cumulative.

Source: Vergo TJ Jr, Papas A. Physiological aspects of geriatric dentistry. *J Mass Dent Society* 1988 Fall; 374(4):165–168.[38]

Resorption is greater in the mandible than in the maxilla, and when severe, constitutes a major problem in the wearing of dentures. The residual bony ridge may become thin and knifelike and unable to withstand the downward compressive forces of a conventional denture.

Osteopenia and Osteoporosis. Osteopenia refers to metabolic bone diseases that are characterized by X-ray findings of a subnormal amount of mineralized bone mass (Chapter 14). The most common osteopenia is osteoporosis, generally defined as a decrease in the quantity of bone, with an increased incidence of fractures from minimal trauma.[62] Osteoporosis is observable within the oral cavity as dental osteopenia.

One of the first signs of osteoporosis is alveolar bone loss, followed by loss in the vertebrae and long bones.[63] Indeed, there is a significant correlation between skeletal osteopenia and density of alveolar bone and residual ridges.[63] Radiographically, it appears as diminished bone mass in the mandibular angular cortex, decreased trabeculae, and a diminished alveolar crest.[64] Subsequently, it leads to an inadequate amount of bone mass in the mandible, loss or mobility of teeth, edentulousness, and inability to wear dentures.[65] The loss of teeth and the use of ill-fitting dentures also cause extensive alveolar bone or residual ridge atrophy.[65,66]

Although calcium deficiencies and calcium-phosphorus imbalances are contributing factors in the pathogenesis of osteoporosis,[63] prevention and management include not only increased calcium intake but estrogen therapy, bone-building or antiresorptive agents, dietary vitamin D, and exercise.[67–69] Although fluoride therapy is used extensively in preventive dentistry, its widespread use in the prevention of osteoporosis is still being investigated.[70]

Teeth

Dental Caries (Tooth Decay): Coronal and Root Surfaces. Dental caries has been considered a disease of young people that stabilizes in the mid-20s and remains dormant until periodontal disease or gingival recession exposes the roots of the teeth and caries of the root surfaces occurs.[58,71,72] However, more recent research indicates that a significant increase in caries, including recurrent decay around restorations, cervical caries at the gingival margin, and root caries, is associated with aging.[11,73,74] Most of the recurrent caries are in the proximal regions of the teeth.[75] Root caries occurs following exposure of the tooth root.[74,76–78]

The diagnosis of dental caries is based on X-ray examination and clinical observation, since there is no absolute correlation between the presence or extent of dental decay and symptoms. It is generally recognized that four things are necessary to produce a carious lesion: cariogenic bacteria, a substrate of dietary carbohydrates, a susceptible host (tooth), and time. However, factors that contribute to high caries risk include poor oral hygiene, gingival recession, reduced salivary flow (which increases plaque accumulation), bacterial virulence, and diet.[75]

Conditions that predispose to xerostomia (dry mouth), such as medications, Sjögren's syndrome, and head and neck irradiation, can promote rampant dental caries in all age groups.[79] In fact, the incidence of root surface caries in elderly people is significantly correlated with a low rate of salivary secretion.[80]

Historically, the most effective strategy for preventing dental caries has been increasing tooth resistance to pathogenic plaque through the use of fluorides by systemic introduction (water and diet) and topical application (professional or self-applied).[81,82] Even fluoridation of other vehicles, such as salt, milk, and sugar, has been considered in areas where no reticulated water supplies exist.[83] In patients with xerostomia, the development of caries has been avoided largely by daily topical application of either 0.5% sodium fluoride or 0.5% stannous fluoride solutions.[84]

Unfortunately, there are few clinical data supporting the use of topical fluoride for prevention of dental caries in geriatric patients with adequate salivary flow.[84–87] Newbrun,[88] however, believes that the elderly population would benefit from the use of fluoride dentifrices, mouth rinses, and gels applied by brush, finger applicator, or plastic tray. The method to be used is dictated by the anticipated susceptibility to decay and the ability of the patient to manage the regimen.

Since both coronal and root caries are plaque-related diseases, measures that limit or inhibit plaque formation should be effective in prevention. Mechanical oral hygiene techniques and chemical antimicrobial agents such as chlorhexidine[89] reduce bacterial flora and substrate. Even dietary modification decreases the amount of substrate, acid production, and decalcification of teeth if individuals eliminate or reduce the intake of foods that are soft, sticky, retentive, or high in sugar and if they chew firm foods.[9]

Abrasion and Erosion. An aging population with longer retention of teeth is at increased risk for both abrasion (wear of tooth structure by nonmasticatory mechanical forces) and erosion (wear of tooth structure by chemical dissolution). The incidence of both of these conditions increases with age, simply because any damage to the teeth is cumulative. In patients with xerostomia, the diminution in the mucin level of the oral cavity provides less lubrication and protection, posing an even greater risk for abrasion and erosion.

A major etiologic factor of abrasion is overzealous and improper tooth brushing with a hard-bristle brush or an abrasive dentifrice.[90] The damage appears as transverse scoring of the tooth surface and tends to be asymmetric in its severity, depending on whether the patient is right-handed or left-handed.[90] Prevention is largely a matter of proper tooth brushing and the use of a soft bristle brush and toothpaste with minimal abrasivity. Other forms of abrasion result from holding objects with the teeth, chewing tobacco, and using dental floss and toothpicks improperly.

Erosion is a chemical process that occurs when the concentration of acid in the mouth is too high for the saliva to neutralize. The most common causes are chronic ingestion of fruits, fruit juices, and carbonated beverages; sucking candies containing phosphorus or citric acid; and gastroesophageal reflux.[91–93] Erosion can also result from working in an industry that uses or produces acidic materials.[94,95] To prevent dietary erosion, the use of straws with fruit juices and carbonated beverages and the substitution of sugar-free candies or gums are indicated.

The lesions of abrasion and erosion look different: The lesions of abrasion are characteristically narrow in relation to depth, and areas of erosion are usually saucer shaped.[22,96] Generally, these lesions do not require restorative treatment unless they are extensive or symptomatic.[96]

Hypersensitive Dentin and Cementum. Exposure of dentin or cementum from abrasion, erosion, acute or chronic trauma, or various restorative treatment procedures can lead to hypersensitive dentin and cementum. The teeth are exquisitely sensitive with exposure to any chemical, thermal, tactile, or osmotic stimulus. Although there is great individual variation in pain sensation, hypersensitivities to sour, sweet, cold, hot, and mechanical irritations are most common.[97]

Since hypersensitivity may deter a person from establishing or maintaining adequate oral hygiene procedures, decreasing sensitivity is the first step in treatment. One method is "sealing" the exposed tooth surfaces by applying agents or dentifrices such as fluoride gels and rinses.[98] In some cases, dental restoration and even endodontic therapy may be necessary to arrest the progress of the lesion, restore the function and shape of the tooth, and relieve pain.[98]

Tooth Loss and Edentulousness. Tooth loss is an irreversible, cumulative process that is no longer considered a natural consequence of aging. Instead, it is known to be the ultimate sequela of the two most common dental diseases, which are dental caries and periodontal disease. Nevertheless, tooth loss increases in frequency with age. By age 65 years, approximately 40% of Americans have lost all their teeth; another 20% have lost more than half their teeth.

In all age groups, the total loss of teeth is historically related to increased sugar consumption, combined with ignorance of prevention and insufficient dental manpower resources at the time.[26] Tooth loss in adults older than 35 years has been consistently attributed to periodontal diseases.[99] However, recent studies of tooth loss in adult populations indicate that caries is most often the cause for tooth extractions.[100,101]

The rate of edentulousness, or total lack of teeth, is declining in the elderly population of the United States. In 1957, 67.3% of persons older than 65 years were edentulous, whereas only 45.5% were so in 1971.[102] This was largely due to the introduction of preventive and restorative dental procedures. Today, less than 40% of elderly people are edentulous, and this number is rapidly decreasing.

In the recent national survey of employed and older adults, in the group aged 55 to 64 years, less than 15% were edentulous.[11] However, the prevalence of lost teeth was still extensive enough to compromise the employed adults' dentition and to impair function in most of the older adults.[11,103] This means that the fewer missing teeth predicted to occur in the future will lead not only to an increase in tooth-related diseases, but also to the continuing need for regular dental care.

Temporomandibular Joint

Dysfunctions of the TMJ have their primary base in the joint mechanism, even though the actual dysfunction may involve the ligaments, the muscles, or the bone itself. One half of the edentulous and one third of the dentulous older population have signs and symptoms of TMJ disorders,[104] including soreness of the jaw; dull, aching facial pain; severe pain in the joint area; tenderness or pain of the masticatory and facial muscles; dizziness; headaches; impaired hearing or earache; eye pain; chronic fatigue; and popping, clicking, or cracking noises near the ear while opening and closing the mouth.[105] These manifestations are dynamic, characterized by periods of quiescence and exacerbation, and have a wide range of expression among patients.[106] However, elderly individuals appear to have more symptoms than do younger persons.[104]

The causes of TMJ dysfunction may be external, internal, or both. External causes include degenerative joint disease; alveolar bone resorption; and injuries to the head, neck, or mandible. Internally, attrition, malocclusion, and bruxism,

in either natural or artificial teeth, can cause the facial muscles and TMJ to quit working together correctly.[107]

Diagnostic and treatment decisions are based on symptom reports and clinical examination findings. Management therapies advocated for TMJ dysfunction include applying moist heat to the face; using prescribed muscle relaxants or other medications; massaging the muscles; eating soft and nonchewy foods; undergoing counseling; training in biofeedback or relaxation procedures; correcting the "bite" of the teeth; and, in severe cases, undergoing surgery.

Soft Tissues

Mucous Membranes/Epithelium

The oral mucosa is composed of both keratinized and nonkeratinized epithelium. In addition, the mouth has a dark, moist environment that is replete with microorganisms. The oral mucosa also may be subjected to several environmental influences, such as smoking; chewing of the lips and cheeks; eating a variety of foods; and sources of trauma, allergy, and carcinogenesis.[108]

Aphthous Ulcer (Canker Sore, Aphthous Stomatitis, Ulcerative Stomatitis). Aphthous ulcers appear as shallow white macules or papules with flat, fairly even borders surrounded by an intense erythematous halo. Each ulcer often is covered with a pseudomembrane. One or more ulcers may be present. They tend to recur and are usually very painful during their acute phase. The pain may interfere with eating, swallowing, and moving the tongue. Aphthous ulcers occur more frequently in women than in men.

Aphthae are found on oral mucosal surfaces that are not bound to underlying bone, especially the buccal and labial mucosa, dorsum of the tongue, floor of the mouth, soft palate, gingivae, lips, and oropharynx. The diagnosis depends mainly on exclusion of similar but more readily identifiable diseases, a history of recurrence, and inspection of the ulcer.

The etiology is still unclear, as it has never been adequately demonstrated that this lesion is due to a virus or any other specific chemical, physical, psychological, or hormonal cause.[109] Nuts, coffee, chocolate, and citrus fruits often cause flare-ups, but abstinence will not prevent recurrence. Trauma, nutritional deficiencies, stresses of various types, food components, and allergies have been shown to be contributory to the disease.[109,110]

Healing, which usually occurs in 1 to 3 weeks without scarring, may be accelerated slightly by treatment. A film-forming medication, hydroxy-propyl cellulose (Zilactin®), brings impressive pain relief and is able to protect the areas of ulceration from irritants, thus allowing patients to eat and drink more normally.[111] Bland antibiotic or anesthetic mouth rinses, topical steroid-antibiotic therapy, and surface protectants can also reduce pain. Sedatives, analgesics, and vitamins may help indirectly, while good oral hygiene and the minimization of mucosal trauma are helpful. Systemic antibiotics are contraindicated.

Ulcerative stomatitis is a general term for multiple ulcerations on an inflamed oral mucosa. It may be secondary to blood dyscrasias, erythema multiforme, bullous lichen planus, acute herpes simplex infection, pemphigoid, pemphigus, and drug reactions. If the lesions cannot be classified, they are referred to as *aphthae*.

Candidiasis (Moniliasis, Thrush). Candidiasis is the most common opportunistic infection of the mouth, caused by overgrowth of a species of the fungus *Candida*. The species most frequently implicated in oral infections is *C. albicans*. The yeast phase of the fungus is a component of the normal oral flora of most people.[112] It exists in a symbiotic relationship with many of the other oral microorganisms. Because it has such low virulence in the yeast phase, some change must take place in the local environment to produce conditions favorable for its overgrowth and tissue invasion. This change commonly occurs when there is a reduction in host resistance caused by bacterial or viral infection, systemic disease, or medications.

Oral candidiasis generally presents in one of three distinct clinical forms: acute pseudomembranous candidiasis (thrush), acute atrophic candidiasis (antibiotic sore mouth), or chronic atrophic candidiasis (denture sore mouth). Rare forms include chronic hyperplastic candidiasis and chronic mucocutaneous candidiasis.

The lesions of acute pseudomembranous candidiasis consist of either multifocal or diffuse, white, superficial curdlike plaques occurring anywhere in the oral cavity. The infection is called pseudomembranous because the plaques can be scraped off easily, leaving an erythematous or bleeding base whereas most other white mucosal lesions cannot be rubbed off.

Acute atrophic candidiasis often follows prolonged antibiotic or steroid therapy and results, clinically, in a painful erythematous mucosa, particularly involving the tongue. The problem usually resolves with cessation of the medications, but antifungal therapy will hasten recovery. Chronic atrophic candidiasis presents as a slightly granular or irregularly eroded erythematous mucosa under dentures.

Any of these types of candidiasis can be accompanied by angular cheilitis. The diagnosis is based on the varied clinical picture of the surface white patches or erythematous changes and may be confirmed by laboratory culture. Treatment includes elimination of the causative or predisposing factor, if practical, and administration of antifungal agents.[113]

Leukoplakia (Benign Keratosis, White Patch). The term *leukoplakia* is used to describe a thickened, white plaque that will not rub or strip off and is not identifiable clinically or pathologically as any other disease. The lesions may be found on all oral mucous membrane surfaces, varying from a small circumscribed area to an extensive lesion involving a large area of mucosa. They are usually asymptomatic and are discovered during a routine dental examination or by patients who feel the thickened plaques in their mouths. Leukoplakia occurs more often in men, and the highest incidence is in the fifth to seventh age decade.[114]

The most common cause of leukoplakia is epithelial hyperplasia, hyperkeratosis, hyperortho-keratosis, dyskeratosis, or acanthosis. These terms refer specifically to reactive conditions of the oral mucosal epithelium, usually in response to an irritant or chronic irritation. The specific etiology is often unknown, but there are risk factors including tobacco, alcohol, deficiency of vitamin A or B complexes, and chronic irritating conditions or habits.[115,116]

Treatment consists of removing all irritants. Failure of a keratotic lesion to regress within 2 weeks after elimination of the apparent cause should arouse suspicion, and the lesion should be biopsied or surgically excised. About 5% of patients with leukoplakia eventually develop squamous cell carcinoma in the area of the white lesion.

Mucositis (Stomatitis). Mucositis and *stomatitis* are clinical terms describing inflammation, breakdown, and ulceration of the oral mucosal tissues. The disease can vary in its clinical presentation from focal or patchy erythema or ulceration to complete sloughing of the oral mucosa. Secondary hemorrhage is relatively common.

There is a wide variety of causative factors, including chronic mouth breathing, medications, systemic diseases, radiotherapy of the head and neck, and nutritional deficiencies. Patients complain of intense pain, burning, and dysphagia, which all lead to an inability to eat or drink.

Treatment relies heavily on palliation of symptoms, which can be provided by local anesthetic and antacid preparations used singly or in combination. Relief is short-lived, however, since the effect of these agents lasts less than 20 minutes. Benzydamine hydrochloride, a local anesthetic and anti-inflammatory drug, is effective for 1 to 2 hours. The use of any toothpastes or mouthwashes accentuates the problem because of their irritating and desiccating properties.

Radiation-induced mucositis initially appears as reddened and swollen mucosa, but the tissue becomes denuded and ulcerated as therapy continues. The patient experiences pain, burning, and discomfort that is greatly intensified by contact with coarse or highly seasoned foods. Involvement of the pharyngeal mucosa produces difficulties in swallowing and speaking. When therapy ends, spontaneous remission occurs in most patients within several weeks. In the meantime, the use of liquid topical anesthetics in the mouth before mealtime frequently facilitates eating without discomfort.

Oral Cancer. Oral cancer is clearly a disease of older people. Over 98% of cases occur in persons older than 40 years;[117] the average age at the time of diagnosis is about 60 years.[118] The male-to-female ratio is approximately 2:1. It was estimated that in 1997 more than 31,000 new cases of cancer of the lips, tongue, floor of the mouth, palate, gingiva, buccal mucosa, and oropharynx would be diagnosed in the United States.[119] These oral cancers account for about 3.1% of all malignancies.

The most common type of oral cancer is squamous cell carcinoma, accounting for more than 90% of all oral malignancies.[120] The remaining 10% are predominantly malignant tumors of minor salivary gland tissue and (rarely) lymphomas, sarcomas, and melanomas.[117]

Clinically, an early cancer may appear as a small white patch (leukoplakia); a red velvety patch (erythroplakia); an aphthous-like, crusting, or traumatic ulcer; an erythematous plaque; a slightly raised lesion with central ulceration and a raised border; a verruciform growth; or a small swelling.[120] The most common signs and symptoms of oral cancer are listed in Table 8–4.

Frequently, it is impossible to differentiate between squamous cell carcinomas and the benign nonneoplastic lesions seen in aphthous ulceration, herpes simplex infection, or traumatic ulceration. However, the nonneoplastic lesions are usually painful, and most early oral cancers are painless, becoming symptomatic only after they are large enough to impinge on the sensory nerves.[118]

The cause of oral cancer is not known. A genetic factor is not apparent, but there is a definite increased risk with the use of tobacco and alcohol.[118,120,121] Independently, each agent is believed to be associated with an increased incidence of the disease, and the two together may in fact act synergistically.[118,120,121] Oral leukoplakia (benign keratosis) is an important precancerous lesion, turning into oral cancer in about 3% to 5% of cases.[122] Malignant transformations arising from the oral mucosa are mostly observed between ages 40 and 69 years. Although the peak prevalence is between ages 50 and 59 years, decline is gradual thereafter.[123] Other risk factors for oral cancer include exposure to sunlight, chronic

Table 8–4 Oral Cancer Warning Signals

- Swelling
- Lumps, growths, exophytic masses
- White, scaly patches
- Red patches
- Oral ulcers (bleed easily, nonhealing)
- Atypical facial pain
- Persistent numbness or pain
- Persistent bleeding
- Difficulty in chewing
- Restricted jaw movement
- Trismus
- Restricted tongue movement
- Difficulty in swallowing
- Sore throat that does not heal
- Hoarseness
- Change in denture fit
- Loose teeth

trauma, diet, poor dentition, and history of syphilis infection.[118,120,124]

Oral cancer is a devastating disease with significant morbidity and mortality. Curative treatment consists of surgery, radiation, and chemotherapy, alone or in combination. Unfortunately, despite advances in these therapeutic approaches, only about 50% of patients with oral cancer survive the disease.[125] Of course, survival rates vary substantially depending on the site, ranging from 32% for cancer of the oropharynx to 91% for lip cancer, and on how early in the disease treatment is instituted. The reason for poor overall prognosis for oral cancer is that the disease is often detected at advanced stages, after the visual detection of tissue changes or the development of symptoms.

Until the process of carcinogenesis is completely understood and true prevention is possible, early detection and treatment remain the best weapons against malignant disease. However, because there are no reliable methods for early diagnosis of squamous cell carcinoma, biopsy is the only definitive means of diagnosis. A biopsy should be done on any oral lesion that has not responded to therapy or resolved itself in a 2-week period.

Many of the predisposing factors for oral cancer are potentially avoidable. Preventive education should include delineation of the hazards of

tobacco and alcohol and the need for regular dental care to reduce irritation and mechanical injury and for early detection.

Traumatic Ulcers. Acute trauma (mechanical, thermal, or chemical) is probably the most common cause of oral ulceration[126] and is a frequent problem in the geriatric patient. Ulcers can occur on any mucous membrane surface and are variable in size and shape. The ulcers are raised and have yellow-gray centers surrounded by an erythematous halo. Secondary infections with bacteria or *C. albicans* can occur.

The diagnosis is made primarily by history, since most patients can identify the cause of the trauma. The patient typically complains of an isolated intraoral "sore" with pain or tenderness in the area of the lesion. Symptoms rarely exceed 3 or 4 days, and the lesion heals within 10 to 14 days.[127]

Chronic irritation from decayed or broken teeth and inadequate dentures may lead to chronic ulcers that persist indefinitely. Cheek and tongue biting produce a thin, rough, keratotic film in the area traumatized. Fragments of epithelium are often seen in these cases, as a result of the continuous chewing on the same area.

Treatment is instituted by avoiding the cause of the trauma and contact with any irritants. Dental care is usually necessary to relieve sources of irritation. Surgical repair of any extensive laceration may be necessary.

Denture-Related Oral Pathology. Dental prosthetic appliances are intended to restore the health and well-being of patients, but they are responsible for many of the most commonly occurring oral lesions among the elderly. Removable appliances (complete or partial dentures) are implicated with greater frequency than are fixed appliances (bridges) because they may become distorted or broken with use and are frequently abused by the patient.[107] Older patients often do not or cannot comply with instructions for proper removal, placement, maintenance, and cleanliness of their appliances.

Because dentures fit next to teeth and soft tissue, they must be kept clean to maintain oral health. Plaque, food debris, and calculi collect on dentures just as they do on natural teeth. If left uncleaned, the dentures can be a source of irritation, inflammation, infection, or halitosis.

Partial dentures contribute to increased plaque formation around abutment teeth, which increases gingival inflammation over time.[128] Since these appliances can also increase tooth mobility and accelerate bone loss,[128] the reduction of plaque becomes even more important.

Frequently, patients perform their own repairs, relines, or adjustments, which can harm the dentures or oral mucosa. Additionally, all denture wearers should be advised that some servicing or readjustment of dentures is necessary occasionally because of normal changes in the supporting tissues and bone. Common pathologic changes associated with denture wearing include the problems described below.

Candidiasis. Denture-related candidiasis is by far the most common type of oral candidal infection.[129] The characteristic appearance is that of a slightly granular or irregularly eroded erythematous mucosa that corresponds exactly to the area covered by the upper denture. In some cases, the denture fits poorly and serves as a nutrient reservoir to foster fungal growth.[129] In patients with well-fitting dentures, the stability and peripheral seal of the upper denture allow the fungus to flourish in the absence of normal salivary flow. The condition seldom causes any discomfort.

These fungi are capable of growing on denture surfaces, from which they can infect and reinfect the soft tissues. Management therefore requires that both the denture and the mucosal surfaces be treated. Dentures should be kept scrupulously clean and soaked frequently in antifungal agents, germicides, or chlorhexidine.[129,130] The infected tissue is treated with topical antifungal agents.[113]

Denture Stomatitis (Denture Sore Mouth, Stomatitis Prosthetica). The true etiology of denture stomatitis, a generalized inflammation associated with denture wearing, is unknown. It has been ascribed to contact hypersensitivity to dental materials, bacterial and candidal infections, tissue reaction to ill-fitting or unclean dentures, residual denture cleanser, medication use, and systemic diseases.[117,131] It is known to worsen in patients who do not remove their dentures at night or are negligent in denture hygiene.[117,129,130,131]

This disease is characterized by a very discrete erythematous reaction that closely follows the outline of the denture. Resolution of the inflammation may be obtained by thoroughly cleaning the denture if it fits well or by constructing a new one if it is ill-fitting. If candidal organisms are a contributing factor to the stomatitis, the denture may be covered with an antifungal ointment before insertion or soaked in an antifungal solution at night.

Traumatic Ulcers (Denture Sore Spots). An unstable or unretentive denture will cause tissue irritation or ulceration because of excess movement. Overextended denture flanges, bone spicules under the dentures, and foods—especially seeds—trapped between the denture and mucosa can also cause ulcerative lesions. The ulcers are small, painful, irregularly shaped lesions usually covered by a necrotic membrane and surrounded by an inflammatory halo. Treatment consists of correcting the underlying cause. Most lesions usually heal promptly.

Periodontium

Periodontal Disease. The most common disease of the periodontium is periodontal disease, a term generally used to describe specific chronic disorders that affect the gingiva, supporting connective tissue, and alveolar bone.[132] It is a chronic, progressive, and destructive condition, and its incidence and severity typically increase with age.[133–135] There is considerable question, however, about whether the increase in severity with age represents age-dependent pathology or the cumulative effects of a lifetime of intermittent destruction.[1]

Periodontal disease commonly develops in two stages, gingivitis and periodontitis. As with dental caries, the major etiologic factor is plaque, which accumulates more rapidly and heavily in elderly people.[133] If the plaque is not removed daily, it will calcify into calculus (tartar). Accumulation of plaque, food, bacteria, and calculi on the tooth surfaces between the tooth and gingiva produces a low-grade inflammation of the gingiva (gingivitis). This is clinically characterized by gingival redness, enlargement, tenderness, and bleeding. Although gingivitis develops more rapidly and with greater severity in older adults,[135] it is reversible with adequate plaque control.

If the inflammatory process is allowed to progress, there is formation of pus (pyorrhea) with or without discomfort or other symptoms. Without drainage, the accumulation of pus leads to acute swelling (periodontal abscess) and pain. When the inflammation extends to the underlying alveolar bone and connective tissue (periodontitis), it loosens the teeth and causes them to be extruded. However, once the teeth are lost, the inflammatory symptoms subside.

The diagnosis depends on a combination of findings, including localized pain, loose teeth, the presence of periodontal pockets, erythema, and swelling or suppuration. A severe case results in a foul odor, inflamed and ulcerated gums, fibrotic tissue, and bleeding. Roentgenograms may reveal the destruction of alveolar bone. Margins of overextended fillings often play a role as local irritating factors. Occlusal trauma, particularly from grinding and teeth-clenching habits, and systemic factors may contribute to periodontal disease, but they do not initiate the disease.[133,135]

The prevention of periodontal disease depends largely on plaque control through meticulous oral hygiene.[133,135] Although there are indications that periodontal breakdown progresses slowly in elderly persons,[135] progression of the disease can be retarded by oral hygiene[135,136] and use of antimicrobial agents.[127] Local drainage and oxygenating mouth rinses (3% hydrogen peroxide in an equal volume of water) will usually reverse any acute symptoms and allow for routine follow-up procedures. In some cases, surgery to reduce excess gum tissue helps prevent the formation of periodontal pockets that predispose to periodontal infections. In advanced disease, extraction of teeth may be necessary.

Necrotizing Ulcerative Gingivitis (Vincent's Infection, Trench Mouth). Necrotizing ulcerative gingivitis is an acute, recurring, noncommunicable inflammatory disease of the gingiva resulting from local irritation and organisms in the normal oral flora that invade the gingival tissue when its resistance is lowered. The disease is characterized by redness, swelling, ulceration, bleeding, and pain. The yellowish-gray pseudomembrane that usually covers the ulcerated surface can be removed easily, leaving a raw, bleeding base. In severe cases, there is a fetid odor and foul taste in the mouth. Recurrent attacks can lead to bone loss. Treatment includes eliminating local irritants by careful and thorough oral hygiene procedures. Local anesthetics, as well as antibiotic therapy, may serve as adjuncts to treatment. Caustics are contraindicated.

Tongue

Fissured Tongue. The prevalence of fissured tongue, characterized by cracks on the dorsolateral surfaces of the tongue, increases progressively in each decade of adult life. Fissured tongue is found in varying degrees in approximately 5% of the population. It occurs in 60% of persons after age 40 years.

The fissures are deep, tend to collect food debris and microorganisms, and cause the tongue to be inflamed often. However, the tongue is usually pain free or only mildly tender, even if the fissures become secondarily infected from retained debris and microbes.

Fissuring of the tongue sometimes is associated with deficiency of the vitamin B_2 complex, or it may be genetic. Another cause is correlation with long-standing glossitis.

Treatment consists of brushing the tongue or rubbing it vigorously with a moistened washcloth to provide relief. The scarring is irreversible.

Glossitis. Inflammation of the tongue, usually manifested by considerable atrophy of the filiform papillae, creates a red, smooth appearance. It may be secondary to a variety of diseases, such as anemia, nutritional deficiency, drug reactions, systemic infection, and physical or chemical irritations. The diagnosis is usually based on the history and laboratory studies, including cultures as indicated.

Treatment is based on identifying and correcting the primary cause, if possible, and palliating the tongue symptoms as required. When the cause cannot be determined and there are no symptoms, therapy is not indicated.

Glossodynia, Glossopyrosis (Burning Tongue, Chronic Lingual Papillitis). *Glossodynia,* or painful, burning, itching, or stinging tongue, is a distressing symptom that predominantly affects older women.[137] It can accompany atrophy of the tongue papillae and is a prominent feature of the "burning mouth" syndrome. Involvement of the entire tongue or isolated areas, occurring with or without glossitis, may be the presenting symptoms of hypochromic or pernicious anemia, nutritional disturbances, emotional upset, hormonal imbalance, allergies, psychosomatic syndromes (grief, loneliness, despair), or other systemic disorders.[138] Smoking, xerostomia, medication use, and candidiasis may also be causative.

In most cases, a primary cause cannot be identified. Cultures are of no value, since the offending organisms usually are also present in the normal oral flora. Dental prostheses, caries, and periodontal disease are usually of no causative significance. Although certain foods may cause flare-ups, they are not the primary causes. Dentifrice ingredients are rare causes of burning and pain of the tongue.

Treatment is mainly empiric, since causative factors usually are not identified. Important approaches include ruling out systemic conditions associated with these symptoms, changing the individual's drug regimen, and reassuring the patient that there is no evidence of infection or neoplasia. Ointments and mouth rinses are of no value.

Hairy Tongue. Hairy tongue is characterized by elongated, thick, densely matted, and stained filaments on the dorsum of the tongue that resemble hair. The filaments are hypertrophied or hyperplastic filiform papillae that can be stained yellow, brown, or black.

Normally, the developing papillary tissue cells slide off the tongue during mechanical stimulation. When desquamation is diminished, the papillae become elongated and provide a nidus for *materia alba* to accumulate, for stains to collect, and for bacteria and fungi to lodge and produce minor infections.[116] Common causes of staining are coffee, tobacco, medications, foods, and chromogenic microorganisms.

Hairy tongue is not a serious condition and is easily eliminated by improving tongue hygiene and promoting desquamation. If candidal organisms are present, the use of antifungal agents is indicated.

Macroglossia. Macroglossia (large tongue) may be congenital or acquired. It is significant in the elderly population because individuals who have been edentulous for many years may develop this condition. The marked use of the tongue to aid in mastication of food results in muscular hypertrophy, a common type of acquired macroglossia. If the patient is able to wear dentures, the tongue muscle may regress, with reduction in the size of the tongue.

Circumoral Tissues

Lips

Angular Cheilitis (Cheilosis, Pseudocheilosis, or Perleche). Angular cheilitis is a nonspecific inflammation at the oral commissure area bilaterally. It proceeds to a cracking of the angles of the mouth, with well-defined fissures present. The drooling of saliva often aggravates the condition.

The etiology of angular cheilosis is often complex. The combination of bone resorption, muscle atrophy, and tooth loss decreases the distance between the nose and chin, which causes the skin to wrinkle and fold around the mouth. The wrinkling can also accompany a change of bite with old, ill-fitting, or even new dentures. The wrinkled folds collect saliva, *C. albicans,* bacteria, and other contaminants that can cause the infection. Contributing factors include vitamin B complex deficiency, iron deficiency, or both.[3,24,29]

Treatment is directed toward unfolding the skin by the fitting of proper dentures; culturing and treating all infections; initiating measures of local hygiene; and, if necessary, giving iron and vitamin supplements.

Squamous Cell Carcinomas. A high risk of lip cancer is associated with the use of tobacco (particularly pipe tobacco) and exposure to ultraviolet radiation. Almost 95% of these cancers develop in the lower lip, where trauma and heat from the pipestem and exposure to the sun are greatest.[139] Atrophy of the lip, thinning of the lip border, and loss of elasticity are early clinical features. Carcinoma of the lip may appear as a crack in the lip surface, a crusting ulcer, or a tumorous growth. The prognosis is very good unless the lesion is extensive, since metastases develop later and less frequently than from intraoral sites.[117,118]

Oral Musculature

Dysphagia. Dysphagia (difficulty in swallowing) may render a patient vulnerable to aspiration of saliva or oral intake. Indicators that a swallowing problem is likely to be present include dysarthria, poor control of oral secretions, inability to swallow spontaneously, drooling or gurgling aspirations, or regurgitation through the nose, and frequent reflexive coughing.[140,141]

The causes of dysphagia may be neurologic, neuromuscular, or structural. In one study,[142] a significant increase in swallowing dysfunction was seen among older persons taking prescription medications. Conditions that alter the ability to form and prepare a bolus in the oral stage of swallowing can also cause dysphagia.[10]

Dyskinesia. Oral dyskinesia is a movement disorder characterized by severe, dystonic, involuntary movement of the facial, oral, and cervical musculature.[143] The involuntary abnormal contractions, mainly of the tongue, lips, and mandible, occur frequently with age in patients who exhibit disturbances of the cerebral stroma or stromal changes of the extrapyramidal motor system.[143–145] Because the movements disappear when the mouth is opened wide, during sleep, or when the patient's attention is distracted, oral dyskinesia tends to be regarded as a disease of the central nervous system.[143]

Some studies have reported a close correlation between oral dyskinesia and poor oral conditions.[143,144] One study describing the clinical appearance of this disease in the aged[143] found that its occurrence was associated with missing teeth and use of uncomfortable dentures. It has also been demonstrated that the symptoms of oral dyskinesia respond favorably to dental treatment, such as extractions, new dentures, and adjustment of old dentures.[143,144]

Drug-induced oral dyskinesia, or tardive dyskinesia, is a permanent side effect of long-term neuroleptic (antipsychotic) drug therapy that does not resolve on withdrawal of the drug. The most common movements are tongue protrusion, licking and smacking of the lips, puffing of the cheeks, sucking and chewing, and facial grimacing.[146,147]

Trismus. Trismus is a condition in which tonic spasms of the masticatory muscles limit opening of the mouth. It may develop during or after radiation therapy if these muscles are included in the treatment field. Management is directed toward exercises and various prosthetic appliances to increase the opening capacity of the muscles.

Other Changes

Salivary Glands

Sialolithiasis. Sialoliths, or salivary stones, may form in any of the major or minor salivary glands or their excretory ducts. The most common manifestation of ductal stones, which do not generally cause complete obstruction, is enlargement of the gland and subsequent pain during eating. Both the glandular swelling and pain subside between meals as the entrapped saliva is gradually excreted.

Tumors. Benign and malignant tumors of the salivary glands are more common in older patients, and both the major and minor salivary glands are involved.[148] Overall, neoplasms arising from the minor salivary glands are relatively uncommon compared with those arising from the major salivary glands.[118,148] However, most tumors of the minor salivary glands are malignant.[148]

Both elderly men and elderly women appear to have an increased risk of salivary gland malignancies; however, little information about the causative factors exists. Radiotherapy is an infrequent etiologic factor.[149] Trauma, infection, stone formation, and the use of alcohol or tobacco are not associated with these tumors.[150]

The survival rates for patients with malignant salivary gland tumors are generally higher than they are for persons with most other oral cancers. Usually, diagnosis and treatment are rendered early, and metastasis occurs late in the course of the disease. Long-term follow-up is essential, however, because there is a high rate of recurrence.

Xerostomia (Dry Mouth, Decreased Salivary Flow). Xerostomia, although not a disease concomitant with aging, is a symptom that is often evident in older patients. The main cause is use of xerogenic medications; other causes include vitamin deficiencies, dehydration, mouth breathing, stress, and a variety of systemic diseases and their therapies.

Without the antibacterial, cleansing, lubricating, remineralizing, and buffering actions of saliva, the individual with xerostomia is at increased risk of developing coronal and root surface caries; abrasion and erosion of tooth surfaces; periodontal disease; atrophic glossitis; traumatic injuries to the mucous membranes; mucosal lesions; infections of the pharynx and salivary glands; and dysfunctions of speech, chewing, swallowing, and taste.[24,151] In addition to the damage to teeth and supporting structures, problems with prostheses are also magnified when the mouth is dry. Saliva provides a thin, fluid film between the denture base and underlying soft tissues necessary for the retention and stability of dentures during function.[42,152] Additionally, saliva prevents the hard acrylic or metal surfaces from abrading the oral mucosa. Consequently, frequent denture problems and sores arise, and the patient complains of generalized intraoral soreness during mastication.

Patients may express one or all of the signs and symptoms associated with xerostomia in varying degrees of severity. Some of these include mouth dryness; a fissured tongue; glossodynia or glossopyrosis; candidiasis; rampant caries; oral soreness; sticking of food or lips to the teeth; cracking of lips; difficulty in speaking, chewing, and swallowing; a generalized burning sensation; and ageusia, dysgeusia, or hypogeusia.[42,152] The mucosa becomes dry, rough, and sticky; bleeds easily; and is subject to ulceration or infection.

Prevention and management of xerostomia depends on its etiology (Table 8–5). With drug-

---

Table 8–5 Prevention and Management of Xerostomia

Determine etiology

Alter medication regimen
  Eliminate medication
  Reduce dosage or frequency of administration
  Replace current medication with another with less severe oral side effects

Alleviate complaints
  Increase fluid intake (water or low-sugar beverages); avoid caffeinated drinks
  Avoid dry, bulky, spicy, salty, or highly acidic foods
  Avoid tobacco and alcohol intake
  Humidify air
  Use saliva stimulants (local and systemic agents)
    Local agents
      Sugarless hard candy or lozenges
      Sugarless gum
      Systemic agents
    Pilocarpine drops
      Oral pilocarpine (2.5–5.0 mg three times daily before meals)
      Use artificial saliva preparations (containing fluoride)
      Glycerin
      Methylcellulose
      Coat lips and dentures with petroleum jelly
  Increase resistance to dental disease
    Have frequent dental examinations
    Use fluorides frequently
    Modify diet
    Control plaque

induced xerostomia, the responsible drug may be able to be eliminated, reduced in dosage or frequency of administration, or replaced by a substitute drug. Management of xerostomia that is irreversible, such as radiation-induced xerostomia, is essentially palliative and accommodative. Small, frequent mouthfuls of water are palatable and inexpensive and moisten the mouth fairly well. To facilitate chewing and swallowing, most patients with xerostomia moisten and thin foods with sauces, gravies, milk, and other fluids.

Artificial saliva preparations provide relief by coating and lubricating the mucosa. Saliva substitutes containing fluoride and fluoride gels are helpful for patients with xerostomia who are at high risk for dental caries. For the lips and dentures, a constant coating of petroleum or water-based jelly and frequent oral application of artificial salivas should alleviate some of the problems. However, lemon glycerin swabs should be avoided because of their cariogenic and drying effects. Also, commercial mouthwashes should be avoided because they have a high alcohol content and dry the oral mucosa. Similarly, ingestion of alcoholic beverages should be minimized.[153]

Sense of Taste

Taste acuity may be affected by oral pathologic conditions, dental diseases, olfactory deficits, medications, malnutrition, smoking, radiation therapy, neurologic deficits, and other systemic disorders.[5] Cues that may indicate alterations in taste sensitivity include decreased or increased appetite, excessive use of seasoning, and excessive use of sugar.

SYSTEMIC DISEASES AND MEDICATIONS AFFECTING ORAL HEALTH

The elderly population suffers from many concurrent acute and chronic diseases, some of which may have oral manifestations or adversely affect oral health. Since 86% of all elderly persons suffer from at least one chronic disease, oral health problems secondary to these diseases may be important.[154] Systemic diseases that affect the oral and circumoral structures are listed in Table 8–6.

Many of the most commonly experienced chronic disease conditions found in the elderly are symptomatically controlled with the proper

---

Table 8–6 Oral Manifestations of Systemic Diseases

Disease/Condition	Oral Manifestations
Achlorhydria	Tongue-glossitis
Adrenal insufficiency	Oral infections—increased risk Oral mucosa—pigmentation Taste—loss or distortion Wound-healing response—poor
Agranulocytosis	Gingiva-spontaneous bleeding Hemorrhagic tendency—petechiae Periodontal disease—high incidence Ulcerations—painful, persistent, necrotic
Alcoholism	Breath odor of alcohol Dental caries—high incidence Facial neuralgia, edema Hemorrhagic tendency—ecchymoses, petechiae Lips—angular cheilosis Oral cancer—increased risk Oral hygiene—poor

continues

Table 8–6 continued

Disease/Condition	Oral Manifestations
Alcoholism	Oral infections-increased risk Oral mucosa—jaundiced, ulcerated Parotid salivary glands-chronic swelling Periodontal disease—chronic (with frequent acute exacerbations) Taste—decreased sensitivity Teeth—attrition, erosion, loss Tongue—glossitis, ulcerated Wound—healing response—delayed Xerostomia
Alzheimer's disease	Dysphagia Oral hygiene—poor, neglected Taste sensitivity—decreased Xerostomia
Amyotrophic lateral sclerosis	Dysarthria Tongue fasciculations—atrophic
Anemia	Burning/sore mouth—mucositis/stomatitis Filiform papillae—atrophic Oral mucosa—pale, atrophic, thin, tender Tongue—glossitis, glossodynia Xerostomia
Anxiety disorders	Burning/sore mouth Dysphagia Xerostomia
Arthritis	TMJ involvement—limited jaw movement Biliary tract obstruction Bleeding—excessive, spontaneous Hemorrhagic tendency—petechiae, hematomas
Bipolar disorders	Depressive phase—oral hygiene neglected Facial pain syndromes due to mood swings Manic phase—self-inflicted mucosal abrasion
Bleeding disorders	Intraoral bleeding—ecchymoses, hematomas, petechiae Oral mucosa jaundiced
Cerebrovascular accident	Chewing difficulty/inability Dysarthria Dysphagia Facial drooping—affects denture fit Gag reflex—decreased Oral motor apraxia Oral sensation—decreased unilaterally
Chorea	Dysarthria Oral dyskinesia
Congenital heart disease	Cyanosis Intraoral hemorrhages, infections Leukopenia, polycythemia, thrombocytopenia

continues

Table 8–6 continued

Disease/Condition	Oral Manifestations
Congestive heart failure	Intraoral bleeding—ecchymoses, petechiae Lips—cyanosis, thinning of vermilion border Oral infections
Coronary arteriosclerotic heart disease	Oral or facial pain—referred
Crohn's disease	Aphthous ulcers—high frequency Burning/sore mouth Dental caries—high frequency Oral hygiene—poor
Cyclic neutropenia	Mucositis/stomatitis Oral infections—increased risk Periodontal disease—high incidence Ulcerations—aphthous type
Dementia	Bruxism Burning/sore mouth Dysphagia Facial pain—atypical Oral injuries—increased susceptibility Periodontal disease—accelerated Poor oral hygiene—chronic
Depression	Burning/sore mouth Dental caries-rapid progression Facial pain syndromes-numerous Oral hygiene-poor Periodontal disease-accelerated Tongue—glossodynia Xerostomia
Diabetes mellitus	Breath odor of ketone Burning/sore mouth—mucositis/stomatitis Candidiasis Dental caries—rampant Gingiva—inflammation Lips—angular cheilitis Mucomycosis Oral infections—increased susceptibility Oral paresthesias Periodontal disease—accentuated, abscesses Taste sensitivity—decreased Teeth—sensitivity Tongue glossodynia Ulcerations Wound—healing response—delayed Xerostomia
Epilepsy	Gingiva—drug-induced hyperplasia Ulcerations—traumatic

continues

Table 8–6 continued

Disease/Condition	Oral Manifestations
Gonorrhea	Gingivitis Oral abscesses/mucosal lesions/ulcerations Oral mucosa—erythematous Parotitis Pharyngitis/tonsillitis Stomatitis—generalized
Hepatitis	Intraoral bleeding Oral mucosa—pigmentation Taste—loss or distortion
Herpes zoster	Bone—osteoradionecrosis Neuralgia—trigeminal Oral mucosa—lesions, ulcerations, pain Teeth—devitalization, exfoliation
Hypertension	Neuritis
Hyperthyroidism	Dental caries—extensive Periodontal disease—progressive Tongue—tumors (midline of posterior dorsum)
Hypoparathyroidism	Candidiasis
Hypothyroidism	Candidiasis Taste—loss or distortion Teeth—malocclusion Tongue—macroglossia Xerostomia
Immunosuppression	Increased susceptibility to candidiasis; dental caries; infections, local and systemic; intraoral bleeding; periodontal disease; recurrent aphthous ulcers; tumor development
Leukemia	Bone-lesions Burning/sore mouth—mucositis/stomatitis Candidiasis Gingiva—hyperplasia, spontaneous bleeding Hemorrhagic tendency—ecchymoses, hematomas, petechiae Herpetic stomatitis Infections—increased risk Lymphadenopathy Oral mucosa—pallor, lesions Oral paresthesias Ulcerations—painful, persistent, necrotic
Leukopenia	Oral infections—increased risk
Liver disease	Bleeding—excessive, spontaneous Hemorrhagic tendency—ecchymoses, hematomas, petechiae
Lupus erythematosus	Burning/sore mouth Candidiasis

continues

Table 8–6 continued

Disease/Condition	Oral Manifestations
Lupus erythematosus	Mandible immobility Oral lesions—bullae, erosions Oral mucosa—sloughing TMJ deviation, pain with movement or palpation, joint sounds, locking or dislocation Tongue fissuring, atrophic papillae Ulcerations Xerostomia
Lymphomas	Burning/sore mouth Candidiasis Cervical lymphadenopathy Extranodal oral tumors Hemorrhagic tendency—ecchymoses, petechiae Infections-increased risk
Malabsorption syndrome	Bleeding—excessive, spontaneous Candidiasis Hemorrhagic tendency—ecchymoses, hematomas, petechiae
Malignant hypertension	Facial paralysis
Multiple myeloma	Amyloid deposits in soft tissue Bone—lesions, pain Soft tissues—tumors Teeth—unexplained mobility
Multiple sclerosis	Dysarthria TMJ—pain with movement or palpation, joint sounds Trigeminal neuralgia Xerostomia, drug-induced
Muscular dystrophy	Mouth breathing Muscles—weakness, decreased biting force Tongue—hypertrophy
Myasthenia gravis	Chewing difficulty Dysphagia Gingiva—poor health Mouth breathing Muscles—weakness, inability to close mouth Tongue-flaccid
Narcolepsy	Candidiasis Xerostomia
Nephritis	Burning/sore mouth Xerostomia
Neurofibromatosis	Oral neurofibromatous lesions Oral paresthesias Soft tissues—pigmentation Tongue—macroglossia, enlarged lingual papillae

continues

Table 8–6 continued

Disease/Condition	Oral Manifestations
Organ transplants	Intraoral bleeding—increased susceptibility Oral infections—increased susceptibility Tumor development—increased susceptibility
Osteoarthritis	Bone—resorption TMJ—unilateral involvement, dysfunction
Paget's disease	Bone—progressive enlargement
Parkinson's disease	Chewing difficulty Drooling of saliva due to swallowing difficulty (not excessive production) Dysarthria Dysphagia Facial paresthesias, tremors Lips—angular cheilitis, tremors Oral hygiene—poor Oral mucositis—stomatitis Tardive dyskinesia, drug-induced Teeth—involuntary bruxism Tongue—tremors Xerostomia, drug-induced
Pemphigus vulgaris	Burning/sore mouth Candidiasis Halitosis Hypersalivation Oral lesions, erosions—bleed easily, painful Ulcerations—raw, red, eroded
Pneumonia	Aspiration—increased susceptibility with dysphagia, poor dentition, poor oral hygiene
Polycythemia	Oral mucosa—cyanosis
Posttraumatic stress disorder	Bruxism Dental caries—increased incidence Oral hygiene—poor Periodontal disease—increased incidence Tongue—glossodynia
Progressive bulbar palsy	Chewing difficulty Dysarthria Jaw muscles—spastic
Radiation therapy to head/neck	Candidiasis Mucositis Muscles—dysfunction, trismus Oral infections—increased susceptibility Pulp—pain, necrosis Taste—lost or distorted Teeth—hypersensitivity, radiation caries Xerostomia

continues

Table 8–6 continued

Disease/Condition	Oral Manifestations
Renal disease/dialysis/transplants	Breath odor of urea Calculus—increased formation Candidiasis Dental caries—low incidence Gingiva—pale, undefined, bleeds spontaneously Oral infections—frequent retrograde infectious parotitis Oral mucosa—pallor, uremic stomatitis Renal osteomalacia/osteodystrophy Salivary flow—decreased Taste—metallic Teeth—mobility Tongue—macroglossia, glossodynia Ulcerations—ulcerative stomatitis Wound—healing response-poor
Rheumatoid arthritis	Bone—resorption Muscles—atrophic TMJ—dysfunction Xerostomia
Sjögren's syndrome	Burning/sore mouth—mucositis/stomatitis Candidiasis Dental caries—increased susceptibility Lips—angular cheilosis, lesions Oral mucosa—lesions Parotid gland—enlargement Periodontal disease—accelerated Saliva—composition changes; increased sodium, potassium, manganese; decreased calcium Taste—loss, distortion Tongue—glossitis, glossodynia Xerostomia
Smokeless tobacco use	Gingiva—recession Halitosis Oral cancer—increased risk Oral mucosa—leukoplakia Periodontal disease—accentuated Smell sensitivity—decreased Taste sensitivity—decreased Teeth—abrasion; attrition, erosion, loss
Syphilis	Oral lesions—chancre, mucous patch, gums Tongue—interstitial glossitis
Temporal arteritis	Orofacial pain
Thrombocytopenia	Hemorrhagic tendency—ecchymoses, hematomas, petechiae
Tobacco smoking	Calculus—increased Gingivitis—increased Hairy tongue

continues

Table 8–6 continued

Disease/Condition	Oral Manifestations
Tobacco smoking	Halitosis Smell sensitivity—decreased Taste—loss or distortion Teeth—abrasion Wound—healing response—delayed
Tuberculosis	Lymph node involvement (scrofula) Ulcerations, especially on tongue
Urticaria (angioneurotic anemia)	Swelling—soft tissues
von Willebrand's disease	Hemorrhagic tendency—ecchymoses, hematomas, petechiae Intraoral bleeding—spontaneous

use of medications. The increased use of medications with advancing age, therefore, is not surprising. Geriatric patients take more drugs because they have more chronic illnesses than do younger patients. Not only does the problem of multiple drug use among elderly people have serious implications due to pharmacokinetic and pharmacodynamic considerations with aging, but also there are iatrogenic oral manifestations of many drugs (Table 8–7).

Table 8–7 Drug-Induced Oral Manifestations

Candidiasis
- Antibiotics
- Antineoplastics
- Corticosteroids
- Diuretics
- Immunosuppressives
- Steroid inhalers

Contact hypersensitivity
- Iodine
- Menthol
- Topical analgesics
- Topical antibiotics

Erythema multiforme
- Anticonvulsants
- Antimalarials
- Barbiturates
- Busulfan
- Chlorpropamide
- Clindamycin
- Codeine
- Isoniazid
- Meprobamate
- Minoxidil
- Penicillins
- Phenolphthalein
- Phenylbutazone
- Propylthiouracil
- Salicylates
- Sulfonamides
- Tetracyclines

Fixed drug eruptions
- Barbiturates
- Chlordiazepoxide
- Sulfonamides
- Tetracyclines

Gingival hyperplasia
- Cyclosporine
- Nifedipine
- Phenytoin sodium

Glossodynia
- Diuretics

Hairy tongue
- Antibiotics
- Corticosteroids
- Sodium perborate
- Sodium peroxide

Hypersalivation/sialorrhea
- Antianxiety agents
- Anticholinesterases
- Apomorphine
- Iodides
- Lithium
- Mercurial salts
- Nitrazepam

Infections
- Antineoplastics
- Corticosteroids (high dose)
- Immunosuppressives

**Intraoral bleeding/
petechiae/purpura**
- Antiarrhythmics

continues

Table 8–7 continued

Antibiotics (broad
  spectrum)
Anticoagulants
Aspirin
Warfarin sodium

**Lichenoid mucosal
  reactions**
Allopurinol
Antihypertensives
Beta blockers
Chloroquine
Chlorothiazide
Chlorpropamide
Dapsone
Diuretics
Doxorubicin hydrochloride
Gold salts
Mercurial diuretics
Mercury compounds
Minocycline
Nonsteroidal anti-
  inflammatory agents
Penicillamine
Phenolphthalein
Phenothiazines
Phenytoin
Quinidine
Silver compounds
Streptomycin
Sulfamethoxazole
Tetracyclines
Tolbutamide

**Lupus erythematosus
  (oral mucosa) reactions**
Gold salts
Griseofulvin
Hydralazine hydrochloride
Isoniazid
Methyldopa
Penicillin
Phenytoin
Primidone
Procainamide
Streptomycin
Sulfonamides

Tetracyclines
Thiouracil

Mucositis/stomatitis
Antineoplastics
Lithium
Mercurial diuretics

Oral dyskinesias
Buspirone

**Orofacial neuropathies
  (numbness, tingling,
  burning of the face or
  mouth)**
Acetazolamide
Antineoplastics
Beta blockers
Chlorpropamide
Ergotamine
Hydralazine hydrochloride
Hypoglycemics (oral)
Isoniazid
Methysergide
Nalidixic acid
Nitrofurantoin
Phenytoin
Streptomycin
Tolbutamide
Tricyclic antidepressants

Pigmentation (soft tissue)
Antimalarials
Busulfan
Chlorhexidine

Salivary gland enlargement
Antipsychotics
Insulin
Iodides
Isoproterenol
Methyldopa
Phenylbutazone
Potassium chloride
Thiocyanate
Thiouracil
Warfarin sodium

**Salivary gland pain
  and/or swelling**
Antihypertensives
Antithyroid agents
Cytotoxic agents
Ganglion-blocking agents
Insulin
Iodine
Isoproterenol
Oxyphenbutazone
Phenothiazines
Phenylbutazone
Potassium chlorate
Sulfonamides
Warfarin sodium

Spontaneous oral bleeding
Anticoagulants
Antineoplastics

Tardive dyskinesias
Butyrophenone
  antipsychotics
Levodopa
Phenothiazines
Thioxanthene

Taste dysfunction
Amphetamines
Benzodiazepines
Carbimazole
Chlorhexidine
Chlorpromazine
Clofibrate
Ethionamide
Gold salts
Griseofulvin
Levodopa
Lincomycin
Lithium carbonate
Methocarbamol
Metronidazole
D Penicillamine
Penicillin
Phenformin hydrochloride
Phenindione
Propranolol

continues

Table 8–7 continued

Quinidine	Phenylbutazone	Antispasmodics
Tranquilizers	Potassium chloride	Atropine
Vitamins (excessive use)	Propranolol	Barbiturates
	Spironolactone	Benzodiazepines
Tooth decay (rampant)	Thiazide diuretics	Bronchodilators
Tricyclic antidepressants	Tolbutamide	Central nervous system stimulants
Tooth discoloration	**Xerostomia**	Congestive heart failure medications
Chlorhexidine	Amphetamines	Decongestants
Gentian violet	Analgesics	Diuretics
Stannous fluoride	Anorexiants	Ganglion-blocking agents
Tetracyclines	Antiallergics	Hypnotics
	Antianxiety agents	Lithium
Ulcerations	Antiarrhythmics	Monoamine oxidase inhibitors
Antiarrhythmics	Anticholinergics	Muscle relaxants
Antineoplastics	Anticonvulsants	Narcotics
Aspirin	Antidepressants	Nonsteroidal anti-inflammatory agents
Gold salts	Antidiarrheals	
Indomethacin	Antihistamines	Phenylbutazone
Meprobamate	Antihypertensives	Scopolamine
Mercurial diuretics	Antiinflammatory agents	Sympathomimetics
Methotrexate	Antinauseants	Tranquilizers
Methyldopa	Antineoplastics	
Naproxen	Anti-Parkinsonism agents	
D Penicillamine	Antipsychotics	

In addition to the oral signs and symptoms from elderly people's use of properly prescribed and over-the-counter medications, there are oral manifestations of recreational drug abuse, including advanced generalized periodontal disease, bruxism, numerous abscessed or missing teeth, poor oral hygiene, rampant caries, tooth attrition (secondary to bruxism), and xerostomia.[155–157]

IMPACT OF NUTRITIONAL STATUS ON ORAL HEALTH

Nutritional status has an important role in oral health. A sophisticated system of nutrient interaction is essential to the formation of healthy teeth and the maintenance of oral and circumoral tissues throughout life.[158–160] The systemic effects of nutrients on oral health, growth and development, cell integrity and renewal, proper function of the tissues and saliva, tissue repair, and resis-tance and susceptibility to oral diseases (Table 8–8) have been studied by very few researchers and need more attention and understanding. The local effects of food on plaque formation and the resultant oral disease processes, including coronal and root caries, gingivitis, and periodontitis, have been relatively well described.

Plaque Formation

Plaque consists mainly of bacteria and a matrix produced by them that is composed primarily of carbohydrate, protein, salts, and water. From a dietary standpoint, carbohydrates have an important role in initiating plaque formation. Once plaque is present, carbohydrates from food and beverages can diffuse into it and be fermented by the plaque bacteria. The acid produced can dissolve tooth structure; thus leading to carious lesions. Although acids present in food and

Table 8–8 Systemic Effects of Nutrients on Oral Health

Nutrient	Systemic Effect	Nutrient	Systemic Effect
Barium	Tooth decay resistance	Nickel	Wound healing
Boron	Tooth decay resistance	Phosphorus	Bone formation/metabolism
Calcium	Bone formation/maintenance		Tooth decay resistance
	Muscle tone maintenance		Tooth formation/metabolism
	Nerve impulse transmission	Protein	Epithelial integrity
	Tooth formation/maintenance		Taste bud renewal
Calcium-phosphorus			Tooth formation
			Wound healing
balance	Bone maintenance	Selenium	Tooth decay promotion
	Periodontal maintenance	Silicon	Bone formation
Copper	Bone formation/maintenance	Strontium	Tooth decay resistance
	Collagen synthesis	Sulfur	Bone maintenance
	Periodontal maintenance	Vanadium	Bone maintenance
	Wound healing		Tooth decay resistance
Fluorine	Tooth decay resistance	Vitamin A	Epithelial integrity
Folic acid	Epithelial integrity		Tooth formation
	Wound healing		Wound healing
Gold	Tooth decay resistance	Vitamin B$_1$	Wound healing
	(mild)	Vitamin B$_2$	Wound healing
Iron	Epithelial integrity	Vitamin B$_6$	Wound healing
	Periodontal maintenance	Vitamin C	Epithelial integrity
Lead	Tooth decay promotion		Periodontal maintenance
Lithium	Tooth decay resistance		Tooth formation
Magnesium	Bone formation/maintenance		Wound healing
	Tooth decay promotion	Vitamin D	Bone formation/maintenance
	Tooth formation		Tooth formation
	Wound healing	Zinc	Epithelial integrity/
Manganese	Cell membrane formation		metabolism
	Tooth decay resistance		Periodontal maintenance
Molybdenum	Tooth decay resistance		Taste bud renewal
	(mild)		Wound healing

beverages may also diffuse into the plaque, the result is usually erosion of the tooth surface and not dental caries.

If fermentable carbohydrates are not part of the diet, the acid-producing activity of the plaque will be low. Plaque is still demonstrable in subjects eating a diet devoid of fermentable carbohydrates, but the plaque is thin and structure-less.[161] In contrast, subjects eating a sucrose-rich diet have voluminous, turgid plaque formation.

The texture of the diet may also influence dental plaque. Diets containing soft foods increase plaque formation more than those composed of firmer foods. In a study of women on a low-calorie diet, the rate of plaque formation increased.[162]

Plaque initially forms along the tooth–gum margin and gradually spreads across the tooth surface as the bacterial matrix grows. Since dietary carbohydrates contribute to this supragingival plaque formation, they have been implicated as an etiologic agent in the resulting gingival inflammation.[68,163]

Dental Caries

Although dental caries is generally accepted as primarily a microbial disease, diet plays a crucial secondary role. The dietary component contributing most to the initiation and progression of the caries process is fermentable carbohydrates.[163] Biochemical, microbiologic, and animal and human clinical and epidemiologic studies support a causal relationship. Even root surface caries in human populations is enhanced by the ingestion of dietary sugars.[163]

Normally, before eating, the pH of tooth surface plaque exposed to saliva is close to neutrality (pH 6.5–7.0).[164] The ingestion of foods containing fermentable carbohydrates leads to acid production by the cariogenic plaque bacteria on tooth surfaces. The acids cause a rapid drop in pH that can result in demineralization of the tooth substance. If the plaque pH falls below the critical point of about 5.5 and remains there for an appreciable time, the food causing the decrease is likely to support caries initiation and progression.[165,166]

The greatest concentration of acid, or lowest pH, occurs in 5 to 15 minutes,[164] but teeth are attacked by acids for 20 minutes or more. Saliva has a buffering effect that helps to control acid production to some degree, and it contains proteins that act as antibacterial agents. However, in elderly persons, who may have reductions in salivary flow and therefore reduced buffering and antibacterial capacity, each acid attack is significantly prolonged.

Dietary Control

There is compelling evidence that dietary control of dental caries requires modification in the form, quantity, frequency, and timing of consumption of carbohydrates.[167,168] Sucrose traditionally has been regarded as the form of carbohydrate most detrimental to teeth.[167,168] However, recent research indicates that many of the common simple sugars (glucose, dextrose, fructose, maltose, and lactose) can contribute to the rapid formation of acid by dental plaque.[169] Some studies even suggest that complex carbohydrates, such as starches, have the potential to promote caries under certain conditions.[170,171]

Reducing the quantity of fermentable carbohydrates ingested deprives the potentially pathogenic plaque of necessary substrates for growth. It also limits the numbers of cariogenic microorganisms found in the dental plaque.[172,173]

Frequency of consumption is important, since each encounter of bacteria with fermentable carbohydrates can result in acid production, tooth surface demineralization, and the formation of carious lesions.[174] There is a strong association between root caries lesions in adults and the frequency of fermentable carbohydrate intake.[174] Since frequent sugar consumption (especially between meals) is associated with increased dental caries activity, restricting between-meal snacks containing cariogenic carbohydrates is advised.

The best time to ingest fermentable carbohydrates is with meals. Eating these foods at mealtime will produce less caries than eating the same foods between meals. One reason for this may be that saliva, the production of which is increased during meals, helps neutralize acid production and clears food from the mouth. This is not true for between-meal snacks. Recently, however, it has been established that increasing salivary flow rates after meals, as with sugarless gum chewing, helps reduce plaque acids that can cause caries.[175]

Cariogenicity

Cariogenicity refers to the potential that a specific food or diet has for dental caries formation. The local acidogenic activity of the food, regardless of its nutrient content, largely determines its cariogenic potential.[176] Clinical trials to evaluate the cariogenicity of foodstuffs are expensive processes.[166] Studies must last 2 or 3 years, since dental caries develop slowly and are not clinically discernible for many months.

A key determinant of cariogenicity is oral clearance time.[177] When sugar is consumed in foods that adhere to or between tooth surfaces, caries activity has been shown to increase.[176,177] However, if the fermentable carbohydrate source is eaten with a beverage or in liquid form, the time needed for oral clearance is reduced, resulting in a lower net cariogenic potential. Thus, solid or retentive sugar-containing foods are more cariogenic than sugar-containing foods that are liquid or nonretentive.[176] Likewise, fermentable carbohydrates eaten at meals are less cariogenic than the same ones eaten between meals.[168]

Another indication of cariogenicity is the change in plaque pH associated with food consumption.[173] This measure has been used by a number of investigators to monitor the cariogenicity of particular foods and has been found to relate to oral clearance time. Studies have shown that foods that adhere to the teeth depress the plaque pH for longer periods than foods that are removed from the teeth more quickly.[173,174,176,177]

The cariogenic potential of preparations of liquid medications is of particular concern for the geriatric patient. These medications frequently include high levels of sucrose, glucose, or fructose as sweeteners. Studies of patients taking sweetened liquid medications demonstrate a significant increase in dental caries, especially with long-term therapy.[178] Sweetened liquid iron supplements, cough syrups, antibiotics, and anticonvulsants have been shown to decrease plaque pH after ingestion.[178]

Artificial Sweeteners

Research has been focused on identifying and developing substances that serve as taste-competitive, noncariogenic sugar substitutes. Aspartame and saccharin are the two agents currently available. Cyclamate was banned by the Food and Drug Administration in 1970 because of concerns over its safety. That ban currently is being reconsidered.

Aspartame is noncariogenic, but it is not noncaloric.[179] However, because its sweetness is of sufficient intensity (180 times sweeter than sucrose), only small amounts are required. This results in a very significant reduction in calories.

Saccharin is 300 times sweeter than sucrose but is not metabolized by the body and is therefore noncaloric and nonnutritive.[180] Although it has been periodically labeled potentially carcinogenic, studies to date support its safety for human consumption.

Sugar Alcohols

Technically, sugar alcohols are not sugars, but they are closely related both chemically and biochemically. Since their degrees of sweetness are similar, they are used as sugar substitutes.

Sorbitol, mannitol, and xylitol are used in sugarless chewing gums and candies. Sorbitol- and xylitol-sweetened products appear to be noncariogenic in clinical trials.[166,181] Apparently, xylitol is not metabolized by plaque microorganisms at all, and sorbitol is not metabolized rapidly enough to support an active carious process.

In one study, chewing sorbitol gum after consuming potentially cariogenic snacks helped counteract the adverse plaque pH measurements.[181] The investigator postulated that the gum not only stimulated salivary flow, which is known to have a high buffering capacity, but allowed the saliva to penetrate between the tooth surfaces to neutralize acid production by plaque microorganisms.

Periodontal Disease

Nutrition has never been implicated as a primary etiologic agent in gingivitis or periodontitis. However, it does play a secondary role by influencing or altering the resistance of the periodontium to the noxious agents and irritants that have a primary etiologic role.[182] The importance of both diet and nutrition in maintaining effective host defense mechanisms to withstand periodontal microbial challenge is well established.[182]

Nutrient deficiencies can affect the rate and degree of periodontal disease rather than its initiation. Research suggests that the disease progresses faster and is more severe in patients whose diets do not supply the necessary nutrients.[182,183] However, there is insufficient evidence at this time to justify nutritional therapy as part of periodontal treatment.[160]

Other Oral Conditions

The role, if any, of diet and nutrition in edentulous ridge resorption, mucosal lesions, glossodynia, and taste perception is poorly defined,[160] although research is evolving in the area of diet as a risk factor for oral cancer.[124] Positive associations have been found with increasing consumption of meats, liver, sodium, and retinol.[184,185] Intakes of vitamins A, C, and E, as well as consumption of raw fruits and vegetables, are associated with a reduced risk of oral cancer.[124,184–189]

A major reason for poor adaptation to dentures by elderly persons is reduced tissue tolerance resulting from an inadequate diet.[190] Thin and friable epithelium covering the edentulous area may not tolerate the forces imposed on it by the hard, unyielding base of the denture.

The composition of saliva is critically dependent on flow rate from the glands, and numerous studies have demonstrated that both the physical consistency and the nutritional quality of the diet influence the structure of the glands, as well as the flow rate of saliva.[191]

Nutrient Intake and Malnutrition

Inadequate amounts of nutrients can result in fragile, friable oral tissues, with a loss of adaptability and tolerance to irritants and a loss of repair potential.[192] For many nutrient deficiencies, the oral cavity serves as an early warning system.

Because of the rapid tissue turnover and easy visibility of the oral mucosa, it is possible to identify signs of inadequate intake or improper absorption before other organ systems are affected.[192] Although not all nutrient deficiencies have oral manifestations, the most common ones are listed in Table 8–9. Oral signs indicative or suggestive of malnutrition are listed in Table 8–10.

IMPACT OF ORAL HEALTH ON NUTRITIONAL STATUS

There is general agreement that poor oral health is a risk factor contributing to malnutrition, weight loss, poor general health, and loss of strength.[193,194] Although the impact of oral health status alone on dietary intake and nutritional status of the elderly is virtually unknown, any alteration in the anatomic structures or physiologic functions of the oral cavity may play an important role in deterring the elderly from attaining or maintaining a proper diet and nutritional state.

Dietary intake, with respect to food selection, chewing, and swallowing, is integral to the health of the geriatric patient. Many factors influence food selection, including social customs, taste preferences, amount of preparation, and cost.[41,195] Chewing is influenced by the status of the oral cavity and the efficiency of the masticatory apparatus. Swallowing depends on adequate lubrication and moisture provided by the salivary glands, as well as sufficient functioning of the oral musculature to form and prepare a food bolus. Clearly, any factor that interferes with food selection, chewing, or swallowing can restrict food intake and thus affect nutritional status.

Dentition Status

Dentition status, inasmuch as it contributes to masticatory efficiency, may exert potent effects on dietary intake. Research suggests that the number of occluding teeth, especially in the posterior segments of the mouth, is correlated with masticatory efficiency.[41,196] Masticatory efficiency is dependent not only on the number and condition of teeth present but also on the length of time spent in chewing a bolus of food and the force exerted when biting.[197]

Impaired masticatory efficiency and biting force have been associated with many oral conditions.[10,14,196,197] These include atrophy of orofacial musculature; oral dyskinesia; trismus; bone loss; tooth attrition, brittleness, mobility, pain, or loss; advanced carious lesions; TMJ dysfunction or dislocation; mucosal atrophy; generalized

Table 8–9 Nutritional Deficiencies and Related Oral Manifestations

Nutrient Deficiency	Oral Manifestations
Vitamin A	Candidiasis Gingiva—hypertrophy, inflammation Oral mucosa—keratosis, leukoplakia Periodontal disease Taste—decreased acuity Xerostomia
Vitamin B complex	Lips—angular cheilosis Oral mucosa—leukoplakia Periodontal disease Tongue—papillary hypertrophy, magenta color, fissuring, glossitis
Vitamin B$_2$ (riboflavin)	Filiform papillae—atrophic Fungiform papillae—enlarged Lips—shiny, red, angular cheilosis Tongue—magenta color, soreness
Vitamin B$_3$ (niacin) *(pellagra)*	Lips—angular cheilosis Mucositis/stomatitis Oral mucosa—intense irritation/inflammation, red, painful, denuded, ulcerated Tongue—glossitis, glossodynia Tongue (dorsum)—smooth, dry Tongue (tip/borders)—red, swollen, beefy Ulcerative gingivitis
Vitamin B$_6$ (pyridoxine hydrochloride)	Burning/sore mouth Lips—angular cheilosis Tongue—glossitis, glossodynia
Vitamin B$_{12}$ (cyanocobalamin) *(pernicious anemia)*	Bone loss Burning/sore mouth—mucositis/lstomatitis Gingiva—hemorrhagic Halitosis Hemorrhagic tendency—petechiae Lips—angular cheilosis Oral mucosa—epithelial dysplasia Oral paresthesias—burning, numbness, tingling Periodontal fibers—detachment Taste—loss or distortion Tongue—beefy red, glossy, smooth; glossitis, glossodynia, loss of papillae Ulcerations—aphthous type Wound—healing response—delayed Xerostomia

continues

Table 8–9 continued

Nutrient Deficiency	Oral Manifestations
Vitamin C *(scurvy or megavitamin C withdrawal)*	Blood vessels—fragility Bone—abnormal osteoid formation, fragility, loss Burning/sore mouth Candidiasis Gingiva—friability, raggedness, swelling, redness hemorrhagic tendency Hemorrhagic tendency—petechiae, subperiosteal Oral infections—decreased resistance Periodontal disease—increased susceptibility Teeth—marked mobility, spontaneous exfoliation Wound—healing response-delayed
Vitamin D	Periodontal disease
Vitamin K	Candidiasis Gingiva-bleeding
Calcium	Bone—excessive resorption, loss of mineral, fragility, osteoporosis Hemorrhagic tendency Periodontal disease Teeth—mobility, early loss, edentulism
Copper	Bone—decreased trabeculae, decreased vascularity, fragility
Folic acid	Burning/sore mouth—mucositis/stomatitis Candidiasis Filiform/fungiform papillae—atrophic, loss Gingiva—inflammation Lip—angular cheilosis Tongue—glossitis Tongue (dorsum)—slick, bald, pale, or fiery Tongue (tip/borders)—red, swollen Ulcerations—aphthous type
Iron	Bleeding complications—increased risk Burning/sore mouth Candidiasis Dental caries—increased susceptibility Dysphagia Filiform papillae—atrophic Lips—angular cheilosis, pallor Oral infections—increased risk Oral mucosa—pallor Oral paresthesias Tongue—atrophic, pale; glossitis, glossopyrosis Ulcerations—aphthous type Xerostomia

continues

Table 8–9 continued

Nutrient Deficiency	Oral Manifestations
Magnesium	Bone—fragility Gingiva—hypertrophy
Phosphorus	Dental decay—increased susceptibility Periodontal disease
Protein	Bone—decreased repair Epithelium—fragility, burning sensation Lips—angular cheilosis Oral infections—decreased resistance Periodontal disease—increased susceptibility Wound—healing response-delayed
Protein-calorie	Bone loss Candidiasis Necrotizing ulcerative gingivitis Periodontal disease
Water	Burning/sore mouth Epithelium—dehydration, fragility Muscle strength—diminished Tongue—glossopyrosis Xerostomia
Zinc	Candidiasis Dental caries—increased susceptibility Epithelial thickening Oral mucosa—atrophic Periodontal disease—increased susceptibility Smell acuity—decreased Taste acuity—loss or distortion Wound—healing response-delayed Xerostomia

periodontal disease; gingival enlargement; and ill-fitting dentures.

One commonly held belief is that optimal masticatory efficiency allows an individual to select a wider variety of foods, which leads to a more nutritionally balanced diet.[196] It is also suggested that the loss of mechanical chewing efficiency leads to a preference for soft, easy-to-chew foods, which may increase the risk of nutritional deficiencies.[16,68,193,195,196–200] These foods tend to be high in carbohydrates, cholesterol, and calories but low in fiber, protein, iron, calcium, and essential vitamins. Such a diet routinely contains salt and saturated fats in unhealthy amounts for persons with heart disease and usually lacks vitamin K, which leads to calcium loss in bone.[201]

Edentulousness can affect masticatory function and dietary choice, but its influence on nutritional status is controversial. Some researchers have found that tooth loss is a strong predictor of inadequate nutrition, resulting from problems with biting, chewing, or swallowing foods.[202] Other investigators have found little evidence to indicate that adequate dentition is necessary for geriatric patients to maintain a satisfactory nutritional state.[203,204]

Table 8–10 Oral Signs Suggestive of Malnutrition

Oral Area	Normal Appearance	Signs Associated with Malnutrition
Teeth	Bright; no caries; no pain	Dental caries; may be missing or erupting abnormally
Gums	Healthy; red; not swollen; no bleeding	Receding; spongy; bleed easily
Tongue	Deep red; not swollen or smooth	Scarlet or magenta color; smooth; raw; swelling; sores; atrophic, hyperemic, or hypertrophic papillae
Lips	Smooth; not swollen or chapped	Redness; swelling of mouth and lips
Face	Uniform color; smooth; pink; healthy appearance; not swollen	Lumpiness or flakiness of skin around mouth
Salivary	Face not swollen in gland areas	Parotid enlargement (swollen glands, cheeks)

Source: Adapted with permission from G. Christakis, *Nutritional Assessment in Health Programs*, 7th printing, p.19, ©1984, American Public Health Association.

Even the incidence of malnutrition, weight loss, and gastrointestinal disturbances in the older adult appears to be unrelated to impaired masticatory function.[197,205] In these studies, the percentage of individuals with significantly reduced or inefficient masticatory ability was similar to the percentage of persons with and without overt signs of malnutrition or undernutrition. In addition, various changes in blood chemistry usually associated with malnutrition have not been routinely found in individuals with significantly reduced masticatory ability.[206]

It would appear that replacing missing teeth with partial or complete dentures would improve chewing and limit the risk of nutritional problems. Indeed, the change from poor natural dentition or edentulousness to complete dentures is generally accompanied by improved chewing efficiency and nutritional status,[203,207] but there are conflicting observations in the literature.[204]

Properly fitted dentures may allow one to choose from a wider selection of food textures. However, denture wearing has been reported to interfere with the ability to eat satisfactorily, talk clearly, and laugh freely.[195,198] Elderly denture wearers also require more time to chew before swallowing than do those with natural teeth.[39]

It is well known that the denture wearer does not have the chewing efficiency enjoyed by the individual with natural teeth. Several studies have shown that significant differences in chewing ability occur among persons with intact natural dentition, individuals with partial prosthetic replacements, and individuals with complete dentures.[196–198,200] Dental studies have established that the chewing efficiency of an average complete denture wearer is only 15% to 25% of that of an individual with natural teeth.[195,196,206–210]

Even so, a chewing efficiency as low as 23%, a level attainable with just the 12 maxillary and mandibular anterior teeth, was sufficient to digest the 28 experimental foods in one study of masticatory efficiency and food assimilation.[211] Since the masticatory efficiency attained by the average denture wearer is in this range, most people with dentures should be able to chew food adequately for proper digestion.

The condition of dentures has a direct bearing on an individual's ability to chew. Well-fitting dentures in a healthy mouth can result in better chewing, swallowing, and digestion.[203,207,212] Problems with denture fit, bone shrinkage, and the gum tissues supporting the denture compromise masticatory function and may negatively alter dietary intake.[39] In fact, many denture wearers avoid foods that tend to slip under dentures or are too difficult to manipulate and chew.[202,203,207,208]

Other studies[213–216] have reported significant variation in the masticatory performance of people who wear dentures. Some individuals are barely able to comminute a test food, whereas others with similar prostheses have a relatively high degree of masticatory proficiency. Furthermore, approximately five times more effort is required for the average person wearing complete dentures to pulverize a test food to the same degree that a person with natural dentition can. This agrees with previous reports that impaired chewing ability is not usually improved by chewing food longer or by increasing the rate of chewing, but rather by ingesting foods that are softer and easier to chew[217] or by swallowing larger particles.[218,219] Therefore, denture wearers may be more prone to accidental choking from improper mastication.[220]

Data from dietary surveys before and after the insertion of new dentures are inconclusive about associated changes in essential nutrient intake.[207,221–226] Before the insertion of new dentures, several essential nutrients were consumed in quantities significantly lower than the recommended daily allowance. After new dentures were placed, shifts in nutrient intake occurred, although the changes were not necessarily beneficial. Subjective evaluations, however, indicated improved chewing efficiency, which aided food digestion, particularly of fibrous foods.

Self-Perceived Chewing Ability

Experimental subjects' evaluations of their own chewing ability have been examined as possible predictors of masticatory efficiency, but most reported results are conflicting.[41,196,208,210,226–229] There appears to be wide individual variation in the subjective assessment of chewing problems that is not always related to dentition status. For those with poor masticatory efficiency, the lack of a perceived problem is probably due in part to the selection of foods that are easy to chew or to preparation of food in such a way as to facilitate chewing. In fact, perceived ease of chewing is related to subjective estimates of food preference.[196,209,210,230] In general, denture wearers give lower preference ratings to hard-to-chew foods than do persons with intact or even compromised natural dentition.

Dietary Control of Chewing Difficulties

For those with chewing problems due to dentures or tooth loss, the key is to modify food selection habits and methods of preparing foods for easier chewing. Specific ways to overcome chewing difficulties are listed in Table 8–11.

Oral Cancer

Neoplasms in the oral cavity can interfere with chewing and swallowing because of both pain and infiltration of tissues. Antineoplastic drugs and radiation therapy can alter the character and volume of saliva. In addition, the balance of the oral flora is disrupted, allowing overgrowth of opportunistic organisms such as *Candida* species.

Many patients who undergo radiation therapy for oral cancer become nutritional casualties. Profound loss of appetite is an early and sustained reaction to radiation-induced soreness, xerostomia, taste loss, dysphagia, and nausea and vomiting.[231] Eating becomes a pleasureless and painful chore, and food selection is restricted to items that do not aggravate the oral discomfort, often at the expense of adequate nutrition. When prolonged and severe enough, lack of nutrients can precipitate a nutritional deficiency stomatitis.

Oral Pain

Oral pain can reduce food intake in both texture and amount. In fact, many patients experiencing dental or facial pain avoid certain foods.[232] As an example, mucositic tissues are sensitive to temperature and pressure, so a semisoft diet that is low in sucrose and citric acid is advised.[233]

Masticatory ability, biting force, and tongue movements are impaired in painful oral conditions, thus influencing the ability to chew many foods. Oral pain can also interfere with swallowing.

Table 8–11 Dietary Control of Chewing Difficulties

- Drink fluids with meals to aid in chewing and swallowing.
- Chop, grind, or mechanically blend foods that are hard to chew.
- Add sources of dietary fiber (stems of vegetables, whole grains, skins of fruits and vegetables, and seeds or berries that can be cooked, shredded, mashed, ground, or softened with liquids without affecting the fiber content.
- Shred or chop raw vegetables and use them in salads.
- Mash or strain cooked vegetables.
- Buy prechopped vegetables and meat.
- Prepare meats and vegetables in soups, stews, and casseroles.
- Trim meats to remove fat and tough fibers.
- Substitute softer, protein-rich foods such as fish, eggs, peanut butter, cheese, baked beans, ground meats, or yogurt for regular meat.

- Use melted cheese as a sauce on vegetables or toast to increase protein intake.
- Add extra nonfat dry milk powder to cream soups, cooked cereals, puddings, custards, creamed vegetables, casseroles, and milk beverages to increase protein and calorie content.
- Use cooked whole-grain cereals such as oatmeal or mixed grains.
- Add bran to hot cereals, baked breads, meatloaf, and casseroles.
- Use fruit juices in place of fruits. Most fruits can be pureed in a blender and the pulp added to juices.
- Avoid sticky foods that adhere to teeth and dentures.
- Use menus from cookbooks written for people with chewing problems.
- Most important, eat a variety of foods from the major food groups each day.

Conditions that can cause oral pain are listed in Table 8–12.

Saliva

Saliva is essential for taste perception, mastication, and swallowing of foods. It provides the environment for optimal functioning of taste buds and contributes to ingestion and digestion by forming a mucin-coated food bolus and adequate fluid volume to allow for ready passage along the chewing and swallowing surfaces. The bolus is then digested in the gastrointestinal tract.

When salivary flow is deficient, it causes various stresses on the hard and soft tissues of the mouth, leading to increased oral disease and dysfunction of chewing, swallowing, and taste.[39] The greater concentration of electrolytes in a diminished amount of saliva can result in a salty or metallic taste in the mouth. In addition, decreased ptyalin levels in the reduced salivary flow may affect digestion of chewed particles.

Most patients with xerostomia have difficulty eating solid and dry foods,[42] which can contribute to changes in nutritional intake patterns.[234–236] Oral pain associated with sialadenitis or sialolithiasis can also impair oral intake. In response, elderly individuals reduce the intake of various foods or switch to foods more easily chewed.

To facilitate chewing and swallowing in severe xerostomia, food must be lubricated with artificial saliva or prepared in liquid or semi-liquid form. Saliva substitutes have been shown to improve both chewing and swallowing.[235,237] Many patients moisten foods with sauces, gravies, milk, and other fluids.

Taste and Smell Sensitivity

For the most part, taste and smell determine the flavor of foods and beverages.[238] Reduced acuity of either of these senses may significantly lessen the ability to enjoy food and thus decrease appetite. Declines in gustation and olfaction,

Table 8–12 Oral Conditions That Can Be Painful

- Angular cheilosis
- Aphthous ulceration
- Benign mucous membrane pemphigoid
- Burning mouth syndrome
- Candidiasis
- Contact stomatitis
- Dental caries
- Denture stomatitis
- Erythema multiforme
- Glossodynia
- Glossopharyngeal neuralgia
- Herpes labialis
- Herpetic stomatitis
- Hypersensitive teeth
- Lichen planus
- Mucositis
- Necrotizing ulcerative gingivitis
- Oral cancer (advanced)
- Periodontal disease
- Pulpal infection
- TMJ dysfunction
- Traumatic ulceration
- Trigeminal neuralgia

whether with age, chronic disease, or drug use, decrease the flavor and palatability of foods and beverages. Because of this, the senses of both taste and smell are important in food selection and nutrient intake.[237,239]

Decreased taste sensitivity is compounded by dental disease or poor oral hygiene.[5] The causes can be physical, such as debris covering the taste buds, or chemical, such as taste fatigue from constant stimulation by decaying matter in the mouth.[45] Also, chronic dental or periodontal infections can result in the continuous discharge of purulent matter into the mouth, creating a constantly unpleasant taste. Routine oral hygiene has been shown to improve sensitivity to salty and sweet tastes and may improve the elderly patient's appetite.[240]

Saliva has modulating effects on taste sensitivity. A salty taste is detected only when the concentration is above salivary levels of sodium chloride. Saliva diminishes the effect of a sour taste as a result of buffering by salivary bicarbonate. Decreased salivation also alters the taste of many foods.[238]

Diminished taste also may result from altered taste perception.[238] It has long been suspected that denture wearers have a lowered ability to taste,[209,238] and edentulous individuals experience a reduction in taste sensitivity after the insertion of complete dentures.[241] Perhaps the taste buds in the hard palate are more insensitive to taste, especially sour and bitter, when covered with dentures.[238]

CONCLUSION

The cumulative effects of aging, disease, and trauma contribute to the wide variety of oral health problems prevalent in the older adult. Although many of these problems can be neither prevented nor cured by diet alone, to ignore nutritional considerations in the oral disease process would be a serious error. Many of the oral problems mentioned previously are associated with dietary deficiencies, excesses, or practices that are detrimental to the oral and circumoral structures. It is imperative that dietary intake provide adequate nutrients to support oral health and function.

There is also a strong association between oral health status and food selection, chewing efficiency, and ability to swallow. Clearly, oral health problems that interfere with any aspects of these factors can restrict food intake and ultimately affect nutritional status.

REFERENCES

1. Somerman MJ, Hoffeld JT, Baum BJ. Basic biology and physiology of oral tissues: overview and age-associated changes. In: Tryon AF, ed. *Oral Health and Aging*. Littleton, MA: PSG Publishing Co Inc; 1986.

2. Baum BJ. Salivary gland function during aging. *Gerodontics* 1986;2:61–64.

3. Baum BJ. Normal and abnormal oral status in aging. *Annu Rev Gerontol Geriatr* 1984;4:87–105.

4. Fox PC, Heft MW, Herrera M, et al. Secretion of antimicrobial proteins from the parotid glands of different aged healthy persons. *J Gerontol* 1987;2:466–469.

5. Spielman AI. Interaction of saliva and taste. *J Dent Res* 1990;69:838–843.

6. Sonies BC, Stone M, Shawker T. Speech and swallowing in the elderly. *Gerodontology* 1984;3:115–123.

7. Kiyak HA. Psychosocial factors in dental needs of the elderly. *Spec Care Dent* 1981;1:22–30.

8. Johnson ES, Kelly JE, Van Kirk LE. *Selected Dental Findings in Adults, by Age, Race and Sex: United States: 1960–1962.* Washington, DC: US Public Health Service; 1965. US Dept of Health, Education, and Welfare PHS publication No. 1000, Series 11.

9. *Basic Data on Dental Examination Findings for Persons 1–74 years, US 1971–1974.* Washington, DC: National Center for Health Statistics; 1979. Vital and Health Statistics series 11, data from National Health and Nutrition Examination Survey (HANES), No. 214.

10. Baum BJ. Characteristics of participants in the oral physiology component of the Baltimore Longitudinal Study of Aging. *Community Dent Oral Epidemiol* 1981; 9:128–134.

11. *Oral Health of United States Adults: National Findings.* Bethesda, MD: National Institute of Dental Research; 1987. National Institutes of Health publication 87-2868.

12. Hand JS, Hunt RJ. The need for restorations and extractions in a non-institutionalized elderly population. *Gerodontics* 1986;2:72–76.

13. Hunt RJ, Srisilapanan P, Beck JD. Denture-related problems and prosthodontic treatment needs in the elderly. *Gerodontics* 1985;1:226–230.

14. Hunt RJ. Periodontal treatment needs in an elderly population in Iowa. *Gerodontics* 1986;2:24–27.

15. Bagramian R, Heller P. Dental health assessment of a population of nursing home residents. *J Gerontol* 1977; 32:168–174.

16. Council on Dental Health and Health Planning, Bureau of Economic and Behavioral Research. Oral health status of Vermont nursing home residents. *J Am Dent Assoc* 1982;104:68–69.

17. Empey G, Kiyak HA, Milgrom P. Oral health in nursing homes. *Spec Care Dent* 1983;3:65–67.

18. Baum BJ. Research on aging and oral health: an assessment of current status and future needs. *Spec Care Dent* 1981;1:156–165.

19. Williams TF. Patterns of health and disease in the elderly. *Gerodontics* 1985;1:284–287.

20. Ramazzotto LJ, Curro FA, Gates PE, et al. Calcium nutrition and the aging process: a review. *Gerodontology* 1986;5:159–168.

21. Somerman MJ. Mineralized tissues in aging. *Gerodontology* 1984;3:93–99.

22. Cohen B. Ageing in teeth and associated tissues. In: Cohen B, Thomson H, eds. *Dental Care for the Elderly*, London, England: Year Book Medical Publishers Inc; 1986.

23. Heeneman H, Brown DH. Senescent changes in and about the oral cavity and pharynx. *J Otolaryngol* 1986; 15:214–216.

24. Langer A. Oral changes in the geriatric patient. *Compend Contin Educ Dent* 1981;2:258–264.

25. Ettinger RL. *Oral Changes Associated with Aging, Module 2.* Iowa City: University of Iowa College of Dentistry; 1982. Geriatric Curriculum Series.

26. Ainamo A, Ainamo J. The dentition is intended to last a lifetime. *Int Dent J* 1984;34:87–92.

27. Hand JS, Beck JD, Turner KA. The prevalence of occlusal attrition and considerations of treatment in a non-institutionalized elderly population. *Spec Care Dent* 1987;7:202–206.

28. Heft MW. Prevalence of TMJ signs and symptoms in the elderly. *Gerodontology* 1984;3:125–130.

29. Klein DR. Oral soft tissue changes in geriatric patients. *Bull NY Acad Med* 1980;56:721–727.

30. Hill MW. The influence of aging on skin and oral mucosa. *Gerodontology* 1984;3:35–45.

31. Breustedt A. Age-induced changes in the oral mucosa and their therapeutic consequences. *Int Dent J* 1983;33: 272–280.

32. Mackenzie IC, Holm-Pedersen P, Karring T. Age changes in the oral mucous membranes and periodontium. In: Holm-Pedersen H, Loe H, eds. *Geriatric Dentistry: A Textbook of Oral Gerontology.* St. Louis, MO: CV Mosby Co; 1986.

33. Gordon SR. Survey of dental need among veterans with severe cognitive impairment. *Gerodontics* 1988;4: 158–159.

34. Weiffenbach JM, Cowart BJ, Baum BJ. Taste intensity perception in aging. *J Gerontol* 1986;41:460–468.

35. Satoh Y, Seluk LW. Taste threshold, anatomical form of fungiform papillae and aging in humans. *J Nihon Univ Sch Dent* 1988;30:22–29.

36. Newton JP, Abel RL, Robertson EM, et al. Changes in human masseter and medial pterygoid muscles with age: a study by computed tomography. *Gerodontics* 1987;3:151–154.

37. Newton JP, Yemm R, Abel RW, et al. Changes in human jaw muscles with age and dental state. *Gerodontology* 1993;10:16–22.

38. Vergo TJ Jr, Papas A. Physiological aspects of geriatric dentistry. *J Mass Dent Society* 1988 Fall; 374(4):165–168.

39. Idowu AT, Graser GN, Handelman SL. The effect of age and dentition status on masticatory function in older adults. *Spec Care Dent* 1986;6:80–83.

40. Elliott JL. Swallowing disorders in the elderly: a guide to diagnosis and treatment. *Geriatrics* 1988;43:95–113.

41. Chauncey HH, Kapur KK, Feller RP, et al. Altered masticatory function and perceptual estimates of chewing experience. *Spec Care Dent* 1981;1:250–255.

42. Massler M. Xerostomia in the elderly. *NY J Dent* 1986;56:260–261.

43. Navazesh M, Brightman VJ, Pogoda JM. Relationship of medical status, medications, and salivary flow rates in adults of different ages. *Oral Surg Oral Med Oral Pathol* 1996;81:172–176.

44. Baum BJ. Evaluation of stimulated parotid saliva flow rate in different age groups. *J Dent Res* 1981;60: 1292–1296.

45. Whitehead MC. Neuroanatomy of the gustatory system. *Gerodontics* 1988;4:239–243.

46. Erickson RI. The elderly patient: a new challenge for dentists. *J Calif Dent Assoc* 1982;10:49–50.

47. Bradley RM. Effects of aging on the anatomy and neurophysiology of taste. *Gerodontics* 1988;4:244–248.

48. Weisfuse D, Catalanotto FA, Kamen S. Gender differences in suprathreshold scaling ability in an older population. *Spec Care Dent* 1986;6:25 28.

49. Kiyak HA. Psychological changes associated with aging: implications for the dental practitioner. In: Tryon AF, ed. *Oral Health and Aging,* Littleton, MA: PSG Publishing Co Inc; 1986.

50. Zegeer LJ. The effects of sensory changes in older persons. *J Neurosci Nurs* 1986;18:325–332.

51. Massler M. Geriatric nutrition. the role of taste and smell in appetite. *J Prosthet Dent* 1980;43:247 250.

52. Baker KA, Didcock EA, Kemm FR, et al. Effect of age, sex and illness on salt taste detection thresholds. *Age Ageing* 1983;12:159–165.

53. Ritchie CS. Oral health, taste, and olfaction. *Clin Geriatr Med* 2002;18:709–717.

54. Weiffenbach JM. Taste and smell perception in aging. *Gerodontology* 1984;3:137–146.

55. Venstrom D, Amoore JE. Olfactory threshold in relation to age, sex or smoking. *J Food Sci* 1968;33: 264–265.

56. Doty RL, Shaman P, Applebaum SL, et al. Smell identification ability: changes with age. *Science* 1984;226: 1441–1443.

57. Ettinger RL. Oral disease and its effect on the quality of life. *Gerodontics* 1987;3:103–106.

58. Mandel ID. Preventive dentistry for the elderly. *Spec Care Dent* 1983;3:157–163.

59. Nystrom GP, Adams RA. Oral hygiene and the elderly. In: Tryon AF, ed. *Oral Health and Aging.* Littleton, MA: PSG Publishing Co Inc; 1986.

60. Kandelman D, Bordeur JM, Simard P, et al. Dental needs of the elderly: a comparison between some European and North American surveys. *Community Dent Health* 1986;3:19–39.

61. Goldberg AF, Gergans GA, Mattson DE, et al. Radiographic alveolar process/mandibular height ratio as a predictor of osteoporosis. *Gerondontics* 1988;4:229 231.

62. Richards M. Osteoporosis. *Geriatr Nurs* (New York) 1982;3:98–102.

63. Kribbs PJ, Smith DE, Chestnutt CH III. Oral findings in osteoporosis, part II: relationship between residual ridge and alveolar bone resorption and generalized skeletal osteopenia. *J Prosthet Dent* 1983;50:719–724.

64. Bras J, van Ouij CP, Abraham-Inpijn L, et al. Radiographic interpretation of the mandibular angular cortex: a diagnostic tool in metabolic bone loss. *Oral Surg Oral Med Oral Pathol* 1982;53:541–545.

65. Shapiro S, Bomberg TJ, Benson BW, et al. Postmenopausal osteoporosis: dental patients at risk. *Gerodontics* 1985;1:220–225.

66. Kribbs PJ, Chesnutt CH. Osteoporosis and dental osteopenia in the elderly. *Gerodontology* 1984;3:101–106.

67. Heaney RP, Gallagher JC, Johnston CC, et al. Calcium nutrition and bone health in the elderly. *Am J Clin Nutr* 1982;36(suppl 5):986–1013.

68. Jakush J. Diet, nutrition, and oral health: a rational approach for the dental practice. *J Am Dent Assoc* 1984; 109:20–32.

69. Goodman CE. Osteoporosis: protective measures of nutrition and exercise. *Geriatrics* 1985;40:59–70.

70. Riggs BL, O'Fallon WM, Lane A, et al. Clinical trial of fluoride therapy in postmenopausal osteoporotic women: extended observations and additional analysis. *J Bone Miner Res* 1994;9:265–275.

71. Banting DW. Epidemiology of root caries. *Gerodontology* 1986;5:5–11.

72. Katz RV. Assessing root caries in populations: the evolution of the Root Caries Index. *J Public Health Dent* 1980;40:7–16.

73. Axelsson P, Lindhe J. Effect of controlled oral hygiene procedures on caries and periodontal disease in adults: results after six years. *J Clin Periodontol* 1981;8: 239–248.

74. Beck JD, Hunt RJ, Hand JS, et al. Prevalence of root and coronal caries in a noninstitutionalized older population. *J Am Dent Assoc* 1985;111:964–967.

75. Goldberg J, Tanzer J, Munster E, et al. Cross-sectional clinical evaluation of recurrent enamel caries, restoration of marginal integrity, and oral hygiene status. *J Am Dent Assoc* 1981;102:635–641.

76. Seichter U. Root surface caries: a critical literature review. *J Am Dent Assoc* 1987;115:305–310.

77. Yanover L. Root surface caries: epidemiology, etiology, and control. *J Can Dent Assoc* 1987;53:842–859.

78. Wallace MC, Retief DH, Bradley EL. Prevalence of root caries in a population of older adults. *Gerodontics* 1988;4:84–89.

79. Slome BA. Rampant caries: a side effect of tricyclic antidepressant therapy. *Gen Dent* 1984;32:494–496.

80. Kitamura M, Kiyak HA, Mulligan K. Predictors of root caries in the elderly. *Community Dent Oral Epidemiol* 1986;14:34–38.

81. Arnold FA Jr. Fluorine in drinking water: its effect on dental caries. *J Am Dent Assoc* 1948;136:28–36.

82. Ripa LW. Professionally (operator) applied topical fluoride therapy: a critique. *Clin Prevent Dent* 1982;4: 3–10.

83. Schamschula RG, Barmes DE. Fluoride and health: dental caries, osteoporosis, and cardiovascular disease. *Annu Rev Nutr* 1981;1:427–435.

84. Swango PA. The use of topical fluorides to prevent dental caries in adults: a review of the literature. *J Am Dent Assoc* 1983;107:447–450.

85. Burt BA, Ismail AI, Eklund SA. Root caries in an optimally fluoridated and a high fluoride community. *J Dent Res* 1986;65:1154–1158.

86. Ripa LW, Leske GS, Forte F, et al. Effect of a 0.05% neutral NaF mouth rinse on coronal and root caries of adults. *Gerodontology* 1987;6:131–136.

87. Sinkford JC. Oral health problems in the elderly: research recommendations. *Gerodontics* 1988;4:209–211.

88. Newbrun E. Prevention of root caries. *Gerodontology* 1986;5:33–41.

89. Tonelli PM, Hume WR, Kenney EB. Chlorhexidine: a review of the literature. *Periodant Abstr* 1983;31:5–10.

90. Hand JS, Hunt RJ, Reinhardt JW. The prevalence and treatment implications of cervical abrasion in the elderly. *Gerodontics* 1986;2:167–170.

91. Reussner GH, Coccodrilli G Jr, Thiessen R Jr. Effects of phosphates in acid-containing beverages on tooth erosion. *J Dent Res* 1975;54:365–370.

92. Linkosalo E, Markkanen H. Dental erosions in relation to lactovegetarian diet. *Scand J Dent Res* 1985;93: 436–441.

93. White DK, Hayes RC, Benjamin RN. Loss of tooth structure associated with chronic regurgitation and vomiting. *J Am Dent Assoc* 1978;97:833–835.

94. Malcolm D, Paul E. Erosion of the teeth due to sulphuric acid in the battery industry. *Br J Ind Med* 1961;26:249–266.

95. ten Bruggen Cate HJ. Dental erosion in industry. *Br J Ind Med* 1968;25:249–266.

96. Levy SM. The epidemiology and prevention of dental caries in adults. *Compend Contin Educ Dent* 1988; (suppl 11):S390–S398.

97. Hong F, Nu Zhong-ying XX. Clinical classification and therapeutic design of dental cervical abrasion. *Gerodontics* 1988;4:101–103.

98. Berman LH. Dentinal sensation and hypersensitivity: a review of mechanisms and treatment alternatives. *J Periodontol* 1985;56:216–222.

99. Pelton WJ, Pennell EH, Druzina A. Tooth morbidity experience in adults. *J Am Dent Assoc* 1954;49:439–445.

100. Niessen LC, Weyant RJ. Causes of tooth loss in a veteran population. *J Public Health Dent* 1989;49:19–23.

101. Johnson TE. Factors contributing to dentists' extraction decisions in older adults. *Spec Care Dent* 1993;13: 195–199.

102. National Center for Health Statistics. *Edentulous Persons, US 1971.* Baltimore, MD: Health Resources Administration; 1974. US Dept of Health, Education, and Welfare publication series 10, No. 29.

103. Brown LJ, Meskin LH. Sociodemographic differences in tooth loss patterns in United States employed adults and seniors, 1985–1986. *Gerodontics* 1988;4:345–362.

104. Budtz-Jorgensen E, Luan WM, Holm-Pedersen P, et al. Mandibular dysfunction related to dental, occlusal and prosthetic conditions in a selected elderly population. *Gerodontics* 1985;1:28–33.

105. Rugh JD, Solberg WK. Oral health status in the United States: temporomandibular joint disorders. *J Dent Educ* 1985;49:398–406.

106. Jeanmonod A. The diagnosis and treatment of temporomandibular dysfunctions in older partially or totally edentulous patients. *Int Dent J* 1982;32:339–344.

107. Richards LC, Brown T. Dental attrition and degenerative arthritis of the temporomandibular joint. *J Oral Rehabil* 1981;8:293–307.

108. Nesbit SP, Gobetti JP. Multiple recurrence of oral erythema multiforme after secondary herpes simplex: report of case and review of literature. *J Am Dent Assoc* 1986;112:348–352.

109. Antoon JW, Miller RL. Aphthous ulcers: a review of the literature on etiology, pathogenesis, diagnosis, and treatment. *J Am Dent Assoc* 1980;101:803–808.

110. Hay KD, Reade PC. The use of an elimination diet in the treatment of recurrent aphthous ulceration of the oral cavity. *Oral Surg Oral Med Oral Pathol* 1984;57: 504–507.

111. Rodu B, Russell CM, Ray KL. Treatment of oral ulcers with hydroxypropyl cellulose film (Zilactin® D). *Compend Contin Educ Dent* 1988;9:420–422.

112. Mackowiak PA. The normal microbial flora. *N Engl J Med* 1982;307:83–93.

113. Gallagher FJ, Taybos GM, Terezhalmy GT. Clinical diagnosis and treatment of oral candidiasis. *J Indiana Dent Assoc* 1985;64:26–28.

114. Waldron CA, Shafer WG. Leukoplakia revisited: a clinicopathologic study of 3256 oral leukoplakias. *Cancer* 1975;36:1386–1392.

115. Gupta PC. Epidemiologic study of the association between alcohol habits and oral leukoplakia. *Community Dent Oral Epidemiol* 1984;12:47–50.

116. Christen AG, McDonald JL Jr, Klein IA. A primer of relevant facts for smokers. *Dent Teamwork* 1989;2: 25–26.

117. Alexander WN. Oral lesions in the elderly. In: Tryon AF, ed. *Oral Health and Aging.* Littleton, MA: PSG Publishing Co Inc; 1986.

118. Silverman S Jr, ed. *Oral Cancer.* 2nd ed. New York, NY: American Cancer Society; 1985.

119. Parker SL, Tong T, Bolden S, et al. *Cancer statistics, 1997.* CA 1997;47:5–27.

120. Little JW, Falace DA. Oral cancer. In: Little JW, Falace DA, eds. *Dental Management of the Medically Compromised Patient.* 3rd ed. St Louis, MO: CV Mosby Co; 1988.

121. Brugere J, Guenel P, Leclerc A, et al. Differential effects of tobacco and alcohol in cancer of the larynx, pharynx, and mouth. *Cancer* 1986;57:391–395.

122. Squier CA. Smokeless tobacco and oral cancer: a cause for concern? *CA* 1984;34:242–247.

123. Shi HB, Xu GQ, Shen ZY. A retrospective study of oral mucosal diseases in three age groups. *Gerondontics* 1988;4:235–237.

124. Hebert JR, London J, Miller DR. Consumption of meat and fruit in relation to oral and esophageal cancer: a cross-national study. *Nutr Cancer* 1993;19:169–179.

125. Silverman S Jr, Gorsky M. Epidemiologic and demographic update in oral cancer: California and national data—1973 to 1985. *J Am Dent Assoc* 1990;120:495–499.

126. Peterson DE. Oral mucosal ulcerative lesions. *Pharmacol Dent* 1986;2:1–4.

127. Greer RO. A problem-oriented approach to evaluating common mucosal lesions in the geriatric patient: a survey of 593 lesions in patients over 60 years of age. *Gerodontics* 1985;1:68–74.

128. Chandler JA, Brudvik JS. Clinical evaluation of patients eight to nine years after placement of removable partial dentures. *J Prosthet Dent* 1984;51:736–743.

129. Lambert JP, Kolstad R. Effect of a benzoic acid detergent germicide on denture-borne *Candida albicans.* *J Prosthet Dent* 1986;55:699–700.

130. Budtz-Jorgensen E, Loe H. Chlorhexidine as a denture disinfectant in the treatment of denture stomatitis. *Scand J Dent Res* 1972;80:457–464.

131. Koopmans ASF, Kippuw N, de Graaff J. Bacterial involvement in denture-induced stomatitis. *J Dent Res* 1988;67:1246–1250.

132. Williams RC. Periodontal disease. *N Engl J Med* 1990; 322:373–382.

133. Anderson DL. Periodontal disease and aging. *Gerodontology* 1982;1:19–23.

134. Douglass CW, Gillings D, Sollecito W, et al. National trends in the prevalence and severity of the periodontal diseases. *J Am Dent Assoc* 1983;107:403–412.

135. Page RC. Periodontal diseases in the elderly: a critical evaluation of current information. *Gerodontology* 1984; 3:63–70.

136. Lindhe J, Haffajee AD, Socransky SS. Progression of periodontal disease in adult subjects in the absence of periodontal therapy. *J Clin Periodontol* 1983;10:433–442.

137. Schmitt RJ, Sheridan PJ, Rogers RS III. Pernicious anemia with associated glossodynia. *J Am Dent Assoc* 1988; 117:838–840.

138. Powell FC. Glossodynia and other disorders of the tongue. *Dermatol Clin* 1987;5:687–693.

139. Hill JH, Deitch RL. Early detection of cancers of the head and neck. *VA Pract* 1986;2:57–72.

140. Venus CA. Interacting with patients who have communication disorders. *Tex Dent J* 1990;107:11–16.

141. Zimmerman JE, Oder LA. Swallowing dysfunction in acutely ill patients. *Phys Ther* 1981;61:1755–175.

142. Baum BJ, Bodner L. Aging and oral motor function: evidence for altered performance among older persons. *J Dent Res* 1983;62:2–6.

143. Watanabe I, Sato M, Yamane H, et al. Oral dyskinesia of the aged, I: clinical aspects. *Gerodontics* 1985;1:39–43.

144. Watanabe I, Yamane G, Yamane H, et al. Oral dyskinesia of the aged, II: electromyographic appearances and dental treatment. *Gerodontics* 1988;4:310–314.

145. Altrocchi PH, Forno LS. Spontaneous orofacial dyskinesia: neuropathology of a case. *Neurology* 1983; 33:802–805.

146. Kamen S. Tardive dyskinesia: a significant syndrome for geriatric dentistry. *Oral Surg Oral Med Oral Pathol* 1975;39:52–57.

147. Nishioka GJ, Montgomery MT. Masticatory muscle hyperactivity in temporomandibular disorders: is it an extrapyramidally expressed disorder? *J Am Dent Assoc* 1988,116:514–520.

148. Eveson JW, Cawson RA. Salivary gland tumours: a review of 2410 cases with particular reference to histological types, site, age and sex distribution. *J Pathol* 1985;146:51–58.

149. Senel SF, Scanlon EF. Irradiation induced salivary gland neoplasia. *Ann Surg* 1980;191:304–306.

150. McKenna RJ. Tumors of the major and minor salivary glands. *CA* 1984;34:24–39.

151. Atkinson JC, Fox PC. Clinical pathology conference: xerostomia. *Gerodontics* 1986;2:193–197.

152. Lloyd PM. Xerostomia: not a phenomenon of aging. *Wis Med J* 1983;82:21–22.

153. Jolly DE, Paulson RB, Paulson GW, et al. Parkinson's disease: a review and recommendations for dental management. *Spec Care Dent* 1989;9:74–78.

154. Kelly JF, Winograd CH. A functional approach to stroke management in elderly patients. *J Am Geriatr Soc* 1985;33:48–60.

155. Rosenbaum CH. Did you treat a drug addict today? *Int Dent J* 1981;31:307–312.

156. Verlander JM, Johns ME. The clinical use of cocaine. *Otolaryngol Clin North Am* 1981;14:521–531.

157. Friedlander AH, Mills MJ. The dental management of the drug-dependent patient. *Oral Surg Oral Med Oral Pathol* 1985;60:489–492.

158. McBean LD, Speckmann EW. A review: the importance of nutrition in oral health. *J Am Dent Assoc* 1974;89:109–114.

159. DePaola DP, Kuftinec MN. Nutrition in growth and development of oral tissues. *Dent Clin North Am* 1976;20:441–459.

160. Alfano MC. Diet and nutrition in the etiology and prevention of oral disease. *J Dent Res* 1980;59:2194–2202.

161. Carlsson J, Egelberg J. Effect of diet on early plaque formation in man. *Odontol Rev* 1965;16:112–125.

162. Johansson I, Ericson T, Steen L. Studies of the effect of diet on saliva secretion and caries development: the effect of fasting on saliva composition of female subjects. *J Nutr* 1984;114:2010–2020.

163. Theilade E, Theilade T. Role of plaque in the etiology of periodontal disease and caries. *Oral Sci Rev* 1976;9:23–63.

164. Englander HR. Anticaries and antiplaque agents. In: Neidel EA, Kroeger DC, Yagiela JA, eds. *Pharmacology and Therapeutics for Dentistry.* St Louis, MO: CV Mosby Co; 1980.

165. Touger-Decker R, van Loveren C. Sugars and dental caries. *Am J Clin Nutr* 2003;78(suppl):881S-892S.

166. Snacks and caries. *Nutr Rev* 1987;45:169–172.

167. Scheinen A, Makinen KK. The Turku sugar studies I–XXI. *Acta Odontol Scand* 1971;32:383–412.

168. Katz S. A diet counseling program. *J Am Dent Assoc* 1981;102:840–845.

169. Sheiham A. Sucrose and dental caries. *Nutr Health* 1987;5:25–29.

170. Mormann JE, Muhlemann HR. Oral starch degradation and its influence on acid production in human dental plaque. *Caries Res* 1981;15:166–175.

171. Jensen ME, Schachtele CF. The acidogenic potential of reference foods and snacks at interproximal sites in the human dentition. *J Dent Res* 1983;62:889–892.

172. de Stoppelaar JD, van Houte J, Backer-Dirks O. The effect of carbohydrate restriction on the presence of *Streptococcus mutans, Streptococcus sanguis* and iodophilic polysaccharide-producing bacteria in human dental plaque. *Caries Res* 1970;4:114–123.

173. Firestone A, Imfeld T, Schmid R, et al. Cariogenicity of foods. *J Am Dent Assoc* 1980;101:443.

174. Papas A, Palmer C, McGandy R, et al. Dietary and nutritional factors in relation to dental caries in elderly subjects. *Gerodontics* 1987;3:30–37.

175. Council on Dental Therapeutics. Consensus: oral health effects of products that increase salivary flow rate. *J Am Dent Assoc* 1988;116:757–759.

176. Hefferren JJ, Harper DS, Osborn JC. Foods, consumption factors and dental caries. *Gerodontics* 1987;3:26–29.

177. Bibby BG, Mundorff SA, Zero DT, et al. Oral food clearance and the pH of plaque and saliva. *J Am Dent Assoc* 1986;112:333–337.

178. Feigal RJ, Jensen ME. The cariogenic potential of liquid medications: a concern for the handicapped patient. *Spec Care Dent* 1982;2:20–24.

179. Matsukobo T, Myake S, Takaesu Y. Evaluation of aspartame as a non-cariogenic sweetener. *Clin Nutr* 1984;65:193–196.

180. Alfin-Slater RB, Pi-Sunyer FX. Sugar and sugar substitutes: comparisons and indications. *Postgrad Med* 1987;82:46–56.

181. Jensen ME. Responses of interproximal plaque pH to snack foods and effect of chewing sorbitol containing gum. *J Am Dent Assoc* 1986;113:262–266.

182. Spolsky VW, Wolinsky L. The relationship between nutrition and diet and dental caries periodontal disease. *J Calif Dent Assoc* 1984;12:12–18.

183. Charbeneau TD, Hurt WC. Gingival findings in spontaneous scurvy: a case report. *J Periodontol* 1983;54:694–697.

184. Marshall JR, Graham J, Haughey BP, et al. Smoking, alcohol, dentition and diet in the epidemiology of oral cancer. *Eur J Cancer B Oral Oncol* 1992;28B:9–15,

185. Day GL, Shore RE, Blot WJ, et al. Dietary factors and secondary primary cancers: a follow-up of oral and pharyngeal cancer patients. *Nutr Cancer* 1994;21:223–232.

186. Marshall J, Graham S, Mettlin C, et al. Diet in the epidemiology of oral cancer. *Nutr Cancer* 1982;3:145–149.

187. McLaughlin JK, Gridley G, Block G, et al. Dietary factors in oral and pharyngeal cancer. *J Natl Cancer Inst* 1988;80:1237–1243.

188. Gridley G, McLaughlin JK, Block G, et al. Diet and oral and pharyngeal cancer among blacks. *Nutr Cancer* 1990;14:219–225.

189. Negri E, Franceschi S, Bosetti C, et al. Selected micronutrients and oral and pharyngeal cancer. *Int J Cancer* 2000;86:122–127.

190. Massler M. Influence of diet on denture-bearing tissues. *Dent Clin North Am* 1984;28:211–221.

191. Buchner A, Screebny LM. Enlargement of salivary glands: review of the literature. *Oral Surg Oral Med Oral Pathol* 1972;34:209–222.

192. Nakamoto T, Mallek HM. Significance of protein-energy malnutrition in dentistry: some suggestions for the profession. *J Am Dent Assoc* 1980;100:339–342.

193. Sullivan DH, Martin W, Flaxman N, et al. Oral health problems and involuntary weight loss in a population of frail elderly. *J Am Geriatr Soc* 1993;41:725–731.

194. Jette AM, Feldman HA, Douglass C. Oral disease and physical disability in community-dwelling older persons. *J Am Geriatr Soc* 1993;41:1102–1108.

195. Epstein S. Importance of psychosocial and behavioral factors in food ingestion in the elderly and their ramifications on oral health. *Gerodontics* 1987;3:23–25.

196. Wayler AH, Chauncey HH. Impact of complete dentures and impaired natural dentition on masticatory performance and food choice in healthy aging men. *J Prosthet Dent* 1983;49:427–433.

197. Mumma RD Jr, Quinton K. Effect of masticatory efficiency on the occurrence of gastric distress. *J Dent Res* 1970;49:69–74.

198. Chen MK, Lowenstein F. Masticatory handicap, socioeconomic status, and chronic conditions among adults. *J Am Dent Assoc* 1984;109:916–918.

199. Sastry RS. Nutrition study, III: nutritional status of edentulous patients subsequent to complete denture treatment. *J Indiana Dent Assoc* 1984;56:145–147.

200. Brodeur JM, Laurin D, Vallcer RE, et al. Nutrient intake and gastrointestinal disorders related to masticatory performance in the edentulous elderly. *J Prosthet Dent* 1993;70:468–473.

201. Ramsey WO. Nutritional problems of the aged. *J Prosthet Dent* 1983;49:16–19.

202. Marshall TA, Warren JJ, Hand JS, Xie XJ, Stumbo PH. Oral health, nutrient intake and dietary quality in the very old. *J Am Dent Assoc* 2002;133:1369–1379.

203. Neill DJ, Phillips HI. The masticatory performance and dietary intake of elderly edentulous patients. *Dent Pract* 1972;22:384–389.

204. Baxter JC. The nutritional intake of geriatric patients with varied dentitions. *J Prosthet Dent* 1984;51:164–168.

205. Horn VJ, Hodge WC, Treuer JP. Dental condition and weight loss in institutionalized demented patients. *Spec Care Dent* 1994;14:108–111.

206. Kapur KK. Optimum dentition in the elderly. In: Chauncey HH, Epstein S, Rose CL, et al., eds. *Clinical Geriatric Dentistry: Biomedical and Psychosocial Aspects,* Chicago, IL: American Dental Association; 1985.

207. Baxter CJ. Nutrition and the geriatric edentulous patient. *Spec Care Dent* 1981;1:259–261.

208. Heath MR. The effect of maximum biting force and bone loss upon masticatory function and dietary selection of the elderly. *Int Dent J* 1982;32:345–356.

209. Chauncey HH, Muench ME, Kapur KK, et al. The effect of the loss of teeth on diet and nutrition. *Int Dent J* 1984;34:98–104.

210. Walls AWG, Steele JG, Sheiham A, et al. Oral health and nutrition in older people. *J Pub Health Dent* 2000;4:304–307.

211. Farrell JH. The effect of mastication on the digestion of food. *Br Dent J* 1956;100:149–155.

212. Idowu AT, Handelman SL, Graser GN. Effect of denture stability, retention, and tooth form on masticatory function in the elderly. *Gerodontics* 1987;3:161–164.

213. Hartsook El. Food selection, dietary adequacy, and related dental problems of patients with dental prostheses. *J Prosthet Dent* 1974;32:324–350.

214. Kapur KK, Soman SD. Masticatory performance and efficiency in denture wearers. *J Prosthet Dent* 1964;14:687–694.

215. Slagter AP, Olthoff LW, Bosman F, et al. Masticatory ability, denture quality, and oral conditions in edentulous subjects. *J Prosthet Dent* 1992;68:299–307.

216. Stagter AP, Bosman F, Va der Bitt A. Comminution of two artificial test foods by dentate and edentulous subjects. *J Oral Rehabil* 1993;20:159–176.

217. Chauncey HH, House JE. Dental problems in the elderly. *Hosp Pract* 1977;12:81–86.

218. Helkimo E, Carlsson GE, Helhmo M. Chewing efficiency and state of dentition: a methodological study. *Acta Odontol Scand* 1978;36:33–41.

219. Oosterhaven SP, Westert GP, Schaub RM-I, et al. Social and psychologic implications of missing teeth for chewing ability. *Community Dent Oral Epidemiol* 1988;16:79–82.

220. Anderson DL. Death from improper mastication. *Int Dent J* 1977;27:349–354.

221. Baxter CI. The nutritional intake of complete denture patients: a computerized study. *J Indiana Dent Soc* 1980;59:14–17.

222. Gunne HS, Wall AK. The effect of new complete dentures on mastication and dietary intake. *Acta Odontol Scand* 1985;43:257–268.

223. Gunne HS. The effect of removable partial dentures on mastication and dietary intake. *Acta Odontol Scand* 1985;43:269–278.

224. Rosenstein DI, Chiodo G, Ho IW, et al. Effect of proper dentures on nutritional status. *Gen Dent* 1988;36:127–129.

225. Elmstahl S, Birkhed D, Christiansson U, et al. Intake of energy and nutrients before and after dental treatment in geriatric long-stay patients. *Gerodontics* 1988;4:6–12.

226. Sebring NG, Guckes AD, Li SH, et al. Nutritional adequacy of reported intake of edentulous subjects treated with new conventional or implant-supported mandibular implants. *J Prosthet Dent* 1995;74:358–363.

227. Lappalainen R, Nyyssonen V. Self assessed chewing ability of Finnish adults with removable dentures. *Gerodontics* 1987;3:238–241.

228. Ekelund R. Dental state and subjective chewing ability of institutionalized elderly people. *Community Dent Oral Epidemiol* 1989;17:24–27.

229. Greksa LP, Parraga IM, Clark CA. The dietary adequacy of edentulous older adults. *J Prosthet Dent* 1995;72:142–145.

230. Gordon SR, Kelley SL, Sybyl IR, et al. Relationship in very elderly veterans of nutritional status, self-perceived chewing ability, dental status, and social isolation. *J Am Geriatr Soc* 1985;33:334–339.

231. Chencharick JD, Mossman KL. Nutritional consequences of the radiotherapy of head and neck cancer. *Cancer* 1983;51:811–815.

232. Locker D, Grushka M. The impact of dental and facial pain. *J Dent Res* 1987;66:1414–1417.

233. Fattore LD, Baer R, Olsen R. The role of the general dentist in the treatment and management of oral complications of chemotherapy. *Gen Dent* 1987;35:374–377.

234. Rhodus NL, Brown J. The association of xerostomia and inadequate intake in older adults. *J Am Diet Assoc* 1990;90:1688–1692.

235. Ernst SL. Dietary intake, food preferences, stimulated salivary flow rate, and masticatory ability in older adults with complete dentitions. *Spec Care Dent* 1993;13:102–106.

236. Lingström P, Moynihan P. Nutrition, saliva, and oral health. *Nutrition* 2003;6:567–569.

237. Vissink A, Schaub RMH, van Rijn LJ, et al. The efficacy of mucin-containing artificial saliva in alleviating symptoms of xerostomia. *Gerodontology* 1987;6:95–101.

238. Moeller TP. Sensory changes in the elderly. *Dent Clin North Am* 1989;33:23–31.

239. Griep MI, Verleye G, Franck AH, et al. Variation in nutrient intake with dental status, age and odour perception. *Eur J Clin Nutr* 1996;50:816–825.

240. Hyde RJ, Feller RP, Sharon IM. Tongue brushing, dentifrice, and age effects on taste and smell. *J Dent Res* 1981;60:1730–1734.

241. Chauncey HH, Wayler AH. The modifying influence of age on taste perception. *Spec Care Dent* 1981;1:68–74.

CHAPTER 9

Swallowing Problems
in Older Adults

Joanne Robbins, PhD and Stephanie Kays, MS

The capacity to effectively and safely swallow in order to eat meets one of the basic human needs. Sustaining oneself nutritionally and maintaining adequate hydration while enjoying the process has become intertwined with satisfying social activities. In fact, as leisure time increases in the United States, and with the anticipated extended retirements of America's baby boomers, older adults look forward to more opportunities to share mealtimes and participate in social activities that include eating and drinking. Ironically, as we grow older, the ability to swallow, a function very much taken for granted, undergoes changes. These changes increase the risk for disordered swallowing, particularly with increasing age and exposure to age-related diseases and conditions. Indeed, the loss of the capacity to swallow can have devastating implications, especially for older individuals.

Dysphagia refers to difficulty swallowing that may include oropharyngeal or esophageal problems. This chapter will address oropharyngeal dysphagia with a focus on the gut discussed in Chapter 10.

Although age-related changes place older adults at risk for dysphagia, an older adult's swallow is not necessarily an impaired swallow. *Presbyphagia* refers to characteristic changes in the swallowing mechanism of otherwise healthy older adults. Clinicians are becoming more aware of the need to distinguish among dysphagia,

presbyphagia (an old yet healthy swallow), and other related diagnoses to avoid overdiagnosing and overtreating dysphagia. Older adults are more vulnerable and with the increased threat of acute illnesses, medications, and any number of age-related conditions, they can cross the line from having a healthy older swallow to being dysphagic. This chapter discusses the swallowing process and aging effects on it. The current state of dysphagia diagnosis and treatment will then be addressed as they relate to nutrition and other health outcomes. Furthermore, the multidisciplinary nature of best patient care in this relatively young and rapidly growing field of dysphagia will be discussed.

THE IMPACT OF DYSPHAGIA

Estimates range from 15% to 40% of individuals over 60 years old have dysphagia. The prevalence depends on the specific populations sampled, with community-dwelling and more independent individuals having rates near 15%.[1] This figure is in agreement with the prevalence rates for several other "geriatric syndromes." Upward of 40% of people living in institutional settings, such as assisted living or nursing homes, are dysphagic.[2] Based on the 15% prevalence rate and the 1998 United States Census data, it is estimated that over 6 million adults have dysphagia. With projected growth in the number of individuals living in nursing homes, there is a clear need to address dysphagia in not only ambulatory and acute care settings, but also in long-term care settings.

The consequences of dysphagia vary from social isolation (because of the embarrassment of choking or coughing at mealtime) and physical discomfort (eg, food sticking in the chest), to potentially life-threatening conditions. The more ominous sequelae include dehydration, malnutrition, and both overt and silent aspiration. For this discussion, aspiration is defined as the entry of material into the airway *below* the level of the true vocal folds. *Silent aspiration* refers to the circumstance in which the bolus comprising saliva, medication, food, liquid, or any foreign material, enters the airway below the vocal folds *without* triggering overt symptoms such as coughing or throat clearing. Both overt and silent aspiration may lead toward pneumonitis, pneumonia, exacerbation of chronic lung diseases, or even asphyxiation and death. Malnutrition and dehydration are other related negative consequences. To gain a better understanding of the effect these consequences have on an older adult and the impact of dysphagia interventions, research in this area has focused on determining more meaningful outcome measures. Assessments focused on pathophysiology, function, and health services are now being conducted to create more evidence-based practice in dysphagia care.

Insofar as dysphagia is a biomechanical disorder of bolus flow, signs of flow abnormality, using videofluoroscopy, have been well detailed.[2,3] These include: (1) the duration, direction, and completeness of the bolus flow; (2) duration and extent (range) of anatomical structural movements; and (3) the relationship between bolus flow and structural movements. Other clinical outcomes of dysphagia have become important endpoints in assessing interventions that aim to make it possible for patients to eat and drink adequately and safely. These include measures of hydration, nutrition, and aspiration episodes. Additionally, pneumonitis, overt aspiration pneumonia, and additional forms of evidence of pulmonary damage are monitored.

Nonetheless, it has been difficult to attribute mortality directly to dysphagia since it often is a secondary rather than a primary diagnosis. Other measures have been developed that target what and how dysphagic adults eat and drink, and most of these scales are directly applicable to older adults. Among the common components of all of these tools are the distinction between oral and non-oral eaters, the time to eat, the need for special techniques or compensations, and the presence of coughing and choking during eating.

Dysphagia is felt to profoundly influence quality of life (QOL). Patients who have swallowing difficulties (especially those who relinquish oral eating) manifest significant changes in psychosocial status, functional status, and emotional well-being. Eating and drinking are social events that relate to friendships, acceptance, entertainment, and communication. As such, major adjustments in the process of feeding and eating can lead to distressing responses such as shame, anxiety, depression, and isolation. Only recently have dysphagia-specific, comprehensive, QOL measures been developed. SWAL-QOL is a 44-item tool that assesses 10 dysphagia-specific QOL concepts, and the SWAL-CARE is a 15-item tool that assesses quality of care and patient satisfaction.[4-6] By monitoring functional outcomes with tools like the SWAL-QOL in clinical practice, physicians and other health care providers may be able to better assess and adjust their treatment of dysphagia.

NORMAL SWALLOWING

The oropharyngeal swallowing mechanism is the natural inroad to the gastrointestinal tract. A basic understanding of the relationship of the anatomic components and functional interactions of the normal swallowing mechanism is essential to understand the effects of age and age-related diseases.

Swallowing is an integrated neuromuscular process that combines volitional and relatively automatic movements. The process of deglutition can be described as occurring in two, three, or four phases or stages,[2] or horizontal versus vertical subsystems related to the direction of bolus flow (Figure 9–1).[7]

The horizontal subsystem is largely volitional and comprises anatomically structures within the oral cavity. Within this subsystem, food is accepted, contained, and manipulated. Labial, buccal, and lingual actions, in combination with enzyme-rich intraoral fluids allow manipulation of the texture of food to mechanically formulate a bolus. The cohesive bolus is moved posteriorly (and horizontally when the subject is in a normal upright seated posture) to the inlet of the superior aspect of the pharynx (Figure 9–2). To accomplish this, the intrinsic and extrinsic tongue muscles change the shape and the position of the tongue, and stimulate oropharyngeal receptors that trigger ensuing portions of the swallow sequence.[8–10]

The pharyngeal and laryngeal components, in conjunction with the tongue dorsum, comprise the superior aspect of the vertical subsystem where gravity begins to assist in the transport of the

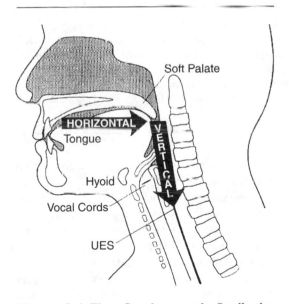

Figure 9–1 The Oropharyngeal Swallowing Mechanism
The oropharyngeal swallowing mechanism may be divided into two basic structural subsystems, horizontal and vertical, that mirror direction of bolus flow. (Adapted from Robbins JA: Normal swallowing and aging. *Semin Neurol* 16(4):309–317, Dec., 1996). Reprinted by permission of Thieme.

bolus. The anatomical juxtaposition of the entrance to the airway (laryngeal vestibule) and the pharyngeal aspect of the upper digestive tract demand biomechanical precision to ensure simultaneous airway protection and bolus transfer or propulsion through the pharynx. As lingual-palatal contact sequentially moves the bolus against the posterior pharyngeal wall, the contact contributes to the positive pressures imparted to the bolus propelling it downward.[11] Simultaneously, the pharyngeal constrictors begin contracting in a descending sequence,[12] first elevating and widening the entire pharynx to engulf the bolus (Figure 9–2d–e). A descending peristaltic wave then cleanses the pharynx of residue. The tongue is the primary propulsive mechanism responsible for plunging the bolus into the vertical subsystem, but other mechanisms, such as velopharyngeal closure, also contribute to pressure gradients facilitating the bolus transfer.

Airway protection is ensured during the swallow by 3 levels of sphincteric closure. (1) aryepiglottic folds, (2) the false vocal folds, and (3) the true vocal folds. The hyolaryngeal complex is also lifted upward and forward by the combined contraction of the suprahyoid and thyrohyoid muscles and pharyngeal elevators. This hyolaryngeal elevation and anterior movement, coupled with tongue base retraction, covers the laryngeal vestibule, diverts the bolus laterally around the airway, and also provides the traction pull on the cricoid cartilage, moving it anteriorly, an important aspect of upper esophageal sphincter (UES) opening.[13]

Timely relaxation and opening of the UES permits continuous vertical passage of the bolus into the esophagus, and the pharyngeal transport stage of the swallow terminates when the UES returns to its hypertonic, closed "resting state."

NEUROPHYSIOLOGY OF OROPHARYNGEAL SWALLOWING

Sensorimotor control of swallowing requires the coordinated activity distributed across both cranial and spinal nerve systems, including peripheral nerves, their central nuclei, and their

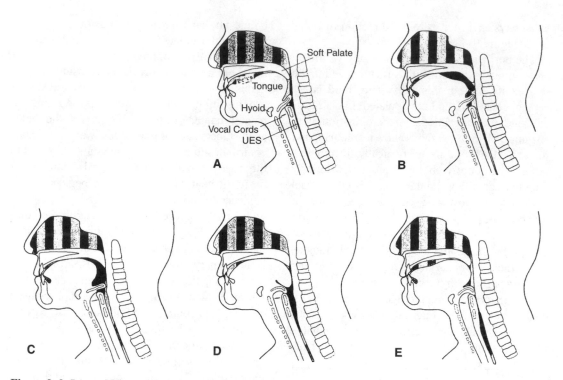

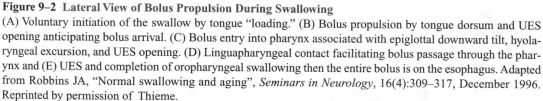

Figure 9–2 Lateral View of Bolus Propulsion During Swallowing
(A) Voluntary initiation of the swallow by tongue "loading." (B) Bolus propulsion by tongue dorsum and UES opening anticipating bolus arrival. (C) Bolus entry into pharynx associated with epiglottal downward tilt, hyolaryngeal excursion, and UES opening. (D) Linguapharyngeal contact facilitating bolus passage through the pharynx and (E) UES and completion of oropharyngeal swallowing then the entire bolus is on the esophagus. Adapted from Robbins JA, "Normal swallowing and aging", *Seminars in Neurology*, 16(4):309–317, December 1996. Reprinted by permission of Thieme.

neural centers. More specifically, the neural control of swallowing involves five major components: (1) afferent sensory fibers contained in cranial nerves; (2) cerebral and midbrain fibers that synapse with the brainstem swallowing centers; (3) paired swallowing centers in the brainstem; (4) efferent motor fibers contained in cranial nerves and the ansa cervicalis; and (5) muscles. This distributed neural network spans all levels of the neuraxis from the cerebrum superiorly to brainstem and spinal nerves inferiorly and muscles at the periphery to integrate and sequence both volitional and automatic activities of swallowing.

Healthy persons depend on a highly automated neuromuscular sensorimotor process that intricately coordinates the activities of chewing, swallowing, and airway protection. To accomplish a normal swallow, which occurs in 2 seconds or less, the muscles of chewing (masseters, temporalis, pterygoids—innervated by cranial nerve V), the lip and buccal musculature, obicularis oris and buccinator (innervated by cranial nerve VII), and the intrinsic and extrinsic lingual muscles (innervated by cranial nerve XII) interact with 26 pairs of striated pharyngeal and laryngeal muscles. In healthy young individuals, the outcome of optimal structural integrity and precise neural mediation is continuous and rapid bolus flow from the mouth to the esophagus (Figure 9–3a–c) that accommodates variation in bolus size, texture, temperature, and the individual's intent to swallow, chew, or just hold the bolus in the mouth.

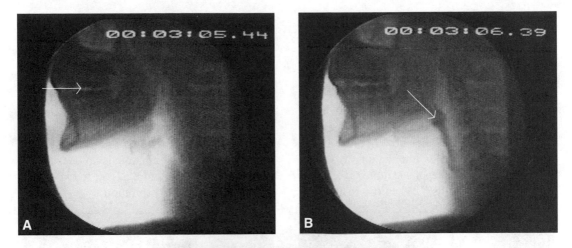

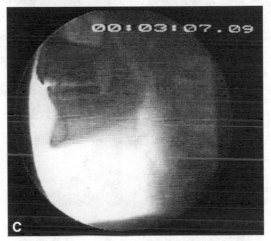

Figure 9–3 Healthy Young Swallowing Documented with Videofluoroscopy
(A) Bolus in mouth initiating swallow. (B) Bolus appears as "column" of material swiftly moving through pharynx. (C) Oropharynx cleared of material when swallow completed. (Adapted from Robbins JA: Normal swallowing and aging. *Semin Neurol* 16(4):309–317, Dec., 1996). Reprinted by permission of Thieme.

SENESCENT SWALLOWING

Changes in swallowing function can occur with healthy aging. A progression of change appears to put members of the older population at increased risk for dysphagia, particularly when they are faced with stressors such as medications that affect the nervous system, mechanical perturbations (eg, nasogastric tubes or tracheostomy), or chronic medical conditions (eg, frailty) that might not elicit dysphagia in a less vulnerable system.

Older healthy swallowing occurs more slowly. Longer swallowing duration occurs in older individuals largely before the more automatic vertical subsystem of the swallow is initiated. Delays in the onset of components that compose the vertical phase are also apparent. In those over age 65, the initiation of laryngeal and pharyngeal events, including laryngeal vestibule closure, maximal hyolaryngeal excursion, and upper esophageal sphincter (UES) opening are significantly delayed relative to durations recorded in adults younger than 45 years.[14–17] In older healthy adults, it is not uncommon for the bolus to be adjacent to an open airway, by pooling or pocketing in the pharyngeal recesses, for a longer time than in younger adults (Figure 9–4a–c). This situation may be associated with greater risk for airway penetration or aspiration.

Aspiration and airway penetration are believed to be the most significant adverse clinical outcomes of misdirected bolus flow. In older adults, penetration of the bolus into the airway occurs more often and to a deeper and more severe level than in younger adults.[18] When the swallowing

mechanism is functionally altered or perturbed in older people, such as with the placement of a nasogastric tube, airway penetration can be even more pronounced. A study examining this issue found that liquid penetrated the airway significantly more frequently when a nasogastric tube was in place in men and women older than 70 years.[15] That study and additional evidence indicates that under stressful conditions or system perturbations, older individuals are less able to compensate and are more at risk to experience airway penetration or aspiration.

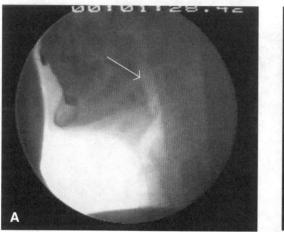

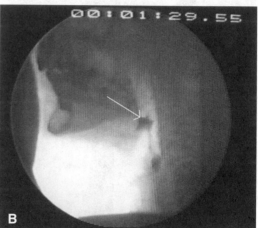

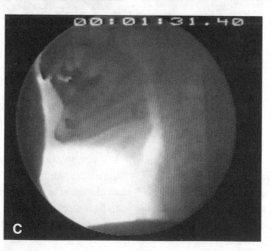

Figure 9–4 Healthy Old Swallowing Documented with Videofluoroscopy
(A) Bolus in mouth initiating swallow. (B) Bolus pooled in vallecula and pyriform sinus during delayed onset of pharyngeal response. (C) Bolus cleared of material when swallow completed. (Adapted from Robbins JA: Normal swallowing and aging. *Semin Neurol* 16(4):309–317, Dec., 1996). Reprinted by permission of Thieme.

Age-related changes in lingual pressure generation also define presbyphagia. Healthy older individuals demonstrate significantly reduced isometric tongue pressures compared with younger counterparts. In contrast, maximal lingual pressure generated during swallowing (which is a submaximal pressure requirement task) remains normal in magnitude. Because peak lingual pressures used in swallowing are lower than those generated isometrically, healthy older individuals manage to achieve pressures necessary to affect a successful swallow, but achieve these peak swallowing pressures more slowly than do young swallowers.[19,20] It has been suggested that as people get older, slower swallowing may permit increased time to recruit the necessary number of motor units for pressures critical for adequate bolus propulsion through the oropharynx. However, it must again be considered that perturbations or functional alterations in the swallowing mechanism, or perhaps general age-related or disease related frailty, may preclude safe swallows in older adults. The compensation of slower swallowing may not be enough. For these individuals, *presbyphagia* crosses over into *dysphagia* at which point there is a need for compensatory or rehabilitative intervention to promote safe swallowing.

Neurophysiologic Correlates of Senescent Swallowing

Slowing of performance in fine and gross motor tasks is well documented in elderly persons. The reaction time to sensory stimuli declines with increasing age.[21,22]

Magnetic resonance imaging (MRI) is highly sensitive in detecting periventricular white-matter hyperintensities (PVHs) in the cerebral white-matter tracts. Neuroimaging studies using cranial MRIs in normal adults show a relationship between slower swallowing and increased number and severity of PVHs in the brain This supports the concept that voluntary control of swallowing is mediated by corticobulbar pathways that travel within the periventricular white matter.[23] The occurrence and degree of these PVHs increase with age and may explain, at least in part, the relatively asymptomatic decline in oropharyngeal motor performance observed in older people. Cerebral atrophy, blood flow changes, and other age-related conditions also must be factored into the process underlying presbyphagia.

Peripheral nervous system changes, as well as central changes, are documented with age and may be related to sarcopenia in muscles of the head and neck. Structurally, sarcopenia is associated with reductions in muscle mass and cross-sectional area (CSA), a reduction in the number or size of muscle fibers, and a transformation or selective loss of specific muscle fiber types.[24] There are reports regarding sarcopenia-like changes in muscles of the upper aerodigestive tract.[25-28] However, most of the work performed in the area of sarcopenia has been in the limb musculature and further work is certainly indicated in cranial-innervated muscles.

Muscle disuse, which may be better termed as "reduction" or "alteration,"[29] has been proposed as the cause of muscular atrophy observed in the aged. This hypothesis has intuitive appeal, due to the assumption that elderly people are less active. However, the fact that muscles of speech, swallowing, and respiration undergo changes associated with aging argues against this hypothesis since aged individuals speak, swallow, and breathe frequently within any given day.[30] Further, "disuse" has not been proven as a simple causative factor in animal studies.[29,31,32] Again, it is clear that mechanisms underlying sarcopenia in muscles of the head and neck must be defined to allow the design and implementation of appropriate treatments.

In summary, the differences in swallowing function for elderly and young individuals appear dependent on age-associated changes of both central and peripheral mechanisms. It can be hypothesized that slowed swallowing that remains coordinated and effective, as found in most healthy old people, may not reflect CNS deterioration as much as it represents a compensatory strategy for generating pressure values that may be critical to successful bolus propulsion.

DIFFERENTIAL CONSIDERATIONS FOR DYSPHAGIA AND ASPIRATION

Etiologies

Older adults are at increased risk for developing dysphagia due to a number of age-associated phenomena.[33] Comorbid processes increase the chances for older adults to suffer the adverse consequences of dysphagia such as dehydration, malnutrition, or aspiration pneumonia. By targeting high-risk groups and intervening with acceptable compensatory and rehabilitative approaches, it is hoped that the ultimate burden of dysphagia on the geriatric population will decline.

Age-related Conditions

Age-related difficulties and comorbidities can develop throughout the upper aerodigestive tract and have the potential of influencing the integrity of the swallow. In the horizontal subsystem, the food bolus may be inadequately prepared due to poor or absent dentition (Chapter 8),[34] periodontal disease, ill-fitting dentures, or inappropriate salivation from xerostomia.[35–37] Older adults are much more likely to be taking medications for multiple medical conditions. Many of these agents can influence salivary flow, intestinal peristalsis, cognition or psychomotor status, thereby interfering with normal oropharyngoesophageal function or altering airway protection. Musculoskeletal factors such as weakness of the muscles of mastication, arthritis of the temporomandibular joint or larynx, osteoporosis of the jaw, changes in tongue strength, and discoordination of oropharyngeal events can deter efficient swallowing. Sensory input for taste, temperature, and tactile sensation changes in many older adults.[38–40] This may impair sensorimotor interaction required for proper bolus formation and timely response of the swallowing sequence. All of these factors may detract from the pleasure of eating.

Age-related Disease

Neurological and neuromuscular disorders are principal risks for dysphagia (Table 9–1). Neu-

Table 9–1 Neurologic Disorders Causing Dysphagia

Stroke
Head trauma
Parkinson's disease and other movement and
    neurodegenerative disorders
Progressive supranuclear palsy
    Olivopontocerebellar atrophy
    Huntington's disease
    Wilson's disease
Torticollis
    Tardive dyskinesia
Alzheimer's disease and other dementias
Motor neuron disease (amyotrophic lateral
    sclerosis)
Guillain-Barre syndrome and other
    polyneuropathies
Neoplasms and other structural disorders
    Primary brain tumors
    Intrinsic and extrinsic brainstem tumors
    Base of skull tumors
    Syringobulbia
    Arnold-Chiari malformation
    Neoplastic meningitis
Multiple sclerosis
Post-polio syndrome
Infectious disorders
    Chronic infectious meningitis
    Syphilis and Lyme disease
    Diphtheria
    Botulism
    Viral encephalitis, including rabies
Myasthenia gravis
Myopathy
    Polymyositis, dermatomyositis, inclusion
        body myositis, and sarcoidosis
    Myotonic and oculopharyngeal muscular
        dystrophy
    Hyper- and hypothyroidism
    Cushing's syndrome
Iatrogenic conditions
    Medication side effects
    Postsurgical neurogenic dysphagia
        Neck surgery
        Posterior fossa surgery
        Irradiation of the head and neck

rological diseases rise in prevalence in older cohorts of the population. Conditions of stroke, head injury, Alzheimer's and other dementia syndromes, and Parkinson's disease all place older adults at increased risk for dysphagia with its incipient consequences. For example, cerebrovascular conditions such as stroke increase steadily with advancing age with incidence ranging from 9–12/1000 individuals by age 75. Between 50% and 75% of acute stroke patients develop eating and swallowing problems with ensuing complications of aspiration in 50%, malnutrition in 45%, and pneumonia in 35% of these individuals. Six clinical features are associated with increased risk for aspiration poststroke.[41] These include: (1) abnormal volitional cough; (2) abnormal gag reflex; (3) dysarthria; (4) dysphonia; (5) cough after trial swallow; and (6) voice change after trial swallow. The presence of any two of these findings has a sensitivity of 92% and specificity of 67% that there would be penetration and aspiration of material as evidenced with videofluoroscopy.

A host of common problems within the head and neck can directly damage effector muscles of swallowing and increase the risk for dysphagia. Head and neck injury, carcinoma, complex infections, thyroid conditions, and diabetes are associated with age-related dysphagia. Head and neck cancer surgeries, some spinal cord surgeries, thyroid surgeries, and any intervention that may jeopardize the recurrent laryngeal nerve may incite dysphagia. A number of chemotherapy and radiotherapy regimens can lead to swallowing impairment, but tend to improve with time posttreatment.[42] The prospective outcome of dysphagia should be incorporated into the risk-benefit discussions of these procedures.

SIGNS AND SYMPTOMS OF A SWALLOWING PROBLEM

Present-day dysphagia care varies dependent upon the clinical setting. Yet, while multidisciplinary dysphagia teams frequently are available only in academic or larger hospital settings, the responsibility for screening and treating swallowing problems inevitably rests on a versatile team of health care professionals and care providers in addition to a swallowing specialist. Speech-language pathologists, who are usually the swallowing therapists, are well trained to conduct bedside or "noninstrumental" examinations that include history taking, oral motor assessment, voice and respiratory measures, and assessment of trial swallows. Because swallowing is not something a patient traditionally considers, it may be necessary to ask related questions until a particular word or phrase triggers association in the patient's experience (eg, swallowing, chewing, moving food to the throat, cough, choke). In some cases, the patient is unaware of the presence of dysphagia, such as when a patient is silently aspirating, has cognitive impairments, or is in a medically fragile state. In these cases, clinicians may rely on a team of primary care providers, nursing staff, family members, and friends, among others, to provide information about the patient's mealtime behavior and medical status. Other times, subtle indications of dysphagia might manifest as a recurring exacerbation of an underlying chronic disease such as chronic obstructive pulmonary disease.

Although certain screening measures are convenient for use at a patient's bedside, even experienced clinicians fail to identify aspiration in a large number of bedside evaluations due to the high presence of silent aspiration.[2] Noninstrumental dysphagia screening tools also provide inadequate information about the underlying pathophysiology of the swallow. Therefore, selection of interventions tailored to treat the "root problem" remains elusive. For these reasons, an oropharyngeal videofluoroscopic swallowing evaluation, which is a radiographic imaging technique, is commonly preferred to assess the integrity of the oropharyngeal anatomy, swallowing physiology, and bolus flow. A variety of other imaging methods is available for studying the swallow, including fiberoptic endoscopy, ultrasound, MRI, CT scans, and scintigraphy. Instrumental evaluation provides information about the underlying movement disorder that results in disordered bolus flow in terms of its direction, duration, and clearance, which must be defined and remediated in order to eliminate or minimize the dysphagia. A list of some typical symptoms described by and observed in patients with swallowing problems follows.

Possible Underlying Oropharyngeal Dysfunction

Signs and symptoms of oropharyngeal dysphagia (Table 9–2) have been organized in relation to the horizontal and vertical phases of swallowing described earlier. That is, symptoms that relate to the oral preparatory phase are first, followed by oral transit (ie, moving the bolus horizontally through the oral cavity to the inlet of the pharynx), the pharyngeal swallow and laryngeal components of the swallow, and upper esophageal sphincter relaxation and opening. Thus, by understanding the relationship between overt signs and symptoms and the underlying dysfunction, the clinician can form well-founded hypotheses about the fundamental disorder and implement appropriate interventions.

Signs and Symptoms of Aspiration and Aspiration Pneumonia

Patients with dysphagia are more likely to develop pneumonia than those without dysphagia.[43,44] Among the evidence to substantiate this is the suggestion that individuals with dysphagia who manifest related nutritional deficiencies are at an increased risk for developing pneumonia. Protein-energy malnutrition can impact dysphagia mortality both by increasing the occurrence of pneumonia and by hindering recovery from aspiration pneumonia.[45] Malnourished patients demonstrate a loss of respiratory muscle strength necessary for clearing aspirants.[46] Certain warning signs can indicate the presence of aspiration of food or liquid into the lungs. If a patient demonstrates any of the following changes, it is important to notify the doctor for a referral to a swallowing specialist immediately.

- Coughing
- Wet, gurgly voice
- Temperature spike or low-grade fever for more than 24 hours
- Changes in lung sounds
- Recurrent upper respiratory infections or pneumonia
- Increased secretions
- Weight loss

Table 9–2 Signs and Symptoms of Oropharyngeal Dysphagia

Sign or Symptom	Possible Underlying Disorder
Material spills from the front of mouth	May indicate reduced labial or lingual strength or coordination to form a bolus.
Patient cuts food into smaller pieces	Difficulty manipulating food and/or moving food posteriorly in the oral cavity.
Changes in or loss of taste	Taste can be affected by normal aging, although certain medications, radiation, or even reflux can leave a bitter or metallic taste in one's mouth. May also indicate sensory loss related to an underlying neurological process or event.
Increase in secretions or phlegm	Certain disease processes (ALS, Parkinson's disease) affect the automaticity of swallowing, giving patients the perception that they are producing more saliva when, in fact, they are not managing their saliva adequately. Reflux can also increase phlegm or mucus, and a productive cough with yellow sputum is a serious sign of aspiration pneumonia.

continues

Table 9–2 continued

Sign or Symptom	Possible Underlying Disorder
Patient is biting his tongue	May indicate ipsilateral weakness, loss of sensation, or reduced coordination in the oropharyngeal musculature.
Patient has difficulty initiating a swallow/food is in the mouth but the patient does not swallow	Typical of patients with Parkinson's disease, who demonstrate a repetitive rocking motion of the tongue when attempting to initiate a swallow. Patients with swallowing apraxia also have extreme difficulty with initiation. Patients with dementia can experience food agnosia thereby failing to recognize food that is placed in the mouth and the subsequent need to swallow.
Food sticks in mouth	Food can collect in the buccal cavities, along the hard palate, or on the tongue after swallowing, often indicating lingual weakness. Residue on one side of the oral cavity indicates ipsilateral weakness.
Patient is taking much longer to eat meals	Primarily due to a reduction in the speed of moving the bolus through the mouth.
Food or liquid comes through the patient's nose	Nasal regurgitation is a sign of velopharyngeal incompetence, or reduced palatal strength or coordination during swallowing. A nasal vocal quality or frequent snoring may also indicate weak palatal muscles.
Coughing or choking when eating or drinking	Immediate coughing, especially on liquids, is a sign of aspiration.
Coughing or choking with or without regurgitation of food/ patient describes food sticking high in throat	Weakness of the base of the tongue musculature, resulting in residue in the vallecula or pyriform sinuses.
Coughing or choking with or without regurgitation of food/ patient describes food sticking at the bottom of the throat	A dysfunctional cricopharyngeus and residue in the pyriform sinuses. Also a sign of esophageal stasis and/or reflux causing a "referred sensation."
Patient is using extra sauces or drinking extra fluids with meals to "wash food down"	Residue in the oropharynx or the esophagus due to a weakness, obstruction, coordination or motility issue.
Patient is avoiding certain foods	Meat and bread tend to be difficult to swallow because of the dry or sticky consistency and increased resistance to flow. Patients may avoid particular foods, such as rice, nuts, or popcorn, which lack cohesiveness and can be aspirated easily.
Patient is leaving food on the plate	A sign of discomfort when eating or drinking due to one of the above. Reduced appetite might signal early satiety due to esophageal stasis or reflux.
Weight loss	Sudden or gradual unexplained weight loss can be a sign of a swallowing disorder related to any of the above etiologies.

Possible Underlying Esophageal Disorder

Patients with oropharyngeal dysphagia may exhibit a concomitant esophageal disorder. On the other hand, patients with an underlying esophageal disorder may experience oropharyngeal symptoms as a result of the closely interrelated nature of the system. In either case, it is advantageous to evaluate both the oropharyngeal and esophageal aspects of the swallow to provide optimal diagnostic and treatment services, and identify an increased risk for aspiration of refluxed contents, which can flow retrograde from the stomach or esophagus into the laryngeal vestibule or trachea. Signs and symptoms of oropharyngoesophageal dysphagia are organized in Table 9–3, with the underlying neurophysiological correlates of the esophagus being best described in other chapters.

Pill Dysphagia

Older patients frequently report difficulty swallowing pills as the first sign of a swallowing problem. The use of multiple medications in old

---

Table 9–3 Signs and Symptoms of Oropharyngoesophageal Dysphagia

Sign or Symptom	Possible Underlying Disorder
Hoarse voice	Irritated or damaged vocal cords and surrounding tissues. It is critical to distinguish vocal hoarseness from a wet, gurgly voice that is a sign of aspiration.
Sore throat	Irritated or damaged pharyngeal, laryngeal, and esophageal tissues.
Frequent belching	May signify that the patient is using a very effortful swallow when eating or drinking, and therefore is pumping extra air into the esophagus, most likely as an adaptive compensatory strategy to overcome a weakness or obstruction.
Coughing or throat clearing, especially after meals or when lying down	The flow of material through the esophagus to the stomach is facilitated by an upright position, which utilizes the pull of gravity. Therefore, symptoms can increase when reclining after a meal or when sleeping in a horizontal position.
Bitter taste in the mouth, especially in the morning	Reflux can flow retrograde into the oropharynx, causing a bitter taste in the mouth. Sometimes referred to as a "globus sensation," patients may sense something is sticking in the throat when in fact an underlying esophageal disorder is present.
Feeling of something sticking in the chest	Residue in the esophagus.
Difficulty swallowing bread, meat, or pills or avoidance of these items	A dry, glutinous bolus does not flow as well as items with more moisture. Decreased esophageal motility and xerostomia can decrease the flow of certain foods (eg, meat, bread) or pills through the system.
Consuming extra fluids to "wash food down" during meals	A compensatory strategy in response to a sensation of something sticking in the throat or esophagus.
Regurgitation or vomiting	Residue in the esophagus or gastroesophageal reflux may be flowing retrograde into the oropharynx.
Heartburn	Many patients with reflux do not experience heartburn or might take an antacid medication to suppress heartburn, but continue to experience additional symptoms listed above.

age is inevitable as the incidence of certain medical conditions increases with age. More than 2000 drugs can cause xerostomia or reduced salivary flow via anticholinergic mechanisms. Swallowing pills presents a challenge to an older swallowing system that lacks the necessary reserve to generate speed and strength for optimal performance under more demanding conditions. Patients with reduced lingual strength may demonstrate poor manipulation of a tablet in the oral cavity or reduced pressure generation for propelling a pill through the oropharynx and cervical esophagus. A number of psychotropic drugs can further influence the tongue and bulbar musculature by delaying neuromuscular responses or inducing extrapyramidal effects. A dysfunctional cricopharyngeus, poor esophageal peristalsis, or an esophageal stricture are all additional sources of pill dysphagia, and certain agents can directly relax the lower esophageal sphincter and increase acid reflux. Recommendations for patients who have difficulty swallowing pills include:

- Moisten the system by taking several sips of liquid before taking medication.
- Place pills as far back on the tongue as possible to minimize the work of transferring the bolus to the back of the mouth.
- Take pills with a spoonful of applesauce, yogurt, or pudding to form a more cohesive bolus.
- Consider crushing large pills. Some pills, such as time-release medications, cannot be crushed without altering the properties of the drug so it is important to consult with a pharmacist first.
- Some medications are available in liquid form. Although slightly more expensive, they can be quite convenient and palatable.

TREAMENT OF SWALLOWING DISORDERS

A Multidisciplinary Approach to Treatment

Multidisciplinary health care teams play an important role in the care of complex older adults with dysphagia.[47,48] This cross-disciplinary focus helps to address not only the medical, but also functional and psychosocial consequences of this problem. The team approach offers the stated advantage of a more efficient comprehensive assessment with shared responsibility for interventions. Although team care has been demonstrated to control costs of at-risk older adults in managed organizations, similar studies relating to dysphagia care have not, to date, been conducted. Formal teams exist across a spectrum of settings and include a wide variety of health care services to meet the multiple needs of dysphagia patients. The prevention of aspiration pneumonia requires the input of primary care providers and geriatricians, pulmonologists, nursing staff responsible for patient feeding as well as oral care and hygiene, dietitians, and swallowing specialists or speech-language pathologists. Treatment of dysphagia also depends upon treatment of the primary disease process, thus requiring a team that is tailored to meet individual needs. For instance, otolaryngologists and oncologists are critical members of a treatment team for patients with head and neck cancer. On the other hand, although dysphagia can be associated with an explicit medical disorder, it is not uncommon for individuals with no isolated disease process to demonstrate dysphagia in response to the interplay of multiple age-related changes in nutrition, muscle composition, and immunity. In this case, a geriatrician would be an influential team member.

Dysphagia teams aim to restore or maximize functional swallowing and nutritional intake. The frail patient will most always be at risk for nutritional deficits, and this risk is significantly increased in dysphagic patients. Therefore, it is critical that the swallowing therapist, dietitian, and feeding staff work together to identify a well-balanced selection of food and liquid that can be swallowed safely. Ideally, patients are reassessed by a swallowing specialist on a regular basis, and diets are upgraded as warranted, often in response to an improvement in the patient's medical status and associated improvements in functional swallowing and nutrition. Dietitians in an acute care or nursing home setting monitor caloric intake, weight, hydration, and other nutritional parameters that document critical outcomes to support the decision to safely progress patients to oral feeding or to upgrade to a new dietary level.

TREATMENT APPROACHES

Treatment for dysphagia usually is either rehabilitative or compensatory in nature. Rehabilitative interventions have the capacity to directly improve the dysphagia at the biologic level. That is, aspects of anatomical structures or neural circuitry are the targets of therapy that may have direct influence on physiology, biomechanics, and bolus flow. On the other hand, compensatory interventions avoid or reduce the effects of the impaired structures or neuropathology and resultant disordered physiology and biomechanics on bolus flow. Dysphagia clinicians and researchers have historically felt most comfortable with physiological outcomes (movement parameters such as range of motion) and the effect on the bolus flow outcomes as an indicator of success of intervention. Attitudes are changing as reflected by increased reference to quality of life in the literature[49,50] and the development of instruments to quantify dysphagia-specific quality of life. The SWAL-QOL[4-6] was created to fill a void in dysphagia care, including understanding how variations in treatment affect the human experience of living with swallowing difficulty. Data addressing patient perceptions on social dining, food selection, and burden help document the effectiveness of any given treatment on QOL. Examples of common dysphagia interventions follow.

Compensatory Dysphagia Interventions

Postural Techniques

Once the underlying anatomical or physiological swallowing disorder is identified, the clinician may try various postural adjustments to change the positioning of the structures and redirect bolus flow to approximate a normal swallow or minimize the dysphagia. Postural adjustments easily are attempted during the instrumental evaluation to directly observe the effects of specific maneuvers on bolus flow outcomes. The clinician

using radiography to assess swallowing must identify online those postures that will correct the underlying movement disorder revealed during the evaluation. Repositioning the patient's head or body can effectively eliminate aspiration of liquids in 75–80% of all dysphagic patients.[51-54] For example, a simple chin tuck posture enhances airway protection by repositioning the hyolaryngeal complex and narrowing the laryngeal entrance while directing the bolus away from the airway. On the other hand, turning the head to the affected side can redirect the flow of the bolus toward the more functional side of the oropharynx in patients who demonstrate unilateral deficits secondary to neurological diseases or head and neck cancer. These techniques are easy to use and applicable for patients with various etiologies, although their usefulness may be limited for patients with cognitive deficits, receptive aphasia, or reduced range of motion in the head and neck.

Behavioral Swallowing Maneuvers

Swallowing maneuvers are compensatory strategies applied by the patient to voluntarily control specific events of the swallow. Some maneuvers are designed to increase airway protection by conscious adduction of the vocal folds,[55] while another prolongs laryngeal elevation to increase the upper esophageal opening.[56] Swallowing with extra effort,[57] performing multiple swallows per bolus, or alternating sips of liquid with solid boluses may also compensate for a weakness in the oropharyngeal mechanism by facilitating bolus clearance. These strategies can be combined with postural techniques for added airway protection, performed alone during swallows of food or liquid, or performed with dry saliva swallows to practice the timing of specific movements and strengthen the mechanism prior to attempting oral intake. As a patient recovers normal swallowing ability, such maneuvers can be gradually discontinued, although some patients may need to apply these techniques long-term. Although each maneuver requires the ability to follow specific multistep instructions, and is therefore inappropriate for patients with limited cognitive performance, most patients will find that after some practice the behavior becomes habitual.

Increasing Sensory Awareness

Older adults can benefit from increased oral sensory input for a number of reasons. For example, age-related reductions in taste, smell, tactile sensitivity, and perception of viscosity can decrease the speed and enjoyment of swallowing and eating in old age.[39] It is hypothesized that sensory enhancement in the oral and pharyngeal areas facilitates a normal swallow by increasing input to the central nervous system.[58] Some therapeutic procedures are designed to provide a preliminary stimulus to prepare the oropharyngeal swallowing mechanism for bolus reception. For instance, a cold spoon can be applied with downward pressure to the tongue or the patient may be instructed to perform a sucking motion prior to swallowing. A program of sensory therapy known as thermal-tactile stimulation involves brushing the anterior faucial pillars in the back of the patient's throat with a cold laryngeal mirror immediately before presenting a bolus.[59] Thermal-tactile stimulation can be performed several times a day to rehabilitate proper timing of the swallow. In addition, sour boluses have been shown to improve the initiation of the pharyngeal swallow[60] and carbonation seems to facilitate swallowing in certain individuals.[61] Patients with oral apraxia, tactile agnosia, or a decreased sense of taste due to aging or radiation therapy may all benefit from changes to the properties of foods and liquids. Much work remains to be done in the area of sensory awareness and swallowing and development possibilities are great. For instance, the value of various taste qualities (eg, tart, metallic), sensations (eg, burning of hot peppers, pungency of horseradish), or concentrations to swallowing outcomes remain largely unexplored.

Environmental Modifications

In contrast to the "fast-food society" in which we live, older individuals (especially those with dysphagia) take longer to eat. Eating an adequate amount of food becomes a challenge, not only because of the increased time necessary to do so, but fatigue frequently becomes an issue. To promote a safe and efficient swallow in most individuals with swallowing and chewing difficulty, the following recommendations are useful:

- Eat slowly and allow enough time for a meal.
- Do not eat or drink when rushed or tired.
- Take small amounts of food or liquid in the mouth; a teaspoon, not a tablespoon.
- Concentrate on swallowing; eliminate distractions like television.
- Avoid mixing food and liquid in the same mouthful.
- Place the food on the stronger side if there is unilateral weakness.
- Add condiments, such as mayonnaise, mustard, butter, or jelly to dry sandwiches and bread.
- Use packaged gravy and sauce mixes to flavor and moisten meats or vegetables.
- Try adding tart sauces and condiments to foods to enhance taste; for example, use orange juice, lemon juice, pickles, seasoned vinegars, balsamic vinegar, and other seasonings as a sauce or marinade for certain foods.

Adaptive Equipment

Eating and drinking aids can assist in placing, directing, or controlling the bolus of food or liquid and maintaining proper head posture while eating. For example, modified cups with cut-out rims (placed over the bridge of the nose) or straws will prevent a backward head tilt when drinking to the bottom of the cup. A backward head tilt, which results in neck extension, should be avoided in most cases because it misdirects food and liquid toward the airway. However, for a postglossectomy patient with known intact airway protection, a posterior head tilt can facilitate bolus propulsion. Spoons with narrow, shallow bowls or glossectomy spoons (a spoon developed for moving food to the back of the tongue) are useful to individuals who require assistance in placing food in certain locations in the mouth. More importantly, these utensils and devices promote independence in eating and drinking.

Whereas a speech-language pathologist can make suggestions regarding appropriate aids to optimize swallowing safety and satisfaction, the occupational therapist is an expert in the area of adaptive equipment and can obtain commercially available products.

Dietary Modifications

Besides enhancing the oral sensory properties of foods, some patients may require a change in the consistency of foods and liquids to prevent aspiration and make swallowing easier. Withholding thin liquids such as water, tea, or coffee, which are most easily aspirated by older adults, and restricting liquid intake to thickened liquids is almost routine in nursing homes. Increasing the viscosity of liquids decreases the rate of flow, allowing patients more time to initiate airway protection and prevent or decrease aspiration. Despite the huge impact these seemingly unappealing practices may have on quality of life, they are commonly implemented in the absence of efficacy data presumably to minimize thin liquid aspiration and avoid the long-term related outcome of pneumonia. Additional diet modifications include recommending soft foods. For example, patients with lingual weakness or limited upper esophageal opening will find it easiest to swallow foods that are very moist, soft, or finely chewed. Adding sauces or gravies to minimize dry particalization, which may easily be misdirected into the airway, is a common recommendation. Since evidence is lacking to support the long-term effectiveness of diet modification on health outcomes, and given the impact on quality of life, patients who are placed on a modified diet should be reassessed on a regular basis. Eliminated items should be reintroduced when the patient demonstrates an improvement in swallowing function.

Unfortunately, no universal standards for dysphagia dietary textures or viscosities exist. Dietary departments in different facilities often create novel lists of foods and liquids representing a continuum of consistency. In fact, a survey of 71 dietitians in 27 states revealed that 40 different names were used to label solid food textures, while 18 different names were used to describe liquid viscosities.[62] Liquids can be thickened using commercial dry starch-based thickeners by following the mixing instructions available on the canister. However, preparation and delivery issues such as the thickener brand, type of base liquid, and thickening time can greatly affect the viscosity of the final product.[63] Some commercially available prethickened products have been introduced in an attempt to solve this dilemma. However, these items are costly, not standardized, have questionable stability over time, and therefore are less practical for both large acute care and long-term care facilities and for community-dwelling adults.

Efforts have been made to standardize the diagnosis and nutritional management of dysphagic patients. The development of barium contrast materials of standard viscosities,[64] including a semisolid pudding-like material (6000 cP), honey-thick liquid (3000 cP), nectar-thick liquid (300 cP), and thin liquid (<15 cP) (EZ-EM Inc., Westbury, NY) have advanced the standardization of videofluorscopic swallowing evaluation. Standardized diagnostic materials ultimately will direct dietary recommendations, thereby allowing for the creation of specific recipes for foods and liquids that match the viscosities of those materials objectively determined to affect bolus flow outcomes of direction, duration, and clearance.

A group of speech-language pathologists, dietitians, a food scientist, and members of the food industry have also joined forces to create the National Dysphagia Diet Task Force (NDDTF).[65] The goal of the NDDTF is to define standardized dietary levels for dysphagic patients, develop common terminology and viscosity standards for thickened liquids, and guide professionals in selecting the diet that best fits patients' diagnostic profile. Although much work still remains, the NDDTF has identified three levels describing solid food textures based upon five properties of food texture (cohesiveness, adhesiveness, tensile, shear, and fracture) (Table 9–4). Separate viscosity ranges for thickened liquids were defined using the nomenclature "thin," "nectar-thick," "honey-like," and "spoon-thick" (Table 9–5). Although

Table 9–4 National Dysphagia Diets

Dietary Level	Description	Rationale	Example Food Items
Level 1: Dysphagia Pureed	Consists of pureed, homogenous, and cohesive foods. Foods should be "pudding-like" with no coarse textures or raw fruits or vegetables. Excludes foods requiring bolus formation, manipulation, or mastication.	Designed for individuals with poor oral control or reduced airway protection.	Cooked farina-type cereals, pudding, yogurt, pureed fruits and vegetables, mashed potatoes with gravy, pureed meats or soufflés.
Level 2: Dysphagia Mechanically Altered Characteristics	Consists of foods that are moist, soft-textured, and easily formed into a bolus. Meats ground to less than one-quarter inch pieces.	Transition between pureed textures to more solid textures. Requires chewing.	Cooked cereal with texture (oatmeal), canned fruit or soft banana, moistened ground meat with gravy or sauce, casseroles without rice, eggs, tofu, baked potato if moist, all soft-cooked vegetables. Some items with mixed textures may be tolerated but should be assessed individually.
Level 3: Dysphagia Advanced	Consists of foods of regular textures except hard, sticky, and crunchy foods. Foods are moist and in bite-size pieces.	Transition to a regular diet. Requires adequate mastication.	Well-moistened breads and cereals, peeled fruits, tender meats, all cooked vegetables and shredded lettuce, rice. Some items with mixed textures may be tolerated but should be assessed individually.

Source: Bulow M, Olsson R, Ekberg O.[61]

the National Dysphagia Diet has not been adopted nationwide, it has created the basis for discussion to control the properties of foods and liquids served to dysphagic patients and ideally could be aligned with diagnostic standardized materials (EZ-EM Inc., Westbury, NY) for meaningful implementation.

Elderly individuals living in the community may also find it easier to eat soft, moist foods whether or not swallowing is determined to be unsafe.

Table 9–5 National Dysphagia Diet Viscosity Borders and Ranges for Thickened Liquids

Thickness Level	Viscosity Range (Centipoise)	Example Liquids
Thin	1–50 cP	Water, apple juice
Nectar-like	51–350 cP	Buttermilk, cold tomato juice
Honey-like	351–1750 cP	
Spoon-thick	>1750 cP	Drinkable yogurt, thick milkshake

For reference: water is 1 cP at 70 degrees Fahrenheit

Note: All measurements are at a shear rate of 50 s-1 and 25 degrees Celsius.

Source: Bulow M, Olsson R, Ekberg O.[61]

Changes in dentition, food preferences, or appetite can all affect the older person's dietary habits in addition to swallowing challenges. Following a diet similar to those mentioned above may make mealtimes easier and more enjoyable for older individuals. There are a number of home cooking and preparation techniques that can be used to alter the properties of difficult-to-chew foods.

Surgical Procedures

Although compensatory and rehabilitative strategies can facilitate normal swallowing, some patients presenting with structural or functional impairments are best managed surgically. For instance, patients with esophageal strictures, a cricopharyngeal prominence, or a large diverticulum may immediately resume normal swallowing function once the structure is repaired. Other times, both swallowing techniques and surgery are combined to provide the best outcomes. For instance, a patient with a limited upper esophageal sphincter opening may undergo dilation to decrease resistance at the distal end of the pharynx and also perform lingual exercises to increase bolus propulsion at the proximal end. All team members should carefully consider the risks and benefits of surgical intervention for elderly patients because these individuals may experience greater complications given their increased age.

Rehabilitative Dysphagia Interventions

Active Exercise

The treatment approaches mentioned thus far are compensatory in nature and do not directly change the function of the swallowing mechanism. Rehabilitative exercises are naturally more active and rigorous. Often, a rehabilitative approach to dysphagia intervention is withheld from the elderly population because such demanding activity is assumed to deplete any limited remaining swallowing reserve, thus potentially exacerbating dysphagia symptomatology. Interestingly, a body of literature has emerged during the past decade that suggests that loss of muscle strength with age is, to a great extent, reversible through rehabilitative exercise. Although this work has shown progressive resistance training to be safe and effective for the limb musculature in older adults,[66,67] it has only begun to be systematically applied to the muscles of swallowing.[68] Recent research on the benefits of lingual resistance exercise suggests that strength-building exercises for the tongue increase lingual muscle strength and mass and improve the timing of the swallowing components in healthy older adults. This implies greater gains and carryover into swallowing-related outcomes in elderly dysphagic patients.[19,20]

Nutritional Support

Elderly patients are often in need of added nutritional or caloric support because of natural age-associated declines in weight, muscle mass, and strength. Depletions in nutritional stores have been cited in up to 50% of older adults living independently,[69] suggesting that elderly people are at risk for demonstrating clinical signs of malnutrition if they encounter increased physiological stress due to a chronic illness or event. Swallowing and eating difficulties heighten the challenge faced by older adults to maintain adequate nutrition and hydration, especially if the dysphagia results from a neurological insult or catabolic illness. At the same time, malnutrition can affect the swallowing musculature and exacerbate dysphagia.[70] This relationship between dysphagia and malnutrition is documented in a study of consecutive hospital admissions with a primary diagnosis of dysphagia over a 1-year period.[71] In this study, 100% of the patients were malnourished, and more than 80% of these patients exhibited clinical signs of severe weight loss and abnormal anthropometrical measures characteristic of dysphagia-induced starvation.

Oral supplements and calorie-dense foods are often recommended for dysphagic patients who are attempting to maintain weight. However, patients in a catabolic state due to stroke or trauma may require nonoral feedings to boost calories and nutrients and to temporarily prevent aspiration during the recovery period. Neurological dysphagia is one of the most common reasons for gastrostomy tube placement.[72–75] Enteral or parenteral feedings are also chosen for longer-term nutritive supplementation or permanent replacement in patients whose disease process results in confirmed or suspected swallowing-related aspiration or malnutrition and dehydration,[76] or those with a progressive disease state or terminal illness.

It is important to note that tube feedings can be recommended as a supplementary means of intake while the patient maintains some degree of oral intake. For instance, patients with neuromuscular diseases characterized by fatigue, or those with restricted diets, may be unable to take in adequate amounts of calories or nutrients during a meal. Nonetheless, these patients may be able to swallow safely with compensatory strategies such that withholding food and liquid would greatly affect quality of life and raise ethical questions. Since eating and drinking have such strong social, cultural, and emotional ties, all attempts are made to optimize oral intake to the highest degree as long as the patient is willing and able.

In other cases, restoring the nutritional status in elderly dysphagic individuals with short-term enteral or parenteral support may increase their prognosis for swallowing rehabilitation. That is, increasing the patient's nutritional reserve may enhance overall physical strength and endurance, including that of the deglutitive musculature, and translate into a better response to therapy.[70]

Feeding tubes are commonly viewed as a safe and cost-effective alternative means of providing nutrition and hydration. In spite of this, there is little conclusive evidence to support the effectiveness of either nasogastric or gastrostomy tubes in preventing aspiration or aspiration pneumonia. Aspiration pneumonia is the most serious complication of feeding tube placement.[72] An 11-month study of 69 patients with nasogastric tubes, 15 of whom were later referred for a gastrostomy tube and 1 patient who received a percutaneous endoscopic gastrostomy tube, found a death rate of 40% due to aspiration and other underlying diseases.[77] Another study of 109 nursing home patients found that 22.9% of gastrostomy tube-fed patients aspirated and a history of previous respiratory infections was present in 40.7% of those who developed aspiration pneumonia.[78] These statistics pose the question of whether or not tube feedings are truly a safer route of intake, especially in older adults.

Based on evidence reported, the decision to undergo feeding tube placement has many ethical considerations that are best approached by a team of care providers with the patient and the family at the forefront. Advance directives or living wills that outline a patient's wishes regarding tube feedings are becoming more prevalent, although many critical questions regarding decision making for patients who are demented or in a vegetative state remain unanswered. Swallowing specialists, dietitians, nursing staff, physicians, social workers, and religious leaders all can participate in the decision to initiate or withdraw tube feedings. Nonetheless, it is ultimately the patient, and the family in certain cases, who determines the plan of action. Therefore, a swallowing specialist can present the information that the patient is at risk for aspirating all consistencies taken orally, warranting enteral or parenteral feedings as an alternative means of obtaining nutrition. Despite this information, if the patient decides to continue to swallow food or liquid for taste experiences and quality-of-life purposes, these wishes must be respected. Although Rabenek et al.[79] wrote, "No explicit guidelines for percutaneous endoscopic gastrostomy (PEG) tube placement are available to guide clinical decision-making. In the absence of such guidelines, the decision to place a PEG tube focuses mainly on the patient's ability to take food by mouth," it would clearly be narrow and short-sighted to make decisions with such impact merely on the basis of empirical swallowing abilities. For an issue that may be a critical source of a patient's sense of autonomy, self-respect, dignity, and quality of life,[80] ability to swallow is merely one factor in the decision-making formula that is yet to be determined (Chapter 19).

CONCLUSION

In summary, although oropharyngeal dysphagia may be life threatening, so are the alternatives, particularly for the elderly population as indicated by the evidence available. Therefore, contributions by all team members are valuable in this challenging decision-making process, with the patient's family or care provider's point of view perhaps the most critical contribution. Furthermore, tube feeding should not solely be viewed as a long-term feeding replacement, but rather the role of feeding tubes as a temporary supplement serving a rehabilitative role should be equally emphasized. Until additional data on the safety and efficacy of tube feeding is collected, the many behavioral, dietary, and environmental modifications described in this chapter are compassionate and preferred alternatives to the always present option of tube feeding.

REFERENCES

1. ECRI Report. *Diagnosis and Treatment of Swallowing Disorders (Dysphagia) in Acute-Care Stroke Patients.* Evidence Report/Technology Assessment No. 8 (Prepared by ECRI Evidence-Based Practice Center under Contract No. 290-97-0020) AHCPR Publication no. 99-E024 Rockville, MD: Agency for Health Care Policy and Research; 1999.

2. Logemann J. *Evaluation and Treatment of Swallowing Disorders.* San Diego, CA: College-Hill Press; 1983.

3. Robbins JA. Old swallowing and dysphagia: Thoughts on intervention and prevention. *Nutr Clin Prac* 1999;14: S21–S26.

4. McHorney CA, Bricker DE, Kramer AE, et al. The SWAL-QOL outcomes tool for oropharyngeal dysphagia in adults: I. Conceptual foundation and item development. *Dysphagia* 2000;15:115–121.

5. McHorney CA, Bricker DE, Robbins JA, Kramer AE, Rosenbek JC, Chignell KA. The SWAL-QOL outcomes tool for oropharyngeal dysphagia in adults: II. Item reduction and preliminary scaling. *Dysphagia* 2000;15: 122–133.

6. McHorney CA, Robbins JA, Lomax K, et al. The SWAL-QOL outcomes tool for oropharyngeal dysphagia in adults: III. Extensive evidence of reliability and validity. *Dysphagia* 2002;17:97–114.

7. Kennedy J, Kent RD. Anatomy and physiology of deglutition and related functions. In: Logemann J, ed. *Seminars in Speech and Language: The relationship between speech and swallowing.* New York, NY: Thieme-Stratton; 1985: 1–12.

8. Kahrilas PJ, Lin S, Chen J, Logemann JA. Oropharyngeal accommodation to swallow volume. *Gastroenterology* 1996;111:297–306.

9. Dodds WJ. The physiology of swallowing. *Dysphagia* 1989;3:171–178.

10. Kier WM, Smith KK. Tongues, tentacles and trunks: the biomechanics of movement in muscular-hydrostats. *Zool J Linn Soc* 1985;83:307–324.

11. McConnel FMS. Analysis of pressure generation and bolus transit during pharyngeal swallowing. *Laryngoscope* 1988;87:71–78.

12. Doty RW, Bosma JF. An electromyographic analysis of reflex deglutition. *J Neurophysiol* 1956;19:44–60.

13. Logemann J, Kahrilas PJ, Cheng J, et al. Closure mechanisms of the laryngeal vestibule during swallow. *Am J Physiol* 1992;262:B338–B344.

14. Tracy F, Logemann JA, Kahrilas PJ, Jacob P, Kobara M, Krugla C. Preliminary observations on the effects of age on oropharyngeal deglutition. *Dysphagia* 1989;4:90–94.

15. Robbins JA, Hamilton JW, Lof GL, Kempster G. Oropharyngeal swallowing in normal adults of different ages. *Gastroenterology* 1992;103:823–829.

16. Shaw DW, Cook IJ, Dent J, et al. Age influences oropharyngeal and upper esophageal sphincter function during swallowing. *Gastroenterology* 1990;98:A390.

17. Shaw DW, Cook IJ, Gabb M, et al. Influence of normal aging on oropharyngeal and upper esophageal sphincter function during swallow. *Am J Physiol* 1995;L68: G389–G390.

18. Robbins JA, Coyle J, Rosenbek J, et al. Differentiation of normal and abnormal airway protection during swal-

lowing using Penetration Aspiration scale. *Dysphagia* 1999;14:228–232.

19. Robbins J, Levine R, Wood J, Roecker E, Luschei E. Age effects on lingual pressure generation as a risk factor for dysphagia. *J Gerontol Med Sci* 1995;50: M257–M262.

20. Nicosia MA, Hind JA, Roecker EB, Carnes M, Robbins JA. Age effects on the temporal evolution of isometric and swallowing pressure. *J Gerontol Med Sci* 2000; 55A:M634–M640.

21. Birren IE, Woods AM, Williams MV. Speed of behavior as an indicator of age changes and the integrity of the nervous system. In: *Brain Function in Old Age*. Berlin: Springer-Verlag; 1979:10–44.

22. Welford AT. Between bodily changes and performances: some possible reasons for slowing with age. *Exp Aging Res* 1984;10:73–88.

23. Levine R, Robbins JA, Maser A. Periventricular white matter changes and oropharyngeal swallowing in normal individuals. *Dysphagia* 1992;7:142–147.

24. Evans WJ. What is sarcopenia? *J Gerontol* 1995;50A: 5–8.

25. Price PA, Darvell BS. Force and mobility in the aging human tongue. *Med J Aust* 1982;1·75–78.

26. Rastatter MP, Maguire A, Bushong L, et al. Speech motor equivalence in aging subjects. *Percept Mot Skills* 1987;64:635–638.

27. Newton JP, Abel RW, Robertson EM, et al. Changes in human masseter and medial pterygoid muscles with age: a study by computed tomography. *Gerondontics* 1987;3: 151 154.

28. Dayan D, Abrahami I, Buchner A, et al. Lipid pigment (lipofuscin) in human perioral muscles with aging. *Exp Gerontol* 1988;23:97–102.

29. Cartee GD. What insights into age-related changes in skeletal muscle are provided by animal models? *J Gerontol* 1995;50A:137–141.

30. Prakash YS, Sieck GC. Age-related remodeling of neuromuscular junctions on type-identified diaphragm fibers. *Muscle Nerve* 1998;21:887–895.

31. Faulkner JA, Brooks SV, Zerba E. Muscle atrophy and weakness with aging: contraction-induced injury as an underlying mechanism. *J Gerontol* 1995;50A:124–129.

32. Brown M, Hasser EM. Differential effects of reduced muscle use (hindlimb unweighting) on skeletal muscle with aging. *Aging (Milano)* 1996;8:99–105.

33. Sonies BC, Stone M, Shawler T. Speech and swallowing in the elderly. *Gerontology* 1984;3:115–123.

34. Slagter AP, Lambertus OW, Bosman F, et al. Masticatory ability, denture quality, and oral conditions in edentulous subjects. *J Prosthet Dent* 1992;68:299–307.

35. Ship JA, Duffy V, Jones JA, et al. Geriatric oral health and its impact on eating. *JAGS* 1996;44:456–464.

36. Rhodus NL, Brown J. The association of xerostomia and inadequate intake in older adults. *Research* 1990;90: 1688–1692.

37. Slagter AP, Olthoff LW, Steen WHA, et al. Communication of food by complete-denture wearers. *J Dent Res* 1992;71:380–386.

38. Fucci D, Petrosini L, Robey R. Auditory masking effects on lingual vibrotactile thresholds as a function of age. *Percept Mot Skills* 1982;54:943–950.

39. Shiffman SS. Perception of taste and smell in elderly persons. *Crit Rev Food Sci Nutr* 1993;33:17–26.

40. Kenshalo DR. Somesthetic sensitivity in young and elderly humans. *J Gerontol* 1986;41:732–742.

41. Daniels SK, Brailey K, Priestly D, et al. Aspiration in patients with acute stroke. *Arch Phys Med Rehabil* 1998; 79:14–19.

42. Eisbruch A, Lyden T, Bradford CR, et al. Objective assessment of swallowing dysfunction and aspiration after radiation concurrent with chemotherapy for head-and-neck cancer. *Int J Radiat Oncol Biol Phys* 2002; 53:23–28.

43. Holas MA, DePippo KL, Reding MJ. Aspiration and relative risk of medical complications following stroke. *Arch Neurol* 1994;51:1051–1053.

44. Marik PE, Kaplan D. Aspiration pneumonia and dysphagia in the elderly. *Chest* 2003;124:328–336.

45. Veldee MS, Peth LD. Can protein-calorie malnutrition cause dysphagia? *Dysphagia* 1992;7:86–101.

46. Aora NS, Rochester DF. Respiratory muscle strength and maximal voluntary ventilation in undernourished patients. *Am Rev Respir Dis* 1982;126:5–8.

47. Robbins J, Priefer B, Gunter-Hunt G, et al. A team approach to ethical management of an elderly patient with dysphagia. In: Sonies BC, ed. *Dysphagia—A Continuum of Care*. Gaithersburg, MD: Aspen; 1997:41–54.

48. Barczi SR, Sullivan P, Robbins J. How should dysphagia care of the older adult differ? Establishing optimal practice patterns. *Semin Speech Lang* 2000;21:347–361.

49. Ellwood PM. Outcomes management: a technology of patient experience. *N Engl J Med* 1988;318:1549–1556.

50. Batalden PB, Nelson EC, Roberts JS. Linking outcomes measurement to continual improvement: the serial "V" way of thinking about improving clinical care. *J Qual Improve* 1994;20:167–180.

51. Horner J, Massey EW, Riski JE, et al. Aspiration following stroke: clinical correlates and outcome. *Neurology* 1988;38:1359–1362.

52. Shanahan TK, Logemann JA, Rademaker AW, Pauloski BR, Kahrilas PJ. Chin-down posture effect on aspiration in dysphagic patients. *Arch Phys Med Rehabil* 1993;74: 736–739.

53. Welch MV, Logemann JA, Rademaker AW, et al. Changes in pharyngeal dimensions effected by chin tuck. *Arch Phys Med Rehabil* 1993;74:178–181.

54. Logemann J, Kahrilas P, Kobara M, et al. The benefit of head rotation on pharyngoesophageal dysphagia. *Arch Phys Med Rehabil* 1989;70:767–771.

55. Martin BJW, Logemann JA, Shaker R, et al. Normal laryngeal valving patterns during three breath-hold maneuvers: a pilot investigation. *Dysphagia* 1993;8(1): 11–20.

56. Jacob P, Kahrilas P, Logemann JA, Shah V, Ha T. Upper esophageal sphincter opening and modulation during swallowing. *Gastroenterology* 1989;97:469–478.

57. Hind JA, Nicosia M, Roecker E, et al. Comparison of effortful and noneffortful swallows in healthy middle aged and older adults. *Arch Phys Med Rehabil* 2001;82: 1661–1665.

58. Fujiu M, Toleikis JR, Logemann J, et al. Glossopharyngeal evoked potentials in normal subjects following mechanical stimulation of the anterior faucial pillar. *Electroencephal Clin Neur* 1994;92:183–195.

59. Lazzara G, Lazarus C, Logemann J. Impact of thermal stimulation on the triggering of the swallowing reflex. *Dysphagia* 1986;1:73–77.

60. Logemann JA, Pauloski BR, Colangelo L, et al. The effects of a sour bolus on oropharyngeal swallowing measures in patients with neurogenic dysphagia. *J Speech Hear Res* 1995;38:556–563.

61. Bulow M, Olsson R, Ekberg O. Videoradiographic analysis of how carbonated thin liquids and thickened liquids affect the physiology of swallowing in subjects with aspiration on thin liquids. *Acta Radiol* 2003;44: 366–372.

62. Giel L, Ryker A. Is there a need for standardization of a dysphagic diet? American Dietetic Association Annual Meeting and Exhibition Poster Presentation; 1996.

63. Mills RH. Increasing the precision of the videofluoroscopic swallowing examination. *Evaluation of Dysphagia in Adults: Expanding the Diagnostic Options.* Austin, TX: PRO-ED; 2000:103–144.

64. Robbins J. Wisconsin Alumni Research Foundation. Standardized compositions which facilitate swallowing in dysphagic subjects. U.S. Patent 6,461,589; 2002.

65. National Dysphagia Diet Task Force. National dysphagia diet: standardization for optimal care. *J Amer Dietet Assoc* 2000;100:1–47.

66. Fiatarone MA, O'Neill EF, Ryan ND, et al. Exercise training and nutritional supplementation for physical frailty in very elderly people. *N Engl J Med* 1994;330: 1769–1775.

67. Fiatarone MA, Marks EC, et al. High intensity strength training in nonagenarians. Effects on skeletal muscle. *JAMA* 1990;263:3029–3034.

68. Robbins J, Gangnon R, Theis S, Kays S, Hewitt A, Hind J. The effects of lingual exercise on swallowing in older adults. *JAGS* 2005;53(9):1483–1489.

69. Goodwin J, Goodwin J, Garry P. Association between nutritional status and cognitive functioning in healthy adult populations. *JAMA* 1983;249:2917–2921.

70. Hudson HM, Daubert CR, Mills RH. The interdependency of protein-energy malnutrition, aging and dysphagia. *Dysphagia* 2000;15:31–38.

71. Sitzmann JV. Nutritional support of the dysphagic patient: methods, risks, and complications of therapy. *JPEN* 1988;14:60–63.

72. Tealey AR. Percutaneous endoscopic gastrostomy in the elderly. *Gastroenterology Nursing* 1994;151–157.

73. Llaneza P, Menedez A, Robert R, et al. Percutaneous endoscopic gastrostomy: clinical experience and follow-up. *Southern Medical Journal* 1988;81:321–324.

74. Mamel J. PEG. *Am J Gastroenterol* 1989;84:703–710.

75. Moran B, Frost R. PEG in 41 patients: indications and clinical outcomes. *J Royal Soc Medicine* 1992;85: 320–321.

76. Feinberg MJ, Knebl J, Tully J. Prandial aspiration in an elderly population followed over 3 years. *Dysphagia* 1996;11:104–109.

77. Ciocan J, Silverstone F, Graver L, et al. Tube-feedings in elderly patients. *Arch Intern Med* 1988;148:429–433.

78. Cogen R, Weinryb J. Aspiration pneumonia in nursing home patients fed via gastrostomy tubes. *Am J Gastroenterol* 1989;84:1509–1512.

79. Rabeneck L, McCullough LB, Wray NP. Ethically justified, clinically comprehensive guidelines for percutaneous endoscopic gastronomy tube placement. *Lancet* 1997;349:496–498.

80. Watts DT, Cassell CK. Extraordinary nutritional support: a case study and ethical analysis. *JAGS* 1984;32: 237–242.

CHAPTER 10

The Aging Gut

David N. Moskovitz, MD, John Saltzman, MD
and Young-In Kim, MD, FRCP(C)

Life expectancy has increased dramatically over the past 10–15 years, and the population of individuals over age 65 years is expected to more than double by the year 2050. The projected rise in the number of Americans over the age of 85 years is expected to increase from 4 to 18 million over a similar period of time. As life span increases, individuals will acquire chronic and debilitating diseases such as osteoarthritis, Parkinson's disease, and other neurological conditions. These conditions are all associated with gastrointestinal (GI) complications, particularly those related to the esophagus and swallowing. Thus, age-related changes in GI functioning can be categorized in terms of those associated with these comorbid conditions of aging or those associated with the aging process itself.

Little work has been done to describe the GI changes associated with aging, largely due to the invasive nature of the procedures required. There is a dearth of normative data on which to base clinical comparisons. For example, very little work has been done to describe normal colonic functioning, and only a few studies have been published that describe normative parameters of esophageal peristalsis and lower esophageal sphincter functioning. Similar limitations apply to gastric and small bowel functioning. Studies that have been done commonly reveal conflicting results due to differences in the technology used (i.e., manometric vs. radiographic).

This chapter provides a practical view of the impact of aging on normal gastrointestinal func-

tion and suggests the implications of common chronic conditions and altered nutritional requirements brought about by these changes. The challenge in caring for older adults includes understanding changes in nutritional needs with aging and providing adequate nutrition. This chapter describes some of the complex interrelationships involved in the care and feeding of older people.

AGING AND THE GASTROINTESTINAL SYSTEM

Little is known about the morphologic and functional changes of the gastrointestinal system with aging. Available information is mostly derived from studies involving institutionalized subjects. Because of technical limitations associated with the clinical evaluation of gastrointestinal function to differentiate wellness and disease, it is difficult to measure smaller changes of function in a general population. Tests designed to diagnose disease may not be sensitive enough for the study of normal aging, whereas others may be too sensitive and have no clinical or nutritional significance. Contrary to several other organ systems, many variables affect optimal function of the gastrointestinal tract. Furthermore, the heterogeneity of the older population in response to aging, disease, and medications makes the evaluations difficult.

Overall, there is little change in gastrointestinal function due to aging in the absence of disease because of the large reserve capacity of this multi-organ system. The functional reserve of the gastrointestinal system is greatest in the mid-gut, pancreas, and liver. Intestinal segments may adapt, and functional reserves tend to buffer change so that only long-term observations may uncover abnormalities. This is less true for the proximal and distal portions of the gut. Esophageal and gastric disorders usually lead to symptoms associated with eating, whereas colon problems cause difficulties with evacuation. Common gastrointestinal symptoms are often nonspecific and do not indicate the exact nature or severity of disease. Clinical skills are necessary to diagnose these disorders, prognosticate, and prescribe treatment.

Genetics and Aging

Recent data support a role for a genetic component in aging. The nature of the genetic component likely involves several mechanisms. The most obvious is a change in gene expression during aging, which results in the production of altered levels and/or forms of relevant regulatory proteins. Age-associated changes in the integrity of DNA itself have been implicated by studies of mitochondria and telomeres. Changes in DNA are likely the culmination of a complex process involving oxidative damage causing mutations in genes, shortening telomeres, and injury to mitochondrial DNA.

Accumulation of random mutations in genomic DNA could contribute to the gradual decline in cellular function observed in a variety of tissues.[1] Telomeres are the physical ends of chromosomes. In mammals, telomeres are composed of tandem repeats of (TTAGGG) and appear to stabilize the structure of chromosomes. DNA replication machinery is unable to completely replicate the ends of linear chromosomes that result in shortening of the telomere with each round of DNA synthesis. Terminal repeats can be polymerized onto the ends of the chromosomes by the ribonucleoprotein telomerase. This enzyme, therefore, plays an important role in replicating cells to maintain telomere length and chromosome integrity. Telomere shortening, caused by

oxidative damage or a problem with end replication, might result in the accumulation of postmitotic cells during aging. This process could impact a number of physiologically important events, such as tissue repair after injury.

Age-dependent accumulation of mutations in mitochondrial DNA may also contribute to the loss of cells in postmitotic tissues, such as muscle or neurons.[2] Accumulation of damage in DNA suggests that there is an imbalance between two opposing processes: the generation of mutations and the removal of these mutations by DNA repair mechanisms. The frequency of mitochondrial DNA damage is very low, calling into question the significance of its role in aging. Nevertheless, the accumulation of abnormal mitochondrial DNA could result in impaired cell function and activation of apoptosis. Presumably, this would be of particular significance in postmitotic tissues, such as muscle and neurons.

Apoptosis and Aging

A number of studies suggest that there is an association between apoptosis (cell self-destruction) and aging. It remains unclear whether age-associated apoptosis is physiological, pathophysiological, or perhaps both, depending on the circumstances. If the apoptosis cascade functions normally throughout an individual's life, then age-associated increases in apoptosis may reflect an appropriate response to the presence of increased numbers of damaged cells that need to be removed from the body. Thus, apoptosis may have a beneficial effect to remove senescent cells. This process could, however, contribute to the decline of function by removal of nonregenerating postmitotic cells. In organs with regenerating cell populations, the increased presence of apoptosis could have a deleterious effect if the ratio of apoptosis to cell replacement shifts significantly in the direction of apoptosis.

Effect of Aging on Peripheral Nerve Function

There is a substantial amount of literature concerning the effect of aging on the peripheral nervous system (PNS).[3] Anatomic changes include loss of myelinated and unmyelinated nerve fibers, demyelination, remyelination, and myelin balloon figures. Generalized functional and electrophysiological changes with age include declining nerve conduction velocity, sensory discrimination, autonomic responses, and endoneurial blood flow. These age-related changes are often not linearly progressive with age and are observed most commonly in advanced senescence.

ESOPHAGUS

Swallowing functions of the oropharynx and esophagus involve the transport of food from mouth to stomach, while preventing nasal reflux, tracheal aspiration, and gastroesophageal reflux. Impaired swallowing is common in older individuals, but available evidence indicates that this is due more to the effects of associated diseases than to the intrinsic effects of aging *per se.* Dysphagia (food sticking with swallowing) and eating dependence can have a profound impact on nutrition. Common disorders result in malnutrition because of oropharyngeal and esophageal dysphagia. Gastroesophageal reflux frequently is symptomatic and also can lead to dysphagia. Symptoms of esophageal dysfunction in older people may be difficult to recognize because they are often atypical and vague and may not suggest an esophageal problem. Shaker et al[4] have recognized that in older adults, the size of the bolus needs to be bigger and that older persons may handle liquids less well than they handle soft foods (such as pudding).

Incidence and Character of Feeding/Swallowing Disorders

The incidence of eating disabilities in older nursing home residents may reach 50%.[5] In such patients, findings of dysphagia are often accompanied by a higher incidence of pneumonia caused by gram-negative microorganisms.[6,7] In a study of nursing home patients, Siebens and colleagues[5] evaluated eating dependence, defined

as an impairment of the five components of eating, including behavioral and cognitive ability to recognize food and eat it, normal upper extremity function, oral phase of swallowing, pharyngeal phase of swallowing, and esophageal phase of swallowing. Dependent patients who required physical assistance with eating made up 32% of the nursing home population. Only 25% ate regular diets, and they demonstrated a higher prevalence of abnormal oral-stage swallowing behavior, including spitting, choking, inability to chew, drooling, nasal regurgitation, squirreling food (retaining food in the buccal pouch), delayed swallowing, and overstuffing of the mouth. Signs of abnormal pharyngeal swallowing included coughing during meals or while drinking, choking during meals, and speaking in a wet-sounding voice. A large portion of the dependent eaters could not be tested for gag reflex or voice quality because they would not or could not follow instructions. Mortality rates were higher in the dependent eaters. These findings, paired with the results of nursing care in these patients, which were not correlated with weight loss during a 3-month period, suggest that simple bedside observations are effective in identifying this basic clinical problem.

Symptoms of dysphagia may occur in diverse older populations in the presence of a cerebrovascular accident (CVA), head and neck surgery, and progressive neurologic disease. Warning signs include a confused mental state that may interfere with the complex sensory and motor functions of eating; dysarthric speech due to weakness or poor control of muscles common to both speech and swallowing; excessive drooling, which can follow neuromuscular impairment of these same mechanisms; coughing and choking on food or sputum; excessive time to consume a meal; unexplained weight loss; difficulty in chewing; pain with swallowing; or lodgment of food. In spite of these correlates, it is important to recognize the extensive differential diagnoses for pharyngeal and esophageal dysphagias, some of which represent reversible, treatable lesions (Table 10–1).

Table 10–1 Causes of Dysphagia

Oropharyngeal
  Cerebrovascular accident
  Neoplasia
  Zenker's diverticulum
  Cricopharyngeal bar
  Parkinsonism
  Neuromuscular disorders
  Local structural lesions
  Thyroid disorders

Esophageal
  Stricture
  Spasm/motility disturbance
  Neoplasia
  Esophagitis
  Rings and webs
  Medication induced

Oropharyngeal Physiology

There are three phases to swallowing: oral, pharyngeal, and esophageal. Together, the first two take less than 2 seconds; the third takes 3 to 7 seconds. The first two phases involve oropharyngeal transfer. The oral phase begins with the lips closed and the tip of the tongue contacting the upper mouth structure. The tongue is then elevated while a slight elevation of the larynx occurs, resulting in a progressive stripping of the bolus against the hard palate and the tongue into the pharynx. This first phase of swallowing is under voluntary control.

The pharyngeal phase is the most complex neuromuscular aspect of swallowing. The bolus is projected into the esophagus while the airway is protected. When pharyngeal sensation is intact, the medullary swallowing center controls cranial nerve motor impulses, which close the velopharyngeal valve, elevate the larynx, and relax the upper esophageal sphincter. As the bolus passes the upper esophageal sphincter, the vocal cords close, and the base of the tongue is forced against the posterior pharyngeal wall. At the conclusion of the pharyngeal phase of swallowing, there is forceful contraction of the pharyngeal constrictors, followed by descent of the larynx and contraction of the upper esophageal sphincter (see Chapter 9).

Assessment of Oropharyngeal Function

Oropharyngeal function is assessed by history and observation. Careful observation of the patient's eating will make the magnitude of the problems clear. Subsequent clinical studies may include direct inspection of the pharyngeal and esophageal anatomy, an X-ray observation of its function by barium, or a cookie swallow with video scintigraphy. Occasionally, esophageal motility studies are necessary for an accurate clinical diagnosis, which permits a proper prescription for diet and eating behavior.

Oropharyngeal Dysphagia

The symptoms of oropharyngeal dysphagia include reflux of fluid out through the nose, persistent cough, a wet hoarseness, overt choking, and a persistent sense of the need to clear the throat. Clinical signs include progressive wasting, dehydration, and recurrent bronchitis. Oropharyngeal dysphagia occurs in older subjects because of underlying neurologic disease, muscle weakness, or atrophy. Even older asymptomatic adults have demonstrated abnormal swallowing due to poor tone of the pharynx, inadequate opening of the cricopharyngeal sphincter, pooling of barium in the adjacent laryngeal folds, and aspiration into the trachea. Typically, liquids are handled less well than soft foods.

The commonly held belief that patients can localize accurately the source of dysphagia is not supported by the medical literature. Patients often point to the neck when dysphagia is caused by distal esophageal disease, so this symptom cannot be used to identify pharyngeal dysphagia. However, if a patient points to the epigastric area, the distal esophagus is usually the location of the stricture. Although coughing and choking can indicate either oral or pharyngeal abnormality, the majority of such patients do not cough. Likewise, although coughing during swallowing usually indicates laryngeal penetration, some patients do not cough even though this occurs.

Dysphagia for solid foods is strongly suggestive of anatomic narrowing. Barium swallow studies may be inadequate because of incomplete distention of all segments. Barium X-rays should be done with the use of a barium pill to detect significant narrowed areas. A lower esophageal ring is the most commonly missed cause of dysphagia for solid foods. Progressive dysphagia to solids eventually results in dysphagia to both solids and liquids due to an anatomic narrowing.

Mixed dysphagia for liquids and solids can occur in patients with pharyngeal dysphagia due to neurologic injury, as well as esophageal motility disorders. Since oropharyngeal dysphagic patients have more difficulty with thin liquids and also have greater airway penetration, dysphagia for water can be a differential feature.

Regurgitation of undigested food may be of either pharyngeal or esophageal origin. Late regurgitation can be caused by Zenker's diverticulum or achalasia of the esophagus. Chest pain and heartburn are not reliable in differentiating pharyngeal and esophageal dysphagia. Drooling and other evidence of oropharyngeal dysfunction are not necessarily accompanied by clinical evidence of more extensive neuromuscular disease. As many as 50% of neurogenic dysphagic patients have no associated abnormalities on screening physical examination, and in many patients no definite neurologic diagnosis can be established at the initial examination.

Combined functional and anatomic abnormalities are common. As many as one-third of patients may have multifactorial dysphagia with coincidental abnormalities in both the pharynx and the esophagus.[8] These observations support an integrated and thorough assessment of dysphagic symptoms to include the pharyngeal and esophageal mechanisms.

Treatment

After CVA it is difficult to predict rehabilitative potential for swallowing despite the considerable evidence to permit prognostication of behavioral patterns for the extremities and for bulbar and higher cortical functions. In a prospective study, Robbins[9] evaluated patients with isolated left and right CVAs and brainstem CVAs by neurologic examination, computed tomography, video fluoroscopy, selected manometry, and magnetic resonance imaging. All patients demonstrated delayed response of the pharyngeal phase and increased penetration of food. Patients with cortical stroke had increased oral-stage durations for liquid and semisolid foods. Patients with unilateral left and right cortical stroke and those with brainstem CVA had the most difficulty with the oral stage of swallowing and lack of coordination of the lips, mandible, and tongue. The right unilateral CVA patients had increased penetration of the vocal folds by food and an increased risk of aspiration, according to video fluoroscopy and history. This aspiration occurred during the delay of the pharyngeal stage of swallowing. Patients with brainstem CVA had relatively normal oral phases, but the most frequent occurrence of aspiration was due to poor airway protection during swallowing and large pharyngeal residuals after swallowing. Manometric studies demonstrated incomplete relaxation of the upper esophageal sphincter as well as delay with respect to pharyngeal contraction.

The different oropharyngeal patterns provide important information for treatment planning, but the general observations, as noted by Siebens and associates,[5] are also important for the selection of appropriate treatment measures. Because patients with left unilateral cortical CVA often demonstrate findings of verbal and oral apraxia, they are not able to swallow on command. This interferes with interpretation of the swallowing study. When these patients were placed in a more natural eating situation, their oral-stage durations were more equivalent to normal, and they used postural changes spontaneously to facilitate swallowing. Only 1 of 20 patients required nonoral feeding techniques because of dysphagia.

Patients with right unilateral CVA did not attempt compensation spontaneously for their difficulty in swallowing, even though aspiration was commonly observed. Defense of the airway was not very forceful, and over one-third of these subjects required nonvolitional feeding.

The group with brainstem CVA demonstrated forceful reflux attempts at coughing, but most required nonvolitional feeding techniques. These observations effectively prognosticate the outcome of therapeutic maneuvers and the need for nonvolitional nutritional support (Table 10–2). Robbins[9] describes three therapeutic categories: compensatory, rehabilitative, and medical. These treatment categories are based on the thorough clinical evaluation described above.

Compensatory therapy involves the introduction of external factors or new combinations of behavior to substitute for defects. These include postural adjustment, supraglottic swallow, food placement, and diet modification. Choices are available in a complex range and are best implemented with speech therapy consultation. They are most effective in the left unilateral CVA group.

Dietary modifications in combination with posturing are frequently used in the treatment of the stroke patients. Liquids initially are eliminated from the diet because of the likelihood of aspiration during the delayed pharyngeal stage. Occasionally food requiring chewing may need to be eliminated. Tilting the head forward at a 45° angle can facilitate vallecular maintenance of material until the pharyngeal contraction stage is initiated. The size of the bolus must be limited to 2 mL. Patients who cannot carry out instructions often require nonvolitional feeding techniques.

A unique postural compensation was beneficial to the brainstem group. Most of the pooling of the food appeared at the level of the piriform sinuses unilaterally, so that turning the head toward the impaired side facilitated the flow of material through the upper esophageal sphincter, reduced residual material, and reduced or eliminated aspiration.

Rehabilitation therapy involves the retraining of a disordered movement or behavior by repetitive practice. Patients selected for rehabilitative therapy often receive nonvolitional nutritional support because food is not introduced in the treatment regimen until significant progress has been demonstrated. These treatment programs involve oromotor exercises, vocal fold reduction exercises, and thermal sensitization. Several medical/surgical and prosthetic treatments available for the treatment of dysphagia, including intracordal injection, cricopharyngeal myotomy, and palatal reshaping prosthesis, did not prove successful in the study by Robbins.[9] The work done at the Johns Hopkins Swallowing Center demonstrates the necessity of careful clinical and specialized assessment of neurologic deficits and speech pathology combined with nutritional assessment and therapeutic maneuvers.

Esophageal Dysphagia

Swallowing disorders occur in 16–22% of those over the age of 50 and up to 60% of nursing home residents.[10–12] Dysphagia with aspira-

Table 10–2 Swallowing Disorders after CVA

CVA Type	Signs and Symptoms	Aspiration	Need for Enteral Nutrition
Left CVA	Verbal and oral apraxia, spontaneous compensation with swallowing	Present	1/20 of patients
Right CVA	No spontaneous compensation with swallowing	Common	1/3 of patients
Brainstem	Normal oral phase	Most frequent	Almost all patients

tion accounts for a 45% 12-month mortality in nursing home residents.[13] Comorbid illnesses and medications also contribute to altered nutritional intake through changes in salivary flow, absorption, utilization, and excretion of nutrients. Dysphagia is a common complaint, especially among older adults. Oropharyngeal dysphagia clearly increases in the adult population and has been noted to occur in 50% of nursing home residents, resulting in a high frequency of aspiration pneumonia.[14] Oropharyngeal dysphagia can result directly from subtle changes in upper esophageal sphincter (UES) functioning associated with aging, but more commonly this symptom is associated with alterations in pharyngeal and UES functioning associated with neuromuscular disorders or central nervous system diseases such as stroke, Parkinson's disease, or multiple sclerosis. Zenker's diverticulum and cervical osteophytes are conditions that uniquely produce oropharyngeal symptoms in older adults. The UES functions as a primary barrier to the aspiration of refluxed gastric contents and is composed primarily of the cricopharyngeus muscle, which is a skeletal muscle, producing a relatively high pressure in this area (60–80 mmHg). Because it is a skeletal muscle, events associated with swallowing are very rapid and difficult to measure with most conventional manometric techniques. As a result, the most accurate means of assessing pharyngeal and UES functioning is via video swallowing studies, not conventional manometry. With the use of both video and manometric techniques, some subtle changes in oropharyngeal functioning have been described in older adults.

Manometric studies must be used to detect pressure, and there are two studies that document that UES pressure is significantly diminished in older adults. A study by Fulp and colleagues[15] shows a correlation of .54 between age and UES pressure in an age range from 24 to 79 years. Shaker et al[16] did not find any alteration in pharyngeal or UES functioning in older adults. On the other hand, the study by Fulp and colleagues[15] also described a somewhat delayed UES relaxation relative to the pharyngeal peak in older adults. In one study, Aviv et al[17] have shown that, as the aging process continues, sensory discrimination in the oral cavity progressively diminishes, consistent with complaints of dysphagia and aspiration. They have demonstrated diminution in pharyngeal and supraglottic sensitivity in older adults, suggesting a contributing factor to the development of dysphagia and aspiration in this population.

Esophageal dysphagia, as opposed to oral pharyngeal dysphagia, in older adults has been commonly attributed to what is referred to as "presbyesophagus"; that is, disorders that are due to endogenous changes in esophageal function with aging. With the advent of more sophisticated technology to measure the parameters of esophageal peristalsis (i.e., amplitude, duration, and transit time), the mythology associated with the existence of presbyesophagus has largely disappeared. Recent studies indicate that the frequency of abnormal esophageal motility is no greater in older adult populations, with the possible exception of individuals over 70 years of age. In this age group, there are data to indicate that there may be a decrease in the amplitude of esophageal contractions and "defective" peristalsis. It appears that cells of the enteric nervous system diminish with age, and this could explain the diminished strength of peristaltic contractions noted in studies of esophageal motility in older adults.

Dysphagia is a common complaint in any age group, but it is estimated to occur in up to 10% of individuals over 50 years of age.[18] In general, there are no data that would indicate that dysphagia is, in and of itself, a complaint associated with aging alone. Primary esophageal motility disorders associated with clinical complaints of dysphagia would include achalasia, diffuse esophageal spasm, "nutcracker" esophagus, and other nonspecific esophageal motor disorders, which would include primarily ineffective peristalsis (peristaltic amplitudes <40 mmHg). Although achalasia is usually encountered in patients between the ages of 20 and 40 years, a secondary peak appears to occur in older adults.[19]

The most common cause of esophageal disorders in older adults is medication-induced esophageal injury. The most common of these are tetracycline, quinidine, alendronate, NSAIDs, and potassium chloride. Diagnosis is by barium swallow and/or endoscopy. Barium swallow can identify esophageal lesions and provides information about the possible existence of extrinsic esophageal compression. Subsequent endoscopy can confirm the diagnosis. Lesions may vary from some erythema to an ulcer or definite stricture.

Methodology has a substantial impact on results of previous studies. For example, radiographic and manometric studies do not always agree, and manometric studies using outdated infusion technology would not produce results that more recent studies would be capable of determining. For example, radiographic studies have shown abnormalities in older adults with regard to esophageal functioning and have identified the retrograde "escape" of barium more commonly in older adults. In a study by Kahrilas and colleagues,[2] this escape phenomenon was generally associated with peristaltic amplitudes <40 mmHg, which can only be determined via manometry. In one of the few studies conducted in which a within-group assessment was accomplished, Kruse-Anderson and colleagues[21] studied a group of individuals over a median interval of time of 8 years with regard to their esophageal functioning. No differences were noted in the LES pressure or acid-clearing parameters. In a study by Adamek and colleagues,[22] distinguished by the fact that it used modern solid-state technology and ambulatory monitoring conditions, no significant differences were noted in esophageal function in younger vs. older adult populations.

In summary, data with regard to the intrinsic changes in esophageal function with aging are conflicting. There are subtle alterations in esophageal function, namely diminished peristaltic amplitude and deficiencies in the ability to generate secondary peristaltic contractions. Some sensory deficits have been noted in oropharyngeal functioning, and decreased UES pressure has also been documented. Aging is associated with a variety of comorbid conditions that clearly affect esophageal functioning that cannot and should not be ignored by the perspicacious clinician.

Gastroesophageal reflux (GERD) is a common problem and may be more common in older people because of underlying disease and their frequent use of medications that may contribute to it. Gastroesophageal reflux is more common in the upright position and after meals, but it is probably more serious when it occurs in the recumbent position and during sleep. Factors that contribute to its cause include delayed gastric emptying, incompetence of the lower esophageal sphincter, failure of the esophagus to generate waves of peristalsis to clear refluxed material, and the injurious nature of the gastric contents. It is unclear whether age-associated changes may contribute to the frequency of this disorder, but common diseases of older adults and commonly used medications are known to affect this esophageal dysfunction.

Gastroesophageal reflux may produce no symptoms, even while causing severe injury to the esophagus, but commonly patients experience pyrosis or heartburn. Regurgitation may occur with heartburn or independently, with changes in posture, after meals, or at other times. When injury to the esophagus is severe, patients may experience esophageal dysphagia due to esophagitis, or stricture formation. Painful swallowing may accompany dysphagia in some patients. It is increasingly recognized that gastroesophageal reflux may result in pharyngeal reflux or tracheal aspiration and may cause the laryngeal and pulmonary symptoms of change in voice, chronic cough, asthma, and recurrent pulmonary infections. Inflammation of the esophagus may also cause iron-deficiency anemia resulting from occult blood loss from the inflamed mucosa.

Although there are data to suggest that heartburn is a more common symptom in older adults, studies that have investigated heartburn prevalence as a function of age have not noted an increased incidence in older adults. In a population survey by Raiha and colleagues,[23] reflux symptoms in general were not noted to be more prevalent with age, but their subjects ranged from 65 to 85 years of age. There was not a younger control group. Other studies have addressed this issue and have not shown significant differences in reflux or esophageal acid defense mechanisms in the older group. A study that used modern technology in a group that would be considered older was performed by Smout and colleagues,[24] in which they addressed the percentage of time the pH was <4 in a group of individuals ranging in age from 45 to 73 years (mean 61 years). They noted a strong relationship between advancing age and esophageal acid contact time.

The prevalence of hiatal hernia does increase with age, but there are few studies to document this.[19] It is now accepted that the main dysfunction associated with the LES as it relates to reflux is the occurrence of the transient LES relaxation. No studies document the occurrence of transient LES relaxation responses in older adults, although at least one study did not document any difference in resting LES pressure.[25]

In summary, then, it would appear that in adults older than 50 years old, there is an increased incidence in reflux and esophageal acid contact time. This is very likely due to a combination of increased incidence of hiatal hernia, diminished peristaltic amplitudes, and reduced salivary response to esophageal acid contact.

For patients presenting with new onset of GERD, the approach is similar in the elderly and younger patient. A more aggressive approach to the evaluation and management of mild GERD symptoms in the elderly patient is warranted because of the increased prevalence of complicated reflux disease. The presence of warning symptoms such as dysphagia, odynophagia, weight loss, or bleeding suggests the presence of complicated GERD or neoplasia and should prompt the physician to aggressively evaluate the patient, rather than considering empiric therapy. The treatment goal for GERD in the elderly patient is the same as in younger individuals. The goals are to treat the symptoms, heal the esophagitis, manage any complications, and maintain remission.

Antacids may be effective for symptomatic control of heartburn, but they should be used with caution in the elderly patient because of the potential for developing diarrhea, constipation, hypercalcemia, and hypermagnesemia. H$_2$-receptor

antagonists and proton pump inhibitors are the primary treatment modalities used in the elderly patient. Prokinetic agents (currently metoclopramide) should be used with caution in the elderly patient because of their increased side effect profile. Proton pump inhibitors are currently the most effective agents in controlling esophageal acid exposure in GERD.[26] No dosing adjustments are needed for proton pump inhibitors due to age-related reductions in hepatic or renal function.

A decision regarding medical vs. surgical therapy for GERD often focuses on the need for long-term therapy to treat a chronic disease. This obviously has different ramifications for those over the age of 65 years. Nevertheless, laparoscopic surgery is rapidly evolving, and anti-reflux surgery may actually be equal or superior to the traditional approach.[27] Age alone should not be the limiting factor in choice of surgical therapy for GERD because elderly patients fare well with laparoscopic anti-reflux surgery.[28] Surgery may be considered appropriate in the otherwise healthy elderly patient.

Nutrient requirements probably do not change with gastroesophageal reflux, except in the case of iron-deficiency anemia and the metabolic stress brought on by recurrent pulmonary infections. However, dietary modifications are considered an important element of the treatment protocol, which includes postural measures, drug restriction, antacids, motility agents, histamine 2 (H$_2$) blockers, and proton pump inhibitors. Fat, chocolate, peppermint, and alcohol decrease lower esophageal sphincter pressure; coffee, both caffeinated and decaffeinated, stimulates gastric acid secretion; alcohol and fruit drinks irritate the mucosa, probably because of their osmotic effect; and large meals, probably by their volume, delay gastric emptying. Avoiding meals before retiring and elevating the head of the bed with blocks may be the two most important measures to take to prevent complications of gastroesophageal reflux disease. A low-fat, high-carbohydrate diet with smaller meals is desirable. Drugs that contribute to delayed gastric emptying or that increase gastroesophageal reflux are nicotine, anticholinergics, calcium-channel blockers, theophylline, diazepam, and β-adrenergic blocker agonists. Antacids used in the treatment of this condition will increase the dietary load of divalent cations and help to alleviate symptomatic constipation.

The above comments about oropharyngeal dysphagia, esophageal dysphagia, and gastroesophageal reflux disease are especially relevant to the nutritionist participating in the care of older patients in acute care hospitals and long-term care facilities, as well as those treated with tube feedings. For older patients with esophageal dysphagia, one must seek a clinical diagnosis, rather than attributing symptoms to old age.[29] For most of these patients, specific treatment for the underlying condition is central to the goal of adequate nutrition through dietary management or nutritional support techniques.

STOMACH

Changes in gastric morphology and function occur with age, but these changes do not seem to be separate and distinct from those of acquired disease. Gastric secretion does not decrease solely due to advanced age, as thought in the early 1900s.[30] Older adults who have low acid and pepsin secretion have associated atrophic gastritis. Chronic atrophic gastritis occurs in 11% to 50% of older persons in various studies, depending on the population, diagnostic tests, and definition of atrophic gastritis.[8,31] Although there are several different classification systems for chronic gastritis, the system by Strickland and Mackay[32] has been most widely used due to its clinical utility and simplicity. Type A gastritis involves the body and fundus of the stomach and is associated with autoimmune findings, including parietal cell antibodies and autoimmune conditions of other organs (Table 10–3). Type A atrophic gastritis may also be associated with an autosomal dominant inheritance pattern and is relatively uncommon in the United States. It is found in less than 5% of persons over the age of 60.[32] Type B gastritis predominantly affects the antrum of the stomach without autoimmune associations and is the most common type seen in older persons.[33] Krasinski et al.[34] showed that in an urban Boston population the prevalence of atrophic gastritis among 60- to 69-year-old people was 24%, among 70- to 79-year-old people was 32%, and among people age 80 years and older was 37%.

The etiologic factor most strongly associated with the development of type B chronic atrophic gastritis is *Helicobacter pylori*,[35] an organism strongly associated with peptic ulcer disease. Initial infection with *Helicobacter pylori* causes a mild, superficial gastritis that affects both the antrum and body of the stomach. The superficial gastritis progresses with time to a chronic inflammatory gastritis of the antrum and/or the body of the stomach. Eventually the progression of gastritis may lead to atrophic gastritis with loss of gastric glands, a condition in which regression with a return of normal gastric epithelium is unusual. Vitamin B_{12} deficiency is commonly associated with atrophic gastritis type A[19] due to decreased intrinsic factor and acid production.

Table 10–3 Differential Features of Atrophic Gastritis

Characteristics	Type A	Type B
Site	Body Fundus	Antrum body (patchy)
Etiology	Autoimmune	*Helicobacter pylori*
Inheritance	Autosomal	Unknown
Antibodies	Parietal cell Intrinsic factor	Unusual
Prevalence	Rare	Common

However, vitamin B_{12} deficiency is much less frequent in type B atrophic gastritis because intrinsic factor production is relatively well preserved and because there is some gastric acid production except in the most extreme cases of gastric atrophy.

Lack or absence of gastric acid due to atrophic gastritis may lead to adverse clinical consequences. One of the major defenses to limit the growth of bacteria in the upper intestines is gastric acid. When gastric acid production is diminished or lost, the bacterial overgrowth syndrome, with symptoms of abdominal discomfort, nausea, diarrhea, and weight loss with malabsorption, may occur. However, this is relatively unusual unless there are other altered host defenses because the bacteria that colonize the upper gastrointestinal tract solely due to lack of gastric acid are usually not anaerobic, bile salt-splitting organisms. The lack of gastric acid may also lead to altered nutrient absorption for those nutrients that have a pH-dependent uptake mechanism. This will be further discussed in the section "Small Intestine," subsection "Micronutrient Absorption."

Although the incidence of peptic ulcer disease is declining for the population at large, evidence suggests that the incidence of gastric ulcer has increased among older adults.[36] The incidence of ulcer perforation is also increasing.[37] Ulcer disease is more often complicated in older patients, possibly because of malnutrition and concurrent illness.[38] Antacids are frequently used by older individuals for dyspeptic symptoms. Chronic or high-dose antacid therapy is associated with multiple side effects, including constipation, obstruction, and osteomalacia with use of aluminum antacids; diarrhea, dehydration, and electrolyte disturbances with use of magnesium antacids; and hypercalcemia, kidney stones, and acid rebound with use of calcium antacids.[39–41]

Nonsteroidal anti-inflammatory drugs (NSAIDs) play a major role in the pathophysiology and complications of gastroduodenal disease in older patients. They are the most commonly prescribed medications for patients older than age 65 years.[42,43] A substantial number of patients experience pain, burning, indigestion, nausea, and vomiting while taking these drugs.[44] A variety of mucosal injuries occur with ingestion of NSAIDs, including mucosal hemorrhages, erosions, and acute or chronic ulcers.[44] NSAIDs have also been associated with increased risk of gastrointestinal bleeding.[45]

Gastric emptying of solids by the antrum and of liquids by the fundus is elegantly controlled by gastroduodenal regulatory mechanisms responsive to the composition of ingested foods, duodenal contents, and multiple external influences.[46] Liquid emptying of the stomach, which is vagally mediated, is slowed. Solid emptying, which is antrally determined, seems to be preserved with aging.[47] In older adults, the gastric emptying of mixed meals is somewhat delayed. A study demonstrated in 25 older adults that the gastric emptying time (T1,2) of a mixed meal was 136 ± 13 minutes compared to 81 ± 4 minutes in younger controls.[48] However, the changes in gastric emptying may be confounded by the presence of atrophic gastritis because delayed emptying may be attributable to underlying atrophic gastritis.[49] Accelerated early gastric emptying of liquids with normal late phases of gastric emptying has been noted.[49] Gastric emptying of a fatty meal may be delayed. However, it is unlikely that these alterations are clinically significant. It has been reported that gastric emptying of liquids or a mixed meal is delayed in elderly patients.[50] Some have suggested that this may be limited to the liquid phase only. Fich et al.[51] have observed that age did not alter fasting and postprandial antral motility, which is believed to play an important role in the emptying of solid food. Conversely, fundic activity may be affected by age, which may account for a disturbance in liquid emptying.[51]

Dyspepsia

The major organic causes of dyspepsia in the elderly patient are gastroduodenal ulcer, atypical GERD, and gastric cancer.[52,53] Up to 60% of patients with dyspepsia have no definite organic explanation and are classified as having functional dyspepsia.[54] Functional gastrointestinal disorders are defined as a "variable combination of chronic or recurrent gastrointestinal symptoms not explained by structural or biochemical abnormalities."[54] These symptoms, when related to upper abdominal discomfort, are called nonulcer or functional dyspepsia. Because of the high prevalence of organic disease, functional disorders can be particularly difficult to diagnose in the elderly patient. It is also difficult to differentiate symptoms due to comorbidities or medication side effects from symptoms of the functional disorder itself.

Epidemiologic studies have shown a high prevalence of symptoms associated with functional gastrointestinal disorders in the elderly patient. In a random sample of 328 noninstitutionalized elderly residents, aged 66–93 years, of Olmsted County, Minnesota, the age and sex adjusted prevalence (per 100 persons) of frequent abdominal pain (>6 episodes in the previous year) was reported at 24.3%.[55] In contrast to other gastrointestinal disorders, the symptoms of functional gastrointestinal disorders may fluctuate over time. A Danish cohort study showed a 50% decline in reporting of functional dyspepsia symptoms 5 years after the initial study revealed similar prevalence figures to those of Olmsted County.[56–58] These same studies revealed that functional dyspepsia and irritable bowel syndrome significantly reduced functional capacity at baseline and 5 years later. Although most investigators have reported a reduction in irritable bowel syndrome in the elderly, Locke et al. reported an annual increase in these symptoms with aging in women, with an annual incidence rate of 180 per 100,000 population in those aged 20–34 years to a rate of 328 per 100,000 in those aged 55–94 years.[59] The causes of functional dyspepsia in the elderly patient are quite varied, and the association with nonsteroidal anti-inflammatory drugs is debated.[60,61]

The evaluation of dyspepsia in the elderly patient typically involves a more aggressive approach than in the younger patients because of the higher prevalence of organic disease, including carcinoma. Endoscopy is the test of choice to exclude ulceration, reflux esophagitis, or carcinoma.

Once the diagnosis of a functional disorder has been established by the exclusion of organic disease, the patient may be reassured regarding the absence of life-threatening disease. Initial therapy with antisecretory therapy is the preferred approach. Patients with documented *H. pylori* infection should undergo eradication therapy, although improved dyspeptic symptoms will occur in only about 20%. Nonpharmacologic measures may supplement the use of medications in treating functional abdominal pain, but they have not been studied in the elderly population. When managing functional abdominal symptoms in the elderly patient, it is important to provide symptomatic relief for other symptoms, such as constipation and diarrhea.

PANCREAS

Pancreatic Changes with Age

Intraluminal digestion is dependent on pancreatic secretion of enzymes, proenzymes, and bicarbonate. Biliary secretion of bile salts is essential for micelle formation, and biliary bicarbonate contributes to acid neutralization. The functional reserve is so great that 90% of secretory capacity must be lost before significant maldigestion occurs. The complex control of pancreatic secretion involves the central nervous system and gastric and intestinal mediators. Intestinal trophic substances, recurrent cycles of pancreatic secretion, and nutritional state are determinants of the ability of the pancreas to secrete (Figure 10–1). Extrapancreatic factors, such as acid hypersecretory states, decreased or diverted biliary secretions, altered anatomy of the proximal gastrointestinal tract, impaired release of intestinal mediators, and bacterial overgrowth in the small intestine, can adversely influence intraluminal digestion.

It might be expected that there would be age-related changes in both the morphology and the function of the aged pancreas, but the clinical significance of these changes is unclear. In older persons, malnutrition, hepatobiliary or gastrointestinal surgery, and other factors affecting di-

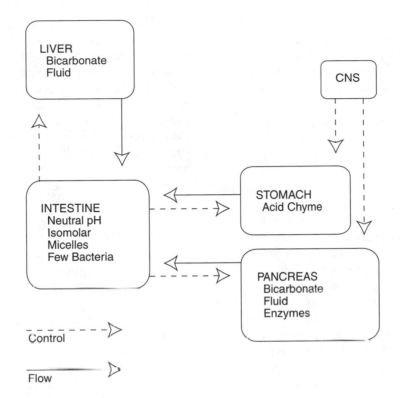

Figure 10 1 Gut Interactions
Control of pancreatic secretion is central to digestion and subject to modulation by the central nervous system (CNS) and intestinal factors.

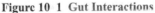

gestion and absorption could exacerbate the effects of these changes.

Beyond age 70 years, the pancreas is smaller and weighs less. Pancreatic ducts are dilated, and there is increased parenchyma fibrosis.[62] The diameter of the pancreatic duct increases with advancing age such that after age 50 it expands an average of 8% per decade.[63] However, the tapered appearance and smooth margins of the pancreatic duct are preserved with aging. The development of ductular ectasia in intralobular and interlobular ducts correlates with the development of pancreatic duct dilatation. These age-related changes can be misinterpreted as chronic pancreatitis during endoscopic retrograde cholangiopancreatography (ERCP).[64]

Clinical pancreatic insufficiency, resulting in loss of fat, protein, minerals, and fluid in the feces, occurs when pancreatic secretion is less than 10% of normal. Lesser decreases in pancreatic function are difficult to detect. Although there is controversy about the presence and extent of pancreatic secretory decline with age, most investigators question its clinical significance. In both human and animal studies, there appears to be a linear decline of enzyme output, while volume and bicarbonate concentration increase to a maximum at about the fourth decade of life and then progressively decline.[45,65,66] Perhaps more insightful is the work by Greenberg and Holt,[67] which demonstrated that the pancreatic enzyme concentrations in aging rats did not adapt to dietary changes as well as they did in younger rats. The enzymes lipase and amylase were studied. The findings suggest that age modifies the effect of gastrointestinal hormones on maintenance of pancreatic mass and enzyme content. Although the clinical significance of these observations is unclear, their potential importance cannot be overemphasized because of the magnification of rather small changes in hormone reactivity or responsiveness, potentially reflecting large changes in secretory rate.[68]

Diseases of the Pancreas in the Aged Population

Acute Pancreatitis

Acute pancreatitis is not uncommon in older people. It is responsible for 5% to 7% of the cases of abdominal pain in older persons.[69] It follows the frequency of gallstone-induced biliary tract disease and occurs most often in women, but drug-induced acute pancreatitis is also frequent.[70] Alcohol is rarely the cause of acute pancreatitis in older adults. Pancreatic cancer is an unusual cause of acute pancreatitis, but must be considered in older persons with acute pancreatitis. Age is a negative prognostic factor because older subjects are more likely to die of shock and sepsis.[71]

The uncomplicated course of this disease usually involves a period of acute illness characterized by pain, nausea, and vomiting. Older adults may initially present with more subtle symptoms and less marked physical symptoms than younger persons. When the disease is more severe, sepsis, pancreatic abscess, and shock complicate the picture. Less-ill patients usually recover in a matter of days with resumption of oral intake, but they may undergo multiple diagnostic and perhaps surgical procedures if retained gallstones are suspected. The management of stress metabolism is the major challenge to the nutritionist. Severely ill patients often face protracted periods of bowel rest. Total parenteral nutrition support is usually provided in patients with moderate or severe pancreatitis (Figure 10–2).

Chronic Pancreatitis

Chronic pancreatitis is of interest to the nutritionist because episodes of symptoms reduce oral intake, while late stages of the disease result in maldigestion due to pancreatic insufficiency. The most common cause of chronic pancreatitis is alcoholism; however, onset after age 60 years is uncommon. Idiopathic chronic pancreatitis in general is the second most common cause of chronic pancreatitis (20%). In older persons with the new onset of chronic pancreatitis, idiopathic causes predominate. Chronic pancreatitis can principally involve the large ducts, as from tumor or stones, or the small ducts, as is typical of

ACUTE PANCREATITIS

Occult
    No oral intake
    Usual short time

Complicated course
Sepsis
Drainage has high protein
    content
Usually no residual
    pancreatic insufficiency

CHRONIC PANCREATITIS

Clinical
    Multiple episodes
    Intake reduced by pain
    Chronic course
    Ethanol as carbohydrate

Malnutrition as late
    presentation
Maldigestion
Steatorrhea

Figure 10–2 Nutrition Problems with Pancreatitis

idiopathic chronic pancreatitis. The small duct form may also involve little to no pancreatic calcification, making diagnosis more difficult.[72]

Pancreatic insufficiency in asymptomatic older people may be accounted for by the presence of either painless disease or chronic primary inflammatory pancreatitis. Painless chronic pancreatitis appears to be more frequent in the sixth and seventh decades. These patients frequently have steatorrhea, diabetes, pancreatic calcifications, and weight loss. There is extensive scarring and atrophy of the gland, and response to therapy is unpredictable.

Nutritional Management. The management of pancreatic insufficiency due to chronic pancreatitis is based on the replacement of pancreatic enzymes, dietary modification to minimize the consequences of pancreatic insufficiency, and supplementation of vitamins that may be malabsorbed as a result of this condition. Pancreatic insufficiency most commonly occurs after a long duration of chronic pancreatitis, but it can occur acutely with obstruction of the pancreatic duct by carcinoma and transiently with acute or relapsing acute pancreatitis. It is likely that visceral protein depletion results in pancreatic insufficiency. Steatorrhea is often a more serious problem than creatorrhea because lipase secretion may decrease more rapidly.[73] Carbohydrate malabsorption also occurs, but its quantitative importance has not been established.[74]

Mild steatorrhea may not be associated with any symptoms. Weight loss may be minimal if food intake is adequate. Enzyme replacement is indicated for weight loss, diarrhea, dyspepsia, and fecal fat excretion exceeding 15 g/d. Some patients also experience reduced pain on pancreatic supplementation.[75] Enzyme preparations are usually given with meals, but even in high doses they do not completely resolve the steatorrhea. Pancreatic extracts may form insoluble complexes with folic acid and interfere with its absorption.

In patients with a painful disease, recurrent hospitalizations with reduced or absent oral intake, and intake reduced secondary to pain and analgesic use can contribute to the overall picture of malnutrition. Patients who fail to respond may have complicating factors such as primary intestinal disease, bacterial overgrowth, or inactivation of enzyme by gastric acid. Disproportionate acidification of the duodenum because of impaired bicarbonate secretion from the pancreas also occurs. Aluminum hydroxide is effective in reducing steatorrhea during pancreatic enzyme replacement therapy, and H_2 blockers have produced variable results.

Fat-soluble vitamin deficiency occurs despite adequate control of steatorrhea.[76] Nondiabetic retinopathy is improved by vitamin A therapy in patients with pancreatic insufficiency, but zinc malabsorption may also play a role. Vitamin B_{12} malabsorption occurs in chronic pancreatic insufficiency and may be due to a deficiency of a pancreatic factor or impaired proteolysis of vitamin B_{12} binders. Clinical evidence of vitamin B_{12} malabsorption is rare. Dietary treatment of chronic pancreatitis is based on the rationale that a high-fat diet exacerbates steatorrhea and abdominal pain and therefore that dietary fat should be restricted to 25% or less of total calories. Malabsorption of protein should be treated with a diet rich in protein. In severe symptomatic chronic pancreatitis, medium chain triglycerides, which do not require lipolysis but enter the intestinal mucosa directly, can be used as replacement calories. A high-fiber diet is relatively contraindicated in pancreatic insufficiency because fiber may bind as much as 80% to 95% of pancreatic enzymes.[77]

SMALL INTESTINE

Morphology

Because passive absorption is dependent on the surface area of the small intestine, studies have been made of the morphologic changes in the intestinal villous and microvillous membranes that might occur with aging. Animal studies have demonstrated a decrease in the number of villi, villous atrophy, and abnormal villous shape with advancing age. However, the validity of these early studies is questionable because of a lack of information on the nutritional state of the animals. In humans, there may be minor changes between young adults and older persons, including shorter villi in the older subjects, but this finding has not been consistently demonstrated.[78] Although it is not possible to equate normal appearance with normal function, later studies effectively excluded disease and nutrition-related variables and did not demonstrate abnormal appearance of the absorptive surface, suggesting that well-being and nutritional state are predominant factors in determining morphology and function.[79]

The epithelial surface of the intestinal villous membrane is normally regenerated at a rapid rate. Replication occurs in the intestinal crypt; then, as cells migrate toward the apex of the villous, differentiation and maturation occur. No difference in migration rate has been demonstrated, but the activities of several important enzymes are delayed in aged rats. Although results from older studies conflict with those of more recent studies, current information concludes that otherwise healthy, well-nourished older individuals have no substantial differences in intestinal morphology; however, they may have functional abnormalities because of altered enzyme activity of epithelial cells due to delayed maturation.

Integrity

Integrity and permeability of the small intestine may be altered by a variety of diseases, including Crohn's disease and celiac sprue. If the small intestinal mucosa is disrupted, there may be increased antigen access and abnormal nutrient transport. The lactulose-manitol absorption test measures the relative absorptions of lactulose, a large molecule absorbed paracellularly, to manitol, a relatively small molecule absorbed transcellularly, and provides an assessment of overall small intestinal permeability. When healthy adults older than 60 years are compared with younger adults, there are no significant changes as measured in the lactulose-manitol absorption test.[80] The α_1-antitrypsin clearance mea-

sures intestinal integrity by assessing the "leakiness" of the gut and measuring lost α_1-antitrypsin in the stool. The α_1-antitrypsin clearance is unchanged with advancing age when older adults are compared to younger adults.[81] Thus, small intestinal integrity does not seem to be altered due to the aging process alone.

Function

Carbohydrate Absorption

The potential for malabsorption is suggested by the alteration of enzyme activity of epithelial cells. Dietary carbohydrates, which approximate 40% of ingested calories, require digestion from the constituent polysaccharides to monosaccharides before intestinal absorption. The initial phase of digestion occurs in the intestinal lumen by pancreatic amylase, the secretion of which is well preserved in older people. Further hydrolysis of disaccharides and short-chain polysaccharides is accomplished by mucosal cell enzymes. However, overall carbohydrate absorption seems to remain intact with advancing age.

The absorption of glucose is difficult to study in older subjects because glucose metabolism, body size, and body composition are altered. In vitro studies do not suggest an abnormality of glucose absorption in aged mice.[82,83] One method used to evaluate glucose absorption is to measure hydrogen excretion in the breath. Hydrogen, a product of bacterial fermentation of carbohydrate, is absorbed in the colon and excreted in the breath. Postprandial breath hydrogen excretion studies of older patients consuming meals with different amounts of carbohydrate demonstrate excessive excretion of breath hydrogen in one-third of people older than 65 years given a 100 g carbohydrate meal. Excessive excretion of hydrogen is also seen in some older subjects given as little as 25 to 50 g of carbohydrate.[84] In young adults, ingestion of a 200 g carbohydrate meal is not associated with elevated breath hydrogen excretions, whereas elevated breath hydrogen excretions can be detected in over 60% of older adults.[84] The excess hydrogen produced may be from malabsorption of carbohydrate, with subsequent hydrogen production by colonic bacteria or from bacterial metabolism of carbohydrate in the small intestine due to bacterial overgrowth.

Carbohydrate absorption is often evaluated by the D-xylose test. D-xylose, a pentose sugar, is absorbed mainly by diffusion that parallels intestinal absorptive capacity, and it is excreted in urine. Low values may result from incomplete urine collections, impaired renal function, or malabsorption. Earlier studies suggesting impaired D-xylose excretion in older subjects have been dismissed because of the known reduction in urine clearance rate with advanced age. Overall absorption of D-xylose is not affected by age alone except in the very old (those older than 80 years).[85,86] In the absence of disease, it appears that the aged small intestine has normal carbohydrate absorption within the range of clinically important parameters such as symptoms and evidence of malabsorption. Although dietary carbohydrate has no recommended dietary allowance (RDA), several organizations, including the American Heart Association and the United States Department of Agriculture, recommend dietary carbohydrate (regardless of age) to make up 55% to 60% of calories, as well as an increased proportion of complex carbohydrates to simple sugars.

Fat Absorption

The absorption of dietary fats is biochemically more complex than that of other nutrients. Malnutrition associated with steatorrhea and appropriate laboratory studies confirm the diagnosis of malabsorption. A 72-hour fecal fat collection, while the patient is on a fixed high-dietary fat intake, is the standard measure of fat absorption. The absorption of long-chain triglycerides, fatty acids, monoglycerides, and vitamin D occurs as passive diffusion after intraluminal digestion. The limiting factors are dependent on the concentration of bile salts and the unstirred water layer.[87]

The absorbed triglycerides and vitamin D are transferred from the intestinal cell to the lymphatics as chylomicrons and very-low-density lipoproteins (VLDLs). In aged animals, the absorption of radioactively labeled glycerol and vi-tamin D_3 is decreased, suggesting a defect in the synthesis of chylomicrons and lipoproteins by the enterocyte.[88] This problem may be related to impaired synthesis of essential apoproteins and phospholipids.[89]

In older adults, the capacity for fat absorption is well maintained. Arora et al[90] measured fat absorption in healthy adults aged 20 to 59 years and found fecal fat excretions of 3.3 ± 2.3 g/d compared with 2.5 ± 1.8 g in those aged 60 to 69 years and 2.9 ± 1.9 g in those aged 70 to 91 years. In a Scandinavian population, similar results were found between young and older adults when dietary fat intake was 85 to 90 g/d.[88] Thus, with normal levels of fat consumption, fat digestion and absorption in older adults are equivalent to those in young persons.[91]

At high levels of fat intake (115 to 120 g/d), older adults have less fat absorption than younger adults.[92] In older adults who are institutionalized, there may be even less fat absorption.[91] When fat malabsorption occurs in older adults without an obvious cause, the small intestinal bacterial overgrowth syndrome including bacterial deconjugation of bile acids is often present. Simko and Michael[92] evaluated very high-fat intakes in debilitated older, malnourished hospitalized patients and found that although there was an increase in fecal fat content, these patients were capable of absorbing an average of 329 g of fat per day. Thus, although older persons have a somewhat diminished reserve capacity of the small intestine to absorb dietary fats compared with that of younger adults, it is still significant.

Protein Absorption

Because of the high synthetic activity related to cell renewal and enzyme production, protein turnover in the intestine is very high, with respect to the total protein content of the intestine. Few studies to date provide information in older adults about quantitative absorptive changes for amino acids and peptides. However, older persons may digest and absorb high-protein diets less well than younger adults, as demonstrated by a small increase in fecal nitrogen content after ingestion of a protein load. Although the 1989 RDA for protein is 0.8 g of protein per kilogram of body weight per day, in older adults this may be adequate only with high energy intakes (>40 kcal/kg per day).[93] Older adults typically have intakes of about 30 kcal/kg per day, at which more than half of older persons do not obtain nitrogen balance. In Boston, free-living older persons were noted by Munro et al[94] to have an average protein consumption of 1.05 g/kg per day, with no evidence that protein-energy malnutrition correlated with lower intakes. Daily protein intakes of 1 g of protein per kilogram of body weight in the older person will usually provide adequate nutrition.

Micronutrient Absorption

It is unclear whether deficiency or disease occurs because of vitamin malabsorption in otherwise healthy older people. Research in this area is hampered by the interpretation of blood levels and how they may relate to biochemical effects or tissue stores. Without disease, it is unlikely that malabsorption of vitamins results in significant vitamin depletion.[95] Inadequate dietary intakes are likely responsible for much of the poor vitamin nutriture in older adults.[96] It is now recognized that the RDAs for dietary nutrients established for younger adults cannot be simply extrapolated to older adults. The RDAs are correctly being reevaluated in older adults, not only to provide adequate nutrients such that deficiency states do not occur, but also to prevent chronic disease or treat a marker of chronic disease.

The fat-soluble vitamins may be absorbed more readily by older individuals. This is also true of other lipids.[97–99] In older animals, vitamin A uptake is increased due to a decrease in the thickness of the unstirred water layer. Krasinski et al.[100] studied why older adults have higher vitamin A tolerance curves than younger adults. Using plasmapharesis after ingestion of vitamin A–rich meals with subsequent reinfusion of chylomicrons and chylomicron remnants, they showed that older adults had about half the vitamin A clearance rates of young adults. It is reasonable to recommend to older adults to obtain a large proportion of the vitamin A requirement from the precursor carotene, found in fruits and vegetables, as carotenes may have a beneficial effect on cancer prevention.

The absorption of vitamin D in older persons appears to be impaired. Blood levels of 25-hydroxycholecalciferol are lower in older subjects, and malabsorption of labeled cholecalciferol has been reported. The importance of this observation is emphasized by evidence that calcium absorption appears to be lower in older people than it is in younger people and that osteoporosis and osteomalacia frequently occur in older individuals. The mechanism of this malabsorption and the relationship of circulating vitamin D metabolites are unclear, but it appears that there is a reduced adaptation to low dietary intake of calcium. Decreased intakes of vitamin D by older adults are in part responsible for low vitamin D levels because over three-quarters have vitamin D intakes less than two-thirds of the 1989 RDA of 5 μg/d. In addition, older adults have decreased renal synthesis of 1,25-dihydroxyvitamin D and decreased skin synthesis of vitamin D.[101] The decrease in skin synthesis of vitamin D is due to reduced sunlight exposure (especially common in institutionalized older adults) and decreased efficiency of skin synthesis.[102,103] In older adults who are institutionalized or homebound, it is reasonable to supplement with 400 IU/d.

Vitamin K levels may be altered with advancing age. Plasma phylloquinone (vitamin K_1) concentrations are decreased in older adults compared with younger adults.[104] Small intestinal bacterial overgrowth can result in the synthesis and absorption of menaquinones (vitamin K_2).[105] Although menaquinones may contribute to vitamin K nutriture, they typically are not sufficient to replete vitamin K in a deficient patient.

Water-soluble vitamin absorption is probably normal in older adults. Low plasma levels of vitamin C have been correlated with reduced oral intake. No differences of thiamin excretion have been seen in young or older subjects. The absorption for folate in the small intestine is pH dependent, with an optimal pH of about 6.3.[106] In older adults with atrophic gastritis, the pH of the small intestine is higher than in those with normal acid production, pH 7.1 ± 0.1 vs. pH 6.6 ± 0.1.[107] This small increase in the pH of the small intestine in older adults with atrophic gastritis results in a significant diminution of folate absorption. The administration of dilute acid along with oral folate improves folate absorption in those with atrophic gastritis. But paradoxically, older adults with atrophic gastritis have higher serum folate values than those with normal gastric acid production. Folate-synthesizing bacteria in the small intestine of older adults with atrophic gastritis are responsible for the additional folate.[108]

Folate deficiency may also increase serum homocysteine levels because folate is needed to convert homocysteine to methionine. High homocysteine levels are a risk factor for atherosclerotic heart and cerebrovascular diseases. In the Framingham Heart Study, plasma folate levels below 11.6 μmol/L, a value well within the normal range, were associated with elevated homocysteine levels.[107] Future guidelines for folate supplementation will need to take into consideration how much dietary folate is required to reduce homocysteine levels to normal.

Serum and plasma vitamin B_6 values tend to decrease with advancing age. Vitamin B_6 is primarily absorbed in the proximal small intestine, and even with supplementation, up to 40% of older adults may remain vitamin B_6 deficient.[109] The average vitamin B_6 requirement for older adult males and females is about 2.0 mg/d.[110] Low vitamin B_6 levels can also lead to elevated homocysteine values by an altered ability to convert homocysteine to cystathionine.[111]

Age does not seem to be an independent variable for the ileal absorption of vitamin B_{12}. However, vitamin B_{12} absorption is complex and dependent on multiple factors, including salivary R binders, gastric secretion of acid and intrinsic factor, pancreatic exocrine sufficiency, and intact terminal ileal mucosa. Disruptions of any of these factors may lead to decreased vitamin B_{12} absorption. The classic cause of vitamin B_{12} deficiency is autoimmune type A atrophic gastritis (pernicious anemia). Type B atrophic gastritis

also limits the bioavailability of vitamin B_{12} due to diminished protein-bound vitamin B_{12} release from lack of gastric acid.[112,113]

Tests of protein-bound vitamin B_{12} absorption have shown that older adults with type B atrophic gastritis have decreased absorptions.[114] However, when subjects with type B atrophic gastritis are given free (crystalline) vitamin B_{12}, absorption is normalized. Patients treated with potent acid-reducing medications such as the proton-pump inhibitors, such as omeprazole, also malabsorb protein-bound vitamin B_{12}.[115] Ingestion of acidic beverages such as cranberry juice along with protein-bound vitamin B_{12} can normalize vitamin B_{12} absorption. In addition, bacteria that colonize the upper gastrointestinal tract in subjects with type B atrophic gastritis can take up and bind vitamin B_{12}, but antibiotic treatment can normalize vitamin B_{12} absorption.[116]

Vitamin B_{12} is also involved in homocysteine metabolism, with low vitamin B_{12} levels causing elevated homocysteine levels. In the Framingham Heart Study, vitamin B_{12} levels below 296 μmol/L were associated with rising homocysteine levels.[107] Although vitamin B_{12} deficiency often results in anemia, the neuropsychiatric manifestations of vitamin B_{12} deficiency may occur even in the absence of anemia.[117]

Low serum concentrations of iron and transferrin in aged individuals do not seem to be related to malabsorption of iron because no such age-related changes have been demonstrated.[118] Iron deficiency in older subjects is most often accounted for by intestinal blood loss due to malignant or benign disease, although gastric achlorhydria may account for the reduction of the absorption of nonheme iron.[119]

Calcium absorption appears to decline with advancing age.[120] However, decreased calcium absorption in older adults is primarily due to poor vitamin D nutriture and inactivity. Older adults also have poor calcium intakes in the diet, which are partially due to the high prevalence of lactase deficiency. Certain types of calcium, such as calcium carbonate, are poorly absorbed in older adults with atrophic gastritis.[121,122] However, several studies have not shown any significant change in calcium absorption when calcium is ingested from or with food in subjects with atrophic gastritis.[123] Lifetime intake of calcium is a major factor in the development of osteoporosis.

Motility

Small bowel motility appears to be intact in healthy older people.[124] This is not true, however, for the changes seen with medical illness or drug effects. In an intestinal motility study of fasting and fed older subjects, all three phases of the migrating motor complex were present, and there were no differences in the motility index or duration or velocity of phase III contractions. There was a slight decrease in the motility index and the frequency of contractions after feeding, but there were no differences in the mean amplitude of contractions. It is not known whether these latter changes have clinical significance or alter intestinal transit time. Several clinical studies suggest that subclinical pancreatic insufficiency and bacterial overgrowth in the small intestine are a common cause of malabsorption. However, the results are clouded by problems of patient selection and concomitant systemic or gastrointestinal disease. Therefore, when malabsorption is suspected, a specific diagnosis should be pursued because it is unlikely that major clinical problems of malabsorption are unique to older people.[91,115]

INTESTINAL DISORDERS

Disaccharidase Deficiency

Deficiency of the disaccharidase lactase is the most common disorder of carbohydrate digestion. Its appearance with aging and maturation can be considered normal in most people, with the exception of some northern Europeans, because there is a steady decline in brush border enzymes after weaning. Adults retain about 10% to 30% of intestinal lactase activity and develop symptoms only when they ingest sufficient lactose to exceed lactase production. Lactase deficiency also occurs in the presence of primary intestinal diseases such as viral gastroenteritis, tropical and nontropical

sprue, Crohn's disease, bacterial and parasitic infections of the intestine, and cystic fibrosis.

The symptoms of lactase deficiency are nonspecific. Even so, most adults who have this condition are aware of their intolerance to milk because of abdominal cramping, bloating, distention, flatulence, and possible diarrhea. Symptoms are due to the osmotic effect of unhydrolyzed and unabsorbed lactose shifting fluid into the intestinal tract, resulting in a rapid passage of contents through the intestine into the colon. Colonic bacteria hydrolyze the lactose to lactic acid and short-chain fatty acids, lowering the pH of the stool. Hydrogen produced by this fermentation is absorbed and excreted in the breath, which is a useful test for detecting lactose intolerance. The diagnosis can be confirmed by administering an oral dose of lactose, observing symptoms, and measuring blood glucose levels. When 0.75 to 1.5 g of lactose per kilogram of body weight is administered, the presence of symptoms and a rise in blood glucose concentration of less than 20 mg/dL above the fasting level are considered diagnostic of the disorder. Measurement of breath hydrogen after the ingestion of 50 g of lactose is a more sensitive and specific test. Lactase deficiency in older adults is important because of the potential for chronic deficiency of calcium and protein intake. The appearance of lactose intolerance as a new symptom should prompt consideration of other underlying gastrointestinal disease.[125–129]

Although lactase activity commonly declines with advancing age, the concentrations of intestinal sucrase and maltase are unchanged. In the rat, there appears to be an age-related decline in small intestinal glucose transport activity. In humans, small intestinal sodium-glucose transport has not consistently been demonstrated to be altered with aging. There is no known clinical consequence of altered sodium-glucose cotransport with aging.

Celiac Disease (Gluten-Sensitive Enteropathy)

Celiac disease, also known as gluten-sensitive enteropathy, results from small intestinal mucosal injury caused by dietary exposure to wheat gluten. The classic symptoms of this disease include diarrhea, bloating, and weight loss, which are a result of the profound malabsorption and steatorrhea seen in these patients. Celiac disease is more common in females, found in a female-to-male ratio of approximately 3:1.[130] The occurrence of this disease in older adults is not widely recognized, and its manifestations may be atypical. In contrast to earlier descriptions, recent reports suggest that as many as 25% of patients with celiac disease may be first diagnosed in later years.[131,132] Most patients with this disease do not present with the classic symptoms of diarrhea with steatorrhea, osteomalacia, or anemia, but they may have more subtle findings, including nonspecific gastrointestinal complaints that may be transient or acute. In over half the reported cases, abnormalities of the blood count, including macrocytosis and mild anemia, prompted further investigation. In older patients, an abnormally low serum folate level may also indicate the presence of celiac disease.

Cachexia, depression, fatigue, and anemia in older individuals usually lead to consideration of occult malignancy rather than primary gastrointestinal disease. Although the mimicking of malignancy appears to be a more common feature of celiac disease in older patients, other manifestations are typical but often misdiagnosed (eg, edema attributed to heart disease; osteomalacia attributed to osteoporosis; wasting due to occult malignancy elsewhere) Older patients may present with small intestinal ulcerations, a syndrome of splenic atrophy, villous atrophy and cavitation of mesenteric lymph nodes, or subacute intestinal pseudo-obstruction. Occult gastrointestinal bleeding may occur in about half of patients with celiac disease and may result in iron deficiency. The diagnosis of celiac disease is dependent on a small bowel biopsy that demonstrates the typical features of a flat mucosa due to villous atrophy. The presence of antigluten or antireticulin immunoglobulin A or immunoglobulin G antibodies in the plasma has long been used as a screening test in adults.[133] However, more recently it has been recognized that the IgA antien-

domysial antibody test is the most sensitive and specific noninvasive diagnostic test available. The breath hydrogen test differentiates patients with celiac disease from normal subjects but does not identify those who have bacterial overgrowth.[134]

The laboratory features of celiac disease reflect the profound disturbance of absorption in the proximal intestine, resulting in steatorrhea and malabsorption of iron and folic acid but typically preservation of vitamin B_{12} and bile salt absorption. This dysfunction of intestinal digestion and absorption due to enzyme depletion is secondary to the early exfoliation of maturing enterocytes. These abnormal findings return to normal after treatment with a gluten-free diet, although lactase deficiency may persist or be slow to improve.[134]

The treatment of celiac disease in older patients consists of the removal of gluten from the diet. Most patients will respond, but those patients with profound malnutrition and debility are at risk for death due to infection and hemorrhage. In such extreme cases, nutritional support measures may be necessary to facilitate the establishment of adequate oral feeding. Older patients may require additional training to successfully alter their dietary intake. Management of calcium and vitamin D metabolism needs to be attended to and may require oral supplementation. Failure to respond to a gluten-free diet should prompt consideration of underlying complicating diagnoses, such as intestinal lymphoma.

Bacterial Overgrowth

The small intestinal bacterial overgrowth syndrome is one of the most important clinical conditions that more frequently occurs in older adults. The upper gastrointestinal tract is normally considered sterile, with fewer than 103 organisms per milliliter of intestinal secretions. Occult malabsorption caused by bacterial contamination of the small intestine is more common in older individuals than is generally recognized. Of 24 patients with unrecognized malabsorption in the presence of clinical malnutrition, 17 were found to have bacterial contamination associated with duodenal-jejunal diverticula, postgastrectomy syndrome, or otherwise normal gastrointestinal anatomy. This condition of overgrowth of abnormal microflora in the small intestine is variously called the *blind loop syndrome, stagnate loop syndrome,* or *small intestinal stasis syndrome.* The condition can occur in patients who have abnormal bacterial flora without stasis. The overgrowth of microflora disturbs intraluminal digestion and mucosal function and results in malabsorption of fat, protein, carbohydrate, electrolytes, and vitamin B_{12}. Malnutrition due to steatorrhea and macrocytic anemia due to vitamin B_{12} deficiency frequently develop.

The normal human jejunum is populated by a variable number of transient organisms derived from oral pharyngeal sources. Ileal bacterial populations are somewhat higher and reflect a colonic origin. Protective mechanisms in the proximal gut include acidity of the stomach and the normal cleansing activity of proximal small intestinal motility. Diseases, operations, or medications that reduce gastric acidity are correlated with high levels of bacterial contamination, as are conditions that reduce small intestinal motility, such as scleroderma, diabetes, and pseudo-obstruction. Older adults are at increased risk to develop small intestinal bacterial overgrowth due to the high prevalence of atrophic gastritis with hypochlorhydria or achlorhydria. Immunologic secretions (from the intestines, liver, and pancreas), the mucous barrier, and bile acids probably play a lesser role in protecting against or reducing bacterial overgrowth. When bacterial contamination of the proximal intestine occurs, anaerobic organisms form a large proportion of the total and result in multiple disturbances of intraluminal digestion and mucosal absorption. The contaminating bacteria deconjugate bile acids, reducing their concentration, and thus interfere with fat digestion. Malabsorption of the fat-soluble vitamins (vitamins A, D, E, and K) may occur in association with generalized fat malabsorption. Bacterial overgrowth also contributes to denaturation of ingested protein, disturbed function of brush border enzymes, and

probable protein loss from injured mucosa. In adults, the D-xylose tolerance test may become abnormal because of bacterial fermentation and impaired mucosal absorption. As a result of malabsorption, the end products of bacterial metabolism contribute to diarrhea and water and electrolyte losses.

Although pathogenic bacteria in the upper gastrointestinal tract cause the bacterial overgrowth syndrome, not all bacteria that can grow in the upper gastrointestinal tract result in adverse clinical conditions. Coliforms and anaerobes are the typical organisms responsible for the bacterial overgrowth syndrome. However, bacterial colonization of the upper gastrointestinal tract that occurs solely from a lack of gastric acid, whether due to atrophic gastritis or medications, may have few adverse clinical manifestations.[135] Thus, "simple" colonization of the upper gastrointestinal tract is clinically silent and is not typically detected. However, most older persons with steatorrhea of unclear etiology will have occult intestinal bacterial overgrowth.

The clinical symptoms of the bacterial overgrowth syndrome include abdominal pain, bloating, diarrhea, and weight loss. Older adults often have nonspecific symptoms such as bloating and nausea with manifestations of weight loss or malnutrition, and because of this, a high index of suspicion is required to diagnose the bacterial overgrowth syndrome in older adults who present in a subtle manner.

Clinical investigation of these patients is directed toward defining anatomic defects or disturbed motility that would contribute to stasis and identifying conditions that reduce bacterial defenses. In addition to the usual diagnostic studies for malabsorption (such as stool examination for fecal fat and D-xylose absorption studies), hydrogen breath tests, small bowel biopsy, and collection of intestinal contents for microbiologic analysis may be done. However, the diagnosis may be difficult because the noninvasive tests are not totally accurate and the invasive tests are rarely performed. The most widely accepted noninvasive tests are the glucose- and lactulose-hydrogen breath tests, with sensitivities of about 80%. The most accurate noninvasive test is the I-g ^{14}C D-xylose breath test, with a sensitivity of 95%, but unfortunately it is not available at most centers.[136] However, the gold standard test is considered to be intestinal intubation using a sterile tube, with aspiration of intestinal contents and subsequent microbiologic quantitative assays. Typically, this is done at the time of upper endoscopy. It is relatively expensive and has potential side effects. Thus, most clinicians will empirically diagnose the bacterial overgrowth syndrome and initiate a diagnostic trial of antibiotics.

The underlying cause of the small intestinal bacterial overgrowth syndrome should be corrected if possible. Because most conditions that cause this syndrome are not easily correctable, antibiotics are the mainstay of treatment. Antibiotics are typically given in 2-week courses that may have to be repeated at varying intervals, or rotating antibiotic courses may be necessary depending on the situation. Nutrition support is also important with appropriate therapy for micronutrient deficiency, fat malabsorption, lactose maldigestion, and fat-soluble vitamin deficiency.

Inflammatory Bowel Disease

Ulcerative colitis and Crohn's disease represent two diagnostic categories of inflammatory diseases of the bowel of unknown etiology. Ulcerative colitis is a mucosal disease limited to the colon and involves the rectum and contiguous parts of the colon proximally to varying degrees. Crohn's disease more typically affects the ileum and proximal portions of the colon and tends to be more segmental, with skipped areas of normal-appearing bowel. Because of the involvement of the small intestine and the propensity for perforation of the bowel with fistula and abscess formation, Crohn's disease has, for most patients, a greater negative impact on nutritional state than does chronic ulcerative colitis. Both diseases occur more frequently in young patients, with onset during the teenage years and the 20s. Onset after age 60 years probably accounts for less than 10% of patients. Published studies of

the epidemiology of inflammatory bowel disease may underestimate the true prevalence by 27% to 38%; examination of asymptomatic patients between the ages of 50 and 75 years during a screening study for colorectal cancer uncovered 8 people with previously undiagnosed inflammatory bowel disease among approximately 18,000 participants.[137] Many patients diagnosed with inflammatory bowel disease after age 60 years are probably suffering from ischemic colitis or infectious colitis instead.[138]

There is a suggestion that some features of late-onset ulcerative colitis distinguish it from early-onset disease. Late-onset disease is less extensive, being more frequently limited to the rectum and the left colon rather than involving the entire colon. Diarrhea is more severe and is accompanied by less bleeding. At the onset of the disease, the illness is more protracted, is perhaps less responsive to treatment, and has shorter remissions. Of great importance in older patients is that significant weight loss, anemia, and frequent hospitalizations are more common.[139]

In older adults, many of the symptoms of Crohn's disease, including diarrhea, cramping abdominal pain, fatigue, weight loss, and low-grade fever, might easily be attributed to underlying malignancy. Features that usually alert the clinician to the presence of Crohn's disease include the anorectal manifestations of fistulas and abscesses. Anemia, hypoproteinemia, and malnutrition are caused by the chronic inflammatory process, poor oral intake, increased gastrointestinal losses, and malabsorption. Older patients with Crohn's disease are more likely to have left-sided colonic involvement than are younger cohorts, who more commonly have isolated ileal disease.

The treatment of inflammatory bowel disease in older patients does not differ substantially from that in younger patients. 5-Aminosalicylate medications, corticosteroids, and metronidazole are commonly used drugs. Other immunosuppressants are used for patients with intractable disease. Sulfasalazine has an anti-folate effect and may contribute to gastrointestinal side effects that include epigastric discomfort and chronic headache. Corticosteroids can exacerbate diabetes mellitus, cause hypertension, accelerate osteoporosis, and complicate conditions marked by salt and water retention, such as congestive heart failure and renal failure. As in younger patients, older patients with late onset disease often require surgery.[140]

Radiation Enteritis

Radiation enteritis results from a dose-related injury to the intestine, most commonly associated with radiation treatment of cancer of the cervix, uterus, prostate, rectum, sigmoid, and bladder. As the population ages and more patients become candidates for radiation therapy, this side effect will become more prevalent. In the acute form, radiation enteritis typically causes diarrhea but is usually self-limited; when severe, it may be sufficient to interrupt treatment. When the disease has continued beyond 3 months, it is considered chronic, and its importance probably is underestimated. Most patients do not seek medical help until serious complications occur.[141,142]

Radiation therapy typically injures cells that divide rapidly, so crypt cells in the small intestine are particularly vulnerable. The chronic form of the disease is thought to be due to a progressive, irreversible ischemia that results in a fibrinous peritonitis in which loops of intestine are bound together. Fibrosis, submucosal edema of the bowel wall, and perforation occur. Ulceration of the mucosa is common; deeper ulcerations are associated with perforation. Mucosal areas of atrophy are also present, and scarring results in luminal narrowing.

The severity of radiation injury based on findings and symptoms is categorized as mild, consisting of diarrhea controlled by diet and reassurance; marked, noted by diarrhea and rectal pain and relieved by medications; or severe, characterized by fistulization, perforation, and stricture. Patients with diabetic vascular disease and atherosclerosis are at greatest risk of developing severe radiation enteritis.

The latent period between radiation therapy and the onset of symptoms can be years. Initial symptoms include postprandial fullness, nausea, and cramping, which progress to distention and vomiting. In a retrospective review of 3900 patients at risk for chronic radiation enteritis, O'Brien and colleagues[143] documented the typical course of these patients. Patients with early symptoms were hospitalized and treated with nasogastric suction and intravenous fluids; there were clinical findings of incomplete bowel obstruction. Diets were advanced as tolerated, and patients were discharged on a soft diet. Repeated episodes of partial small bowel obstruction followed, and patients continued to deteriorate over time. Once this cycle of recurrent small bowel obstruction occurred, all patients ultimately required surgical treatment. Bowel obstruction was due to narrowed, thickened bowel wall rather than to associated adhesions. Resection and anastomosis of bowel often were not possible, and bypass of affected segments was required.[144]

Multiple factors contribute to the risk of chronic radiation injury to the bowel, including adhesions due to prior surgery, pelvic inflammatory bowel disease, extremely low body weight, diabetes mellitus, cardiovascular disease, preexisting vascular compromise of the bowel, and combined chemotherapy and radiation therapy.[145] Some surgeons advise wide excision of affected bowel rather than bypass.[146]

Acute Radiation Enteritis

The treatment of acute radiation enteritis consists of the symptomatic use of antidiarrheal agents, including opiates and anticholinergic drugs. Cholestyramine, a bile salt–binding agent, is used on the basis of the hypothesis that injured distal small bowel fails to resorb bile salts. Bile salts entering the colon have a profound secretory effect; binding the salts reduces these effects.[147] The use of elemental diet therapy to prevent radiation injury has led to conflicting results. McArdle and associates[148] studied the effect of elemental diets before and during radiation therapy for invasive bladder cancer, using retrospective controls. A peptide-based formula was given orally, by nasoenteric tube, or by needle jejunostomy; symptoms improved, and small bowel function returned promptly with early passage of flatus and feces. Patients treated with nutritional support had no microscopic damage to the ileum. On electron microscopic examination, there was preservation of the normal glycocalyx, preservation of cell microstructure and tight cell junctions, and greater preservation of brush border enzymes. It is not certain what role, if any, other factors, such as pancreatic biliary secretions or mechanical effects of regular diet, have in the pathophysiology of intestinal injury.

Chronic Radiation Enteritis

Unfortunately, the lesions of chronic radiation enteritis, including mucosal injury, evidence of stricture with bowel stasis, and perforation with fistula formation, are probably not reversible. A variety of treatment programs has been tried, with a mixture of results. These include treatments for bile salt diarrhea and bacterial stasis syndrome, and the use of a variety of anti-inflammatory agents. Unfortunately, many pathophysiologic factors are probably operating, so the efficacy of low-fat diets, low-residue diets, gluten-free or lactose-deficient diets, and elemental diets remains to be established. Parenteral nutrition has been used to induce weight gain, to correct hypoproteinemia, and to close fistulas.[149]

As noted above, many of these patients eventually have surgical treatment. Resection and bypass often result in short bowel syndrome. During the management of the patient with radiation enteritis, it is important to recognize that premorbid malnutrition often is present. Radiated tissues heal poorly, and dehiscence of wounds and infection are common complications. Nutritional rehabilitation must await metabolic recovery from surgery and the initiation of the convalescent phase.

LIVER

Significant morphologic and functional changes in the liver due to aging are of interest to the clinician because alterations in synthetic, excretory, or metabolic processes can affect the response to disease and the disposition of drugs. However, most hepatic changes are due to systemic disease and the liver diseases commonly seen in older individuals.

Liver weight decreases after age 50 years, parallel to the anthropometric changes of decreased body weight and muscle mass. In advanced age, the liver becomes disproportionately small.[150] On the basis of microscopic observations, these changes appear to be due to diminished numbers of hepatocytes. Other changes in liver morphology are nonspecific and may be due to extrahepatic processes. There is an increase in portal and periportal fibrosis, and liver cells tend to be larger, with larger or multiple nuclei and nucleoli. Enlargement of the liver cells may be due to compensatory hypertrophy. An increased amount of lipofuscin pigment is present in the Kupffer cells,[151] and changes in the Golgi apparatus and rough and smooth endoplasmic reticulum may parallel hepatic functional changes seen in older subjects.[152]

Liver Function and Aging

Decreases in liver blood flow from 0.3% to 1.5% per year occur with age.[153] Alterations in serum bilirubin, transaminases, alkaline phosphatase, dye tests of hepatic excretion (sulfobromophthalein sodium), and radioactive labeled excretion tests (Rose Bengal) do not occur in older people with histologically normal livers.[154] Levels of albumin, a product of hepatic synthesis, are frequently reduced in the older adults. Although albumin metabolism is influenced by many factors, it appears that the rate of albumin synthesis in older people is not sensitive to changes in protein intake, suggesting an altered set point in synthetic rate.[151]

The potential for changes in drug metabolism in the aging liver is of greater concern to clinicians than the apparent minor and probably insignificant changes in morphology and function.[155] The reduction of lean body mass and total body water alters the distribution of water-soluble and fat-soluble drugs. The disposition and side effects of drugs in older patients are of concern.[155] Contrary to conventionally held views, impaired clearance of drugs may not be due to reduced hepatic microsomal enzyme activity. Further study is required to understand this important subject.[156] No generalizations can be made about drug disposition with respect to altered blood flow, drug distribution, and principal metabolic pathways. Nutritional factors can be important, however, because levels of vitamin C and folic acid have been associated with decreased antipyrine clearance in older people.[157]

The rate of total-body protein synthesis is decreased in older individuals; much of this decrease is presumed to be in the liver.[158] In animal studies, synthesis of nucleic acids and proteins in old liver cells is diminished. There is an increase in the synthesis of faulty proteins; such "junk" proteins may account for disturbed drug disposition and function.

Liver Disease in the Older Population

Little has been written about the influence of multisystem disease on the liver, which may be of great importance in older adults. For cardiac, renal, diabetic, stroke, and arthritic patients, among others, the poorly understood intertwining effects of disease, treatment, and complications on nutrition and hepatic function must be considered rationally.

Chronic or acute alcohol use, starvation, protein-energy malnutrition, obesity, diabetes mellitus, and hypothyroidism can alter hepatic lipoprotein metabolism and cause fatty liver. Fatty liver can be associated with some element of liver cell necrosis when alcohol or drugs are involved. Fat in liver cells results from an imbalance of oxidation, esterification, or excretion of fatty acids that accumulate from a flux of fatty acids from adipose tissue to the liver. Generally, fatty liver does not interfere with hepatic function but results only in enlargement of the liver. Advanced cases may be associated with cholestasis, portal hypertension, and ascites. Liver cell necrosis accom-

panying fatty liver is a precursor of a progressive fibrotic process that may lead to cirrhosis.

Nonhepatitis causes of jaundice predominate in older patients. Drugs account for 20% of causes of jaundice in this group.[159] Although adverse drug reactions are more common in older subjects, and although systemic and hepatic alterations exist that can affect drug disposition, there is little evidence that the older liver is more susceptible to drug injury. There is some evidence to suggest that when injury occurs it may be more severe, as in the case of fatal anesthesia-induced liver disease. Commonly used drugs that may have an adverse effect on the liver include NSAIDs, anesthetic agents, antibiotics, antimetabolic agents, antihypertensives, cardiac drugs, and psychotropic drugs.[160]

Viral hepatitis is most often due to hepatitis C associated with blood transfusions before testing for hepatitis C was available. The clinical course of patients older than 60 years is not different from that of younger patients, although the illness may progress more rapidly in older adults.[161] However, acute type B hepatitis, especially when associated with other illness, has a higher risk of severe disease and hepatic failure.[162] In older patients with severe liver disease, age adversely affects prognosis.[161]

Primary biliary cirrhosis represents a model of cholestatic liver disease. There is chronic destruction of the bile ducts that results in cirrhosis and eventual liver failure. Although it is usually considered a disease of middle age, the age range of presentation is actually 20 to 80 years.[163] Fatigue and pruritus are the usual presenting symptoms. Since there is no specific treatment for this disease, symptomatic relief and prevention of the nutritional complications are the current treatment aims. Late in the disease, when hepatic cirrhosis and its complications develop, liver transplantation is indicated.

Older cirrhotics often are asymptomatic. The cirrhosis is caused by multiple factors and is not an inherent characteristic of aging. The peak incidence of cirrhosis due to alcoholism occurs beyond age 60. There may be few clinical indicators of this disease.[160] Patients with primary biliary cirrhosis who are survivors of early-onset disease have associated long-standing metabolic complications in old age.[164,165]

Nutrition in Liver Disease

It is unlikely that there are unique nutritional factors in the cause or treatment of liver disease in older patients, but changes that occur in digestion, absorption, and intermediary metabolism as a result of acute or chronic liver cell injury or cholestasis do affect nutrition.

Fatty Liver

Hepatic lipid metabolism can be disturbed at many points and can result in fat accumulation. Alcohol increases lipolysis, causing a flow of fatty acids to the liver; increases intrahepatic lipid synthesis; decreases fatty acid oxidation in the liver; increases triglyceride formation; and decreases the release of lipoprotein in the form of VLDLs. It is uncertain where alcohol exerts its greatest effect, but a direct hepatotoxic effect of alcohol is favored.[166] Nutritional deficiency is not essential for the formation of acute fatty liver, but it does seem to have some modifying effect, perhaps increasing the severity of the condition when serious levels of nutritional deficiency exist.[167] The source of fatty acids that accumulate as triglyceride in the liver cell differs depending on the fed state of the individual. Under fasting conditions, the source is adipose tissue. During the fed state, triglycerides are of intestinal origin. Stress hormones in acute alcohol intoxication may play a role.[168] It is unclear whether alcohol-induced hepatic fatty acid synthesis, decreased oxidation, or decreased secretion of triglycerides is most important. It is generally accepted that alcohol-induced fatty liver is reversible. As many as one-third of asymptomatic alcoholics may have fatty liver.

Fatty liver can also have features of cholestasis with jaundice and abnormal liver-associated enzymes. Some patients with fatty liver due to alcohol ingestion actually develop hepatitis with evidence of liver cell necrosis. These patients often have anorexia, nausea, vomiting, fever, and jaundice.

The treatment of acute alcoholic fatty liver is abstinence from alcohol. Principles of general nutrition dictate a well-balanced diet, adequate protein and calorie intake without overfeeding, and supplementation with vitamins. Prolonged fasting and starvation can produce fatty liver; this is especially true when the classic adaptation to starvation, which involves the change from peripheral oxidation of glucose to oxidation of fatty acid products, is blocked by carbohydrate feeding. In the classic form of starvation disease, kwashiorkor, fatty liver is a feature. It is treated with a high-protein diet.[169] It is probable that the fat in the livers of these patients arises not from mobilization of peripheral fat stores but rather from glucose administration, resulting in intrahepatic lipid synthesis.[168] Low serum levels of albumin and of VLDLs suggest an impairment of hepatic lipoprotein and protein synthesis that is reversible with protein feeding. In fatty liver associated with obesity, insulin resistance and increased levels of free fatty acids are probably secondary to increased adipose tissue mass.[170] Fatty infiltration is potentially reversible by weight reduction. Fatty liver and diabetes are often associated. Obesity, occurring in about 45% of diabetics older than 60 years, may be a more important factor in type 2 diabetics. Recommendations for treatment include weight reduction and a low-carbohydrate, high-protein diet. Fatty liver seen with total parenteral nutrition is probably due to excessive calorie infusion.

Acute Hepatitis

Whatever the primary cause of acute hepatitis, extensive liver cell necrosis leads to fulminant hepatic failure and impairment of nearly all hepatic functions, including carbohydrate, protein, and lipid metabolism; the catabolic rate is also increased. Hypoglycemia is a common feature of fulminant hepatic failure due to impaired hepatic gluconeogenesis and reduced liver glycogen content. These effects are exacerbated by hyperinsulinemia caused by increased insulin production and increased peripheral insulin resistance.

Characteristic derangements in amino acid metabolism occur in severe liver disease with altered plasma amino acid patterns. More than 85% of the liver must be nonfunctional before these patterns develop. Increased levels of tyrosine, phenylalanine, glutamine, and methionine and decreased levels of valine, leucine, and isoleucine are seen in chronic hepatic encephalopathy. However, in fulminant hepatic failure, branched-chain amino acids are either normal or slightly depressed, while there is a marked elevation of all others. This probably represents amino acid release from dying liver cells. The urea cycle, which is responsible for the clearance of metabolic nitrogen, is depressed in fulminant hepatic failure and leads to low urea levels and hyperammonemia.

For patients who have severe hepatic failure, hypoalbuminemia and edema are due to a substantial loss of hepatic protein synthetic activity (to less than 10% of normal). Reduced synthesis of vitamin K–dependent clotting factors can contribute to increased prothrombin time. If patients are unresponsive to vitamin K supplementation, bleeding complications are exacerbated. Low levels of total cholesterol, triglycerides, and esterified cholesterol are seen in fulminant hepatic failure.

For most patients who have acute hepatitis of various etiologies, no specific nutritional treatment measures are necessary unless anorexia, nausea, or vomiting becomes protracted. The anorexia seen in acute liver disease is best managed by a high-carbohydrate diet, with the greatest number of calories provided in the morning meal. If oral intake is poor or not possible, intravenous fluids containing glucose should be provided. In patients who have fulminant hepatic failure, continuous infusions of concentrated glucose sufficient to maintain normal serum glucose levels may be necessary. The negative nitrogen balance seen in fulminant hepatic failure makes the use of protein infusions at the rate of 0.8 to 1 g/kg of body weight rational. However, this often works out to be a practice of compromises because of limited protein tolerance and fluid overload. Lipid emulsions are not recommended in fulminant hepatic failure when hepatic enceph-

alopathy is present. Supplemental vitamins, especially folic acid and vitamins B_6 and B_{12}, should be provided.

Cholestasis

Because of the chronic course of primary biliary cirrhosis, this cholestatic disease has the most profound nutritional consequences. The decreased secretion of conjugated bile salts into the intestine leads to steatorrhea and bone disease.[171–173] Diarrhea, weight loss, and muscle wasting occur in patients when steatorrhea is significant. Reduced intake of neutral triglycerides and substitution of medium chain triglycerides for calories can be effective in the treatment of this condition, since bile salts are not necessary for medium chain triglyceride absorption.

Although osteomalacia has been assumed to be the principal bone disease of primary biliary cirrhosis, osteoporosis appears to be more important. Nevertheless, treatment is directed toward correcting calcium and vitamin D metabolism, although the results are mixed. Despite normal 25-hydroxyvitamin D_3 levels achieved by monthly intramuscular injections of vitamin D_3, bone disease continues. Vitamin K deficiency has been demonstrated, and vitamin E deficiency is common in primary biliary cirrhosis.[174] Vitamin A levels are low in primary biliary cirrhosis, but symptoms are not commonly noted. Zinc deficiency has also been reported in association with symptomatic vitamin A deficiency. Cholestyramine, which is used to bind and increase the elimination of bile salts in cholestatic liver disease, contributes to steatorrhea and the malabsorption of fat-soluble vitamins, as well as vitamin C.

Cirrhosis

Inadequate dietary intake is the most likely principal cause of malnutrition in patients with liver disease.[175] Decreased sensitivity to taste and smell may contribute to decreased or altered oral intake in the cirrhotic patient.[176] Factors that contribute to malnutrition include anorexia, nausea, poor palatability of special diets, and the indirect effects of chronic alcohol use and its social consequences. The alcoholic cirrhotic may have both pancreatic insufficiency and injury to the small intestinal mucosa. These changes are probably mediated to some extent by nutritional deficiency.[177,178] Steatorrhea, usually of mild extent, is also seen in cirrhotics; whether it is due to the effects of portal hypertension on gut congestion and lymphatic drainage or to diminished bile salt secretion is unclear.

Changes in glucose, amino acid, and fat metabolism that occur in cirrhosis resemble those of normal adaptation to prolonged starvation. Calorie requirements of stable alcoholic cirrhotics are no different from those of normal subjects. Ketogenesis and gluconeogenesis are increased, probably reflecting the mobilization of peripheral fats and amino acids and resulting in the typical wasted appearance of patients with advanced cirrhosis.[179] Abnormally high insulin levels due to hypersecretion and reduced hepatic clearance are not associated with the usual inverse relationship and peripheral branched-chain amino acid levels in cirrhotics. Peripheral insulin resistance may account for this abnormality.[180] A protein intake of 0.8 to 1 g/kg of body weight with branched chain or branched chain–enriched formulas by oral or parenteral means is appropriate. Lipoprotein metabolism is disturbed in severe hepatic insufficiency. The major defects appear to be due to impaired triglyceride release by the liver rather than to disturbances of peripheral fat oxidation; lipid emulsions therefore are probably contraindicated in patients who have advanced, severe, acute liver disease. Supplementation with folic acid, vitamins B_6 and B_{12}, and multivitamins is rational. A trial of parenteral vitamin K administration when low prothrombin levels exist is common.

Clinically significant vitamin B deficiency has been demonstrated in alcoholic patients with macrocytosis, megaloblastic changes, or microcytic anemia associated with low serum folate levels, and peripheral neuropathy is often associated with low thiamine levels; nicotinic acid and riboflavin deficiencies are often seen.[181] Septi-cemia frequently may accompany end-stage cirrhosis, resulting in metabolic stress.[180]

Hepatic Encephalopathy

Hepatic encephalopathy occurs as a syndrome of impaired mental function in the setting of severe, acute, or chronic liver disease. Factors that contribute to it are multiple, and they differ depending on the clinical circumstances. The diagnosis is based on clinical features, including disturbed consciousness, which ranges from sleepiness to coma and occasionally delirium. Personality changes are most remarkable in patients who have chronic liver disease. It may be difficult to differentiate the effects of alcohol from those of hepatic encephalopathy. Specialized testing may be needed in mild cases. With advanced disease, there is gross confusion, disturbed speech, and a flapping tremor. Hepatic coma is graded on a scale of 1 through 5:

- grade 1, confused state with altered mood and behavior with psychometric defects
- grade 2, drowsiness and inappropriate behavior
- grade 3, stupor, inability to obey simple commands, inarticulate speech, marked confusion
- grade 4, coma
- grade 5, deep coma, no response to painful stimuli

In fulminant hepatic failure, the syndrome is due to liver cell necrosis. In cirrhosis, it is due to portosystemic shunting with other precipitating factors. In fulminant hepatic failure, the finding of hepatic encephalopathy indicates a very poor prognosis, although the symptoms are reversible if the liver recovers. In cirrhosis, the reversibility depends on the inciting factors. These findings suggest that a metabolic agent or agents interfere with normal cerebral activity. The specific nature and mechanism of action is unknown.

Current theories of hepatic encephalopathy are based on the hypotheses that the agent is nitrogenous; arises from the colon as a result of intestinal bacterial action; is present in the portal venous system; normally would be metabolized by the liver; and, under the clinical circumstances of hepatic encephalopathy, is able to enter the brain and impair function. In fulminant hepatic failure, the liver cells are unable to metabolize the agent. In cirrhotic liver, blood bypasses the liver by portal-systemic shunting. Candidate toxins include amino acids (eg, methionine), aromatic amino acids, and gamma-aminobutyric acid. The production of these agents and their transport to and into the brain, as well as brain function, can be modified by serum amino acid imbalance, alkalosis, and hypoxemia.

Treatment of hepatic encephalopathy is pragmatic. Medical measures are directed at precipitating factors and at identifying and treating sources of infection, gastrointestinal bleeding, and electrolyte disturbances. Toxic medications and alcohol are withdrawn. Sources of nitrogen load are eliminated or reduced. If excess nitrogen is suspected in the intestines, they are purged; diuretics are discontinued, and antibiotics may be administered to decrease bacterial ammonia production. The synthetic disaccharide lactulose is not digested by the human intestinal mucosa but is broken down by colonic bacteria to produce fatty acids, yielding a low fecal pH; it alters colonic bacterial populations to reduce ammonia production. Although the mechanism of action is uncertain, total fecal output is increased, as well as fecal nitrogen.

While these measures are undertaken, dietary protein is discontinued, and calories are provided in carbohydrate form intravenously or by enteral feeding tube. As the patient improves, protein is added in 20 g increments on alternate days in divided doses of four meals. In chronic encephalopathic patients, it may be necessary to restrict protein intake. The appropriateness of vegetable instead of meat protein diets is controversial, but some authors have demonstrated advantages.[183,184] The ratio of branched-chain to aromatic amino acids is reduced in hepatic encephalopathy, and infusions of branched-chain acids have been used in its treatment, but it is difficult to justify their use except in patients with encephalopathy re-

fractory to all other forms of treatment, given their high cost.

Ascites

The formation of cirrhotic ascites is another serious manifestation of liver failure. The accumulation of a protein-rich fluid in the peritoneal cavity occurs as a result of venous outflow obstruction in the liver. This results in an elevated hydrostatic pressure of the liver sinusoid, transudation of plasma into the space of disse, and increased liver lymph flow. When the capacity of the lymphatic system is exceeded, fluid begins to accumulate in the peritoneal cavity. Factors contributing to the shift of fluid include low levels of plasma albumin, resulting in a low plasma oncotic pressure. In response to baroreceptors in the liver, the kidney is less able to excrete a salt load, which results in a net retention of sodium. A second alteration in renal function is impaired excretion of water loads. This multiple-organ-system dysfunction in patients with advanced cirrhotic ascites makes patient management and dietary treatment complex.

Although the presence of ascites dictates the need to determine its exact cause and to exclude other treatable disorders, the presence of ascites *per se* does not demand treatment. When ascites is massive or tense, it can interfere with respiration, can cause discomfort, and (when extreme) can contribute to herniation and necrosis of the umbilicus, resulting in spontaneous rupture and death. A traditional approach to the treatment of ascites involves a therapeutic trial of bed rest and sodium restriction. When a careful history reveals a recent substantial increase in salt intake or exacerbation of a reversible liver disease, the prognosis for response is quite good. However, patients with cirrhotic ascites require a more substantial restriction of sodium intake than do typical patients with heart disease. Restrictions as low as 250 to 500 mg of sodium per day are often required. This represents a significant challenge to meeting other dietary goals.

If diuresis is not evident within several days, the diuretic spironolactone may be effective in nonazotemic patients. In addition to azotemia, hyper-

kalemia may limit the usefulness of spironolactone, and often furosemide is given as well to
decrease hyperkalemia and promote diuresis.
Patients taking spironolactone should not use
potassium-containing salt substitutes because of
this potential complication. Weight loss should be
limited to 1 kg/d. Patients with peripheral edema
can tolerate a large volume. In addition to the dietary restriction of salt, at least 50 g of high-
biologic protein and a 2000 kcal/d diet are usually
recommended. Fluid restriction is not required unless serum sodium levels are below 130 mmol/L.

One treatment that is regaining popularity is
large-volume paracentesis. A volume of 4 to 6 L of
fluid (and perhaps much more) can be withdrawn
safely with fewer complications than occur with
standard diuretic programs. In patients without peripheral edema, albumin infusions are necessary
to prevent volume contraction and azotemia. Fluid
is withdrawn over 20 to 30 minutes and is followed
by an infusion of 6 to 8 g of salt-poor albumin per
liter of ascites fluid removed. The advantages of
this approach are that it can be accomplished in an
outpatient setting with less utilization of hospital
resources. The goals of nutritional management
are to ensure adequate dietary intake with salt restriction to avoid recurrence, although some patients are able to eliminate salt and water loads
more effectively as treatment progresses.

COLON

Like the gallbladder and the appendix, the
colon is not essential for health and well-being.
However, for many older people, the colon is a
major source of symptoms and disease. The most
important function of the colon is its role as a
reservoir and final processor of fecal residue.
Water, electrolytes, bile salts, and short-chain
fatty acids are absorbed. Of the physiologic
processes of motility, secretion, and absorption,
movement disorders predominate.

Little is known about age-related alterations
in structure and function of the colon. Biopsy
specimens from healthy older subjects have
demonstrated mucosal atrophy, alteration of mucosal glands, muscularis mucosa hypertrophy,

increased connective tissue, and changes of atherosclerosis.[185] Electron microscopic cytologic
changes in nuclei, cytoplasm, and cell organelles
have also been noted but are of questionable significance. The most significant functional
change that occurs with aging is constipation;
the most important morphologic change is diverticular disease.

Constipation

Two mechanisms of chronic constipation are
known: colon dysmotility and disordered defecation. Contributing causes include drug effects,
neurologic disease, structural abnormalities, and
systemic disease. Although constipation often is
attributed to diet, behavior, and inactivity, it is a
condition of multiple causes. It is a symptomatic
disease with decreased frequency of bowel movements, difficult passage, passage of hard stools,
or a sensation of incomplete evacuation. In nonconstipated adults, intestinal transit time does not
appear to be increased with advancing age.[185]
However, colonic transit times may be increased
in older adults.[186] Normal bowel habits range
from two per day to three per week.[187] Overall
bowel habits and stool outputs of older adults are
not significantly different than in the young.[188]
About 30% of aged women use laxatives regularly. Frequent laxative use has been attributed to
social attitudes brought about by popular mis-
conceptions in the early part of the 20th century.
Older people who chronically consume laxatives
have demonstrated prolonged transit time as well
as electromyographic and physiologic changes in
colorectal and anal function.[189,190]

Postprandial sigmoid, rectosigmoid, and rectal
motility in healthy older people are not altered.[191]
Abnormalities of anorectal function in older persons include decreased maximal basal and squeeze
pressures of the anal canal; higher rectal pressures
with distention; reduced tolerance for rectal distention; and progressive neuropathic damage to the
nerves of the anal sphincters, which occurs most
frequently in women and is probably related to
childbirth. Many of these factors also contribute to
the risk of incontinence in older people.[192]

A strategy for the effective treatment of chronic constipation involves a careful diagnostic classification and search for underlying and complicating factors. Patients with slow-transit constipation, established by a prolonged colonic transit study, and normal colonic anatomy have either colonic atonia with retention of markers in the right colon or outlet dysfunction with delay of rectosigmoid emptying.[193] Some of these patients may actually suffer from a neuropathic disorder similar to the functional abnormalities found in the esophagus, proximal gastrointestinal tract, and bladder.[194] Patients with outlet dysfunction due to impaired sensory perception or disturbances of anatomy that cause impaired expulsion do not respond to laxatives. These patients may respond to biofeedback or surgical procedures. If transit studies suggest outlet obstruction, further diagnostic evaluation of anorectal physiology is necessary. Patients with normal-transit constipation have either a defecatory disorder or a misperception of what normal bowel function should be.[195,196]

Dietary treatment of constipation invariably involves the addition of dietary or supplemental fiber.[197] An increase of 25% to 40% in fiber intake is accompanied by prevention or elimination of constipation in up to 60% of patients; transit time is also reduced. An intake of 10 to 20 g of bran daily usually is required; initially this almost invariably causes altered bowel habits, distention, and occasional discomfort. Stool bulking is contraindicated in patients who are severely debilitated or who have obstruction as an element of their disease. Coarse bran has a greater laxative effect than fine bran. The concept that the water-holding capacity of bran is the mechanism by which it works may not be true because similar modifications of stool consistency, weight, and ease of passage were experienced by subjects taking indigestible plastic particles. For older patients who have taken laxatives for years, it is not reasonable to adhere slavishly to a concept of fiber supplementation without laxatives when results of therapeutic efforts dictate otherwise.

When bran supplementation is impractical, preparations containing psyllium seed at a dosage of 1 teaspoon twice daily as a hydrophilic agent are effective when accompanied by generous amounts of fluid. The dosage may be slowly increased and titrated to the desired effect. Since these agents can obstruct the esophagus, they should be avoided in patients with dysphagia or known esophageal strictures. Sugar-containing supplements may alter diabetic control. Many other laxatives commonly used may lead to a cathartic colon or toxic systemic effects. Lactulose may be used, but mineral oil is not recommended because of its interference with fat-soluble vitamin absorption and its potential for pulmonary aspiration. Anthracine purgatives are known to cause degeneration of the myoneural chains of the colon. Nonabsorbable osmotic agents such as lactulose are preferable agents to use if a laxative is needed.

Diverticulosis

Diverticulosis is a common disorder of older individuals, occurring in 30% of those older than 60 years and 60% of those older than 80 years.[198] The disease is usually asymptomatic. Symptomatic uncomplicated diverticulosis is thought to be essentially the same as irritable bowel syndrome. Diverticulitis is an inflammatory disease that causes obstruction, abdominal pain, and/or bleeding. Most pathophysiologic concepts have included the idea of a specific motility disorder resulting in increased intraluminal pressure. Although diverticulosis increases in frequency with age, among active older people there is no difference in fecal output.[199] There has been no demonstrated increased sigmoid colon pressure with age. Although muscular layers are greatly thickened in diverticular disease, the morphology of muscle cells is normal. There is no evidence that intrinsic changes in muscle cells account for the thickening associated with diverticulosis. There is a progressive elastosis of the taeniae coli compared with normal structures, which supports the concept of a shortening or contracture of the colon as an initiating factor in the development of diverticulosis. This results in a greater cross-section mass of both longitudinal and circular muscle fibers of the muscularis propria. The luminal dimensions are decreased, and therefore higher pressures can be developed with contraction of these circular muscle folds. The length of the taeniae do respond to fecal bulk. Rural Africans consuming a high-fiber diet have a redundant sigmoid colon with a generous lumen.

The usual dietary measures prescribed in diverticulosis are identical with those used in the treatment of irritable bowel syndrome or chronic constipation. Small, undigestable foods such as seeds or nuts are not recommended, as they may obstruct the orifice of a diverticulum and contribute to diverticulitis. Patients with high levels of sigmoid colon obstruction or stenoses, like their constipated cohorts, may be intolerant of usual amounts of dietary or supplementary fibers, so that symptoms of constipation may need to be treated somewhat independently.

Anorectal Functioning and Fecal Incontinence

Few studies in the literature address issues of anorectal functioning in healthy older adults. As is the case with the evaluation of GI motility in this population, the results are conflicting due to differences in methodology as well as the number and composition of elderly subjects. Evidence would support the presence of a decrease in both resting and squeeze pressures in the anal canal. In a study by McHugh and Diamant,[200] 157 healthy volunteers ranging in age from 20 to 89 years were evaluated, with 74 subjects over the age of 50 years. This is perhaps the most comprehensive study that has been published, and it shows a decline in both resting and anal canal squeeze pressures with age. Similar results have been reported by Akervall and colleagues.[201] There are conflicting data with regard to whether or not there is a loss of rectal sensation with aging. In a study by Loening-Baucke and Anuras[192] and in another study by Read and colleagues[196] using rectal infusion of saline until the first sensation and the first leak occur, no differences were found in older adults with regard to sensory functioning.[192,196]

However, it has been noted that the threshold sensation for rectal filling does increase with age.[201]

Anorectal dysfunction is commonly noted in patients with fecal incontinence, and this is a very common problem in older adults. Estimates of the prevalence of incontinence in the older adult population vary widely, but clearly this is more common in older adults.[202] It is a common cause of institutionalization and is a symptom in nursing homes. The prevalence of fecal incontinence in institutionalized older adults has been estimated to be between 30% and 60%.[203] It is likely that the aforementioned alterations in anal functioning and the reported deficits in the ability of these patients to detect rectal filling would contribute substantially to the development of anal incontinence in older adults.

CONCLUSION

Although changes in structure and function of the gastrointestinal tract do occur with aging, they do not seem to be clinically significant in the healthy older population. Enzyme and bicarbonate secretions by the pancreas are diminished; whether this is a result of lessened or faulty enteral stimulation or intrinsic age-related pancreatic insufficiency is not clinically relevant because of the huge pancreatic secretory reserve. Mucosal regeneration of the small bowel is accompanied by functional enzyme-related differentiation, which has been noted to be reduced in laboratory animals, but it does not approach clinical significance, nor has it been demonstrated to be important in human studies. Alteration in motility could have far-reaching effects, but to date clinical problems appear to be caused by disease rather than aging. Alterations resulting from disease have to be the focus for the diagnosis and treatment of malnutrition in the setting of gastrointestinal dysfunction in the older adult.

Chewing and swallowing problems are the most easily recognized causes of nutritional failure because of poor intake, notwithstanding the frequent drug-induced alterations of taste, nausea, or disturbed mood or attention, which also reduce intake. Simple clinical observations can identify these disorders and lead to appropriate diagnostic studies to enable treatment plans. Disturbances of digestion and absorption in the midgut are more occult and difficult to differentiate. A knowledgeable diagnostic approach based on pathophysiologic principles often requires treatment by trial and error when multiple problems exist. Here the collaboration of the dietitian and physician is most important.

The effects of functional gastrointestinal disorders, such as constipation, on dietary intake are difficult to quantify. A lifetime of learned behavior can exasperate attempts at a very scientific approach and necessitate a practical and compromising plan for successful management to include good nutrition goals. In the care of the very old, ethical and spiritual issues may come to dominate the theme of respectful care.

REFERENCES

1. Goyns MH. Genes, telomeres and mammalian ageing. *Mech Aging Dev* 2002;123:791–799.

2. Elson JL, Samuels DC, Turnbull DM, Chinnery PF. Random intracellular drift explains the clonal expansion of mitochondrial DNA mutations with age. *Am J Hum Genet* 2001;68:802–806.

3. Verdu E, Ceballos M, Vilches JJ, Navaroo X. Influence of aging on peripheral nerve function and regeneration. *J Peripher Nerv Syst* 2000;5:191–208.

4. Shaker R, Ren J, Zamir Z, Sarna A, Liu J, Sui Z. Effect of aging, position, and temperature on the threshold volume triggering pharyngeal swallows. *Gastroenterology* 1994;107:396–402.

5. Siebens H, Trupe MA, Hilary A, et al. Correlates and consequences of eating dependency in institutionalized elderly. *J Am Geriatr Soc* 1986;34:192–198.

6. Dorff GL, Rytel MW, Farmer SG, et al. Etiologies and characteristic features of pneumonias in a municipal hospital. *Am J Med Sci* 1973;266:349–358.

7. Ebright JR, Rytel MW. Bacterial pneumonia in the elderly. *J Am Geriatr Soc* 1980;28:220.

8. Ravich WJ. Classification of dysphagia on the basis of the clinical examination. In: *Second Symposium on Dysphagia*. Baltimore, MD: Johns Hopkins Swallowing Center; March 1988.

9. Robbins J. Approaches to rehabilitation of neurogenic dysphagia. In: *Second Symposium on Dysphagia*. Baltimore, MD: Johns Hopkins Swallowing Center; March 1988.

10. Bloem BR, Lagaay AM, van Beek W, Haan J, Roos RA, Wintzen AR. Prevalence of subjective dysphagia in community residents aged over 87. *Br Med J* 1990;300: 721–722.

11. Lindgren S, Janzon L. Prevalence of swallowing complaints and clinical findings among 50–79 year old men and women in an urban population. *Dysphagia* 1991;6: 187–192.

12. Siebens H, Trupe E, Siebens A, Cook F, Anshen S, Hanauer R, Oster G. Correlates and consequences of eating dependency in institutionalized elderly. *J Amer Geriatr Soc* 1986;34:192–198.

13. Croghan JE, Burke EM, Caplan S, Denman S. Pilot study of 12-month outcomes of nursing home patients with aspiration on videofluoroscopy. *Dysphagia* 1994; 9:141–146.

14. Hollis JB, Castell DO. Esophageal function in elderly men. A new look at "presbyesophagus." *Ann Intern Med* 1974;80:371–374.

15. Fulp SR, Dalton CB, Castell JA, Castell DO. Aging-related alterations in human upper esophageal sphincter function. *Am J Gastroenterol* 1990;85:1569–1572.

16. Shaker R, Ren J, Podvrsan B, et al. Effect of aging and bolus variables on pharyngeal and upper esophageal sphincter motor function. *Am J Physiol Gastrointestinal Liver Physiol* 1993;264:G427–G432.

17. Aviv JE, Martin JH, Jones ME, et al. Age related changes in pharyngeal and supraglottic sensation. *Ann Otol Rhin Laryngol* 1994;103:749–752.

18. Shaker R, Staff D. Esophageal disorders in the elderly. *Gastroenterology Clin N Amer* 2001;30:335–361.

19. Castell DO. Esophageal disorders in the elderly. *Gastroenterology Clin N Amer* 1990;19:235–254.

20. Kahrilas PJ, Dodds WJ, Hogan WJ. Effect of peristaltic dysfunction on esophageal column clearance. *Gastroenterology* 1988;94:73–80.

21. Krue-Anderson S, Wallin L, Madsen T. The influence of age on esophageal acid defense mechanism and spontaneous acid gastroesophageal reflux. *Am J Gastroenterol* 1988;83:637–639.

22. Adamek RJ, Wegener M, Weinbeck M, Gielen B. Long term esophageal manometry in healthy subjects. Evaluation of normal values and influences of age. *Dig Dis Sci* 1994;39:2069–2073.

23. Raiha I, Impivaara O, Seppala M, Sourander LB. Prevalence and characteristics of symptomatic gastroesophageal reflux disease in the elderly. *J Amer Geriatr Soc* 1992;40:1209–1211.

24. Smout A, Breedijk M, van der Zouw C, Akkermans LM. Physiological gastro-esophageal reflux and esophageal motor activity studied with a new system for 24-hour recording and automated analysis. *Dig Dis Sci* 1989;34:372–378.

25. DeVault KR, Castell DO. Updated guidelines for the diagnosis and treatment of gastroesophageal reflux disease. The Practice Parameters Committee of the American College of Gastroenterology. *Am J Gastroenterol* 1999;94:1434–1442.

26. Vigneri S, Termini R, Leandro G, et al. A comparison of five maintenance therapies for reflux esophagitis. *N Engl J Med* 1995;333:1106–1110.

27. Brunt LM, Quasebarth MA, Dunnegan DL, et al. Is laparoscopic antireflux surgery for gastroesophageal reflux disease in the elderly safe and effective? *Surg Endosc* 1999;13:838–842.

28. Trus TL, Laycock WS, Wo JM, et al. Laparoscopic antireflux surgery in the elderly. *Am J Gastroenterol* 1998; 93:351–353.

29. Kekki M, Sipponen P, Siurala M. Age behavior of gastric acid secretion in males and females with a normal antral body and body mucosa. *Scand J Gastroenterol* 1983;18:1009–1016.

30. Hurwitz A, Brady DA, Schaal E, Samloff IM, Dedon J, Ruhl CE. Gastric acidity in older adults. *JAMA* 1997; 278:659–662.

31. Ekberg O, Feinberg MJ. Altered swallowing function in elderly patients without dysphagia. *Am J Roentgenol* 1991;156:1181–1184.

32. Strickland R, Mackay IR. A reappraisal of the nature and significance of chronic atrophic gastritis. *Dig Dis Sci* 1973;18:426–437.

33. Siurala M, Isokoski M, Varis K, et al. Prevalence of gastritis in a rural population: bioptic study of subjects selected at random. *Scand J Gastroenterol* 1968;3:211–223.

34. Krasinski SD, Russell RM, Samloff IM, et al. Fundic atrophic gastritis in an elderly population: effect on hemoglobin and several serum nutritional indicators. *J Am Geriatr Soc* 1986;34(11):800–806.

35. Saltzman JR, Kowdley KV. The consequences of *Helicobacter pylori* infection and gastritis. *Contemp Intern Med* 1994;6:7–16.

36. Sonneberg A. Changes in physician visits for gastric and duodenal ulcer in the United States during 1958–1984 as shown by National Disease and Therapeutic Index. *Dig Dis Sci* 1987;32:1–7.

37. Walt R, Katschinski B, Logan R, et al. Rising frequency of ulcer perforation in elderly people in the United Kingdom. *Lancet* 1986;1:489–492.

38. Myren J. The natural history of peptic ulcer views in the 1980s. *Scand J Gastroenterol* 1983;18:993–997.

39. Gerbino PP, Gans JA. Antacids and laxatives for symptomatic relief in the elderly. *J Am Geriatr Soc* 1982;30: 581–585.

40. Girotti MJ, Ruddan J, Cohanim M. Amphojeloma: antacid impaction in critically ill patients. *Can J Surg* 1984;27(4):379–380.

41. Godsall JW, Baron R, Insogna KL, et al. Vitamin D metabolism in bone histomorphometry in a patient with antacid induced osteomalacia. *Am J Med* 1984;77: 747–750.

42. Baum C, Kennedy DL, Forbes MB, et al. Drug utilization in the geriatric age group. In: Moore SR, Teal TW, eds *Geriatric Drug Use: Clinical and Social Perspectives,* New York: Pergamon Press; 1985:63–69.

43. Baum C, Kennedy DL, Forbes MB. Utilization of nonsteroidal anti-inflammatory drugs. *Arthritis Rheum* 1985;28:686–692.

44. Coles LS, Fries JK, Kraines RG, et al. From experiment to experience: side effects of nonsteroidal anti-inflammatory drugs. *Am J Med* 1983;74:820–828.

45. Silvoso GR, Ivey KJ, Butt JH, et al. Incidence of gastric lesions in patients with rheumatic disease on chronic aspirin therapy. *Ann Intern Med* 1979; 91:517–520.

46. Bartle WR, Gupta AK, Lazor J. Nonsteroidal anti-inflammatory drugs and gastrointestinal bleeding: a case-control study. *Arch Intern Med* 1986;146:2365–2367.

47. Minami H, McCallum RW. The physiology and pathophysiology of gastric emptying in humans. *Gastroenterology* 1984;86:1592–1610.

48. Moore JG, Tweedy C, Christian PE, et al. Effect of age on gastric emptying of liquid solid meals in man. *Dig Dis Sci* 1983;28:340–344.

49. Frank EB, Lange R, McCallum RW. Abnormal gastric emptying in patients with atrophic gastritis with or without pernicious anemia. *Gastroenterology* 1981;80: 1151.

50. Kupfer RM, Heppell M, Haggith JW, et al. Gastric emptying and small bowel transit rate in the elderly. *J Am Geriatr Soc* 1985;33:340–343.

51. Fich A, Camilleri M, Phillips SF. Effect of age on human gastric and small bowel motility. *J Clin Gastroenterol* 1989;11:416–420.

52. Firth M, Pranterh CM. Gastrointestinal motility problems in the elderly patient. *Gastroenterology* 2002;122: 1688–1700.

53. Agreus L, Talley N. Challenges in managing dyspepsia in general practice. *Br Med J* 1997;315:1284–1288.

54. Talley N, Silverstein MD, Agreus L, Nyren O, Sonnenberg A, Holman G. AGA Technical review: evaluation of dyspepsia. American Gastroenterological Association. *Gastroenterology* 1998;114:582–595.

55. Drossman D, Corazziari E, Talley N. Rome II: A multinational consensus document on functional gastrointestinal disorders. *Gut* 1999;45:II1–II81.

56. Talley NJ, O'Keefe EA, Zinsmeister AR, Melton LJ III. Prevalence of gastrointestinal symptoms in the elderly: a population-based study. *Gastroenterology* 1992;102: 895–901.

57. Kay L. Prevalence, incidence and prognosis of gastrointestinal symptoms in a random sample of an elderly population. *Age Ageing* 1994;23:146–149.

58. Kay L, Avlund K. Abdominal syndromes and functional ability in the elderly. *Aging (Milano)* 1994;6:420–426.

59. Locke G, Yawn B, Wollan P, Wydick E. The incidence of clinically diagnosed irritable bowel syndrome in the community (abstr). *Gastroenterology* 1999;116:GO325.

60. Talley NJ, Evans JM, Fleming KC, Harmsen WS, Zinsmeister AR, Melton LJ III. Nonsteroidal antiinflammatory drugs and dyspepsia in the elderly. *Dig Dis Sci* 1995;40:1345–1350.

61. Jones RH, Tait CL. Gastrointestinal side-effects of NSAIDs in the community. *Br J Clin Pract* 1995;49:67–70.

62. Laugier R, Sarles H. The pancreas. *Clin Gastroenterol* 1985;14:749–756.

63. Kreel L, Scandin B. Changes in pancreatic morphology associated with aging. *Gut* 1973;14:962–970.

64. Schmitz-Moorman P, Himmelmann GW, Brandes JW, et al. Comparative radiological and morphological study of the human pancreas: pancreatitis like changes in post-mortem ductograms and their morphological pattern. *Gut* 1985;26:406–414.

65. Snook JT. Effect of age and long-term diet on exocrine pancreas of the rat. *Am J Physiol* 1975;228:262–268.

66. Kim SK, Weinhold PA, Catkins DWI, et al. Comparative studies of the age-related changes in protein synthesis in the rat pancreas and parotid gland. *Exp Gerontol* 1981;16:91–99.

67. Greenberg RE, Holt PR. Influence of aging upon pancreatic digestive enzymes. *Dig Dis Sci* 1986;31:970–977.

68. Greenberg RE, McCann PP, Holt PR. Trophic responses of the pancreas differ in aging rats. *Pancreas* 1988;3:311–316.

69. Fenyo G. Acute abdominal diseases in the elderly: experience from two series in Stockholm. *Am J Surg* 1982;143:751–754.

70. Bourke JB, Mead GM, McIllmurray MB, et al. Drug associated primary acute pancreatitis. *Lancet* 1978;1:706–708.

71. Ranson JH, Pasternack BS. Statistical methods for quantifying for severity of clinical acute pancreatitis. *J Surg Res* 1977;22:79–91.

72. Walsh TN, Rode J, Theis BA, Russell RC. Minimal change chronic pancreatitis. *Gut* 1992;33:1566–1571.

73. DiMagno EP, Malagelada JR, Go VL. Relationship between alcoholism and pancreatic insufficiency. *Ann NY Acad Sci* 1975;252:200–207.

74. Mackie RD, Levine AS, Levitt MD. Malabsorption of starch in pancreatic insufficiency. [Abstract]. *Gastroenterology* 1981;80:1220.

75. Toskes PP, Greenberger NJ. Acute and chronic pancreatitis. *Dis Mon* 1983;29:1–81.

76. Dutta SK, Bustin MP, Russell RM, et al. Deficiency of fat-soluble vitamins in treated patients with pancreatic insufficiency. *Ann Intern Med* 1982;97:549–552.

77. Lankisch PG, Creutzfeldt W. Therapy of exocrine and endocrine pancreatic insufficiency. *Clin Gastroenterol* 1984;13:985–999.

78. Lipski PS, Bennett MK, Kelly PJ, James OFW. Aging and duodenal morphometry. *J Clin Pathol* 1992;45:450–452.

79. Holt PR, Kotler DP, Pascal RR. Delayed enterocyte differentiation: a defect in aging rat jejunum. *Clin Res* 1982;30:496A.

80. Saltzman JR, Kowdley KV, Perrone G, Russell RM. Changes in small-intestine permeability with aging. *J Am Geriatr Soc* 1995;43:160–164.

81. Saltzman JR, Russell RM. The aging gut: nutritional issues. *Gastroenterol Clin N Am* 1998;27:309–324.

82. Klimas JE. Intestinal glucose absorption during the life-span of a colony of rats. *J Gerontol* 1968;23:529–532.

83. Calingaert A, Zorzoli A. The influence of age on 6-deoxy-D-glucose by mouse intestine. *J Gerontol* 1965;20:211–214.

84. Feibusch JM, Holt PR. Impaired absorptive capacity for carbohydrate in the aging human. *Dig Dis Sci* 1982;27:1095–1100.

85. Hollander D, Ruble PE Jr. Beta-carotene intestinal absorption: bile, fatty acid, pH and flow rate effects on transport. *Am J Physiol* 1978;235:E686–E691.

86. Holt PR, Dominguez AA. Intestinal absorption of triglyceride and vitamin D3 in aged and young rats. *Dig Dis Sci* 1981;26:1104–1115.

87. Geokas MC, Conteas CN, Majumdar AP. The aging gastrointestinal tract, liver and pancreas. *Clin Geriatr Med* 1985;1:177–205.

88. Werner I, Hambraeus L. The digestive capacity of elderly people. In: Carlson LA, ed. *Nutrition in Old Age.* Uppsala, Sweden: Almquist & Wiksell; 1972:55.

89. Southgate DAT, Durnin JVGA. Calorie conversion factors: an experimental reassessment of the factors used in the calculation of the energy value of human diets. *Br J Nutr* 1970;24:517–535.

90. Arora S, Kassarjian Z, Krasinski S, Croffey B, Kaplan MM, Russell RM. Effect of age on tests of intestinal and hepatic function in healthy humans. *Gastroenterology* 1989;96:1560–1565.

91. Pelz KS, Gottfried SP, Soos E. Intestinal absorption studies in the aged. *Geriatrics* 1968;23:149.

92. Simko C, Michael S. Absorptive capacity for dietary fat in elderly patients with debilitating disorders. *Arch Intern Med* 1989;149:557–560.

93. Cheng AHR, Gomez A, Bergan JG, et al. Comparative nitrogen balance study between young and aged adults using three levels of protein intake from a combination wheat-soy-milk mixture. *Am J Clin Nutr* 1978;31:12–22.

94. Munro HN, McGandy RB, Hartz SC, Russell RM, Jacob RA, Otradovec CL. Protein nutriture of a group of free-living elderly. *Am J Clin Nutr* 1987;46:586–592.

95. Sklar M, Krisner JB, Palmer WL. Gastrointestinal disease in the aged. *Med Clin North Am* 1956;40:223–337.

96. Suter PM, Russell RM. Vitamin requirements of the elderly. *Am J Clin Nutr* 1987;45:501–512.

97. Hollander D, Morgan D. Increase in cholesterol intestinal absorption with aging in the rat. *Exp Gerontol* 1979;14:301–305.

98. Hollander D, Morgan D. Aging: its influence on vitamin A intestinal absorption *in vivo* by the rat. *Exp Gerontol* 1979;14:301–305.

99. Hollander D, Dadufalza VD, Sletten EG. Does essential fatty acid absorption change in aging? *J Lipid Res* 1984;25:129–134.

100. Krasinski DS, Cohn JS, Schaefer EJ, Russell RM. Postprandial plasma retinyl ester response is greater in older subjects compared with younger subjects. *J Clin Invest* 1990;85:883–892.

101. Webb AR, Kline L, Holick MF. Influence of season and latitude on the cutaneous synthesis of vitamin D3: exposure to winter sunlight in Boston and Edmonton will not promote vitamin D3 synthesis in human skin. *J Clin Endocrinol Metab* 1988;67:373–378.

102. McLaughlin J, Holick MF. Aging decreases the capacity of human skin to produce vitamin D3. *J Clin Invest* 1985;76:1536–1538.

103. Webb AR, Pilbeam C, Hanafln N, Holick MF. An evaluation of the relative contributions of exposure to sunlight and of diet to the circulating concentrations of 25-hydroxyvitamin D in an elderly nursing home population in Boston. *Am J Clin Nutr* 1990;51:1075–1081.

104. Sadowski JA, Hood SJ, Dallal GE, Garry PJ. Phylloquinone in plasma from elderly and young adults: factors influencing its concentration. *Am J Clin Nutr* 1989;50:100–108.

105. Paiva SAR, Sepe TE, Booth SL, et al. The interaction between vitamin K nutriture and bacterial overgrowth in hypochlorhydria induced by omeprazole. *Am J Clin Nutr* 1998;68:699–704.

106. Russell RM, Dhar GJ, Dutta SK, Rosenberg I. Influence of intraluminal pH on folate absorption: studies in control subjects and in patients with pancreatic insufficiency. *J Lab Clin Med* 1979;93:428–436.

107. Selhub J, Jacques PF, Wilson PWF, Rush D, Rosenberg IH. Vitamin status and intake as primary determinants of homocysteinemia in an elderly population. *JAMA* 1993;270:2693–2698.

108. Camilo E, Zimmerman J, Mason JB, et al. Folate synthesized by bacteria in the upper intestine is assimilated by the host. *Gastroenterology* 1996;110:991–998.

109. Kirsh A, Bidlack WR. Nutrition and the elderly: vitamin status and efficiency of supplementation. *Nutrition* 1987;3:305.

110. Ribaya-Mercado JD, Russell RM, Sahyoun N, et al. Vitamin B6 requirements of elderly men and women. *J Nutr* 1991;121:1062–1074.

111. Verhoef P, Stamfer MJ, Buring JE, et al. Homocysteine metabolism and risk of myocardial infarction: relation with vitamin B_6, B_{12} and folate. *Am J Epidemiol* 1996;143:845–859.

112. Carmel R, Sinow R, Siegel M, Samloff M. Food cobalamin malabsorption occurs infrequently in patients with unexplained low serum cobalamin levels. *Arch Intern Med* 1988;148:1715–1719.

113. King C, Leibach J, Toskes P. Clinically significant vitamin B_{12} deficiency secondary to malabsorption of protein-bound vitamin B_{12}. *Dig Dis Sci* 1979;24:397–402.

114. Saltzman JR, Kemp JA, Golner BB, Pedrosa MC, Dallal GE, Russell RM. Effect of hypochlorhydria due to omeprazole treatment or atrophic gastritis on protein-bound vitamin B_{12} absorption. *J Am Coll Nutr* 1994;13:584–591.

115. Serfaty-Lacrosniere CS, Wood RJ, Voytko D, et al. Hypochlorhydria from short-term omeprazole treatment does not inhibit intestinal absorption of calcium, phosphorus, magnesium or zinc from food in humans. *J Am Coll Nutr* 1995;14;364–368.

116. Suter PM, Golner BB, Goldin BR, et al. Reversal of protein-bound vitamin B_2 malabsorption with antibiotics in atrophic gastritis. *Gastroenterology* 1991;101:1039–1045.

117. Nelson, JB, Casteli DO. Effects of aging on gastrointestinal physiology. *Pract Gastroenterol* 1988;12:28–35.

118. Marx JJM. Normal iron absorption and decreased cell iron uptake in the aged. *Blood* 1979;53:204–211.

119. Jacobs P, Bothwell T, Charlton RW. Role of hydrochloric acid in iron absorption. *J Appl Physiol* 1964;19:187–188.

120. Gallagher JC, Riggs BL, Eisman J, Hamstra A, Arnaud SB, DeLuca HF. Intestinal calcium absorption and serum vitamin D metabolites in normal subjects and osteoporotic patients. *J Clin Invest* 1979;64:729–736.

121. Dawson-Hughes B, Jacques P, Shipp S. Dietary calcium intake and bone loss from the spine in healthy postmenopausal woman. *Am J Clin Nutr* 1987;46:685–687.

122. Dawson-Hughes B, Dallal GE, Krall EA, Sadowski L, Sahyoun N, Tannenbaum S. A controlled trial of the effect of calcium supplementation of bone density on postmenopausal women. *N Engl J Med* 1990;323:878–883.

123. Knox TA, Kassarjian Z, Dawson-Hughes B, et al. Calcium absorption in elderly subjects on high and low fiber diets: effect of gastric acidity. *Am J Clin Nutr* 1991;53:1480–1486.

124. Husebye E, Engedal K. The patterns of motility are maintained in the human small intestine throughout the process of aging. *Scand J Gastroenterol* 1992;27:397.

125. Montgomery RD, Hainey MR, Ross IN, et al. The aging gut: a study of intestinal absorption in relation to nutrition in the elderly. *Q J Med* 1978;47:197–211.

126. Price HL, Gazzard BG, Dawson AM. Steatorrhea in the elderly. *Br Med J* 1977;1:1582–1584.

127. Bayless TM, Rothfeld B, Massa C, et al. Lactose and milk intolerance: clinical implications. *N Engl J Med* 1975;292:1156–1159.

128. Bond JH, Levitt MD. Use of breath hydrogen (H_2) in the study of carbohydrate absorption. *Am J Dig Dis* 1977;22:379–382.

129. Vincenzini MT, Iantomasi T, Stio M, et al. Glucose transport during aging in human intestinal brush-border membrane vesicles. *Mech Aging Dev* 1989;48:33–41.

130. Trier JS. Celiac sprue. *N Engl J Med* 1991;325:1709–1719.

131. Hallett C, Gothard R, Norrby K, et al. On the prevalence of adult coeliac disease in Sweden. *Scand J Gastroenterol* 1981;16:257–261.

132. Fine KD. The prevalence of occult gastrointestinal bleeding in celiac sprue. *N Engl J Med* 1996;334:1163–1167.

133. Friis SU, Gudmand-Hoyer E. Screening for coeliac disease in adults by simultaneous determination of IgA and IgG antibodies. *Scand J Gastroenterol* 1986;21:1058–1062.

134. Pena AS, Truelove SC, Whitehead R. Disaccharidase activity and jejunal morphology in coeliac disease. *Q J Med* 1972;41:457–476.

135. Saltzman JR, Kowdley KV, Pedrosa MC, et al. Bacterial overgrowth without clinical malabsorption in elderly hypochlorhydric subjects. *Gastroenterology* 1994;106:615–623.

136. Isaacs PET, Kim YS. The contaminated small bowel syndrome. *Am J Med* 1979;67:1049–1057.

137. Brandt LJ, Boley S, Goldberg L, et al. Colitis in the elderly: a reappraisal. *Am J Gastroenterol* 1981;76:239–245.

138. Mayberry JF, Ballantyne KC, Hardcastle JD, et al. Epidemiologic study of asymptomatic inflammatory bowel disease: the identification of cases during a screening program for colorectal cancer. *Gut* 1989;30:481–483.

139. Tedesco FJ, Hardin RD, Harper RN, et al. Infectious colitis endoscopically simulating inflammatory bowel disease: a prospective evaluation. *Gastrointest Endosc* 1983;29:195–197.

140. Brandt LJ, Boley SJ, Mitsudo S. Clinical characteristics and natural history of colitis in the elderly. *Am J Gastroenterol* 1982;77:382–386.

141. Joslin CA, Smith CW, Malik A. The treatment of cervix cancer using high activity cobalt-60 sources. *Br J Radiol* 1972;45:247–270.

142. Yeoh EK, Horowitz M. Radiation enteritis. *Surg Gynecol Obstet* 1987;165:373–379.

143. O'Brien PH, Jenrette JM III, Garvin AJ. Radiation enteritis. *Am Surg* 1987;53:501–504.

144. Cox JD, Byhardt RW, Wilson F, et al. Complications of radiation therapy and factors in their prevention. *World J Surg* 1986;10:171–188.

145. Galland RB, Spencer J. Surgical management of radiation enteritis. *Surgery* 1986;99:133–138.

146. Harling H, Balslev IB. Radical surgical approach to radiation injury of the small bowel. *Dis Colon Rectum* 1986;29:371–372.

147. Arlow FL, Dekovich AA, Priest RJ, et al. Bile acids in radiation-induced diarrhea. *South Med J* 1987;80:1259–1261.

148. McArdle AH, Reid EC, Laplante MP, et al. Prophylaxis against radiation injury. *Arch Surg* 1986;121:879–885.

149. Miller DH, Ivey M, Young J. Home parenteral nutrition in treatment of severe radiation enteritis. *Ann Intern Med* 1979;91:858–860.

150. Galloway NO, Foley CF, Lagerbloom P. Uncertainties in geriatric data, II: organ size. *J Am Geriatr Soc* 1965;13:20–28.

151. Thomas FB, Clausen KP, Geenberger NJ. Liver disease in multiple myeloma. *Arch Intern Med* 1973;132:195–202.

152. Tauchi H, Sato T. Effective environmental conditions upon age changes in the human liver. *Mech Aging Dev* 1975;4:71–80.

153. Bender AD. The effect of increasing age on distribution of peripheral blood flow in man. *J Am Geriatr Soc* 1965;13:192–198.

154. Kitani K. Hepatic drug metabolism in the elderly [Editorial]. *Hepatology* 1986;6:316–319.

155. Crooks J, O'Malley K, Stevenson IH. Pharmacokinetics in the elderly. *Clin Pharmacokinet* 1976;1:280–296.

156. Woodhouse KW, Mutch E, Williams FM, et al. The effect of age on pathways of drug metabolism in human liver. *Age Ageing* 1984;13:328–334.

157. Smithard DJ, Langman MJ. The effect of vitamin supplementation upon antipyrine metabolism in the elderly. *Br J Clin Pharmacol* 1978;5:181–185.

158. Young VR, Steffee WP, Pencharz PB, et al. Total human body protein synthesis in relation to protein requirements at various ages. *Nature* 1975;253:192–194.

159. Geokas MC, Conteas CN, Majumdar AP. The aging gastrointestinal tract, liver, and pancreas. *Clin Geriatr Med* 1985;1:177–205.

160. James OFW. Gastrointestinal and liver function in old age. *Clin Gastroenterol* 1983;12:671–691.

161. Gibinski K, Fajt E, Suchan L. Hepatitis in the aged. *Digestion* 1973;8:254–260.

162. Ludwig J, Baggenstoss AH. Cirrhosis of the aged and senile cirrhosis: are there two conditions? *J Gerontol* 1970;25:244–248.

163. Kaplan M. Primary biliary cirrhosis. *N Engl J Med* 1987;316:521–528.

164. Hislop WS, Hopwood D, Bouchier IA. Primary biliary cirrhosis in elderly females. *Age Ageing* 1982;11:153–159.

165. Lehman AB, Bussendine MF, James OF. Primary biliary cirrhosis: a different disease in the elderly? *Gerontology* 1985;31:186–194.

166. Alpers DH, Sabesin SM. Fatty liver: biochemical and clinical aspects. In: Schiff L, Schiff ER, eds. *Diseases of the Liver,* 6th ed. Philadelphia, PA: JB Lippincott Co; 1987.

167. Lieber CS. Alcohol-nutrition interaction: 1984 update. *Alcohol* 1984;1:151–157.

168. Katz J, McGarry JD. The glucose paradox: is glucose a substrate for liver metabolism? *J Clin Invest* 1984;74:1901–1909.

169. Flores H, Pak N, Maccioni A, et al. Lipid transport in kwashiorkor. *Br J Nutr* 1970;24:1005–1011.

170. Flatt JP. Role of increased adipose tissue mass in the apparent insulin insensitivity of obesity. *Am J Clin Nutr* 1972;25:1189.

171. Atkinson M, Nordin BE, Sherlock S. Malabsorption and bone disease in prolonged obstructive jaundice. *Q J Med* 1956;25:299–312.

172. Ros E, Garcia-Puges A, Reixach M, et al. Fat digestion and exocrine pancreatic function in primary biliary cirrhosis. *Gastroenterology* 1984;87:180–187.

173. Lanspa SJ, Chan AT, Bell JS III, et al. Pathogenesis of steatorrhea in primary biliary cirrhosis. *Hepatology* 1985;5:837–842.

174. Epstein O. Nutritional therapy in women with primary biliary cirrhosis. *Geriatr Med Today* 1983;2(10):48–60.

175. Mezey E. Progress in hepatology: liver disease and nutrition. *Gastroenterology* 1978;74:770–783.

176. Burch RE, Sackin DA, Ursick JA, et al. Decreased taste and smell acuity in cirrhosis. *Arch Intern Med* 1978;138:743–746.

177. Mezey E, Jow E, Slavin RE, et al. Pancreatic function and intestinal absorption in chronic alcoholism. *Gastroenterology* 1970;59:657–664.

178. Mezey E, Potter JJ. Changes in endocrine pancreatic function produced by altered dietary protein intake in drinking alcoholics. *Johns Hopkins Med J* 1976;138(1):7–12.

179. Mezey E. Intestinal function in chronic alcoholism. *Ann NY Acad Sci* 1975;252:215–227.

180. Owen OE, Trapp VE, Reichard GA Jr, et al. Nature and quantity of fuels consumed in patients with alcoholic cirrhosis. *J Clin Invest* 1983;72:1821–1832.

181. Marchesini G, Bianchi G, Zoli M, et al. Plasma amino acid response to protein ingestion in patients with liver cirrhosis. *Gastroenterology* 1983;85:283–290.

182. Leevy CM, Baker H, TenHove W, et al. B complex vitamins in liver disease of the alcoholic. *Am J Clin Nutr* 1965;16:339–346.

183. Uribe M, Marquez MA, Ramos GG, et al. Treatment of chronic portal systemic encephalopathy with vegetable and animal protein diets: a controlled crossover study. *Dig Dis Sci* 1982;27:1109–1116.

184. Jonung T, Jeppsson B, Ashland U, et al. A comparison between meat and vegan protein diet in patients with mild chronic hepatic encephalopathy. *Clin Nutr* 1987;6:169–174.

185. Yamajata A. Histopathological studies of the colon due to age. *Jpn J Gastroenterol* 1965;62:224–235.

186. Melkerson M, Anderson H, Bosaeus I, et al. Intestinal transit time in constipation and nonconstipated geriatric patients. *Scand J Gastroenterol* 1983;18:593–597.

187. Madsen JL. Effects of gender, age and body mass index on gastrointestinal transit times. *Dig Dis Sci* 1992;37:1548–1553.

188. Connell AM, Hilton C, Irvin C. Variations in bowel habit in two population samples. *Br Med J* 1965;2:1095–1099.

189. Marchesini G, Bianchi G, Zoli M, et al. Plasma amino acid response to protein ingestion in patients with liver cirrhosis. *Gastroenterology* 1983;85:282–290.

190. Frieri G, Parisi F, Corazziari E, et al. Colonic electromyography in chronic constipation. *Gastroenterology* 1983;84:737–740.

191. Shoulder P, Keighley MRB. Changes in colorectal function in severe idiopathic chronic constipation. *Gastroenterology* 1986;90:41420.

192. Loening-Baucke V, Apuras S. Sigmoidal and rectal motility in healthy elderly. *J Am Geriatr Soc* 1984;32:887–891.

193. Bannister JJ, Abouzekry L, Read NW. Effect of aging on anorectal function. *Gut* 1987;28:353–357.

194. Martelli H, Devroede G, Arhan P, et al. Mechanisms of idiopathic constipation: outlet obstruction. *Gastroenterology* 1978;75:623–631.

195. Watier A, Devroede G, Duranceau A, et al. Constipation with colonic inertia: a manifestation of systemic disease? *Dig Dis Sci* 1983;28:1025–1033.

196. Read MW, Timms JM. Defecation in the pathophysiology of constipation. *Clin Gastroenterol* 1986;15:937–965.

197. Wald A, Stoney B, Hinds JP. Physiological profiles in patients with constipation associated with normal and slow colonic transit [Abstract]. *Gastroenterology* 1988;95: 892.

198. Hull C, Greco RS, Brooks DL, et al. Alleviation of constipation in the elderly by dietary fibre supplementation. *J Am Geriatr Soc* 1988;28(9):41–44.

199. Parks TG. Natural history of diverticular disease of the colon. *Clin Gastroenterol* 1975;4:53–69.

200. Eastwood MA, Watters DAK, Smith AN. Diverticular disease: is it a motility disorder? *Clin Gastroenterol* 1982;11:545–561.

201. Akervall S, Nirdgren S, Fasth S, et al. The effects of age, gender, and parity on rectoanal functions in adults. *Scan J Gastroenterol* 1990;25:1247–1256.

202. Johanson JF, Lafferty J. Epidemiology of fecal incontinence: the silent affliction. *Am J Gastroenterol* 1996;91: 33–36.

203. Roberts RO, Jacobsen SJ, Reilly WT, et al. Prevalence of combined fecal and urinary incontinence: a community-based study. *J MA Geriatr Soc* 1999;47:837–841.

CHAPTER 11

Aging and the
Cardiovascular System

Jeanne P. Goldberg, PhD

Our understanding of the role of diet in cardiovascular disease prevention has grown considerably over the past several decades. Nutrition interventions are now used as both an initial and adjunct therapy for the treatment of cardiovascular disease (CVD) risk factors including hypertension, diabetes, and lipid disorders. However, only 50% of adults over age 65 reported receiving nutrition-related guidance from their health care provider to lower their risk.[1] Diseases of the heart and blood vessels are by far the most important cause of morbidity and mortality among elderly individuals, and their incidence increases with age. Americans over age 65 make up 40% of the people with one or more types of CVD. The incidence of a first time coronary event increases from 26 per 1000 in men ages 65 to 74 to 39 per 1000 in men ages 85 to 94, and doubles among women, from 12 per 1000 to 24 per 1000.[2] Women are more likely to die from a CHD event than men. About 84% of CVD deaths occur in people older than 65.[3] Among those individuals who reach age 65 years, more than half will suffer a cardiovascular catastrophe. By 2050, it is expected that one in five Americans will be 65 years of age or older.[4] As the population ages, the challenge for health professionals is to help their patients delay the onset of diseases and the resulting disabilities.[5]

CVD in elders may go unrecognized because symptoms might be attributed to "normal aging."[6] For example, a decline in physical activity that is indicative of ischemia might be attributed to "slowing down" with age. Whereas the modifiable risk factors for CHD are the same for older and younger adults, the prevalence of these risk factors increases with age. It is widely agreed that primary efforts to prevent cardiovascular disease should begin with altering lifestyle habits during middle age; many experts believe that these efforts should begin considerably earlier. Prevention activities include maintaining ideal body weight, detecting and treating hypertension, maintaining a blood lipid profile consistent with minimizing risk, stopping smoking, and increasing physical activity. Most of these modifiable risk factors are closely linked to dietary factors (Table 11–1).[7] However, the benefit of risk factor modification among older populations remains a matter of conjecture, based to a great extent on extrapolation of findings from studies conducted on younger populations. This chapter considers the best current evidence for recommendations for disease prevention and modification of risk where it exists.

Dietary recommendations for elderly people must be based on our knowledge of the benefits of risk factor modification in older populations and on appropriate modifications for individuals with frank disease. Recommendations must be made within a framework that acknowledges the universal importance of a nutritionally adequate diet and the unique constellation of constraints that might make it difficult to achieve that goal. Moreover, interventions that will reduce risk should take into account the potential for dimin-

Table 11–1 Risk Factors for Cardiovascular Disease

Major modifiable risk factors

- Cigarette smoking
- Hypercholesterolemia
- Hypertension
- Obesity and overweight, especially abdominal adiposity
- Diabetes mellitus

Other recognized risk factors

- Advancing age
- Being male
- Positive family history
- Physical inactivity and sedentary lifestyle
- Hypertriglyceridemia
- Hypoalphalipoproteinemia

Emerging risk factors and proatherothrombotic conditions

- Elevated concentrations of lipoprotein(a)
- Lipoprotein profiles relatively enriched in small, dense low-density lipoprotein particles
- Inflammation (e.g., as indicated by increased concentration of C-reactive protein)
- Elevated concentrations of coagulation factors including fibrinogen
- Chronic infection
- Hyperhomocysteinemia
- Oxidative stress

Source: Reprinted with permission from Tribble DL, Krauss RM, Atherosclerotic Cardiovascular Disease, *Present Knowledge in Nutrition,* 8e, Copyright (2001) International Life Sciences Institute

ishing morbidity and disability that result from cardiovascular disease.[8]

THE DISEASE PROCESSES

Decline in cardiovascular function is a major physical impairment associated with aging from middle age onward. Loss of cardiovascular reserve capacity can be attributed to three factors: age-associated changes, physical deconditioning associated with an increasingly sedentary lifestyle, and changes associated with atherosclerotic cardiovascular disease. The relative contribution of each of these factors is unclear.[9] It is clear, however, that environmentally induced atherosclerotic changes play a major role in this process.

Atherosclerosis, thickening and hardening of the intima (the lining of the coronary arteries), underlies most cardiovascular disease in elderly individuals; hypertension and diabetes act as im-

portant contributing factors. The development of atherosclerosis is believed to result from years of interaction between intrinsic aging processes and environmental factors including diet, superimposed on unknown, predisposing genetic factors.[10] At least two lines of evidence suggest that atherosclerosis is not simply the result of unmodified biologic aging processes. The first is that some mammalian species age without developing atherosclerosis; second, there are populations that realize the human life span without clinical evidence of the disease.[11]

Changes do occur in the arteries during normal aging. A slow, apparently continuous, symmetric increase in the thickness of the interior walls of the arteries results from the gradual accumulation of smooth muscle cells from the middle layer of the vessels, surrounded by additional connective tissue. In addition, there is a progressive accumulation of both sphingomyelin and cholesterol ester. These age-associated changes result in a gradual increase in the rigidity of the vessels. Larger arteries may become dilated, elongated, and tortuous. Aneurysms (balloonings of the arterial wall) may form in areas of expanding arteriosclerotic plaques. These wear-and-tear changes often depend on the diameter of the vessel and tend to occur where vessels branch and curve and at anatomic attachment points.[11]

Although these structural changes are considered to be a normal part of the aging process, atherosclerotic changes are believed to be strongly influenced by environmental factors, especially diet. The lesions of atherosclerosis are generally classified into three categories: fatty streaks, fibrous plaques, and complicated lesions. Fatty streaks are characterized by an accumulation of lipid-filled smooth muscle cells and are surrounded by lipid in the lining of the vessels. Whether they are the earliest lesions is a matter of debate. They are universal, appearing in the aorta by age 10 years, and occupying as much as 50% of the aortic surface by age 25 years. The age-related increase in the surface area of coronary arteries involved with fatty streaks is believed to be readily reversible.[12]

Fibrous plaques, which are not ubiquitous among populations, are elevated areas of thickening in the lining of the arteries. They represent the most characteristic lesions of progressive atherosclerosis, appearing first in the intima of the abdominal aorta, coronary arteries, and carotid arteries during the third decade and gradually increasing with advancing age. A fibrous plaque is firm, elevated, and dome shaped, with an opaque, glistening surface that bulges into the lumen of the affected artery. It consists of an accumulation in the arterial intima of smooth muscle cells rather heavily laden with cholesterol and surrounded by other lipids, collagen, elastic fibers, and other substances. The protrusion of fibrous plaques into the lumina of arteries reduces their diameter. The cholesterol in these plaques closely resembles that in plasma lipoproteins. Raised lesions are thought to develop in the setting of a disruption of the endothelial cell continuity overlying fatty streaks. Evidence suggests that the progression of raised lesions continues into very old age.[13]

Complicated lesions are calcified fibrous plaques exhibiting various degrees of necrosis, thrombosis, and ulceration. Increasing necrosis, accumulation of cell debris, and weakening of the arterial wall increase the likelihood of rupture of the interior wall, causing hemorrhage. Arterial emboli may occur when fragments of plaque dislodge into the lumen. The thickening of plaque and the formation of thrombi (clots) lead to narrowing of blood vessels, reduced blood flow, and impaired organ function.[11] Arteries narrowed by raised lesions are more vulnerable to occlusion or blockage than normal arteries.

The extent of the surface area of coronary arteries involved with fatty streaks increases in men during the second and third decades of life and remains constant through the remainder of their lives. However, the development of raised lesions, which gradually impair blood flow, continues. In women, the extent of fatty streaks increases to about age 50 years, but the development of raised lesions lags nearly 20 years behind that for men.

Interventions designed to prevent clinical complications of raised, atherosclerotic lesions have focused on men aged 40 to 50 years for several reasons. First, raised lesions generally appear earlier in men than in women. Second, the risk of death from CHD increases in men at an earlier age than in women. Finally, the greatest likelihood of reversing the atherosclerotic process focuses on the smaller, less mature plaques.[14] However, several studies have demonstrated significant regression of larger fatty lesions.[15–18] Fibrous, calcified lesions may be prevented from further progression, but they probably do not regress.

RISK FACTORS AND THEIR MODIFICATION IN ELDERLY SUBJECTS

Coincidentally with the increased publicity focused on CHD as a cause of death, death rates from CHD began to decline. This decline began in 1950, with dramatic decreases observed in the 1960s and 1970s and slower declines during the 1980s and 1990s.[19] Heart disease is still the leading cause of death, but the death rate from heart disease decreased by 3.8% between 1999 and 2000.[20] The most recent figures show a decline in CHD death rates in people over 65 years from 595,406 in 1980 to 582,730 in 2001.[4] The decline in the CHD death rate is partly responsible for the increase in life expectancy. The average life expectancy of someone born in the United States now is 77.2 years. According to Centers for Disease Control and Prevention, National Center for Health Statistics, if all forms of major CHD were eliminated, there would be a 7-year increase in life expectancy. A key question is whether this decline is associated only with better survival rates attributable to improved medical management or whether a decline in incidence is also a contributing factor, perhaps related to better preventive strategies.

A number of risk factors predict the likelihood of developing a clinical atherosclerotic event, but only some of them can be altered (Table 11–1). Research conducted over several decades has identified a series of diet-related factors associated with the incidence of cardiovascular disease and the development and progression of the underlying atherosclerosis. The role of dietary fats (particularly saturated and trans-fatty acids) in regulating circulating lipoprotein levels is of particular importance, as is the role of body weight in affecting both blood lipoprotein levels and blood pressure. Dietary sodium also has a role in hypertension.[21] Research has elucidated possible roles of other micronutrients in CHD. Vitamin E, with its antioxidant function, has been shown to have protective effects on risk for CHD.[22] Vitamin B_6, vitamin B_{12}, and folate may act to lower levels of plasma homocysteine.[23,24] Elevated homocysteine levels have been associated with increased risk of myocardial infarction[25] and mortality in patients with CHD.[26]

Metabolic syndrome, syndrome x, and insulin resistance syndrome refer to a cluster of risk factors, including obesity, hyperinsulinemia, dyslipidemia, hypertension, and diabetes, all of which are associated with atherosclerosis and CHD. The Expert Panel on Detection, Evaluation, and Treatment of High Blood Cholesterol in Adults (ATP III) define metabolic syndrome as the presence of at least three of the following symptoms:

- Abdominal obesity (waist circumference)
  Men   >102 cm
  Women   >88 cm
- Triglycerides   ≥150 mg/dL
- HDL cholesterol
  Men   <40 mg/dL
  Women   <50 mg/dL
- Blood pressure   ≥130/≥85 mmHg
- Fasting glucose   ≥110 mg/dL

About 44% of people over age 50 years meet at least three of these, and the prevalence seems to be growing in the United States as obesity and lack of physical activity increase. According to the Third National Health and Nutrition Examination Survey (NHANES III), the prevalence of CHD among older adults with diabetes and metabolic syndrome is 19.2% compared to less than 10% in those without metabolic syndrome, regardless of diabetes status.[27] Women increase their risk of developing metabolic syndrome by 60% after menopause. This may partially explain the rise in CVD among this group.[28]

C-reactive protein (CRP), a marker of inflammation that is predictive of CHD, has received much attention in recent years.[29–31] Increased CRP levels are associated with hypertension, obesity, triglycerides, fasting glucose, endothelial dysfunction, and impaired fibrinolysis.[29] In fact, the Women's Health Study found C-reactive protein to be a better predictor of CVD events than LDL cholesterol.[32] It is still unclear whether routine screening to identify patients with elevated CRP or interventions aimed at lowering CRP will actually reduce CHD events.[33]

Mild to moderate elevations in homocysteine increase the risk of CHD by promoting platelet activation, oxidative stress, endothelial dysfunction, hypercoagulability, vascular smooth muscle cell proliferation, and endoplasmic reticulum stress.[34–36] Several B vitamins (folate, B_{12}, and B_6) act as substrates and cofactors in the metabolism of homocysteine. A number of studies have shown an inverse relationship between homocysteine concentrations and plasma/serum levels of folate, B_{12}, and B_6.[37] These could provide an inexpensive and safe means of lowering homocysteine levels.[33] In a sample of 689 adults in the

United States without diabetes, those with the lowest serum folate levels had twice the risk of CHD mortality than those with the highest levels, after adjusting for age and sex.[38] The 1998 decision by the U.S. Food and Drug Administration to fortify all enriched cereal grains with folic acid was estimated to increase folic acid intake by 70 to 130 micrograms per day, depending on age and consumption patterns.[39] However, a 2002 analysis of studies that measured serum or plasma folate within the same population before and after fortification determined that increases in folic acid from fortified foods ranged from 215 to 240 µg.[40] It remains to be seen whether increased levels of B vitamins will lower CHD risk, and the American Heart Association (AHA) currently suggests meeting the RDA for folate, B_{12}, and B_6 through an adequate intake of vegetables, fruits, legumes, meats, fish, and fortified grains and cereal. The effectiveness of screening for elevated homocysteine is unknown.[33,37]

BLOOD LIPIDS

Patterns of atherogenic blood lipid levels and their relationship to risk of CHD differ among older men and women. Data from NHANES 1999 to 2000 show that total serum cholesterol level tends to peak in men between 45 to 54 years of age and then decrease; in women, serum cholesterol levels peak at 55 to 64 years of age and actually exceed those seen in men. High-density lipoprotein (HDL) cholesterol levels are substantially higher in women and remain higher than HDL cholesterol levels in men. HDL cholesterol is inversely correlated with weight and is likely to be lower in individuals with impaired glucose tolerance.[41] It is also lower among individuals who have suffered a coronary event.[41]

In the Framingham study, the relative predictive power of the major cardiovascular risk factors weakened with age for both men and women.[42] Among men age 35 years with total cholesterol levels of 310 mg/dL, the risk of suffering a coronary event was 5.2 times greater than among those with total cholesterol levels of 185 mg/dL. However, by age 65 years the relative risk at the higher cholesterol level was only 1.1. Among

women age 45 years with total cholesterol levels of 310 mg/dL, the risk of a coronary event was 2.5 times that of women with total cholesterol levels of 185 mg/dL. However, by age 65 years, that risk diminished to 1.1.

Barrett-Connor and colleagues[43] found a significant predictive effect of total cholesterol in groups of men and women aged 65 to 79 years who were followed for 9 years. Data from the Framingham study confirm the long-term predictive power of serum cholesterol levels in individuals aged 65 years and older. For each 1% increase in total cholesterol, there is a 2% increase in the incidence of CHD among those aged 60 to 70 years old.[44]

Elevated LDL-cholesterol concentrations and decreased HDL-cholesterol concentrations are independent risk factors for CHD, and studies indicate a benefit in CHD risk reduction from both lowering LDL cholesterol and increasing HDL cholesterol.[45] In the Framingham study, fractioning serum cholesterol into atherogenic LDL and protective HDL cholesterol restores the predictive power of total cholesterol demonstrated at younger ages.[41] A ratio of either LDL cholesterol to HDL cholesterol or total cholesterol to HDL cholesterol is highly predictive of CHD in elderly people. In men, this atherogenic lipid ratio plateaus at age 54 years; in women, it continues to rise until age 80 years but still remains lower than for men. Until recently, studies of lipid lowering have not included elderly adults.[6] Early findings in primary and secondary prevention studies have indicated that older adults can benefit from lipid-lowering therapy.[6,46]

A number of dietary factors affect blood lipid levels. LDL cholesterol is elevated by saturated fat, trans-unsaturated fatty acids, and to a lesser degree, cholesterol. LDL cholesterol is lowered when polyunsaturated fatty acids and monounsaturated fatty acids are substituted for saturated fatty acids. Soluble fiber, plant stanol/sterol ester-containing foods, and soy protein also lower LDL cholesterol, although to a lesser degree. In some individuals, losing weight and maintaining the loss will lower LDL levels.[47,46] Low HDL cholesterol and elevated serum triglycerides are independent risk factors for CHD. Low HDL levels are caused by elevated triglycerides, over-weight and obesity, physical inactivity, type 2 diabetes, cigarette smoking, a very high carbo-hydrate intake (more than 60% of calories), and certain drugs. These same elements contribute to hypertrigylceridemia as do excess alcohol intake, dietary intake of trans-fatty acids, and genetic disorders (familial combined hyperlipidemia, familial hypertriglyceridemia, and familial dysbetalipoproteinemia).[46,48]

The National Cholesterol Education Program (NCEP) was developed by the National Heart, Lung, and Blood Institute in 1985[49] as a means to reduce coronary morbidity and mortality re-lated to elevated blood cholesterol levels. The NCEP Expert Panel on Detection, Evaluation, and Treatment of High Blood Cholesterol in Adults (Adult Treatment Panel, or ATP) produces clinical updates as advances in science and the understanding of cholesterol management war-rant. The third and most recent of the reports (ATP III) focuses on intensive LDL-lowering therapy in certain groups of people, but was built on ATP I and ATP II, which outlined a method for preventing CHD in people with elevated LDL cholesterol levels and other CHD risk factors.[46]

The new ATP III guidelines identify an LDL cholesterol level of <100 mg/dL as "optimal" and raise the definition of low HDL cholesterol from <35 mg/dL to <40 mg/dL (Table 11–2).[46] Total cholesterol cutoff points for relative risk for CHD are uniform for men and women of all ages. The panel acknowledged that there were limited clin-ical trial data available for the elderly population but stated that extrapolation of data from trials showing reduction in CHD risk in middle-aged patients seemed reasonable. Since older age in-creases the risk of CHD, lowering total cholesterol levels in elderly individuals could result in sub-stantial reductions in morbidity and mortality rates. Modifications of this general approach may be warranted, especially in extreme old age.[50]

All adults should have their fasting lipoprotein profile—total cholesterol, LDL and HDL cho-lesterol, and triglycerides—tested every 5 years. If the values are nonfasting, the total and HDL cholesterol values should be used and a total cho-lesterol of ≥200 mg/dL or a HDL of <40 mg/dL warrants a follow-up lipoprotein profile for ap-propriate therapy based on LDL cholesterol. Because elevated LDL cholesterol continues to be the primary target for cholesterol-lowering therapy, the goals of therapy and the levels for be-ginning treatment are stated in terms of LDL.

The ATP III takes into account other CHD risk factors such as the presence or absence of CHD, or other forms of atherosclerosis that might mod-ify LDL target goals (Table 11–3).[46] The highest category of risk includes current CHD and CHD risk equivalents. Diabetes is regarded as a CHD risk equivalent because it confers a high risk of new CHD within the next 10 years, in part, be-cause diabetes is often associated with other CHD risk factors. Those in this highest category

Table 11–2 ATP III Classification of Total, LDL, and HDL Cholesterol

Total Cholesterol (mg/dL)		LDL Cholesterol (mg/dL)		HDL Cholesterol (mg/dl)	
<200	Desirable	<100	Optimal	<40	Low
		100–129	Near optimal Above optimal		
200–239	Borderline High	130–159	Borderline High		
≥240	High	160–189	High	≥60	High
		≥190	Very High		

Source: Executive Summary of the Third Report of the National Cholesterol Education Program (NCEP) Expert Panel on Detection, Evaluation, and Treatment of High Blood Cholesterol in Adults (Adult Treatment Panel III).

Table 11–3 Risk Factors That Modify LDL-Cholesterol Goals

- Age (men ≥45 years; women ≥55 years)
- Family history of premature CHD (definite myocardial infarction or sudden death in male first-degree relative <55 years, or in female first-degree relative <65 years)
- Current cigarette smoking
- Hypertension (≥140/90 mmHg, or on antihypertensive medication)
- Low HDL cholesterol (<40 mg/dL)*

*HDL cholesterol ≥60 mg/dL is considered a "negative" risk factor; its presence subtracts one risk factor from the total count.

Source: Executive Summary of the Third Report of the National Cholesterol Education Program (NCEP) Expert Panel on Detection, Evaluation, and Treatment of High Blood Cholesterol in Adults (Adult Treatment Panel III).

of risk, which means their risk of a major coronary in the next 10 years is more than 20%, have the lowest recommended LDL-cholesterol goal of <100 mg/dL. The second risk category is defined as risk of a major coronary event in the next 10 years as equal to or less than 20% and corresponds to a goal LDL of <130 mg/dL. The third category consists of people with 0–1 risk factors and corresponds to a 10-year risk of developing CHD as less than 10%. Their LDL goal is <160 mg/dL (Table 11–4).[46]

The approach recommended by the ATP III is a multifaceted therapeutic lifestyle change (TLC). Its primary components are:

1. Reduced saturated fat intake to less than 7% of total calories and cholesterol to less than 200 mg/day (Table 11–5[46] has a complete TLC diet composition)
2. Enhance LDL lowering with plant stanols/sterols (2 g/day) and increased soluble fiber (10–25g/day)

Table 11–4 LDL-Cholesterol Goals and Initiation Points for Therapeutic Lifestyle Changes (TLC) and Drug Therapy in Different Risk Categories

10-year Risk	LDL Goal (mg/dL)	LDL Level to Initiate TLC	LDL Level at Which to Initiate Drug Therapy
<10%:			
0–1 risk factors	<160	≥160	≥190 (160–189: drug therapy optional)
Multiple (2+) risk factors	<130	≥130	≥160
10–20%	<130	≥130	≥130
>20%	<100	≥100	≥130 (100–129, consider drug options*)

*Some authorities recommend LDL-lowering drugs in this category if an LDL cholesterol 100 mg/dL cannot be achieved by TLC. Others prefer drugs that primarily modify other lipoprotein fractions, eg, nicotinic acid and fibrate. Clinical judgment may also call for withholding drug therapy in this category.

Source: Executive Summary of the Third Report of the National Cholesterol Education Program (NCEP) Expert Panel on Detection, Evaluation, and Treatment of High Blood Cholesterol in Adults (Adult Treatment Panel III).

Table 11–5 Nutrition Composition of the Therapeutic Lifestyle Changes (TLC) Diet

Nutrient	Recommendation
Total fat	25–35% of total calories
Saturated fat*	<7% of total calories
Polyunsaturated fat	Up to 10% of total calories
Monounsaturated fat	Up to 20% of total calories
Carbohydrate†	50–60% of total calories
Dietary fiber	20–30 g/day
Protein	Approximately 15% of total calories
Dietary cholesterol	<200 mg/day
Total calories	Balance total calorie intake to maintain desirable weight/ prevent weight gain

* Trans-fatty acids are another LDL-raising fat that should be kept at a low intake.
† Carbohydrate should be derived predominately from foods rich in complex carbohydrates including grains—especially whole grains, fruits, and vegetables.

Source: Executive Summary of the Third Report of the National Cholesterol Education Program (NCEP) Expert Panel on Detection, Evaluation, and Treatment of High Blood Cholesterol in Adults (Adult Treatment Panel III).

3. Weight reduction
4. Increased physical activity

The TLC diet is in keeping with the 2000 Dietary Guidelines for Americans with the exception of a slightly more lenient fat intake (25–35% of total calories compared to <30% as suggested in the Dietary Guidelines) if saturated and trans-fatty acid intake remain low. Trans-fatty acids, found naturally in meat and dairy products and formed during hydrogenation of fats and oils, appear to affect the total-cholesterol-to-HDL-cholesterol ratio even more negatively than saturated fats because trans-fatty acids do not affect HDL cholesterol and saturated fats tend to increase HDL-cholesterol levels.[48] Unsaturated fats can help lower LDL and total cholesterol while raising HDL cholesterol when substituted for saturated fats and trans-fatty acids.[51] Data from the Nurses Health Study demonstrate that replacing 5% of energy from saturated fat with unsaturated fats would reduce the risk of coronary disease by 42%, and replacing 2% of energy from trans fat with energy from unhydrogenated, unsaturated fats would reduce risk by 53%.[52] Results from the DASH-Sodium Trial show that a reduced fat/low cholesterol diet was less effective in lowering total and LDL cholesterol in the presence of high CRP levels.

A meta-analysis of 41 studies showed that 2 g/day of plant stanols or sterols lowered LDL cholesterol by 10%. Combining their use with a diet low in saturated fat and cholesterol can reduce LDL cholesterol by 20%.[53] Although there is some concern that plant stanol/sterol ester-containing foods may lower plasma levels of fat-soluble vitamins, this same meta-analysis found a significant decrease only in beta-carotene. Alpha-carotene and lycopene were also lowered, but in part from the reduction in LDL. The AHA recommends continued monitoring for those using stanol/sterol ester-containing foods and reserving their use for adults requiring lowering of total and LDL-cholesterol levels due to hypercholesterolemia or those trying to prevent a second CHD event.[47]

The ATP III TLC diet is consistent with the American Heart Association's individualized guidelines for specific subgroups (those with lipid disorders, diabetes, or CHD). These more targeted dietary recommendations replace the AHA's Step 2 diet for higher risk patients. The American Heart Association has replaced its Step 1 diet with guidelines for the general population with an emphasis on foods, an overall eating pattern, and the importance of all Americans to achieve and maintain a healthy body weight. The guidelines are appropriate for anyone over 2 years old. The goal is an "overall" healthy eating pattern including the following major points:

- Consume a variety of fruits, vegetables, and grain products, including whole grains.
- Include fat-free and low-fat dairy products, fish, legumes, poultry, and lean meats.
- Match energy needs to overall calorie needs and make appropriate changes to achieve weight loss when indicated.
- Modify food choices to reduce saturated fats (<10% of calories), cholesterol (<300 mg/day), and trans fatty acids by substituting grains and unsaturated fatty acids from fish, vegetables, legumes, and nuts.
- Limit salt intake to <6 g/day.
- Limit alcohol intake (≤2 drinks/day for men and ≤1 drink/day for women) among those who drink.

The AHA recommends that all adults eat at least two servings of fish, particularly fatty fish, a week. Fish is low in saturated fat and a good source of omega-3 fatty acids, 20-carbon eicosapentaenoic acid (EPA), and 22-carbon docosahexaenoic acid (DHA), which epidemiological and clinical studies suggest are beneficial for people at risk for CHD. And, although the mechanism for protection is not entirely known, omega-3 fatty acids appear to lower triglycerides and blood pressure, decrease platelet aggregation, and reduce arrhythmias.[54] The Nurses Health Study found that women who ate fish 2 to 4 times per week lowered their risk of CHD by almost 30% compared to those who rarely ate fish.[55] A review of dietary interventions for CHD protection cites the Diet and Reinfarction Trial and GISSI-Prevention trial as evidence that eating fish twice per week or taking fish oil (1–1.5 g/day) lowered CHD events and mortality rates.[56]

For patients with CHD, the AHA recommends consuming ~ 1 g/day of combined EPA and DHA obtained from fatty fish or omega-3 fatty acid supplements. Patients with elevated triglycerides might benefit from 2 to 4 g/day of EPA and DHA capsules taken under the supervision of a physician.[57] Omega-3 fatty acids are also contained in some nut and plant oils including canola, walnut, soybean, and flaxseed. However, the 18-carbon α-linolenic acid (ALA) they contain appears to be less potent than the EPA and DHA in fish. Some species of fish may contain high levels of environmental contaminants (methyl mercury, polychlorinated biphenyls [PCBs], and dioxins), prompting the Environmental Protection Agency and the FDA to issue advisories for some populations (women who are pregnant, may become pregnant, or breastfeeding, and young children) to limit their intake of certain fish. But for middle-age and older men and postmenopausal women, the benefits of fish outweigh the risks within the EPA and FDA guidelines. Eating a variety of types of fish is the best way to minimize exposure to a particular contaminant.

In 1999, the FDA approved a health claim that recognizes the heart health benefits of soy protein. The claim states that 25 g/day of soy protein as part of a diet that is low in saturated fat and cholesterol may reduce the risk of heart disease. A meta-analysis of 38 studies concluded that daily soy consumption decreased total cholesterol by 9.3%, LDL cholesterol by 12.9%, and triglycerides by 10.5%. There was no adverse effect on HDL cholesterol.[58] The AHA supports the FDA's claim, noting that 25 to 50 g/day is safe and effective, although the benefits are greater in those with hypercholesterolemia.[59] Replacing animal products that are higher in saturated fat and cholesterol with soy foods can result in an overall eating pattern that may reduce CVD. There are an increasing number of soy foods available to consumers, but in the United States, soy intake remains relatively low at less than 5 g/d.[60]

Epidemiologic evidence has shown a protective effect of antioxidant nutrients (vitamin E, vitamin C, and beta carotene) on CHD risk.[61–64] Antioxidants decrease the formation of atherosclerosis by preventing oxidation of LDL cholesterol. Some cohort studies have shown an association between vitamin supplement use and reduced CVD risk. The Nurses Health Study found a lower MI risk associated with higher intakes of vitamin E, and the Health Professionals Study found vitamin E, and multivitamin supplements to lower CHD risk among men. NHANES data show vitamin C reduced the standard mortality ratio for CVD by 48%. However, randomized, controlled studies of specific supplements including the Alpha-Tocopherol, Beta-Carotene Cancer Prevention (ATBC) Study, and the Beta-Carotene and Retinal Efficacy Trial (CARET) have not shown a consistent or significant effect of any single vitamin or combination of vitamins.[65] The most prudent recommendation for the general public is to consume antioxidant-rich fruits, vegetables, and whole grains according to the AHA.[64]

Diet alone may not provide the levels of vitamin E that have been associated with secondary prevention of CHD. Although the RDA can often be easily met with dietary sources, NHANES III data show that elderly Americans do not consume enough vitamin E to meet this recommended level.[66] However, the clinical relevance of this is unclear and vitamin E deficiency is rare. Few studies of vitamin E supplements and CHD have focused on the elderly, though some have found a protective effect of vitamin E supplementation in the elderly, consistent with that observed in younger populations.[22,67] The benefits of supplementation may be long term, as those in the Nurses' Health and the Health Professionals' Follow-Up studies were seen only after 2 years of using supplements.[68] Lack of data from randomized controlled trials has prevented an established recommendation regarding the use of supplements. The use of vitamin E supplements

for primary prevention of CHD has not been definitively demonstrated. Large-scale randomized intervention trials currently under way will contribute to clarifying specific recommendations regarding vitamin E supplementation.

The goal of dietary therapy is to reduce elevated cholesterol levels while maintaining a nutritionally adequate diet. Once the LDL-cholesterol goal has been met, attention can be placed on other lipid and nonlipid risk factors (hypertension, elevated triglycerides, low HDL, and use of aspirin to reduce the prothrombotic state). Patients should be monitored every 4 to 6 months or more to evaluate response to treatment (Figure 11–1).[46]

BLOOD PRESSURE

Despite the high prevalence of hypertension among older adults, high blood pressure classifications are the same for all adults, regardless of age.[69] The Seventh Report of the Joint National Committee on Prevention, Detection, Evaluation, and Treatment of High Blood Pressure (JNC 7 Report) adds a new stage to the classification of blood pressure (BP) (Table 11–6).[70] Patients with prehypertension, a systolic BP of 120 to 139 mmHg or a diastolic BP of 80 to 89 mmHg, are at twice the risk for developing hypertension as those with lower values. Those who are prehypertensive require health and lifestyle modifications to prevent CVD. This new classification calls for education of health professionals, their patients, and the public to take appropriate measures to prevent the development of hypertension.[70]

The prevalence of hypertension is increasing in the United States. In 1999 to 2000, almost 30% of NHANES participants had hypertension, which is almost a 4% increase from 1988–1991.[71] Hypertension is the most powerful predictor of stroke and the risk factor most readily amenable to treatment. It accelerates atherogenesis and imparts a two- to threefold increased risk of cardiovascular disease events, including CHD.[72] Multiple United States prospective population studies demonstrate that systolic blood pressure and diastolic blood pressure relate strongly and

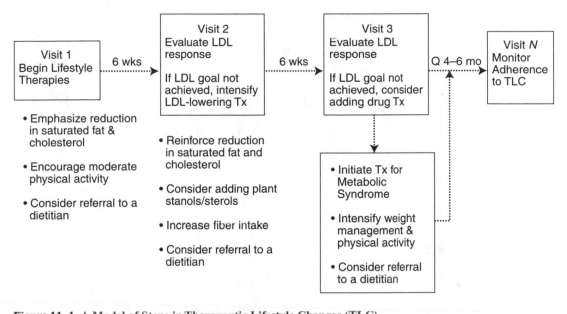

Figure 11–1 A Model of Steps in Therapeutic Lifestyle Changes (TLC)
Source: Executive Summary of the Third Report of the National Cholesterol Education Program (NCEP) Expert Panel on Detection, Evaluation, and Treatment of High Blood Cholesterol in Adults (Adult Treatment Panel III)

independently to risk of cardiovascular events.[73] Hypertension is also extremely common among elderly people, doubling the overall mortality and tripling cardiovascular mortality.[74]

Despite the severe health consequences of high blood pressure, the goal of the U.S. Department of Health and Human Services that 50% of Americans with high blood pressure have it controlled by the year 2000 was not met. A review of NHANES III data showed that in 1999–2000, only 31% of those with hypertension had it controlled.[71]

Individuals at age 55 who are normotensive have a 90% lifetime risk of developing hypertension.[75] Over a period of 38 years of follow-up to the Framingham study, increasing cardiovascular morbidity and mortality rates with increasing blood pressure levels were observed in both men and women, aged 75 to 94, who were initially free of cardiovascular disease.[76] An age-adjusted increased risk of death from all causes and from cardiovascular causes during 24 years of follow-up in the Framingham study was at least twice that of subjects with blood pressure at or below 140/95 mmHg.

Longitudinal observations from the Framingham study show different patterns for systolic and diastolic pressures in men and women. In men, systolic pressure peaks in middle age and then levels off, whereas diastolic pressure rises until the mid-50s and then declines.[77] In women, systolic pressure continues to increase with age and to a greater degree.[69] According to data from the Framingham Heart Study, among those aged 65 to 89 years with hypertension, 65% of the women compared with 57% of the men had isolated systolic hypertension.[69] Both the Framingham Heart Study and NHANES III show a similar pattern of increasing isolated systolic blood pressure with age.[78]

Isolated systolic hypertension (ISH) was once widely viewed as a benign disease of older persons thought to be a physiologic adaptation necessary for the perfusion of aging organ systems. Antihypertensive therapy was commonly believed by practicing physicians to be of little value and too dangerous in individuals older than 65 years. Now, the JNC 7 Report cautions that in people over age 50, systolic blood pressure of

Table 11–6 Classification and Management of Blood Pressure for Adults

BP Classification	Systolic BP,* mmHg	Diastolic BP,* mmHg	Lifestyle Modifications	Management — Initial Drug Therapy	
				Without Compelling Indication	*With Compelling Indications*
Normal	<120	and <80	Encourage		
Prehypertension	120–139	or 80–89	Yes	No antihypertensive drug indicated	Drug(s) for the compelling indications
Stage 1 Hypertension	140–159	or 90–99	Yes	Thiazide-type diuretics for most. May consider ACEI, ARB, BB, CCB, or combination	Drug(s) for the compelling indications‡ Other antihypertensive drugs (diuretics, ACEI, ARB, BB, CCB as needed)
Stage 2 Hypertension	≥160	or ≥100	Yes	Two-drug combination for most† (usually thiazide-type diuretic and ACEI or ARB or BB or CCB)	Drug(s) for the compelling indications‡ Other antihypertensive drugs (diuretics, ACEI, ARB, BB, CCB as needed)

Drug abbreviations: ACEI, angiotensin-converting enzyme inhibitor; ARB, angiotensin-receptor blocker; BB, beta-blocker; CCB, calcium channel blocker.

* Treatment determined by highest BP category.

† Initial combined therapy should be used cautiously in those at risk for orthostatic hypotension.

‡ Treat patients with chronic kidney disease or diabetes to BP goal of <130/80 mmHg.

Source: The Seventh Report of the Joint National Committee on Prevention, Detection, Evaluation, and Treatment of High Blood Pressure. The National Heart, Lung, and Blood Institute.

more than 140 mmHg is a much more important cardiovascular disease risk factor than diastolic blood pressure.[70] Evidence from the Framingham study indicates that no measure is superior to systolic pressure in predicting cardiovascular events in general and stroke, the hypertensive event most closely related to blood pressure elevation, in particular.[10]

ISH, usually a reflection of diminished distensibility of the aorta, accounts for 65–75% of hypertension in the elderly in the Framingham study, occurring as the endpoint of several contributing factors.[72,74] These include the effects of systolic hypertension on arterial wall compliance, inducing a gradual reduction in diastolic pressure and increased pulse pressure. The disproportionate rise in systolic pressure is consistent with a progressive loss of elasticity. The Systolic Hypertension in the Elderly Program (SHEP) was the first intervention trial to show that antihypertensive therapy could reduce cardiovascular events in individuals with ISH.[79] SHEP, a double-blind, placebo-controlled, randomized clinical trial of antihypertensive therapy in subjects with ISH, observed a significant 36% reduction in the combined incidence of fatal and nonfatal stroke, a 27% reduction in nonfatal myocardial infarction or coronary death, and a 32% reduction in all major cardiovascular events.[79]

The National High Blood Pressure Education Program (NHBPEP) Coordinating Committee advises elderly people, including those with systolic hypertension, to follow the same principles for the general treatment of hypertension with the ultimate objective of reducing cardiovascular and renal morbidity and mortality.[70] Since most people with hypertension will achieve the diastolic BP goal once the systolic goal is met, the primary focus should be on achieving the systolic BP goal.[70] A decrease in cardiovascular disease complications is associated with BP goals of less than 140/90 mmHg and less than 130/80 mmHg for hypertensive patients with diabetes or renal disease.[70]

All hypertensive patients should adopt a healthy lifestyle that includes achieving and maintaining a healthy weight, reducing dietary sodium, adopting a DASH Diet eating pattern, limiting alcohol intake, and ceasing smoking, where applicable. Drug therapy should be initiated for those with Stage 1 or Stage 2 hypertension (Table 11–6).[70] The choice of medication is based on the coexistence of both risk factors and disease. Most patients will require at least two types of medication to reach a blood pressure goal of less than 140/90 or 130/80 mmHg.[70]

Thiazide-type diuretics should be the initial therapy for most patients and may be used alone or in combination with other classes of drugs including angiotensin-converting enzyme (ACE) inhibitors, angiotensin-receptor blockers (ARBs), beta-blockers (BB), and calcium channel blockers (CCBs).[70] The Antihypertensive and Lipid-Lowering Treatment to Prevent Heart Attack Trial (ALLHAT) found thiazide-type diuretics more effective than ACE inhibitors and ARBs in preventing CVD outcomes and lowering systolic blood pressure in older adults and less expensive.[80] The possibility of particular sensitivity to the hypokalemic effects of diuretics among elderly people suggests that serum potassium should be monitored closely and that extra emphasis should be placed on including generous amounts of potassium-rich foods in the diet. Although potassium supplements reportedly can help offset the effects of a high sodium intake, cost and the potential hazards associated with their use make them impractical.[81]

The Dietary Approaches to Stop Hypertension (DASH) trial demonstrated that a diet rich in fruits, vegetables, and low-fat dairy foods; that includes whole grains, poultry, fish, and nuts; that contains small amounts of red meat, sweets, and sugar-containing beverages; and that contains decreased amounts of total and saturated fat and cholesterol lowers blood pressure in people with and without hypertension. The approximate reduction in systolic blood pressure from the DASH diet is 8 to 14 mmHg.[70,82] Adopting the DASH diet is one of the lifestyle modifications recommended by the NHBPEP to manage hypertension.

The sodium level in the original DASH diet was kept at 3000 mg, slightly less than the 3300 mg consumed by many Americans. A second study compared the effects of different levels of sodium (high: 3300 mg, intermediate: 2400 mg, and low: 1500 mg per day) in conjunction with the DASH diet and also with a typical American diet. Lowering sodium levels reduced blood pressure in both eating plans, although blood pressure was lower at each sodium level when combined with the DASH diet. Compared to the American diet with high sodium, the DASH diet with low sodium reduced systolic blood pressure by 7.1 mmHg in patients without hypertension and 11.5 mmHg in participants with hypertension.[83]

Although subjects in the DASH study were younger (ages 37–59), it is reasonable to extrapolate the findings to the elderly, given the high prevalence of hypertension in older cohorts, and to recommend modification of the Step 1 diet described earlier to reflect the DASH low-sodium combination diet. Other lifestyle modifications recommended by the NHBPEP include reducing weight when indicated, engaging in regular physical activity (at least 30 minutes a day on most, preferably all, days of the week), restricting alcohol to 2 drinks per day for men and 1 drink a day for women (one drink equals 12 ounces of beer, 5 oz of wine, or 3 oz spirits), and stopping smoking.

OBESITY

The relationship of obesity to increased risk for cardiovascular disease in elderly individuals remains controversial, with some studies indicating increased risk at both extremes of the weight distribution curve.[84] Much of the controversy is explained by the confounding effects of smoking, coexisting disease, and inadequate follow-up.[77] However, the preponderance of evidence suggests that obesity heightens other atherogenic risk factors[85] and thereby contributes to increased risk.

Data from the Framingham study at 30-year follow-up demonstrate a continuous relationship between obesity and coronary morbidity and mortality (stronger in men than in women). Obesity is associated with both blood pressure

and serum lipoprotein levels. In the Framingham study,[86] correlation between relative weight and either systolic or diastolic pressure declined steadily over adult life. Havlik and colleagues,[87] using the body mass index (BMI) (weight/height^2) and blood pressure, reported similar declines in men over the age range of 30 to 70 years. Harlan and associates[88] showed a reduction in association between BMI and systolic blood pressure in older women. The weaker association at older ages remains significant for men but not for women.

In the Framingham study, the correlation between relative body weight and total plasma cholesterol is not significant in men older than 50 years; in women, it is significant only among 35- to 39-year-olds.[89] After age 50 years, BMI is no longer significantly associated with LDL cholesterol in either sex. However, the strong inverse relationship between HDL cholesterol and BMI remains statistically significant, even among subjects aged 70 to 79 years.[89] Therefore, the benefits of maintaining optimal weight for height are associated with a positive effect on HDL cholesterol levels.[9] Lamon-Fava et al[90] found that BMI increased with age in men until the age of 50 and then plateaued, while in women it increased with age through the seventh decade of life. BMI was significantly associated with systolic blood pressure, fasting glucose levels, total cholesterol, and LDL cholesterol and was inversely associated with HDL cholesterol, leading the authors to conclude that "elevated BMI is associated with adverse effects on all major CHD risk factors."

National surveys have found that the incidence of overweight among U.S. adults has increased. Between 1988 and 1994, 56% of U.S. adults were overweight or obese. That increased to 64% by the years 1999 and 2000 (Figure 11–2).[4] Extreme obesity (a BMI of 40 or more) increased as well, from 2.9% to 4.7%.

More effective control of obesity, and especially the prevention of weight gain in middle adult life, is of potentially great value in further reducing CHD mortality. One of the most profound impacts of obesity on cardiovascular health is its link to hypertension.[91] Population studies

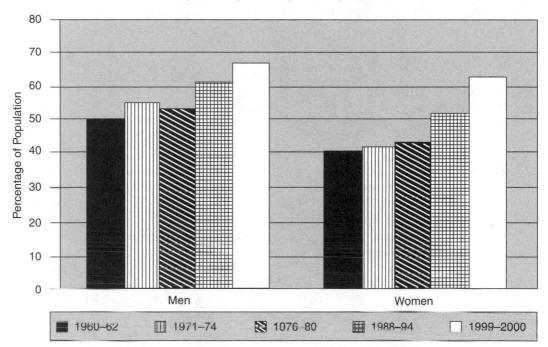

NHES, NHANES I, NHANES II, NHANES III, NHANES IV:
1960–62, 1971–74, 1976–80, 1988–94, 1999–2000

■ 1960–62   ▥ 1971–74   ▨ 1976–80   ▦ 1988–94   ☐ 1999–2000

Figure 11–2 Age-Adjusted Prevalence of Overweight (BMI equal to or greater than 25) in Americans Ages 20–74

Source: U.S. Department of Health and Human Services, Centers for Disease Control and Prevention, National Center for Health Statistics. Health, United States, 2003.

suggest that 75% of hypertension is due to obesity. There is also a strong association between obesity, particularly abdominal obesity, and metabolic syndrome.

The inability to achieve and maintain sustained weight loss is widely documented.[92] Moreover, it is impractical to conduct a controlled trial with random assignment of subjects to a weight reduction program. In the Framingham study, weight at younger ages has been found to be an important predictor of cardiovascular disease.[93,94] Relative weights at the time of initial examination predicted a 26-year incidence of CHD and cardiac failure in men, independent of risk factors associated with increased fatness. In women, there was an independent association between relative weight and CHD, stroke, cardiac failure, and cardiovascular mortality.

Few data compare the relative risks associated with weight fluctuation and sustained obesity. The relative risk of CHD 25 years later in a group of men ranging in age from 45 to 57 years at time of entry into the study who reported weight fluctuation during young adulthood was double that of men whose weight remained stable or increased.[95]

Weight reduction has been shown to confer substantial improvement in the cardiovascular risk profile. The U.S. Clinical Guidelines on the Identification, Evaluation, and Treatment of Overweight and Obesity in Adults have set the upper limit of ideal weight for all adults at a BMI of 25. However, it is controversial as to whether this cutoff is applicable to those aged 65 and over. A meta-analysis by Heiat et al[96] concluded that the federal guidelines for ideal weight (BMI 18.7

to <25) might be too restrictive for older adults and the optimal BMIs regarding all-cause and CVD mortality and CHD incidence ranged from 27 to 30.

PHYSICAL ACTIVITY

Regular physical activity can prevent CVD and treat and prevent many CHD risk factors, including hypertension, insulin resistance, glucose intolerance, elevated triglycerides, low HDL-cholesterol levels, and obesity.[97] The relative risk of CHD associated with lack of physical activity ranges from 1.5 to 2.4, an increase that is similar to that of high blood pressure, high cholesterol levels, or smoking.[3] When exercise is done in conjunction with weight loss it can lower LDL cholesterol and limit the reduction in HDL cholesterol that often accompanies a reduction in dietary saturated fat.[98] Intervention studies have generally found that exercise results in positive cardiovascular changes in older adults.[99] The Cardiovascular Health Study found that physical activity was associated with remaining healthy during 7 years of follow-up of 5,888 men and women over age 65.[100] Yet recent data show that almost 50% of Americans over age 18 never engage in any vigorous physical activity. In those over age 65, 80% report no vigorous activity.[4]

An exercise program should include all aspects of physical conditioning including aerobic capacity, muscular endurance and strength, range of motion, and flexibility. The program should not be limited to structured exercise, but should consider varying levels of abilities, needs, socialization, and diverse activities.[97]

DIETARY MODIFICATION FOR CARDIOVASCULAR RISK REDUCTION

NHANES III shows that 86% of U.S. adults age 65 years and older have at least one nutrition-related CVD risk factor (hypertension, elevated LDL cholesterol, and diabetes). The decline in CHD mortality that began in the 1960s coincided with considerable changes in the American diet. Red meat and dairy foods, which include butter, whole milk, and cheese, are the major sources of saturated fat in the diet and intake of these foods has fallen considerably since 1965. The reduction in saturated fat intake is mostly due to the decline in whole milk consumption, from over 21 gallons in 1972–1976 to 8.2 in 1997.[101] Diet surveys show that among U.S. adults average caloric intake fell from 2,049 in 1965 to 1,807 in 1991, but then increased to 2,000 in 1996. Total daily fat intake also increased between 1991 and 1996, from 70.9 grams to 74.8 grams.[102] The intake of trans-fatty acids has decreased over the past 10 years in developed countries due to the reformulation of hydrogenated fat for low-trans and trans-free margarines and for commercial frying and baking.[48]

Information about changes in dietary intake in elderly people is limited. However, elderly individuals (age 60 and over) surveyed in the NHANES III were found to have fat intakes of 31% to 34% of total calories and cholesterol intakes of 200 to 225 mg for men and 132 to 150 mg for women.[102] A study of free-living elderly subjects aged 60 to 100 years found higher values. Men consumed 35% of calories from fat, 16.5% of calories from saturated fat, and 350 mg/d of cholesterol. Women consumed 35.4% of calories from fat, 16.3% of calories from saturated fat, and 265 mg/d of cholesterol.[103] Studies of secular trends in blood lipid levels have shown that serum total cholesterol began to decline in the late 1950s across the broad age span from 20 to 74 years. Data from the large national health surveys and from the Framingham study have shown substantial decreases among individuals of both sexes.[9] Data from the Baltimore Longitudinal Study extend this observation to men in their 70s and 80s. Therefore, the decline in blood total cholesterol over the past 25 years is consistent with dietary changes, even among older age groups.[9]

Consideration of further dietary modifications for elderly persons must address two questions. First, are the dietary modifications of value for older people? Second, are the proposed changes feasible? A consistent observation in elderly people has been their extremely low energy intakes. Since intake of essential nutrients is closely related to calorie intake, the risk of nutrient deficiencies rises in older groups. Further calorie restriction carries with it the potential danger of increasing the risk of nutrient deficiencies. For weight reduction and maintenance, it is perhaps more reasonable to suggest increased physical activity rather than further decreases in calorie intake.

Any dietary modification in older individuals should begin with a careful assessment to determine both the nutritional adequacy of the diet and the level of intake of nutrients to be modified. In particular, current and usual levels of sodium intake should be assessed before dietary modifications are made. To succeed, the diet plan should be developed in cooperation with the patient, allowing for differences in cultural patterns and taste preferences. The concept that only 30% of calories should come from fat and no more than 10% from saturated fat is difficult for many individuals to apply to their diets. To be effective, the nutrition counselor must develop unique methods of communicating simple concepts to older individuals who are expected to modify their diets. A nutrition counselor who prescribes diets modified in calories, fat, and sodium to older subjects and neglects to teach them how to select and prepare the diets is likely to see failure and noncompliance.

CONCLUSION

Recommendations for cardiovascular disease prevention for older people are extensions of recommendations for younger age groups. The majority of older Americans have one or more cardiovascular disease risk factors that require nutrition therapy, and nutrition-based interventions have demonstrated benefits in older adults. The focus of primary cardiovascular disease prevention is adopting healthful habits, including diet, physical activity, weight management, and avoidance of tobacco. A role of health care providers is to encourage and reinforce healthy life habits for all adults. The continual development of more effective nutrition interventions for elderly people requires a series of steps. It is essential, first, to define appropriate risk factors and effective modifiers for the natural history of disease; second, to define outcomes meaningful to elderly individuals in terms of the burden of illness; and third, to identify critical points of intervention to prevent disability.

REFERENCES

1. Erlinger TP, Pollack H, Appel LJ. Nutrition-related cardiovascular risk factors in older people: results from the Third National Health and Nutrition Examination Survey. *JAGS* 2000;48:1486–1489.

2. Kannel WB. Coronary heart disease risk factors in the elderly. *Am J Geriatr Cardiol* 2002;11:101–107.

3. American Heart Association. *Heart Disease and Stroke Statistics–2004 Update.* American Heart Association; Dallas, TX: 2003.

4. U.S. Department of Health and Human Services, Centers for Disease Control and Prevention, National Center for Health Statistics. *Health,* Washington, DC: 2003.

5. Bierman EL, Hazzard WR. Preventive gerontology: strategies for attenuation of the chronic diseases of aging. In: Hazzard WR, Andres R, Bierman EL, Blass JP, eds. *Principles of Geriatric Medicine and Gerontology,* 2nd ed. New York, NY: McGraw-Hill,1990.

6. Fair JM. Cardiovascular risk factor modification: is it effective in older adults? *J Cardiovascular Nurs* 2003; 18:161–168.

7. Tribble DL, Krauss RM. Atherosclerotic cardiovascular disease. In: Bowman BA, Russell RM, eds. *Present Knowledge in Nutrition* 8th ed. Washington, DC: ILSI Press; 2001.

8. Fried LP, Bush TL. Morbidity as a focus of preventive health care in the elderly. *Epidemiology Rev* 1988;10: 48–64.

9. McGandy RB. Nutrition and the aging cardiovascular system. In: Hutchinson ML, Munro HN, eds. *Nutrition and Aging.* Orlando, FL: Academic Press Inc; 1986.

10. Lakatta EG. Health, disease and cardiovascular aging. *Cardiovasc Med.* March 1985;38.

11. Lakatta EG. Heart and circulation. In: Schneider EL, Rowe JN, eds. *Handbook of the Biology of Aging.* San Diego, CA: Academic Press; 1990.

12. McGandy RB. Atherogenesis and aging. In: Chernoff R, Lipschitz DA, eds. *Health Promotion and Disease Prevention in the Elderly.* New York, NY: Raven Press; 1988.

13. Waller BF, Roberts WC. Cardiovascular disease in the very elderly. *Am J Cardiol* 1983;51:403–421.

14. Hennerici M, Rautenberg W, Trockel U, et al. Spontaneous progression and regression of small carotid atheromata. *Lancet* 1985;1:1415–1419.

15. Blankenhorn DH. Prevention or reversal of atherosclerosis: review of current evidence. *Am J Cardiol* 1989; 63:38H–41H.

16. Cashin-Hemphill L, Sanmarco ME, Blankenhorn DH. Augmented beneficial effects of colestipolniacin therapy at four years in the CLAS trial. Presented at: The American Heart Association Annual Meeting; New Orleans, LA; November 1989.

17. Ornish D, Scherwitz W, Brown SE, et al. Adherence to lifestyle changes and reversal of coronary atherosclerosis. Presented at: The American Heart Association Annual Meeting; New Orleans, LA; November 1989.

18. Gould KL, Ornish D, Scherwitz L, et al. Changes in myocardial perfusion abnormalities by positron emission tomography after long-term, intense risk factor modification. *JAMA* 1995;274:894–901.

19. *CDC Fact Sheet: Facts about Cardiovascular Disease.* Atlanta, GA: Centers for Disease Control and Prevention, Office of Communication, Division of Media Relations; June 27, 1997.

20. Minino AM. Smith BL. Deaths: preliminary data for 2000. *National Vital Statistics Reports.* Vol 49, no 12. Hyattsville, MD: National Center for Health Statistics; 2001.

21. Corry DB, Tuck ML. Nutritional interventions as antihypertensive therapy in the elderly. In: Morley JE, Glick Z, Rubenstein LZ, eds. *Geriatric Nutrition: A Comprehensive Review*, 2nd ed, New York, NY: Raven Press; 1995.

22. Losonczy KG, Harris TB, Havlik RJ. Vitamin E and vitamin C supplement use and risk of all-cause and coronary heart disease mortality in older persons: the Established Populations for Epidemiologic Studies of the Elderly. *Am J Clin Nutr* 1996;64:190–196.

23. Selhub J, Jacques PF, Wilson PF, et al. Vitamin status and intake as primary determinants of homocysteinemia in an elderly population. *JAMA* 1993;270:2693–2698.

24. Tucker KL, Selhub J, Wilson PWF, et al. Dietary intake pattern relates to plasma folate and homocysteine concentrations in the Framingham Heart Study. *J Nutr* 1996;126:3025–3031.

25. Stampfer MJ, Malinow MR, Willett WC, et al. A prospective study of plasma homocyst(e)ine and risk of myocardial infarction in US physicians. *JAMA* 1992; 268:877–881.

26. Nygård O, Nordrehaug JE, Refsum H, et al. Plasma homocysteine levels and mortality in patients with coronary artery disease. *N Engl J Med* 1997;337:230–236.

27. Ford ES, Mokdad AH, Giles WH, Brown DW. The metabolic syndrome and antioxidant concentrations: findings from the Third National Health and Nutrition Examination Survey. *Diabetes* 2003;52:2346–52.

28. Carr MC. The emergence of the metabolic syndrome with menopause. *J Clin Endocrinol Metab* 2003;88: 2404–2411.

29. Ridker PM. Clinical application of C-reactive protein for cardiovascular disease detection and prevention. *Circulation* 2003;107:363–9.

30. Wang TJ, Nam BH, Wilson PW, Wolf PA, Levy D, Polak JF, D'Agostino RB, O'Donnell CJ. Association of C-reactive protein with carotid atherosclerosis in men and women: the Framingham Heart Study. *Arterioscler Thromb Vasc Biol* 2002;22:1662–7.

31. Erlinger TP, Miller ER 3rd, Charleston J, Appel LJ. Inflammation modifies the effects of a reduced-fat low-cholesterol diet on lipids: results from the DASH-sodium trial. *Circulation* 2003;108:150–154.

32. Ridker PM, Rifai N, Rose L, Buring JE, Cook NR. Comparison of C-reactive protein and low-density lipoprotein cholesterol levels in the prediction of first cardiovascular events. *N Engl J Med* 2002;347:1557–1565.

33. Hackam DG, Anand SS. Emerging risk factors for atherosclerotic vascular disease: a critical review of the evidence. *JAMA* 2003;290:932–940.

34. Mangoni AA, Jackson SH. Homocysteine and cardiovascular disease: current evidence and future prospects. *Am J Med* 2002;112:556–565.

35. De Bree A, Verschuren WM, Kromhout D, Kluijtmans LA, Blom HJ. Homocysteine determinants and the evidence to what extent homocysteine determines the risk of coronary heart disease. *Pharmacol Rev* 2002;54: 599–618.

36. Werstuck GH, Lentz SR, Dayal S, Hossain GS, Sood SK, Shi YY, Zhou J, Maeda N, Krisans SK, Malinow MR, Austin RC. Homocysteine-induced endoplasmic reticulum stress causes dysregulation of the cholesterol and triglyceride biosynthetic pathways. *J Clin Invest* 2001;107:1263–1273.

37. Malinow MR, Bostom AG, Krauss RM. Homocyst(e)ine, diet, and cardiovascular diseases: a statement for healthcare professionals from the Nutrition Committee, American Heart Association. *Circulation* 1999; 99:178–182.

38. Loria CM, Ingram DD, Feldman JJ, Wright JD, Madans JH. Serum folate and cardiovascular disease mortality among US men and women. *Arch Inter Med* 2000;160: 3258–3262.

39. Food and Drug Administration. Food labeling: health claims and label statements; folate and neural tube defects. *Fed Regist* 1993;58:53254–53295.

40. Quinlivan EP, Gregory JF. Effect of food fortification on folic acid intake in the United States. *Am J Clin Nutr* 2003;77:221–225.

41. Castelli WP, Doyle JT, Gordon T, et al. HDL cholesterol and other lipids in coronary heart disease. *Circulation* 1977;55:767–772.

42. Kannel WB, Gordon T, eds. *The Framingham Study: An Epidemiological Investigation of Cardiovascular Disease.* Washington, DC: US Public Health Service; 1971. US Dept of Health, Education, and Welfare publication NIH 1740–0320.

43. Barrett-Connor E, Suarez L, Kjaw K, et al. Ischemic heart disease risk factors after 50. *J Chronic Dis* 1984; 27:103–114.

44. Castelli WP, Wilson PWF, Levy D, et al. Cardiovascular risk factors in the elderly. *Am J Cardiol* 1989;63: 12H–19H.

45. Schaefer EJ, Lichtenstein AH, Lamon-Fava S, et al. Lipoproteins, nutrition, aging, and atherosclerosis. *Am J Clin Nutr* 1995;61(suppl):726S–740S.

46. Expert Panel on Detection, Evaluation, and Treatment of High Blood Cholesterol in Adults. Executive Summary of the Third Report of the National Cholesterol Education Program (NCEP) Expert Panel on Detection, Evaluation, and Treatment of High Blood Cholesterol in Adults (Adult Treatment Panel III). *JAMA* 2001; 285:2486–2497.

47. Krauss RM, Eckel RH, Howard B, et al. AHA Dietary Guidelines: revision 2000: A statement for healthcare professionals from the Nutrition Committee of the American Heart Association. *Circulation* 2000;102: 2284–2299.

48. Lichtenstein AH. Trans fatty acids: where are the dietary recommendations? *Curr Opin Lipidol* 2003;14: 1–2.

49. Lenfant C. New national cholesterol education program. *Cardiovasc Med* 1985;10:39–40.

50. Blum CB, Levy R. Current therapy for hypercholesterolemia. *JAMA* 1989;261:3582–3587.

51. Kris-Etherton PM, Daniels SR, Eckel RH, et al. Summary of the scientific conference on dietary fatty acids and cardiovascular health: conference summary from the Nutrition Committee of the American Heart Association. *Circulation* 2001;103:1034–1039.

52. Hu FB, Stampfer MJ, Manson JE, et al. Dietary fat intake and the risk of coronary heart disease in women. *N Engl J Med* 1997;337:1391–1399.

53. Katan MB, Grundy SM, Jones P, et al. Efficacy and safety of plant stanols and sterols in the management of blood cholesterol levels. *Mayo Clin Proc* 2003;78: 965–978.

54. Kris-Etherton PM, Harris WS, Appel LJ. American Heart Association Nutrition Committee. Fish consumption, fish oil, omega-3 fatty acids, and cardiovascular disease. *Circulation* 2002;106:2747–2757.

55. Hu FB, Bronner L, Willett WC, et al. Fish and omega-3 fatty acid intake and risk of coronary heart disease in women. *JAMA* 2002;287:1815–1821.

56. Hu FB, Willett WC. Optimal diets for prevention of coronary heart disease. *JAMA* 2002;288:2569–2678.

57. Kris-Etherton PM, Harris WS, Appel LJ, AHA Nutrition Committee, American Heart Association. Omega-3 fatty acids and cardiovascular disease: new recommendations from the American Heart Association. *Arterioscler Thromb Vasc Biol* 2003;23:151–152.

58. Anderson JW, Johnstone BM, Cook-Newell ME. Meta-analysis of the effects of soy protein intake on serum lipids. *N Engl J Med* 1995;333:276–282.

59. Erdman JW Jr. AHA Science Advisory: Soy protein and cardiovascular disease: a statement for healthcare professionals from the Nutrition Committee of the AHA. *Circulation* 2000;102:2555–2559.

60. Hasler CM. The cardiovascular effects of soy products. *J Cardiovasc Nurs* 2002;16:50–63.

61. Manson JE, Gaziano JM, Jones MA, Hennekens CH. Antioxidants and cardiovascular disease: a review. *J Am Coll Nutr* 1993;12:426–432.

62. Rimm EB, Stampfer MJ. The role of antioxidants in preventive cardiology. *Curr Opin Cardiol* 1997; 12:188–194.

63. Gaziano JM. Antioxidant vitamins and coronary artery disease risk. *Am J Med* 1994;97(3A):18S–21S.

64. Tribble DL, AHA Science Advisory. Antioxidant consumption and risk of coronary heart disease: emphasis on vitamin C, vitamin E, and beta-carotene: a statement for healthcare professionals from the American Heart Association. *Circulation* 1999;99:591–595.

65. Morris CD, Carson S. Routine vitamin supplementation to prevent cardiovascular disease: a summary of the evidence for the U.S. Preventive Services Task Force. *Ann Inter Med* 2003;139:56–70.

66. Meydani M. Nutrition interventions in aging and age-associated disease. *Ann N Y Acad Sci* 2001;928:226–235.

67. Paolisso G, Gambardella A, Giugliano D, et al. Chronic intake of pharmacological doses of vitamin E might be useful in the therapy of elderly patients with coronary heart disease. *Am J Clin Nutr* 1995; 61:848–852.

68. Emmert DH, Kirchner JT. The role of vitamin E in the prevention of heart disease. *Arch Fam Med* 1999;8: 537–542.

69. Supiano MA. Hypertension. In: Cassel CK, Cohen HJ, Larson EB, Meier DE, Resnick NM, Rubenstein LZ, Sorenson LB, eds. *Geriatric Medicine.* 3rd ed. New York, NY: Springer-Verlag;1997.

70. National Heart, Lung, and Blood Institute Joint National Committee on Prevention, Detection, Evaluation, and Treatment of High Blood Pressure, National High Blood Pressure Education Program Coordinating Committee. The Seventh Report of the Joint National Committee on Prevention, Detection, Evaluation, and Treatment of High Blood Pressure: the JNC 7 report. *JAMA* 2003;289:2560–2572.

71. Hajjar I, Kotchen TA. Trends in prevalence, awareness, treatment, and control of hypertension in the United States, 1988–2000. *JAMA* 2003;290:199–206.

72. Kannell WB. Blood pressure as a cardiovascular risk factor. *JAMA* 1996;275:1571–1576.

73. Stamler J, Stamler R, Neaton JD. Blood pressure, systolic and diastolic, and cardiovascular risks. *Arch Int Med* 1993;153:598–615.

74. Wilking SVB, Belanger A, Kannel WB, et al. Determinants of isolated systolic hypertension. *JAMA* 1988; 260:3451–3455.

75. Vasan RS, Beiser A, Seshadri S, Larson MG, Kannel WB, D'Agostino RB, Levy D. Residual lifetime risk for developing hypertension in middle-aged women and men: the Framingham Heart Study. *JAMA* 2002;287: 1003–1010.

76. Kannel WB, D'Agostino RB, Silbershatz H. Blood pressure and cardiovascular morbidity and mortality rates in the elderly. *Am Heart J* 1997;134;758–763.

77. Kannel WB. Nutrition and the occurrence and prevention of cardiovascular disease in the elderly. *Nutr Rev* 1988;46:68–78.

78. Franklin SS, Jacobs MJ, Wong ND, L'Italien GJ, Lapuerta P. Predominance of isolated systolic hypertension among middle-aged and elderly US hypertensives: analysis based on National Health and Nutrition Examination Survey (NHANES) III. *Hypertension* 2001;37:869–874.

79. National High Blood Pressure Education Program Working Group. National High Blood Pressure Education Program Working Group report on hypertension in the elderly. *Hypertension* 1994; 23:275–285.

80. ALLHAT Officers and Coordinators for the ALLHAT Collaborative Research Group. The Antihypertensive and Lipid-Lowering Treatment to Prevent Heart Attack Trial. Major outcomes in high-risk hypertensive patients randomized to angiotensin-converting enzyme inhibitor or calcium channel blocker vs diuretic: the Antihypertensive and Lipid-Lowering Treatment to Prevent Heart Attack Trial (ALLHAT). *JAMA* 2002; 288:2981–2997.

81. Pell S, Fayerweather WE. Trends in the incidence of myocardial infarction and in associated mortality and morbidity in a large employed population. *N Engl J Med* 1985;312:1005–1011.

82. US Department of Health and Human Services, National Institutes of Health National Heart, Lung, and Blood Institute. *Facts about the DASH eating plan.* Washington, DC; 2003.

83. Sacks FM, Svetkey LP, Vollmer WM, et al. DASH-Sodium Collaborative Research Group. Effects on blood pressure of reduced dietary sodium and the Dietary Approaches to Stop Hypertension (DASH) diet. DASH-Sodium Collaborative Research Group. *N Engl J Med* 2001;344:3–10.

84. Manson JE, Willett WC, Stampfer MJ, et al. Body weight and mortality among women. *N Engl J Med* 1995;333:677–685.

85. Willett WC, Manson JE, Stampfer MJ, et al. Weight, weight change, and coronary heart disease in women: risk within the "normal" weight range. *JAMA* 1995;273: 461–465.

86. Kannel WB, Gordon T. *An Epidemiologic Investigation of Cardiovascular Disease.* Washington, DC: US Public Health Service; 1968. US Dept of Health, Education, and Welfare publication.

87. Havlik RJ, Hubert HB, Fabsitz RR, et al. Weight and hypertension. *Ann Intern Med* 1983;98:855–859.

88. Harlan WR, Hull AL, Schmouder RL, et al. High blood pressure in older Americans: the first national health and nutrition examination survey. *Hypertension* 1984;6: 802–809.

89. Kannel WB, Gordon T, Castelli WP. Obesity, lipids, and glucose intolerance: the Framingham study. *Am J Clin Nutr* 1979;32:1238–1245.

90. Lamon-Fava S, Wilson PW, Schaefer EJ. Impact of body mass index on coronary heart disease risk factors in men and women: the Framingham Offspring Study. *Arterioscler Thromb Vasc Biol* 1996;16:1509–1515.

91. Krauss RM, Winston M, Fletcher RN, Grundy SM. Obesity: impact of cardiovascular disease. *Circulation* 1998;98:1472–1476.

92. Brownell KD. Public health approaches to obesity and its management. In: Breslow L, Fielding JE, Lave LB, eds. *Annual Review of Public Health.* Palo Alto, CA: Annual Reviews Inc; 1986.

93. Dannenberg A, Drizd T, Horan M, et al. CVD [Abstract]. *Epidemiol Newslett* January 1985;68.

94. Higgins M, Kannel WB, Garrison R, et al. Hazards of obesity: the Framingham experience. *Acta Med Scand* 1987;723(suppl):23–26.

95. Hubert HB, Feinleib M, McNamara PM, et al. Obesity as an independent risk factor for cardiovascular disease: a 26-year follow-up of participants in the Framingham Heart Study. *Circulation* 1983;67:968–977.

96. Heiat A, Vaccarino V, Krumholz HM. An evidence-based assessment of federal guidelines for overweight and obesity as they apply to elderly persons. *Arch Intern Med* 2001;161:1194–203.

97. American Heart Association Council on Clinical Cardiology Subcommittee on Exercise, Rehabilitation, and Prevention. American Heart Association Council on Nutrition, Physical Activity, and Metabolism Subcommittee on Physical Activity. Exercise and physical activity in the prevention and treatment of atherosclerotic cardiovascular disease: a statement from the Council on Clinical Cardiology (Subcommittee on Exercise, Rehabilitation, and Prevention) and the Council on Nutrition, Physical Activity, and Metabolism (Subcommittee on Physical Activity). *Circulation* 2003;107:109–116.

98. Stefanick ML, Mackey S, Sheehan M, et al. Effects of diet and exercise in men and postmenopausal women with low levels of HDL cholesterol and high levels of LDL cholesterol. *N Engl J Med* 1998;339:12–20.

99. Houde SC, Melillo KD. Cardiovascular health and physical activity in older adults: an integrative review

of research methodology and results. *J Adv Nurs* 2002;38:219–234.

100. Burke GL, Arnold AM, Bild DE, et al. CHS Collaborative Research Group. Factors associated with healthy aging: the cardiovascular health study. *J Am Geriatr Soc* 2001;49:254–262.

101. Marwick C. NHANES III health data relevant for aging nation. *JAMA* 1997;277:100–102.

102. Popkin BM, Siega-Riz AM, Haines PS, Jahns L. Where's the fat? Trends in U.S. diets 1965–1996. *Prev Med* 2001;32:245–254.

103. Lamon-Fava S, Jenner JL, Jacques PF, Schaefer EJ. Effects of dietary intakes on plasma lipids, lipoproteins, and apolipoproteins in free-living elderly men and women. *Am J Clin Nutr* 1994;59:32–41.

CHAPTER 12

The Aging Renal System

Robert D. Lindeman, MD

The increasing number and proportion of the population that are considered elderly, combined with an increasing awareness of the clinical importance of age-related changes in organ function, have stimulated the need for a more precise knowledge of these changes in the kidney. Kidney function can be easily, accurately, precisely, and noninvasively quantified using clearance techniques that require only the collection of timed urine samples and blood samples obtained at the midpoints of the urine collection periods. These tests have made the kidney a model system to study the changes with aging in humans.

The following is an overview of the changes in kidney function that occur during adult life with discussions covering the pathophysiology of the decline in renal function observed with advancing age in cross-sectional and longitudinal studies.[1-4] Is this decline all due to superimposed, often undetected, pathology, or is there a progressive involutional loss of function that is inevitable? Another possibility discussed is that age-related glomerular sclerosis develops only when a threshold of environmental and genetic factors is reached that initiates the process. This would explain why many, but not all persons, show a decrease in renal function with age.

It is important to understand the nutritional implications involved in the development of this age-related loss of renal function. Patients with abnormal carbohydrate metabolism (diabetes mellitus), dyslipidemias, atherosclerosis, and hypertension all have accelerated development of renal lesions similar to those observed with age-related glomerular sclerosis. All of these conditions can be treated effectively by dietary modifications and/or with medications with resultant beneficial effects on the kidney.

This chapter will not attempt to cover the spectrum of renal diseases that can afflict the elderly, but rather will focus on several issues that have nutritional implications. The studies, for example, remain inconclusive about whether or not protein restriction at any point in the development of chronic renal disease prior to the need for dialysis or transplantation is of sufficient value to warrant the efforts involved. Management of an elderly patient who forms stones or has recurring infections in the kidney and urinary tract also, at times, warrants dietary interventions.

CHANGES IN RENAL MORPHOLOGY WITH AGE

The weight of both kidneys, about 50 grams at birth, increases to 270 grams during the third and fourth decades, and thereafter decreases to 185 grams in the ninth decade.[5] The loss of renal mass is primarily from the cortex and is mostly vascular in origin, with the most significant changes occurring at the capillary level. The numbers of glomerular and tubular cells decrease, and the size of individual surviving cells increases with age.[6] The glomerular changes occurring with age-related glomerular sclerosis have been studied more extensively in animal models than in man, but consist initially of a progressive increase in mesangial cells and matrix, thickening of the glomerular basement membrane, an increase in interstitial fibrosis, and atrophy and loss of tubular cells. Ischemic obsolescence of the cortical glomerulus results in resorption and disappearance of the entire glomerulus; ischemic obsolescence of the juxtamedullary glomerulus results in the hyalinization of the glomerular capillary bed with development of a shunt between the afferent and efferent arteriole.[7] The outer cortex is more severely involved than the juxtamedullary portion of the kidney.

These changes are accelerated in individuals with diabetes, hypertension, dyslipidemia, and atherosclerotic disease. A direct correlation exists between the number of obsolete (hyalinized) glomeruli observed and the severity of atherosclerosis elsewhere in the body.[8] Some sclerotic glomeruli were observed in all kidneys studied, eg, 60-year-old subjects with the least atherosclerotic disease still had 5% of their glomeruli obsolete. Eighty-year-olds had 10% to 30% of their glomeruli completely hyalinized. The functional loss associated with this anatomical loss might be hard to detect as functional adjustments (hypertrophy, hyperperfusion, and hyperfiltration) in the remaining nephrons may be compensating.

CHANGES IN RENAL FUNCTION WITH AGE

Glomerular Filtration Rate

A number of cross-sectional studies have shown an age-related decline in renal function after age 30 years.[1–3] (Figure 12–1.) The rate of decline in the glomerular filtration rate (GFR) approximates 1 mL/minute/year. Rowe et al.[3] reported a 10-year analysis of the first large-scale longitudinal study of renal function. Serial true creatinine clearances were obtained on 884 community-dwelling volunteers at 12- and 18-month intervals (Baltimore Longitudinal Study on Aging). Their cross-sectional analysis pro-

vided results similar to those observed in previous studies. A longitudinal analysis of the serial creatinine clearances showed an accelerating decline similar to that observed in cross-sectional studies suggesting that selective mortality and cohort differences could be excluded as responsible for the changes observed.

Although mean creatinine clearance rates fell from 140 mL/min per 1.73 m^2 at age 25–34 years to 97 mL/min per 1.73 m^2 at age 75–84 years, mean serum creatinine concentrations rose insignificantly from 0.81 to 0.84 mg/100 mL (72 to 74 μmol/L) (Table 12–1).[3] This indicates that the mean creatinine production decreases at nearly the same rate as the mean renal clearance of creatinine, reflecting the decrease in body muscle mass that occurs with age. The practical implication is that serum creatinine concentration in the older patient must be interpreted with this in mind when used to determine or modify dosages of drugs cleared totally (eg, aminoglycoside antibiotics) or partially (eg, digoxin) by the kidney. The Cockcroft-Gault formula is used commonly to estimate creatinine clearance rates (CCR) in older individuals.[9] It is corrected for age as follows:

$$\text{For men,}\ C_{CR} = \frac{(140 - \text{age in years})\,(\text{weight in Kg})}{72 \times \text{serum creatinine (mg/100 mL)}}$$
$$\text{For women,}\ C_{CR} = C_{CR\ \text{for men}} \times 0.85$$

A subsequent publication from the Baltimore Longitudinal Study on Aging reported the mean decrease in GFR in 446 volunteers followed over a 23-year period with at least 5 measures of creatinine clearance was 0.87 mL/min/year, close to that previously reported in cross-sectional studies (this value decreased to 0.75 mL/min/year if individuals with potential renal or urinary tract disease and/or treated or untreated hypertension were eliminated).[4] However, one-third of these subjects had no decline in creatinine clearance rates over the period of time followed. Figure 12–2 shows the serial plots of six representative volunteers followed for periods up to 15–21 years who showed no decrease in the slopes of creatinine clearances plotted over time (positive slopes). These observations suggest

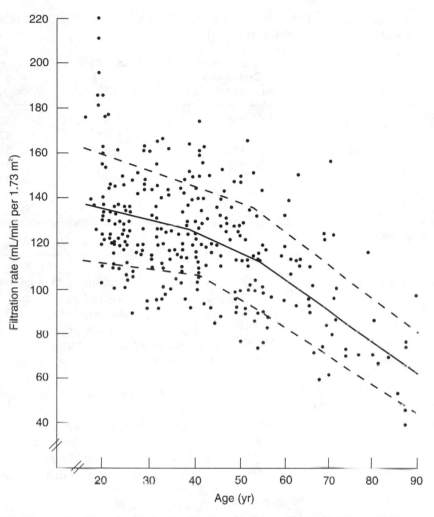

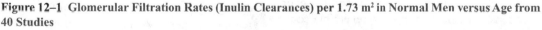

Figure 12–1 Glomerular Filtration Rates (Inulin Clearances) per 1.73 m² in Normal Men versus Age from 40 Studies
The solid line represents the mean and broken lines one standard deviation (from Wesson,[2] with permission).

that the decline in renal function observed with age may be the result of intervening pathologic processes, eg, vascular occlusions with resultant ischemic injury from atherosclerotic and/or hypertensive processes; undetected glomerulonephritis or interstitial nephritis secondary to drugs, infections, immunologic insults, or other toxic exposures; or urinary tract infection or obstruction, as opposed to any chronic involutional process occurring in all individuals, albeit at different rates. Another more likely possibility is

that there is an age-related glomerular sclerosis that occurs in some, but not all, individuals only when a combination of environmental factors such as hypertension, abnormal carbohydrate metabolism, dyslipidemia, etc., and genetic factors reach a threshold sufficient to initiate the process. This would be consistent with what has been observed in the Baltimore Longitudinal Study on Aging patients,[4] and in some rat models apparently free of any age-related evidence of kidney damage.[10]

Table 12–1 Cross-Sectional Age Differences in Mean Creatinine Clearances, Serum Creatinine Concentrations, and 24-hour Urine Creatinine Excretions

Age Group (years)	No. Subjects	Creatinine Clearances (mL/min/1.73 m²)	Serum Creatinine (mg/100 mL)	Creatinine Excretions (mg/24 hr)
25–34	73	140.1	0.81	1862
35–44	122	132.6	0.81	1746
45–54	152	126.8	0.83	1689
55–64	94	119.9	0.84	1580
65–74	68	109.5	0.83	1409
75–84	29	96.9	0.84	1259

Source: Adapted from Rowe JW, Andres R, Tobin JD, et al.[3] Copyright © *The Gerontological Society of America.* Reproduced by permission of the publisher.

Renal Blood (Plasma) Flow

The quantity of blood perfusing the kidney, generally estimated by using p-amino-hippuric acid (PAH) clearances, decreases with age at a rate slightly greater than that of GFR (inulin clearance). The mean PAH clearance has been reported to fall from 649 mL/min in the fourth decade to 289 mL/min in the ninth decade.[1] The decrease in renal blood flow (RBF) with age without a proportionate decrease in blood pressure is indicative of vascular impedance due to intraluminal pathology (atheromata, sclerosis) or an increase in renal vascular resistance due to vasoconstriction. Since RBF can be increased transiently by administration of vasodilators or pyrogens, a vasoconstrictive or reversible component must be implicated in the regulation of the renal circulation in both age groups.[11,12] Administration of a pyrogen produced a greater vasodilatation of the arteriolar system in the kidneys of older subjects than in the kidneys of young subjects, suggesting that a greater resting vasoconstriction exists in older subjects.[11] This potentially could explain some or all of the decrease in RBF and GFR observed with age.

Hollenberg et al.[12] provided conflicting information showing that the vasodilator acetylcholine increased renal blood flow in both young and old subjects, but the effect was much more striking in the young subjects. In contrast, the vasoconstrictor responses to angiotensin were similar in the young and old subjects. These studies suggest that the renal vasculature in the older subject is in a relatively greater state of baseline vasodilatation compared with the vasculature of the younger subject. These investigators also found, using Xenon washout studies, that the perfusion of the outer cortical nephrons decreased more with age than did the perfusion of the juxtamedullary nephrons. Since the juxtamedullary nephrons have a higher filtration fraction (GFR divided by effective renal plasma flow as measured by PAH clearance) than the cortical nephrons, a selective loss of the latter could explain the increase in this filtration fraction observed with age. An alternative explanation for the increase in filtration fraction is that the efferent arteriole is disproportionately vasoconstricted compared with the afferent arteriole, thereby increasing the filtration pressure in the glomerular capillary bed.

Maximum Tubular Transport Capacity

The tubular maximum for secretory transport (as measured by clearance of PAH given in amounts exceeding the ability to secrete this compound in a single pass through the kidneys) decreases with age at a rate nearly parallel to the decrease in GFR (inulin clearance).[1] The tubular maximum for glucose resorption also decreases

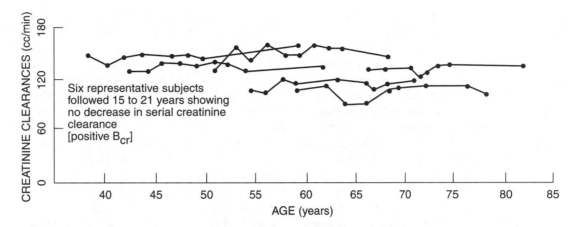

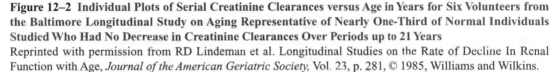

Figure 12–2 Individual Plots of Serial Creatinine Clearances versus Age in Years for Six Volunteers from the Baltimore Longitudinal Study on Aging Representative of Nearly One-Third of Normal Individuals Studied Who Had No Decrease in Creatinine Clearances Over Periods up to 21 Years
Reprinted with permission from RD Lindeman et al. Longitudinal Studies on the Rate of Decline In Renal Function with Age, *Journal of the American Geriatric Society,* Vol. 23, p. 281, © 1985, Williams and Wilkins.

at a rate closely paralleling the decrease in inulin clearance.[13] Reduction in the secretory and re-sorptive tubular maximums with age then could be explained by a progressive loss of functional nephrons. However, animal studies suggest aging produces changes in the basic biochemistry of the tubular cell. Tissue slice studies show fewer energy producing mitochondria,[14] lower enzyme concentrations,[14,15] lower concentrations of aden-osine triphosphatase (ATPase),[16] and decreased tubular transport capacity[14] in tubular cells of old compared to young kidneys.

Concentrating and Diluting Ability

A decrease in the concentrating ability of the kidney with age is well documented.[17–19] This means a loss in ability to conserve body water in the face of dehydration in older individuals (Chapter 5). Rowe et al.[18] suggested that the rel-ative increase in medullary blood flow per neph-ron with age, as demonstrated by Hollenberg et al,[12] would result in enhanced removal of med-ullary solute (washout) and decreased osmolal-ity in the medullary interstitium. Maximum urine osmolality after infusion of large amounts of va-sopressin (Pitressin) is significantly decreased in

older subjects undergoing a water diuresis.[20] In contrast, the kidneys of older subjects respond normally to graded doses of vasopressin insuffi-cient to maximally concentrate the urine.[19] This suggests that the decrease in concentrating abil-ity of older subjects in the first study is the result of a decrease in medullary tonicity rather than any defect in the ability of the tubule to respond to vasopressin.

Maximum diluting ability, as measured by the minimum urine osmolality achieved with water loading, also decreases with age.[19,21] Since free water clearance per unit of GFR is similar in young and old, it does not appear that there is any water-handling defect in tubular function with aging.

Urine Acidification

Despite the decrease in renal function with age, blood pH, pCO_2, and bicarbonate values of aged individuals without renal disease in early studies did not differ significantly under basal conditions from the values observed in young subjects.[22] More recent studies, however, showed that healthy elders develop a low-grade diet-dependent metabolic acidosis, the severity of which increases with age when endogenous acid production is maintained constant.[23]

The decreases in blood pH and serum bicarbonate concentrations after ingestion of an acid load are prolonged in elderly persons.[24,25] The minimum urine pH values achieved after an acid load are similar in young and old persons.[24] However, a much larger percentage of the ingested acid load, as measured by total acid excretion (ammonium plus titratable acid minus bicarbonate), is excreted over an 8-hour period by young subjects when compared to the older individuals. When total acid excretion is factored by GFR, similar rates of excretion are obtained in young and old subjects. The young subjects excreted a greater percentage of their total acid as ammonium, whereas the older subjects excreted more as titratable acid. This was because older subjects had an increase in their urinary buffers, eg, phosphates, creatinine, responsible for titratable acids per unit of GFR. A subsequent report found that elderly subjects had a small pH gradient defect and ammonium excretion was significantly reduced even after factoring by GFR.[25]

Glomerular Permeability

Most older patients do not have significant proteinuria (albuminuria) suggesting there is not a clinically significant increase in glomerular permeability with age. There does appear to be some increase in the prevalence of proteinuria in older individuals, probably as a result of pathological processes. Glomerular permeability to free hemoglobins and a spectrum of dextrans of varying molecular weights was not different in normal young versus old subjects.[26,27]

AGE-RELATED CHANGES IN RENAL RESPONSE TO ENVIRONMENT

Epstein and Hollenberg[28] found that older individuals failed to conserve sodium as avidly or efficiently as younger subjects when placed on a sodium-restricted diet. Many of the determinants of renal sodium conservation, eg, GFR, the renin-angiotensin-aldosterone system, atrial natriuretic peptide, and physical factors determined in part by hemodynamics, vary significantly with age. As an example, the elderly have lower plasma renin activities and urinary aldosterone excretions both on an unrestricted salt diet and after 3 to 6 days of salt restriction.[29,30] Whether this is due to a renal defect or extrarenal adaptation remains unclear. This change might not only explain the decreased ability of elderly subjects to conserve sodium when salt depleted, but it could account for the propensity of elderly subjects to develop hyperkalemia when faced with a potassium load (Chapter 5). Elderly individuals also are more prone to the development of extracellular fluid volume overload when challenged with an increased sodium intake or intravenous sodium load.[31]

Similarly, there is a decrease in the ability of the elderly to convert 25-hydroxyvitamin D_3 to 1,25-dihydroxyvitamin D_3.[32] This appears to be due to a deficiency of 1 α-hydroxylase enzyme activity in old compared to young kidneys. This contributes to deficient vitamin D activity in older persons, in turn contributing to the development of osteoporosis.

PATHOPHYSIOLOGY OF THE AGE-RELATED DECLINE IN RENAL FUNCTION

It remains unclear whether the mean decrease in renal function observed with aging is all due to superimposed pathology, eg, vascular occlusion with resultant ischemic injury, undetected glomerulonephritis caused by immunologic injury after an infection, or acute tubular injury or interstitial nephritis after an infection or exposure to drugs or other toxins, or rather is due to a progressive involutional process with loss of nephron units (glomerular obsolescence), albeit at different rates in different individuals. The sequence of glomerular loss in the absence of overt lesions in the large and small vessels suggests nephron loss can occur normally without overt vascular lesions.[7] On the other hand, one-third of volunteers in the Baltimore Longitudinal Study on Aging followed between 1958 and 1981 showed no decrease in creatinine clearance supporting the concept that the mean decrease in renal function with age might all be due to intervening pathologic processes, rather than any relentless involutional process that affects all individuals.[4]

Another possible explanation is that age-related glomerular sclerosis develops only when a threshold of environmental and genetic factors is reached that initiates the process. This would explain why many, but not all persons, show a decrease in renal function with age. Findings from animal models of age-related nephropathy help to understand the processes in man, although they do not explain the mechanisms (biochemistry) responsible for these changes. The roles of reactive oxygen intermediates (ROIs) (eg, hydroxyl radicals), advanced glycosylation end products (AGEs), angiotensin II, nitrous oxide synthesis and response, endothelin, and a variety of growth factors, cytokines, vasoactive peptides, and lipid mediators all have been implicated as having a role in the development of age-related glomerular sclerosis. For those interested in more information related to this topic, a recent Nephrology Forum provides an excellent review.[33]

ROLE OF HYPERPERFUSION, HYPERFILTRATION, AND RENAL RESERVE

When the population of normal glomeruli is reduced by surgical ablation or renal disease in the rat model, the remaining glomeruli react with an "adaptive" hyperperfusion and hyperfiltration.[34] This glomerular hyperfiltration disrupts the integrity of the capillary membrane, resulting in proteinuria, accumulation of mesangial deposits, and initiation or acceleration of the loss of renal function through a process of developing glomerular sclerosis. The phenomenon of hyperfiltration also is seen in the remaining kidney after uninephrectomy, in uncontrolled diabetes, and after the ingestion of large amounts of protein or infusions of amino acids. Brenner et al[35,36] have suggested that the protein-rich diet charac-

teristic of modern Western society itself induces chronic renal hyperperfusion and hyperfiltration, thereby contributing to the structural and functional deterioration of the aging kidney. Presumably, the high glomerular pressures and flow rates created by the high protein intake contribute to the development of glomerular sclerosis, resulting in a progressive decline in renal function with age alone, as with primary renal disease, diabetes mellitus, hypertension, and renal ablation (Figure 12–3).[36]

In early diabetes mellitus, both kidney size and GFR are increased, producing changes in humans similar to those observed in the remnant kidney of animal models.[37] With long-standing hyperperfusion and hyperfiltration, diabetics develop glomerular sclerosis with declining renal function. Hypertension also produces hyperperfusion and hyperfiltration, compounding the effect in diabetics. The ACE inhibitors have been effectively employed to reduce the hyperfiltration in diabetics working by vasodilating the efferent arteriole of the glomerulus more than the afferent arteriole, thereby decreasing the pressure in the glomerulus.[38] Not all evidence, however, favors the theory that hyperfiltration leads to glomerulosclerosis in humans. Transplant donors do not show an accelerated decline in renal function after uninephrectomy even though they develop hyperperfusion and hyperfiltration.[39] It may be that the glomerulus can tolerate some increase in perfusion pressure and hyperfiltration without damage, but once a threshold, determined by both environmental and genetic factors, is surpassed, injury occurs.

Bosch et al.[40] quantified the increase in GFR and RPF after an oral protein load and termed this increase "renal functional reserve capacity." An 80-gram protein meal increased GFR from a mean of 105 mL/min to 171 mL/min in four normal subjects. They theorized that this represented the ability of the kidney under stress to increase flow and filtration rates. These same investigators[41] showed that patients with underlying renal disease lost some to all of this ability to increase their GFR, meaning that they were continuously hyperfiltrating, presumably subjecting their kidneys to the

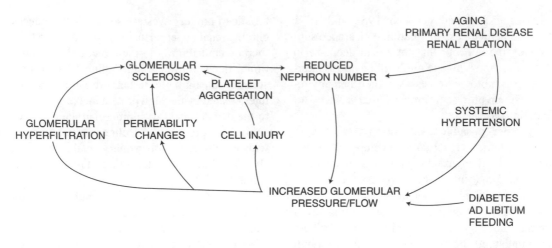

Figure 12–3 Proposed Role of Hyperperfusion and Hyperfiltration in the Development of Age- and Disease-Related Glomerular Sclerosis
From Anderson S and Brenner BM. Effects of aging on the renal glomerulus. *American Journal of Medicine*, Vol. 80, p. 435, © 1986, Cahners Publishing. Reprinted with permission from Excerpta Media, Inc.

development of glomerular sclerosis and a progressive decline in renal function. Others have demonstrated that limitation in protein intake to patients with chronic renal disease reduces the rate of progression of renal insufficiency.[42,43] One can speculate that a low protein diet might restore renal functional reserve and provide protection to the kidneys of elderly with reduced GFR.

Rodriquez-Iturbe et al.[44] found the mean increases in GFR after a high protein meal were 18% in two groups of patients with acute nephritis and postuninephrectomy (kidney donors) compared to 58% in normal control subjects. This suggests the first two groups had a diminished renal reserve and were chronically in a state of hyperfiltration. Infusions of amino acids and dopamine have been used to increase GFR and quantify renal reserve, but offer no advantages other than a more rapid onset of action.[45]

The studies by Hollenberg et al.[12] reported earlier suggest that older persons may be in a relative state of renal vascular vasodilatation. This would suggest they might have lost some of their "renal reserve" and already be hyperperfusing and hyperfiltering. Fliser et al.[46] compared the increases in GFR in young and old subjects after an amino acid infusion and found GFR increased significantly and similarly in both groups. They

concluded that the renal reserve or residual vasodilatory capacity of the kidney was not impaired in normal elderly subjects (mean age 70 years). In contrast, Fuiano et al[47] found the percentage increase in GFR and RBF was less in older subjects after infusions of amino acids and dopamine compared to young subjects, suggesting there was a defect in the vasodilatory capacity of the aging kidney.

RISK FACTORS FOR AGE-RELATED GLOMERULAR SCLEROSIS

Both diabetes and hypertension have long been recognized as frequent causes of glomerular sclerosis and chronic renal failure, both accelerating the decline in renal function observed in patients with underlying renal disease. Treatment of both conditions will delay the relentless progression of kidney disease.

More recently, the dyslipidemias, either an increase in total or LDL cholesterol, or a decrease in HDL cholesterol, also have been implicated as being a cause or contributor to the development of chronic renal failure.[48–50] Furthermore, a meta-analysis of the effects of lipid reduction on the rate of progression of renal disease showed a significant slowing with treatment.[51]

RENAL DISEASES IN THE ELDERLY

The most common presenting manifestations of renal disease in the elderly, as in younger persons, are acute and chronic renal insufficiency (azotemia), proteinuria (nephrotic and non-nephrotic), and hematuria. Most of the causes of these diseases are similar in young and old subjects, but the prevalences (incidences) of these vary. As examples, renal vascular disease, obstructive disease, and acute renal failure due to postischemic acute tubular necrosis are more common in older persons, whereas acute post-infectious glomerulonephritis and nephrotic syndrome due to minimal change disease and focal glomerulosclerosis are more commonly seen in younger persons. For those wanting more information on this topic, there are various geriatric medicine and nephrology texts available.[52]

ROLE OF PROTEIN RESTRICTION IN CHRONIC RENAL DISEASE

Until the availability of dialysis and transplantation became more widely available, protein restriction was the primary means of managing patients with end-stage renal disease having uremic symptoms (anorexia, nausea, vomiting, fatigue, etc.) because it could be used effectively to lower the blood urea nitrogen level and reduce symptoms. It also was reported that protein restriction earlier in the course of chronic renal disease slowed the progression of the disease process. The Modification of Diet in Renal Disease (MDRD) study was a large multicenter clinical trial designed to test the hypothesis that dietary protein restriction and strict blood pressure control would delay the progression of chronic renal disease. The primary analysis in 1994 was inconclusive regarding the benefits of a low protein diet,[53] however, a later analysis of the study suggests that the balance of evidence was more consistent with a beneficial effect of protein restriction than the contrary hypothesis of no beneficial effect.[43]

One also has to be concerned that an adequate protein and energy intake be maintained to ensure a positive nitrogen balance in these patients with chronic renal disease. This can be difficult especially if the patient continues to lose substantial amounts of protein in the urine. The usual prescribed protein intake for patients with chronic renal insufficiency is 0.6 grams per kg of body weight per day, which is less than the Recommended Dietary Allowances (RDA) of the Food and Nutrition Board of 0.8 grams per kg of body weight per day. Studies from the MDRD study revealed no clinically meaningful changes in weight, anthropometry, or serum proteins, lipids, or amino acids from this level of dietary restriction.[54] Since adherence to such a low protein intake can be challenging, regular follow-up with a skilled dietitian to monitor protein and energy intake and nutritional status is necessary to ensure malnutrition does not develop and compliance is achieved.

As serum phosphate increases, phosphate-binding antacids should be given to prevent the development of secondary hyperparathyroidism. Calcium carbonate and acetate antacids are the phosphate binders of choice because toxicity may result from aluminum-containing (bone demineralization, dementia, anemia) and magnesium-containing (respiratory depression) antacids. If serum calcium remains below normal, vitamin D or its active metabolite, 1,25-dihydroxycholecalciferol (Caltriol), should be added to normalize the serum calcium concentration.

RENAL CALCULI

Often the constituents of renal calculi, most notably calcium, are normally present in the urine as supersaturated solutions and are maintained in solution by protective colloids. A delicate balance is maintained, and precipitation results if an infectious nidus or a change in urine concentration or pH occurs. Calcium phosphate or oxalate becomes insoluble at an alkaline pH; an acid pH favors precipitation of uric acid and cystine. Triple phosphates generally indicate infection with a urea-splitting organism.

Calcium Stones

Identification of calcium on stone analysis should lead one to suspect hypercalciuria as an underlying cause. On a normal diet, a normal person excretes approximately 150 mg/day of calcium. More than 250 mg/day is considered evidence of hypercalciuria. Most of these patients have an absorptive defect; in some, there is a renal defect. Serum calcium, phosphorus, and alkaline phosphatase can be used to screen for hyperparathyroidism, but hypercalciuria can result from hypercalcemia of any cause. Immobilization, particularly that resulting from paralysis or extensive casting, greatly increases urinary calcium excretion (>500 mg/day), which in turn can lead to stone formation. In older persons, there often is an increase in urinary oxalate related to increased intestinal absorption and dehydration.

Idiopathic hypercalciuria (normal serum calcium without an underlying cause of hypercalciuria) can be treated with a high fluid intake (2 to 3 liters per day), restriction of calcium intake (dairy products), urinary acidification, and thiazides. The last decreases urinary calcium excretion, but may cause hypercalcemia.

Uric Acid Stones

Uric acid stones develop when urinary uric acid excretion exceeds 1,000 mg/day or when pH falls to the range of 5.5. Therapy is directed at raising the urine pH level using an alkali such as potassium citrate and decreasing production of uric acid with allopurinol. Dietary restriction of foods high in uric acid content (eg, proteins) may be effective, but usually are unnecessary if allopurinol is given. Often calcium oxalate precipitates with the uric acid stone so that treatment with a thiazide may be indicated.

URINARY TRACT INFECTIONS (UTIs)

In frail elderly individuals, especially women, there is a tendency for the bladder to become colonized with bacteria, generally from the gastrointestinal tract. Determining whether or not this bacteriuria represents true infection or rather asymptomatic colonization becomes problematic. Often there is associated pyuria (defined as 5–10 WBC per high-power field or more on urine microscopic examination). Typical symptoms of UTIs are dysuria, suprapubic or flank pain, fever, and cloudy or foul-smelling urine. However, the frail elderly may present atypically with altered mental status, nausea and vomiting, and/or a new onset of urinary incontinence or retention.

Treatment of UTIs consists of an antibiotic, eg, trimethoprim sulfa or fluroquinolone, following collection of a urine sample for culture and sensitivities. The recommendation for patients with asymptomatic bacteriuria is that they not be treated with antibiotics. Treatment is often followed by evidence of recolonization with more resistant organisms. The problem is that many patients have varying degrees of pyuria indicating inflammation, but no symptoms. It remains controversial whether or not these patients should be treated with antibiotics.

Cranberry juice has been proposed as a preventative measure for individuals with recurrent UTIs. It contains the urinary antiseptic, hippuric acid. Substances in the juice also appear to inhibit adherence of bacteria to urinary epithelium. Two recent randomized controlled trials suggest that cranberry juice has a modest effect in preventing UTIs.[55,56]

CONCLUSION

Cross-sectional population studies document the progressive decline in renal function that occurs with age. Most other renal functions decline with age at a rate similar to the glomerular filtration rate. Some individuals followed longitudinally, however, go for decades with no decrease in renal function, suggesting that there is not an inevitable involutional senescence that affects all individuals, albeit at different rates. Rather, it appears there is an age-related glomerular sclerosis that develops in aging individuals only when a combination of environmental and genetic factors reaches a threshold to initiate the process. Environmental factors include those conditions that create hyperperfusion and hyperfiltration in the glomerulus including diabetes, hypertension, dyslipidemia, and primary renal disease, all conditions that accelerate the development of disease-related glomerular sclerosis.

It is important to recognize this age-related decline in renal function. Failure to appropriately adjust dosages of medications cleared by the kidney can result in serious toxicity and even death. Nutritional issues arise in dealing with the chronic renal insufficiency patients. It remains unresolved whether or not dietary protein restriction accomplishes enough to outweigh the adverse impact on quality of life. Finally, dietary modifications may be helpful in managing the elderly patient with chronic stone formation or recurrent urinary tract infections.

REFERENCES

1. Davies DF, Shock NW. Age changes in glomerular filtration rate, effective renal plasma flow, and tubular excretory capacity in adult males. *J Clin Invest* 1950;29: 496–507.

2. Wesson LG Jr. Renal hemodynamics in physiologic states. In Wesson LG Jr, ed. *Physiology of the Human Kidney* Orlando, FL: Grune and Stratton: 1969:98.

3. Rowe JW, Andres R, Tobin J, et al. The effect of age on creatinine clearance in men: a cross-sectional and longitudinal study. *J Gerontol* 1976;31:155–163.

4. Lindeman RD, Tobin JD, Shock NW. Longitudinal studies on the rate of decline in renal function with age. *J Am Geriatr Soc* 1985;33:278–285.

5. Roessle R, Roulet F. *Mass and Zahl in der Pathologie.* Berlin, Germany: F. Springer; 1932.

6. Goyal VK. Changes with age in the human kidney. *Am J Anat Exp Gerontol* 1982;17:321–331.

7. Takazakura E, Wasabu N, Handa A, et al. Intrarenal vascular changes with age and disease. *Kidney Int* 1972; 2:224–230.

8. Kasiske BL. Relationship between vascular disease and age-associated changes in the human kidney. *Kidney Int* 1987;31:1153–1159.

9. Cockcroft DW, Gault MH. Prediction of creatinine clearance from serum creatinine. *Nephron* 1976;16:31–41.

10. Dodane V, Chevalier J, Bariety J, et al. Longitudinal study of solute excretion and glomerular ultrastructure in an experimental model of aging rats free of kidney disease. *Lab Invest* 1991;64:377–391.

11. McDonald RF, Solomon DH, Shock NW. Aging as a factor in the renal hemodynamic changes induced by a standardized pyrogen. *J Clin Invest* 1951;5:457–462.

12. Hollenberg NK, Adams DF, Solomon HS, et al. Senescence and the renal vasculature in normal man. *Circ Res* 1974;34:309–316.

13. Miller JH, McDonald RK, Shock NW. Age changes in the maximum rate of renal tubular reabsorption of glucose. *J Gerontol* 1952;7:196–200.

14. Barrows CH Jr, Falzone JA Jr, Shock NW. Age differences in the succinoxidase activity of homogenates and mitochondria from the livers and kidneys of rats. *J Gerontol* 1960;15:130–133.

15. Burich RJ. Effects of age on renal function and enzyme activity in male C57 BL/6 mice. *J Gerontol* 1975;30: 539–545.

16. Beauchene RE, Fanestil DD, Barrows CH Jr. The effect of age on active transport and sodium-potassium activated ATPase activity in renal tissue of rats. *J Gerontol* 1965;20:306–310.

17. Lindeman RD, Van Buren HC, Raisz LG. Osmolar renal concentrating ability in healthy young men and hospitalized patients without renal disease. *N Engl J Med* 1960; 262:1306–1309.

18. Rowe JW, Shock NW, DeFronzo RA. The influence of age on the renal response to water deprivation in man. *Nephron* 1976;17:270–276.

19. Lindeman RD, Lee TD Jr, Yiengst MJ, Shock NW. Influence of age, renal disease, hypertension, diuretics and calcium on the antidiuretic response to suboptimal infusions of vasopressin. *J Lab Clin Med* 1966;68: 206–223.

20. Miller JH, Shock NW. Age differences in the renal tubular response to antidiuretic hormone. *J Gerontol* 1953;8: 446–450.

21. Ledingham JGG, Crowe MJ, Forsling ML, et al. Effect of age on vasopressin secretion, water excretion, and thirst in man. *Kidney Int Suppl* 1987;21:S90–S92.

22. Shock NW, Yiengst MJ. Age changes in the acid-base equilibrium of the blood of males. *J Gerontol* 1950;5: 1–4.

23. Frassetto LA, Morris RC Jr, Sebastian A. Effect of age on blood acid-base composition in humans: role of age-related renal functional decline. *Am J Physiol* 1996;271: F1114–F1122.

24. Adler S, Lindeman RD, Yiengst MJ, et al. Effect of acute acid loading on urinary acid excretion by the aging human kidney. *J Lab Clin Med* 1968;72:278–289.

25. Agarwal BH, Cabebe FG. Renal acidification in elderly subjects. *Nephron* 1980;26:291–293.

26. Lowenstein J, Faulstick DA, Yiengst MJ, et al. The glomerular clearance and renal transport of hemoglobin in adult males. *J Clin Invest* 1961;40:1172–1177.

27. Faulstick D, Yiengst MJ, Ourster DA, et al. Glomerular permeability in young and old subjects. *J Gerontol* 1962; 17:40–44.

28. Epstein M, Hollenberg NK. Age as a determinant of renal sodium conservation in normal man. *J Lab Clin Med* 1976;87:411–417.

29. Crane MG, Harris JJ. Effect of aging on renin activity and aldosterone excretion. *J Lab Clin Med* 1976;87: 947–959.

30. Weidman P, DeMyttenaere-Burztein S, Maxwell MH, et al. Effect of aging on plasma renin and aldosterone in normal man. *Kidney Int* 1975;8:325–333.

31. Epstein M. Aging and the kidney. *J Am Soc Nephrol* 1996;7:1106–1122.

32. Armbrecht HJ, Zenser RV, Davis BB. Effect of age on the conversion of 25-hydroxyvitamin D_3 to 1,25 dihydroxy-vitamin D_3 by kidney of rats. *J Clin Invest* 1980;66: 1118–1123.

33. Rodriguez-Puyol D. Nephrology Forum. The aging kidney. *Kidney Int* 1998;54:2247–2265.

34. Hostetter TH, Olson JL, Rennke HG, et al. Hyperfiltration in remnant nephrons: a potentially adverse response to renal ablation. *Am J Physiol* 1981;9:F85–F93.

35. Brenner MM, Meyer TH, Hostetter TH. Dietary protein intake and the progressive nature of kidney disease: the role of hemodynamically mediated glomerular injury in the pathogenesis of progressive glomerular sclerosis in aging, renal ablation, and intrinsic renal disease. *N Engl J Med* 1973;307:652–659.

36. Anderson S, Brenner BM. Effects of aging on the renal glomerulus. *Am J Med* 1986;80:435–442.

37. Mogensen CE, Andersen MJF. Increased kidney size and glomerular filtration rate in early juvenile diabetes. *Diabetes* 1973;22:706–712.

38. Giatras I, Lau J, Levey AS. Effect of angiotensin-converting-enzyme inhibitors on the progression of non-diabetic renal disease: a meta-analysis of randomized trials. *Ann Intern Med* 1997;127:337–345.

39. Miller IJ, Suthanthiran M, Riggio RR, et al. Impact of renal donation: long term clinical and biochemical follow-up of living donors in a single center. *Am J Med* 1985; 79:201–208.

40. Bosch JP, Saccaggi A, Lauer A, et al. Renal functional reserve in humans: effect of protein intake on glomerular filtration rate. *Am J Med* 1983;75:943–950.

41. Bosch JP, Lauer A, Glabman S. Short-term protein loading in assessment of patients with renal disease. *Am J Med* 1984;77:873–879.

42. Barsoni G, Morelli E, Giannoni A, et al. Restricted phosphorus and nitrogen intake to slow the progression of chronic renal failure: a controlled trial. *Kidney Int* 1984; 24(suppl 16):278–284.

43. Levey AS, Greene T, Beck GJ, et al. Dietary protein restriction and the progression of chronic renal disease: what have all of the results of the MDRD study shown? *J Am Soc Nephrol* 1999;10:2426–2439.

44. Rodriquez-Iturbe B, Herrera J, Garcia R. Response to acute protein load in kidney donors and in apparently normal post-acute glomerulonephritis patients: evidence for glomerular hyperfiltration. *Lancet* 1985;2:461–464.

45. Ter Wee PM, Rosman JB, VanDerGiest S, et al. Renal hemodialysis during separate and combined infusions of amino acids and dopamine. *Kidney Int* 1986;29:870–874.

46. Fliser D, Zeier M, Nowack R, et al. Renal functional reserve in healthy elderly people. *J Am Soc Nephrol* 1993; 3:1371–1377.

47. Fuiano G, Sund S, Mazza G, et al. Renal hemodynamic response to maximal vasodilating stimulus in healthy older adults. *Kidney Int* 2001;59:1052–1058.

48. Keane WF, Mulcahy WS, Kasiske BL, et al. Hyperlipidemia and progressive renal disease. *Kidney Int* 1991; 39 (suppl 31):S41–S48.

49. Grone EF, Walli AK, Grone HJ, et al. The role of lipids in nephrosclerosis and glomerulosclerosis. *Atherosclerosis* 1994;107:1–13.

50. Attman PO, Alaupovic P, Samuelsson O. Lipoprotein abnormalities as a risk factor for progressive non-diabetic renal disease. *Kidney Int* 1999;56(suppl 71):S14–S17.

51. Fried LF, Orchard TJ, Kasiske BL for the Lipids and Renal Disease Progression Meta-analysis Study Group. Effect of lipid reduction on the progression of renal disease: a meta-analysis. *Kidney Int* 2001;59:260–269.

52. Lindeman RD. Renal and electrolyte disorders. In: Duthie EH Jr, Katz PR, eds. *Practice of Geriatrics*. 3rd ed. Philadelphia, PA: WB Saunders Co;1998:546–561.

53. Klahr S, Levey AS, Beck GJ, et al. for the Modification of Diet in Renal Disease Study Group. The effects of dietary protein restriction and blood pressure control on the progression of chronic renal disease. *N Engl J Med* 1994;330:877–884.

54. Kopple JK, Levey AS, Chumlea WC, et al. for the Modification of Diet in Renal Disease Study Group. Effect of dietary protein restriction on nutritional status in the MDRDS. *Kidney Int* 1997;52:778–791.

55. Kontiokari T, Sundqvist K, Nuutinen M, et al. Randomized trial of cranberry-ligonberry juice and *Lactobacillus* GG drink for the prevention of urinary tract infections in women. *BMJ* 2001;322:1571.

56. Strothers L. A randomized trial to evaluate the effectiveness of naturopathic cranberry products as prophylaxis against urinary tract infection in women. *Can J Urol* 2002;9:1558–1562.

CHAPTER 13

Impact of Nutrition on the Age-Related Declines in Hematopoiesis

Gurkamal S. Chatta, MD and Linda Barry Robertson, RN, MSN

The production of hematopoietic cells involves a complex interaction between proliferating marrow stem cells, a unique stroma, and a series of diffusible molecules that regulate the production of erythroid, myeloid, and megakaryocytic elements. The high cellular turnover makes the bone marrow particularly susceptible to nutritional deprivation, leading to significantly compromised function. The aging hematopoietic system is characterized by a decline in reserve capacity that makes it particularly susceptible to environmental insults that are known to affect the bone marrow adversely. This chapter discusses the effects of age on the hematopoietic system and the role of nutrition in the common hematologic problems seen in elderly people.

EFFECT OF AGE ON THE HEMATOPOIETIC SYSTEM

Pluripotent Stem Cells

All immunohematopoietic elements are derived from a small pool of pluripotent stem cells that are characterized by a unique self-renewal capacity.[1] They have the ability to divide and yield a progenitor cell committed to differentiating into a specific cell lineage and an identical daughter cell, thus maintaining the pluripotent stem cell pool size. These morphologically unidentifiable cells are referred to as colony-forming unit-spleen (CFU-S) because they form colonies when marrow is injected into lethally irradiated mice recipients. One of the major questions about the aging of the hematopoietic system is whether or not CFU-S has a finite replicative capacity. Studies using serial transplantation to assess finite replicative capacity have yielded conflicting results. When cells are subjected to in vivo serial transfer by repeated injection into lethally irradiated recipients, they gradually lose their ability to replicate.[2,3] Recent evidence has suggested that results of serial transplantation may well be the result of methodologic artifact.[4,5] Even if their life span is finite, it is clear that CFU-S have a vastly redundant reserve capacity, enabling production of hematopoietic cells in numbers that far exceed the maximal life expectancy of the animal.[6] This point is further highlighted by the observation that as few as 20 CFU-S are able to reconstitute the bone marrow of lethally irradiated mice.[7]

The effect of age on CFU-S senescence has been studied in long-term bone marrow culture. Several studies have shown an inverse relationship between donor age and maintenance of hematopoiesis in this long-term bone marrow culture system.[8,9] Additional studies using this in vitro culture system have shown that CFU-S with high replicative histories are more likely to be recruited into the committed cell compartments than are CFU-S that have divided fewer times.

Additional evidence for a finite life span comes from a series of elegant studies that examined stem cell kinetics in long-term marrow culture subjected to various doses of irradiation.[10–12]

Effect of Age on Normal Marrow Function

The CFU-S divide into an identical daughter cell and progenitor cells committed to differentiation, and in the case of hematopoiesis, into myeloid, erythroid, megakaryocytic, and macrophage precursors (Figure 13–1). There are two forms of erythroid progenitor cells. The first is a more primitive precursor, which requires high concentrations of erythropoietin and is referred to as a burst-forming unit-erythroid (BFU-E). This precursor is thought to give rise to a more mature progenitor cell that requires lower erythropoietin concentrations. It is referred to as a colony-forming unit-erythroid (CFU-E) and is the immediate precursor of the proerythroblast, which is the first morphologically identifiable erythroid element. Committed myeloid progenitors include the colony-forming unit-culture (CFU-C), which is the immediate precursor of the myeloblast. A primitive progenitor cell that gives rise to megakaryocytes (CFU-MEGG) and to macrophages (CFU-M) can also be identified under appropriate culture conditions. Morphologically recognizable hematopoietic cells proliferate and mature in a transit or amplification compartment, eventually giving rise to terminally differentiated cells that continually enter the peripheral blood. Recent studies have examined the effect of age on committed hematopoietic progenitor cell number and on the number of differentiated cells in the various marrow compartments. In both animals and humans, no age-related declines in any bone marrow element can be demonstrated when carefully selected subjects are examined in the basal state.[13,14] These observations strongly suggest that marrow function can be adequately maintained, and that no measurable declines occur as a consequence of age per se. However, the aging process is characterized by a significant reduction in reserve capacity, so that abnormalities not present in the basal state become apparent when the response

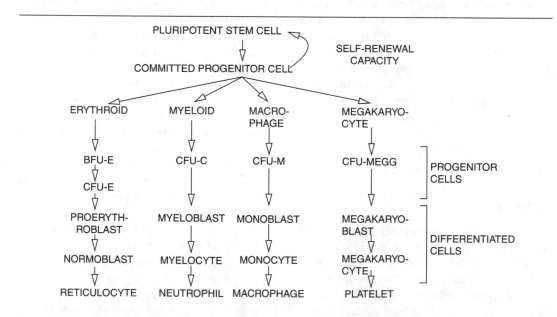

Figure 13–1 The Production of Terminally Differentiated Cells of Various Lineages Is Derived from a Small Pool of Pluripotent Stem Cells (CFU-S) with a Unique Self-renewal Capacity
They give rise to progenitor cells of specific lineages that divide and differentiate, resulting in the daily production of the required amounts of hematopoietic elements.

to maximal stimulation is examined. Udupa and Lipschitz[15,16] have undertaken a number of studies in which they examined hematopoietic function in animals exposed to increased stimulation. Both in vivo and in vitro studies have shown that the hematopoietic response to increased stimulation in old mice is blunted and more variable. Furthermore, greater pathologic abnormalities are noted in response to infection or protein deficiency.

DOES ANEMIA OCCUR AS A CONSEQUENCE OF NORMAL AGING?

It is generally recognized that anemia is a common clinical problem in the elderly. Studies have shown a high prevalence in hospitalized older subjects, patients attending geriatric clinics, and institutionalized older individuals. A series of epidemiologic studies from the United States, Canada, and Europe[17-19] demonstrated a high prevalence of anemia in the elderly. In women older than age 59 years, anemia occurs as frequently as in women of childbearing age. In men, a definite increase in the prevalence of anemia is found in older age groups. Studies from Great Britain are important because they have determined the prevalence of anemia in large numbers of subjects older than age 60 years. In both men and women, the prevalence of anemia increased significantly with each successive decade.

An analysis of the second National Health and Nutrition Examination Survey (NHANES II) demonstrated a significant reduction in hemoglobin levels with advancing age in apparently healthy males and a minimal, though significant, decrease in elderly females.[20] Based upon a lower normal limit of 14 g/dL for hemoglobin concentration, a very large percentage of elderly males would be found to be anemic. This study proposed that the reduction in hemoglobin in males was a consequence of aging, and most likely secondary to a decline in the serum testosterone. Hence, age-specific reference standards for hemoglobin concentration should be adopted and used for diagnosing anemia in the elderly.

There are few reports on the incidence of new cases of anemia in the elderly population. In the general population, the annual incidence of anemia is estimated to be 1–2%.[21,22] Compared to this, the incidence of anemia in a well-defined population of elderly (over age 65 years) Caucasians attending the Mayo Clinic[23] was reported to be four- to sixfold higher; the incidence of anemia was 13% per year in the "oldest-old" (over age 85 years). Anemia was diagnosed in accordance with World Health Organization (WHO) criteria, if the hemoglobin concentration was less than 13 g/dL in men and less than 12 g/dL in women, then they were anemic. In this study, in every age group over age 65 years, the incidence of anemia in men was higher than in women. At the time of diagnosis, less than 50% of the men had a hemoglobin concentration lower than 12 g percent. Significantly, despite an exhaustive workup, in 16% of the elderly the etiology of the anemia was uncertain.

The above data are consistent with an evaluation of apparently healthy elderly subjects with mild anemia, which also fail to uncover an obvious cause of the anemia.[24] A careful assessment of hematopoiesis in these individuals reveal mild marrow failure, as evidenced by reductions in bone marrow progenitor cell numbers and modest decreases in peripheral leukocyte counts.[25] A major unanswered question is whether this decline in hemoglobin with advancing age is a consequence of the normal aging process or if it reflects some yet to be defined abnormality. Of particular importance in this regard is the finding that anemia is extremely rare in an affluent, healthy elderly population examined in New Mexico.[26] None of the elderly males and females in this group were anemic. Furthermore, longitudinal monitoring of these subjects over a 5-year period failed to demonstrate an increased prevalence of anemia. Based upon this observation and animal studies of hematopoiesis, it seems highly likely that the decrease in hemoglobin seen commonly with advancing age is not a consequence of the normal aging process and is related to some extrinsic variable that remains to be determined.

Inflammation or chronic disease is one likely etiology of apparent age-related anemia.[27] A second possibility is that the anemia has a nutritional basis. This is suggested by a closer examination of data obtained in epidemiologic surveys in which anemia has been shown to be most prevalent in populations in a low socioeconomic level, where the prevalence of nutritional deficiencies is high.

We performed a comprehensive nutritional and hematologic evaluation of a group of 73 elderly veterans living in a domiciliary facility. A high prevalence of anemia was present in this population. A close evaluation demonstrated that iron deficiency, folate deficiency, and other commonly described causes of anemia were rare. We then performed a multivariate analysis of the data using age, hematopoietic indices, and nutritional factors as covariants. We demonstrated that although age appeared to be the major variable accounting for the decline in immunologic measurements observed in this elderly population, age did not appear to be an important factor in the prevalence of anemia. In contrast, serum albumin, transferrin, and prealbumin, which assess nutritional status, appeared to be excellent predictors of anemia. This information provides indirect evidence that a nutritional variable may contribute to the anemia seen in these elderly populations. Further evidence suggesting that a nutritional factor may contribute to the anemia comes from the observation that there is a marked similarity between the alterations in immunologic and hematopoietic function that occur with aging and those that occur with protein deprivation. This raises the possibility that protein deprivation, in some form, may contribute to the hematopoietic changes normally ascribed to aging.

There is evidence that correction of protein-energy malnutrition in the hospitalized elderly can markedly improve hematopoietic function.[28] In these subjects, interpretation of improvements in hematologic status is extremely difficult. Any hospitalized elderly individual has coexisting diseases that can affect hematopoietic function. Thus, the overall improvement seen with nutritional rehabilitation may reflect an overall improvement of the patient's medical status. The effect of increased feeding on hematopoietic status has been examined in relatively healthy elderly individuals who lived at home, were ambulatory but were underweight, and had marginal evidence of protein-energy deprivation. By providing polymeric dietary supplements to these subjects between meals, it was possible to correct nutritional deficiencies and obtain weight gain. However, despite a positive impact on nutritional status, the anemia, invariably present in this population, did not improve.

Some conclusions can be drawn from these observations. It is clear that significant nutritional deficiencies reversibly aggravate the hematologic abnormalities in the elderly. Even in apparently healthy older individuals, it is possible that nutritional factors contribute to hematopoietic changes, but alternative mechanisms other than simple nutritional deficiency must be considered. Marginal reductions of one or more nutrients acting alone or in combination over a prolonged period of time may modulate hematopoietic change usually ascribed to aging. Alternatively, nutrient delivery to the target organ may be altered with aging or changes in nutrient target interaction may occur. These possibilities could account for the higher prevalence of anemia reported in epidemiologic studies. They remain no more than potential hypotheses that will require further research.

In contrast to healthy older persons, in whom the prevalence of anemia is relatively low, anemia is extremely common in hospitalized patients in both acute and chronic care settings. In a recent survey of hospitalized patients in a Department of Veterans Affairs hospital, 56% of patients over age 75 years had a significant anemia (Rothstein et al, personal communication) (Table 13–1).

HEMATOLOGIC MANIFESTATIONS OF PROTEIN-ENERGY MALNUTRITION IN THE ELDERLY

A high incidence of protein-energy malnutrition (PEM) has been reported in hospitalized elderly patients. The incidence is also very high in nursing homes and in other long-term care

Table 13–1 Anemia in Patients over Age 75 in an Acute Care Veterans Hospital

Diagnosis	Percentage
Multiple diagnoses	53
No diagnosis	17
Single diagnosis	30
Anemia of chronic disease	10
Malnutrition	9
Infection	4
Post-op bleeding	3
Alcoholism	1
Iron deficiency	1

settings.[29] PEM is a metabolic response to the release of cytokines and hormones and is characterized by an increase in the energy and protein requirements. The increased catabolism, however, is not matched by an increased intake because of anorexia or other limitations to ingestion. When exogenous energy is not provided, endogenous protein stores are mobilized and depleted in order to meet the demands of the body. The disorder is characterized by hypoalbuminemia, increased protein and energy requirements, and declines in immune and hematologic function. Anemia is invariably present in patients with PEM, the features being identical to those that occur as the "anemia of chronic disease," and with inflammatory processes.[28] In both men and women, the hemoglobin concentration ranges from 100 to 120 g/L. The disorder is associated with an impaired ability of the reticuloendothelial system to recycle iron from senescent red cells. As a result, serum iron concentrations are low and the transferrin saturation is less than 20%. These findings indicate the presence of iron-deficient erythropoiesis, which also occurs in iron deficiency anemia that most commonly results from blood loss. In this disorder, iron stores are absent and, as a result, the serum ferritin level, which is a relatively accurate measure of iron stores, is reduced (usually less than 50 mg/L) and total iron-binding capacity (TIBC) is increased.

In contrast, iron stores are normal or increased in the anemia associated with chronic disease and in the anemia associated with PEM. This is reflected in a normal to elevated serum ferritin level (<60 mg/L) and a low TIBC (<45 mmol/L). In elderly people, the immunohematopoietic sequelae of PEM tend to be more severe than they are in younger individuals. This may relate to the diminished reserve capacity that is believed to exist in elderly individuals. Furthermore, the effects of age on the immune and hematologic systems are remarkably similar to the declines in function noted in PEM. The effects of age and PEM on declines in function may be additive, resulting in more severe abnormalities in older individuals.

An example of this additive effect is provided by the observations made of the effect of age and protein deficiency on neutrophil function in mice. Lipschitz and Udupa[30] showed that, although neutrophil function was compromised in aged mice and in young mice fed a low-protein diet, the reduction was not sufficient in either case to compromise the neutrophil's ability to phagocytose or kill bacteria. In contrast, the reserve capacity of the neutrophil was markedly compromised when aged mice were fed a low-protein diet. Neutrophils obtained from these animals had a marked impairment of their ability to phagocytose and kill bacteria. These results may explain the high prevalence of severe bacterial infections in hospitalized, malnourished elderly people. They also emphasize that the reduced reserve in cellular function as a consequence of aging results in increased susceptibility to external stress.

The most appropriate definition of PEM is that it is a metabolic response to stress associated with increased requirements for calories and protein.[31] It may be that elderly people are more susceptible to PEM and develop pathologic conditions more rapidly, and with less stress than do younger subjects. The stresses that result in this disorder include trauma, infection, and other acute or chronic inflammatory conditions. Considering these pathophysiologic facts, it is likely that the hematologic changes noted in these patients reflect the underlying disease and only indirectly relate to a nutritional problem.

Clinical studies have shown that the initial responses to stress that characterize PEM are beneficial and assist the patient in developing an optimal response to the underlying primary pathology. Since acute stress is associated with severe anorexia, patients rarely, if ever, consume sufficient calories or protein to meet their daily needs. In young subjects, inadequate nutrient intake for a period of up to 10 days usually does not affect outcome adversely. Thereafter, inadequate protein and calorie intake results in further lowering of serum albumin and worsening of hematologic, immunologic, and hepatic function, which can affect outcome adversely. In elderly subjects, the time period before PEM exerts a negative effect is likely to be much shorter than that observed in younger subjects. In elderly individuals, failure to meet nutrient needs after a period as brief as 2 to 3 days can lead to the further decrease of serum albumin, worsening immunohematologic function, and increased morbidity. Therefore, it is essential that the presence of PEM be appropriately diagnosed and managed in elderly people.

Lipschitz and Mitchell[28] have studied the effects of nutritional rehabilitation on the hematologic system in elderly subjects with PEM who did not have terminal disease. They confirmed previous reports that adequate nutritional support improved delayed cutaneous hypersensitivity and increased lymphocyte count. In addition, marked improvements in the hematologic system were demonstrated. Correction of the nutritional deficits resulted in a highly significant increase in the hemoglobin concentration, which was accompanied by a return of both serum iron levels and TIBC to normal ranges. Simultaneously, serum ferritin levels fell, presumably as a result of redistribution of iron from stores to the circulating erythrocyte mass (Figure 13–2).

In selected individuals, Lipschitz and Mitchell also demonstrated that improved nutritional status was accompanied by significant increases in the number of bone marrow–differentiated cells and immature cells. The observation that deliv-

ery of adequate nutrition resulted in a prompt rise in both serum iron level and TIBC is of great interest, particularly since these changes occurred long before any other improvement in the clinical status was noted. This observation provides the strongest evidence for a nutritional role in the hematopoietic alterations occurring in PEM.

The overall interpretation of the improved immunohematopoietic function in malnourished elderly subjects is extremely difficult. Any hospitalized elderly patient who has PEM also has coexisting medical conditions (including infection, dehydration, and psychoneurologic changes) that will affect immune and hematologic function. Therefore, the overall improvement seen with nutritional rehabilitation may reflect an overall improvement of the medical status of the patient.

To examine this possibility more closely, Lipschitz et al[32] studied the effects of increased feeding on the immune and hematologic status of mildly malnourished, elderly, homebound subjects. These individuals were underweight, had evidence of inadequate food intake, were invariably anemic, and had diminished immune function. By providing polymeric dietary supplements between meals, it was possible to increase total calorie and protein intake by 50% for a total of 16 weeks. A significant improvement in nutritional status occurred: weight gain, increased serum albumin and transferrin, and significant increases in selected vitamins and minerals were seen. Despite this improved nutritional profile, immune function and hematologic status remained unchanged. No anergic subject demonstrated improved delayed cutaneous hypersensitivity, T and B cell function remained abnormal, and the hemoglobin concentration did not increase.

This study, and one on more severely malnourished elderly, suggests that nutritional deficiencies aggravate immune and hematopoietic function in elderly subjects. Correction of coexisting disease and nutritional rehabilitation in the severely malnourished are associated with measurable improvements in host defense parameters. Mildly malnourished elderly individuals who had changes in immune and hematopoietic

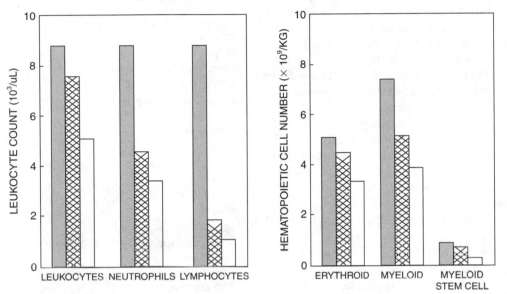

QUANTITATION OF HEMATOPOIESIS IN ELDERLY SUBJECTS WITH UNEXPLAINED ANEMIA

Figure 13–2 **Peripheral Blood Counts (left panel) and Hematopoietic Precursor Number (right panel) in Groups of Healthy Young Subjects and Groups of Carefully Selected Elderly Subjects With or Without an Unexplained Anemia**
Source: Reprinted with permission from Lipschitz et al, *Blood,* Vol. 63, p. 502, © 1984, Grune & Stratton, Inc.

function similar to those seen in healthy elderly did not show an improvement in their function despite an obviously improved nutritional status. A reasonable conclusion from these studies is that neither protein nor calorie deprivation entirely accounts for the immune and hematologic changes seen in elderly people. However, the prevalence and incidence of anemia in the elderly is a concern because of the associated complications and impact on the individual's quality of life and possibly survival. Therefore, it is important that the cause and pathophysiology be determined so that intervention can occur as early as possible.

IRON DEFICIENCY ANEMIA

Throughout the world, iron deficiency as a result of blood loss is the most common nutritional problem and accounts for significant morbidity in Third World countries. In both men and women, a progressive increase in iron stores oc-

curs with advancing age. This has been demonstrated in numerous studies that have shown an age-associated increase in serum ferritin in both men and women (Figure 13–2). In older men, tissue iron stores average 1,200 mg. In older women, iron stores increase from an average of 300 mg to 800 mg in the decade after menopause. The rise in iron stores clearly relates to improved iron balance because of cessation of menstruation.[33] Consequently, in contrast to younger women, iron deficiency is not the most common cause of anemia in ambulatory, healthy elderly people.[24,25]

In the hospital setting, however, iron deficiency anemia is more common in elderly patients. In a number of studies of elderly hospitalized subjects, the prevalence of anemia ranged from 6.4–41%.[34–36] In 21–90% of the patients, the etiology of the anemia was thought to be caused by iron deficiency. This information must be interpreted with a lot of caution because the criteria for the diagnosis of anemia varied, and in many cases only serum iron concentration and TIBC were used to make the diagnosis. Factors such as comorbid conditions and different cut-off values in the above studies for diagnosing anemia contribute to the significant variation of these prevalence rates. However, it is apparent that iron deficiency is a common problem in hospitalized people.

In the United States, the prevalence rates for iron deficiency anemia were recently reported in the third National Health and Nutrition Examination Survey (NHANES III; 1988–1994).[37] In this large, nationally representative survey, the prevalence rates of iron deficiency state and iron deficiency anemia were relatively higher in toddlers, adolescent girls, and women of childbearing age. The prevalence rates of iron deficiency state and iron deficiency anemia in the 50- to 69-year age group for females was reported to be 5% and 2% of the U.S. population, while in the age group older than 70 years it was 7% and 2%, respectively. For males, the reported figures in the age group of 50 to 69 years were 2% and 1%, while in the older than 70 years they were 4% and 2%, respectively. Although this points to relatively low prevalence rates in the elderly U.S. population, emerging aging trends in the U.S. population would translate relatively low rates to high numbers over the next few years. Screening strategies, therefore, should be evolved to pursue work-up for preventable etiologies of iron deficiency states in the elderly (Table 13–2), which will translate into early diagnosis and treatment, as well as low health care costs for the elderly.

Epidemiological studies have generally focused on the prevalence of anemia and few data exist regarding the frequency or etiology of newly diagnosed anemia in the elderly. Ania et al.[22,23] assessed the incidence and clinical spectrum of anemia in the elderly in a predominantly Caucasian, affluent community with excellent access to health care facilities. In this community-based survey, the incidence of anemia among older people was 4 to 6 times greater than that suspected clinically and rose higher with age, with the highest incidence being recorded in el-

Table 13–2 Major Causes of Iron Deficiency in the Elderly

Gastrointestinal Blood Loss
Tumors
Polyps
Carcinoma of the colon
Carcinoma of the stomach
Peptic Ulcer Disease
Gastric
Duodenal

Drugs
Nonsteroidal anti-inflammatory drugs
Aspirin
Indomethacin
Anticoagulants

Miscellaneous Causes
Angiodysplasia of the large bowel
Hiatal hernia
Hemorrhoids
Diverticulosis

Other Sources of Blood Loss
Genitourinary blood loss
Carcinoma of the uterus and cervix
Hematuria (rare)

derly males. In half of the cases, the apparent cause of newly diagnosed anemia in this population base survey was blood loss. Even mild anemia was associated with reduced survival.

The role of nutrition in contributing to iron deficiency anemia and other nutritional deficiencies in the elderly depends on cultural, regional, and socioeconomic factors. There is no strong evidence to suggest that poor diet and/or poor bioavailability of dietary iron are causes for iron deficiency anemia in large segments of the population in industrialized nations. Small cross-sectional and longitudinal studies have attempted to underscore the role of diet in developing iron deficiency states along with deficiencies of elements, such as zinc and copper. In a small longitudinal study of healthy elderly vegetarians, the long-term consequences of ovo-lacto or lacto-vegetarianism were assessed.[38] The results indicated that in comparison to omnivorous elderly, the vegetarian elderly population is at a higher risk for a marginal iron, zinc, and vitamin B_{12} status.

Recently, Fleming et al.[39] reported on the role of dietary factors modulating iron bioavailability in the elderly population. Based on the elderly cohort from the Framingham Heart Study, five significant dietary factors were found to be associated with iron stores. Heme iron, supplemental iron, dietary vitamin C, and alcohol were positively associated with serum ferritin after correcting for other causes of raised ferritin. On the other hand, coffee consumption was found to have a negative association.

When iron deficiency does occur in elderly individuals, it is almost always secondary to gastrointestinal blood loss. The common causes of blood loss anemia in elderly patients are listed in Table 13–2. The etiology of this blood loss in both elderly men and elderly women must be assumed to be gastrointestinal malignancy until proved otherwise. Depending on the patient's medical condition, an aggressive attempt to define the cause of the anemia should be undertaken, whether or not occult blood is detected in the stool. Comprehensive evaluation of the gastrointestinal tract, including radiography and endoscopy, frequently will identify a malignancy or the presence of polyps that accounts for the blood loss. Other common causes of blood loss from the gastrointestinal tract include atrophic gastritis, gastrointestinal ulcers, diverticuli, and angiodysplasia of the large bowel.

Primarily, iron deficiency anemia must be distinguished from other disorders that are characterized by the presence of iron-deficient erythropoiesis. These include the anemia of chronic disease, the anemia associated with inflammation, and, as described previously, protein-energy malnutrition.[40] Older individuals may be more susceptible to anemia of chronic disease due to the age-associated hematopoietic restrictions.[41] Data show that age may be associated with relative erythropoietin insufficiency, which makes these individuals susceptible to anemia.[41] In addition, the increased concentrations of inflammatory cytokines, such as tumor necrosis factor and interleukin-6, which are common in

elderly people, may also inhibit the responses to erythropoietin.[41] The major defect in these disorders appears to be an impaired ability of the reticuloendothelial cells to recruit the iron derived from previously phagocytosed erythrocytes. Therefore, serum iron levels are low, iron supply to the marrow is inadequate, and iron deficient erythropoiesis develops. In contrast to iron deficiency, tissue iron stores are normal or increased rather than absent. The mechanism accounting for the reticuloendothelial abnormality is not well understood. Other factors contributing to this anemia include a modest reduction in erythrocyte survival. The erythropoietin response to the level of the anemia is frequently reduced, but in some circumstances has been shown to be normal or increased.

Figure 13–3 lists an approach to distinguishing whether iron deficiency is caused by iron deficiency anemia, chronic disease, or inflammation. In all three, there is evidence of iron-deficient erythropoiesis characterized by a low serum iron level and low transferrin saturation. Transferrin saturation is the percentage of circulating transferrin that is saturated with iron; it is calculated by dividing the serum iron value by the TIBC and expressing the result as a percentage. The free erythrocyte protoporphyrin is also elevated in iron-deficient erythropoiesis. However, saturation below 15% favors iron deficiency. Although microcytosis does occur in the anemia of chronic disease, a mean corpuscular volume below 75 fL is very unusual.

The major distinguishing feature between the two disorders is the absence of iron stores in iron deficiency and its presence in chronic disease or inflammation. In classic iron deficiency anemia, the serum ferritin level is less than 20 μg/L and the TIBC is greater than 72 μmol/L. In the anemia of inflammation, serum ferritin is usually greater than 100 μg/L provided that iron stores are adequate. In this circumstance, TIBC is usually less than 45 μmol/L. Frequently, the serum ferritin and the TIBC yield equivocal results. This is particularly likely in patients with inflammatory disorders complicated by iron deficiency. For example, a patient with active rheumatoid

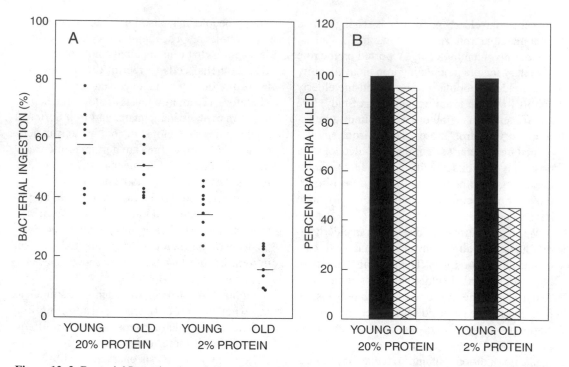

Figure 13–3 Bacterial Ingestion (panel A) and Percentage Bacteria Killed (panel B) in Neutrophils Obtained from the Peritoneal Cavity of Young (Aged 6 Months) or Old Mice (Aged 24 Months) Fed a 20% (normal) or 2% Protein Diet for 3 Weeks
The results demonstrate that phagocytosis and bacterial killing are significantly compromised only in the old animals fed the low-protein diet. *Source*: Reprinted with permission from *Journal of Gerontology*, Vol. 41, p. 690, © 1998, The Gerontology Society of North America.

disease and iron deficiency caused by drug-induced gastrointestinal blood loss may demonstrate confusing blood chemistries. In a patient like this, the serum ferritin level is usually above 12 μg/L but less than 100 μg/L. Despite the presence of inflammation, this type of patient will respond to oral iron therapy with a significant increase in hemoglobin.

A reasonable recommendation for subjects with anemia and inflammatory disorders is to consider a trial of oral iron when the ferritin level is less than 100 μg/L. Alternatively, the diagnosis of iron deficiency can be made definitively by demonstrating absent hemosiderin iron in a bone marrow aspirate. In the anemia of chronic disease, sideroblasts are absent, but hemosiderin iron is readily seen in marrow macrophages.

Once the diagnosis has been made, initial therapy should be directed at correcting the underlying pathologic process that resulted in the iron deficiency. In most cases, the iron deficiency can be corrected by oral administration of an iron salt. Ferrous sulfate in either tablet form or as an elixir should be given 3 times per day with meals;[42] the usual dose contains 60 mg of elemental iron. An adequate response to iron therapy is an increase in the hemoglobin concentration of approximately 0.5 g weekly. Elderly patients appear to respond as rapidly to oral iron as do younger individuals.[43]

Side effects, which include nausea, vomiting, epigastric discomfort, constipation, and diarrhea, are common causes for cessation of medication. The best approach to minimize these complications is to reduce the dose and assure that iron therapy is administered with meals. In some elderly subjects, there may be value in prescribing one tablet daily to diminish polypharmacy and aid with compliance. A slow-release iron preparation may be more appropriate when prescribing iron on a daily basis. Reticulocytosis usually starts within a week following the initiation of the iron therapy.

Failure to respond is not uncommon and usually results from noncompliance, inadequate iron absorption, or continued bleeding. Once these possibilities have been excluded, an incorrect diagnosis or a contributing condition such as renal impairment, infection, or neoplasia should be considered. In the rare patient who does not respond to oral iron, parenteral iron therapy may be considered. This should be reserved for those individuals proven to have iron malabsorption or when noncompliance is a serious problem. The importance of treating with oral iron only when indicated cannot be overemphasized. There is evidence that as many as 83% of elderly subjects have received oral iron therapy unnecessarily.[44] Anemia of chronic disease such as rheumatoid arthritis and cancer may also respond to erythropoietic therapy.[41]

In conclusion, anemia is a common problem in the elderly and, therefore, it is important that it be diagnosed early to decrease the severity, slow disease progression, and potentially improve the outcomes.[45] Since the elderly often have a number of comorbidities as well as decreased sensory perception and activity limitations, the symptoms of anemia may be masked. Therefore, periodic screens for anemia in this population may be beneficial, particularly if there is any evidence of symptomology. The screen should include a complete blood count and a reticulocyte count and index. The reticulocyte index is generally increased in anemia. If it is adequate, then blood loss or red blood cell destruction should be suspected and further evaluation is indicated to determine the cause and develop a treatment plan.

Iron Deficiency and Immune Function

Aging is often associated with a decline in T-cell mediated functions, which is associated with immunocompetence.[46] There have been several studies that have focused on nutrient deficiencies in the elderly and the role it plays in impairment of the immune function.[46] However, the effects of iron deficiency on immune response in the elderly has not been fully examined, despite indications of a fairly high prevalence of iron deficiency among the homebound and institutionalized elderly.[46] In a study conducted by Fulop et al.[47] institutionalized elderly who were nonresponsive to the influenza vaccine had lower hemoglobin, hematocrit, and serum iron concentrations. This suggests that iron-deficient elderly may have a lower cell-mediated immune response.

The findings have generally been inconsistent regarding the relationship between impaired cell-mediated immunity and bactericidal function in iron-deficient individuals.[46] These differences may be due to the differences in ages of the subjects, underlying infections, and coexisting nutritional deficiencies. In a study of 72 elderly homebound women, conducted by Ahluwalia et al.[46] these confounding factors were adjusted through a rigid screening process. The results for the nutritional status and inflammation were in normal ranges for both iron-sufficient and iron-deficient groups. The iron-deficient group did have significantly lower ($P < .05$) values for all body iron compartments.[46] Approximately half the iron-deficient group was also anemic. There were no differences noted in the total lymphocytes, monocytes, or granulocytes in either of the groups. T-cell proliferation in response to stimulation with various concentrations of Con A and PHA was significantly less in the iron-deficient group.[46] Phagocytosis and respiratory burst on ingestions of *E coli* did not differ between groups. However, the magnitude of the oxidative burst expressed by granulocytes was significantly less (28%) in the iron-deficient women.[46] This may place the iron-deficient elderly at risk for bacterial infections. This finding is consistent with those of a randomized controlled study of young children in Sri Lanka, in which an improvement in iron deficiency by the use of iron supplementation reduced the incidence and duration of upper respiratory infections.[47]

The role of iron in maintaining immune response is considered important at the biochemical and cellular levels.[46] For example, iron is a component of DNA production and cell division and it is also necessary to the activity of myeloperoxidase, which is involved in killing bacteria by neutrophils. Reports on iron deficiency and immune function are often confounded by the presence of poor nutritional status and underlying infection or inflammation. This makes it difficult to evaluate the study outcomes. These current findings suggest that the diagnosis, treatment, and prevention of iron deficiency in the elderly may be of public health significance.

FOLIC ACID AND VITAMIN B$_{12}$

Folic acid deficiency in elderly people can result from inadequate intake. The body stores very little folate, generally enough to last 4 to 6 months.[48] It is difficult to distinguish the symptoms of folate deficiency since they are similar to those of vitamin B$_{12}$ deficiency. As a general rule, however, pathologic deficiencies occur only when decreased intake is accompanied by increased requirements, as in alcoholics or in patients with gastrointestinal malabsorption. Epidemiological studies conducted in Great Britain indicate that significant folate deficiency is relatively common, with significantly low erythrocyte folate levels as well as low serum B$_{12}$ levels occurring in 8–14% of subjects examined.[49] Low B$_{12}$ and folate levels reported in this sample population were not associated with any clinical manifestations of their deficiencies.

However, in 1985, Craig et al.[50] presented evidence that the majority of elderly with folate deficiency do not have overt macrocytosis. The actual size of the problem has only recently been unveiled through the use of plasma total homocysteine (tHcy) concentrations as an indicator of folate status.[51] Homocysteine is derived from methionine and is either remethylated back to methionine in a reaction that requires cyanocobalamin (vitamin B$_{12}$) and folic acid as cofactor and substrate, or it is catabolised by pyridoxine 5'-phosphate (vitamin B$_6$) dependent trans-sulphuration pathway.[52]

The use of plasma tHcy concentrations as an indicator for folate status is stimulating re-evaluation of adequate folate nutrition.[51] Hematologic indices or plasma/erythrocyte folate concentrations are insensitive markers that are abnormal only if folate status is severely compromised.[51] A fasting tHcy concentration is a sensitive marker of folate status and its use suggests that relative folate deficiencies are common in the elderly.[53–55]

Increased circulating total homocysteine concentrations are associated with premature vascular disease.[53–55] A recent meta-analysis of published data shows that over 10% of coronary artery disease in the United States is attributable to hyperhomocysteinemia.[56] One of the reasons that homocysteine is of interest is that it is a reversible risk factor.[57] Vitamin B supplementation, particularly with folic acid, appears to be a safe and inexpensive way to lower tHcy.

There is increased evidence that folate deficiencies may be more common than once thought in elderly people and that folate deficiency may contribute to cardiovascular disease and cancer. However, this does not imply that elderly individuals should take folate supplementation. Both cancer and cardiovascular disease are lifestyle diseases and folate supplementation is not likely to reverse the diseases in this population. However, there is a need for controlled clinical intervention studies to assess the possible use of folate supplementation in disease prevention.[51]

In another survey of folate intake among adults in the Netherlands, only 4% of elderly males were found to be deficient per the daily recommended allowance.[58] Physiological and lifestyle variables, such as alcohol and tobacco use, were also important determinants of folate levels. Again, no clear association was found between low folate levels and the clinical manifestations of its deficiency. Potatoes, vegetables, and fruit provided 36% of the dietary folate intake along with bread (18%) and dairy products (16%).

In general, other than special requirements for additional folate, such as pregnancy, hemolysis, or ongoing alcohol abuse, the adult diet in most industrialized countries is adequate in meeting daily recommended folate consumption. Dietary recall information suggests that a large fraction of older individuals consume well below the recommended dietary allowance of 400 pg/d. In three separate studies, intakes ranging from 129 to 300 μg/d have been reported.[47,59,60] In a Canadian study of elderly men, intake averaged 150 pg daily, which is inadequate, coupled with the relatively uncommon incidence of biochemical deficiency, probably relates to the unrealistically high recommended daily intake. It must be emphasized, however, that folate balance in older individuals is marginal and that significant deficiencies are likely to develop rapidly if intake is further compromised by illness or if demand for the vitamin is increased.

Megaloblastic anemia due to folate deficiency in elderly people usually occurs in association with other medical problems. Of these, chronic alcoholism is the most important. In alcoholics, significant folate deficiency results from a combination of inadequate dietary intake combined with decreased absorption and altered folate metabolism.[61,62] Intestinal malabsorption is rare in the elderly but can present or manifest with isolated megaloblastic anemia caused by folate deficiency.

Drugs are another common cause of folate deficiency. Phenytoin (Dilantin) causes folate deficiency through a direct effect on the ability of cells to incorporate thymidine into DNA.[61] The common use of combinations of sulfamethoxazole with trimethoprim in elderly individuals with chronic urinary tract infections can also result in folate deficiency. Trimethoprim inhibits dihydrofolate reductase and hence prevents the formation of the active tetrahydrofolate. Although macrocytosis is common in patients consuming drugs that interfere with folate metabolism, frank anemia is rare. Finally, folate deficiency has been reported in elderly individuals who have hemolytic anemia. The presence of increased erythrocyte production results in increased folate requirements that frequently cannot be met from diet alone.

Significant folate deficiency results in ineffective erythropoiesis and a classic megaloblastic anemia. The disorder should be diagnosed by the detection of features of ineffective erythropoiesis, which include a low absolute reticulocyte count and evidence of intramedullary hemolysis, suggested by an indirect bilirubin level of greater than 0.6 mg/dL and an elevated lactic acid dehydrogenase level. The presence of macrocytosis (mean corpuscular volume greater than 100 fL) suggests either vitamin B$_{12}$ or folate deficiency. The diagnosis is confirmed by the presence of pathologically low serum (less than 2 nmol/L) and erythrocyte (less than 227 nmol/L) folate concentrations. Oral folate is the treatment of choice.

As with iron and folate deficiencies in the elderly, nutritional intake of B$_{12}$ appears to have an association with regional, cultural, and socioeconomic factors. Long-term vegetarian dietary patterns may predispose to a marginal risk of vitamin B$_{12}$ deficiency.[38] Other causes of vitamin B$_{12}$ deficiency in the elderly include malabsorption, gastric surgeries such as stapling procedures performed in the past for treatment of obesity, pernicious anemia, intestinal overgrowth (stasis syndrome), Crohn's disease, resection of terminal ileum, tropical sprue, pancreatic insufficiency, drugs (eg, biguanides, neomycin, cholestyramine, ethanol), fish tapeworm, and acquired abnormality of B$_{12}$ metabolism.[63-65]

The prevalence of low vitamin B$_{12}$ is estimated to be between 12% and 14% among individuals over the age of 60, and 25% among institutionalized elderly.[66] In a survey of elderly subjects in Boston, about 24% of those over age 80 years were found to have atrophic gastritis, using the criteria of pepsinogen I: pepsinogen II ratios as markers of this condition.[67]

An overwhelming majority of cases of vitamin B$_{12}$ deficiency in elderly individuals are due to pernicious anemia, in which impaired secretion of intrinsic factor by gastric parietal cells results in reduction of active vitamin B$_{12}$ absorption in the terminal ileum. The initial diagnostic workup should include a Schilling test, which helps to distinguish vitamin B$_{12}$ deficiency due to lack of intrinsic factor from other causes of B_{12} malabsorption.[68] The presence of serum intrinsic factor and parietal cell antibodies may point toward a diagnosis of pernicious anemia, but the latter are also reported in healthy elderly people. Further investigation of pernicious anemia should include a screen for other autoimmune disorders, especially hypothyroidism. In view of the increased incidence of gastric carcinoma and carcinoid tumors in pernicious anemia, endoscopy should also be considered.

Serum B_{12} levels have been reported in some studies to fall with aging.[63,69] Numerous clinical manifestations of B_{12} deficiency have been well documented in the literature. These include hematological defects such as megaloblastic anemia; neuropsychiatric disorders such as dementia, psychosis, peripheral neuropathies, subacute degeneration of the spinal cord; and gastrointestinal manifestations such as glossitis and malabsorption. Threshold levels of B_{12} below which clinically important manifestations of deficiency are seen are controversial. Patients with pernicious anemia usually have a level less than 90 pmol/L and a megaloblastic marrow is generally found in patients with a serum B_{12} level of less than 115 pmol/L. Patients with neuropsychiatric manifestations of B_{12} deficiency commonly have a level of less than 175 pmol/L. These patients may thus have a normal blood count.

Stott et al[63] recently reported the prevalence and hematopoietic effects of low B_{12} levels in both an outpatient as well as an inpatient elderly population. Of the population sampled prospectively, 13% were found to have serum B_{12} levels less than 175 pmol/L, without any significant reduction of the hemoglobin values. Interestingly, one-third of these vitamin B_{12} deficient patients also were iron deficient, perhaps resulting in normal values of their mean corpuscular volume (MCV). Therefore, some evidence exists to suggest that vitamin B_{12} deficiency is more common in elderly people. However, the clinical manifestations are subtle and may not be reflected in the peripheral complete blood count (CBC). Only about 60% of elderly people with vitamin B_{12} de-

ficiency are anemic.[70] Neurologic symptoms may develop before anemia is present. Anemia due to vitamin B_{12} deficiency is usually macrocytic and megaloblastic, but it can be monocytic or microcytic.[48] In addition, serum B_{12} levels may not reflect tissue B_{12} deficiency. Up to 30% of the older patients with low-normal serum vitamin B_{12} levels have anemia and neurological disease.[48] In a separate, subsequent prospective study, the same authors assessed the hematological response to intramuscular hydroxycobalamin in 34 patients with low serum B_{12} levels. Treatment resulted in a significant fall in MCV and rise in hemoglobin values, even in those patients who had a normal CBC prior to treatment.

The treatment of vitamin B_{12} deficiency is based on the underlying cause. Replacement therapy for severe vitamin B_{12} deficiency consists of intramuscular injections of hydroxycobalamin 1 mg each, initially for a total of 5 to 7 injections at weekly intervals. Once stores are replenished, the dosage frequency can be reduced to once every 3 months for life. Utmost care should be taken to follow the potassium levels during the initial weekly injections since a reduction in plasma potassium of 1 to 2 mEq/dL may occur in the first 48 hours after the first injection of vitamin B_{12}. Although vitamin B_{12} is generally replaced by intramuscular injection, oral replacement with 1 mg daily can be effective. Vitamin B_{12} may also be administered via intranasal gel of 500 μg to 1,500 μg per day of cyanocobalamin or hydroxycobalamin, but this may be a more expensive method of administration.

CONCLUSION

There is compelling evidence that nutritional factors contribute to, or account for, age-related changes in the hematopoietic system. A clear relationship exists between the prevalence of anemia and socioeconomic status, the disorder being common in groups in which poverty is prevalent and rare in affluent elderly people. In low socioeconomic populations a relationship exists between the prevalence of anemia and other nutritional deficiencies. Furthermore, nutritional deprivation reversibly aggravates hematologic changes in the elderly. If nutritional factors do contribute to the anemia seen in relatively healthy elderly individuals, mechanisms other than simple single-nutrient deficiencies must be considered. In older people, erythropoietic reserve is diminished, resulting in abnormalities under less stressful conditions than is likely to occur in younger subjects. A minor nutritional deficit that would cause no abnormality in young people may result in anemia in elderly individuals. Clearly, further research is required to unravel the complex nature of the interrelationships among age, nutrition, disease in general, and hematopoiesis in particular. Iron and folate are common nutritional causes of hematologic abnormalities in elderly subjects. In the case of both nutrients, deficiency that is severe enough to result in anemia occurs only in the presence of an associated pathologic process. Gastrointestinal blood loss is the major cause of iron deficiency. Increased folate requirements, altered metabolism, or decreased absorption invariably accompany the presence of significant folate deficiency. Therefore, systematic periodic screening in the elderly with inexpensive blood tests, particularly if it can be shown that treatment of disease discovered by testing may increase the quality of life, may have the potential to affect survival.

REFERENCES

1. Schofield R. The pluripotent stem cell. *Clin Haematol* 1979;8:221.
2. Schofield R, Lord BI, Kyffin S, et al. Self maintenance capacity of CFU-S. *Cell Physiol* 1980;103:355.
3. Albright JA, Makinodan T. Decline in the growth potential of spleen-colonizing bone marrow stem cells of long lived aging mice. *J Exp Med* 1976;144:1204.
4. Harrison DE, Astle CM, Delaittre JA. Loss of proliferative capacity in immunohemopoietic stem cells caused by serial transplantation rather than aging. *J Exp Med* 1978;147:1526.
5. Ross EAM, Anderson H, Micklem HS. Serial depletion and regeneration for the murine hematopoietic system: implication for hematopoietic organization and the study of cellular aging. *J Exp Med* 1982;155:432.
6. Harrison DE. Normal production of erythrocytes by mouse marrow continues for 73 months. *Proc Natl Acad Sci USA* 1972;70:3184.
7. Spangrude GJ, Heimfeld S, Weissman IL. Purification and characterization of mouse hematopoietic stem cells. *Science* 1988;261:58.
8. Mauch P, Greenberger JS, Sotnick L, et al. Evidence of structured variation in self-renewal capacity within long-termed bone marrow cultures. *Proc Natl Acad Sci USA* 1980;77:2927.
9. Lipschitz DA, McGinnis SK, Udupa KB. The use of long term marrow culture as a model for the aging process. *Age* 1983;6:122.
10. Mauch P, Botnick LE, Hannon EC, et al. Decline in bone marrow proliferative capacity as a function of age. *Blood* 1982;60:245.
11. Hellman S, Botnick L, Hannon EC, et al. Proliferative capacity of murine hematopoietic stem cells. *Proc Natl Acad* 1978;75:490.
12. Reincke U, Hannon EC, Rosenblatt M, et al. Proliferative capacity of murine hematopoietic stem cells in vitro. *Science* 1982;215:1619.
13. Williams LH, Udupa KB, Lipschitz DA. An evaluation of the effect of age on hematopoiesis in the mouse. *Exp Hematol* 1985;19:237.
14. Boggs DR, Patrene KD. Hematopoiesis and aging III. Anemia and a blunted erythropoietic response to hemorrhage in aged mice. *Am J Hematol* 1985;19:327.
15. Udupa KB, Lipschitz DA. Erythropoiesis in the aged mouse, I. Response to stimulation in vivo. *J Lab Clin Med* 1984;103:574.
16. Udupa KB, Lipschitz DA. Erythropoiesis in the aged mouse, II. Response to stimulation in vitro. *J Lab Clin Med* 1984;103:581.
17. McLennan WJ, et al. Anaemia in the elderly. *Q J Med* 1973;52:1.
18. Myers MA, et al. The hemoglobin level of fit elderly people. *Lancet* 1968;2:261.
19. *Nutrition Canada: National Survey*. Ottawa, Canada: Information Canada; 1973.
20. Yip R, et al. Age-related changes in laboratory values used in the diagnosis of anemia and iron deficiency. *Am J Clin Nutr* 1984;39:427.
21. McPhee SJ. The evaluation of anemia. *West J Med* 1982;137:253.
22. Ania BJ, et al. Prevalence of anemia in medical practice: community versus referral patients. *Mayo Clin Proc* 1994;69:730.
23. Ania BJ, et al. Incidence of anemia in older people: an epidemiologic study in a well defined population. *J Am Geriatr Soc* 1997;45:825.
24. Lipschitz DA, et al. The anemia of senescence. *Am J Hematol* 1981;11:47.

25. Lipschitz DA, et al. Effect of age on hematopoiesis in man. *Blood* 1984;63:502.

26. Garry PJ, et al. Iron status and anemia in the elderly. *J Am Geriatr Soc* 1983;31:389.

27. Sears DA. Anemia of chronic disease. *Med Clin North Am* 1992;76:567.

28. Lipschitz DA, Mitchell CO. The correctability of the nutritional, immune and hematopoietic manifestations of protein calorie malnutrition in the elderly. *J Am Coll Nutr* 1982;1:17.

29. Rudman D, Mattson DE, et al. Antecedents of death in the men of a Veterans Administration nursing home. *J Am Geriatr Soc* 1987;35:496.

30. Lipschitz DA, Udupa KB. Influence of aging and protein deficiency on neutrophil function. *J Gerontol* 1986;41:690.

31. McMahon MM, Bistrian BR. The physiology of nutritional assessment and therapy in protein-calorie malnutrition. *Dis Mon* 1990;36(7):373–417.

32. Lipschitz DA, Mitchell CO, Milton KY. Nutritional evaluation and supplementation of elderly participants in a Meals on Wheels program. *J Parenter Enter Nutr* 1985;9:343.

33. Cook JD, Finch CA, Smith NJ. Evaluation of iron status of a population. *Blood* 1976;48:449.

34. Bedford PD, Wollner L. Occult intestinal bleeding as a cause of anaemia in elderly people. *Lancet* 1958;1:1144.

35. Kirkeby OJ, Fossum S, Risoe C. Anemia in elderly patients: incidence and causes of low hemoglobin concentration in a city general practice. *Scand J Prim Health Care* 1991;9:167–171.

36. Joosten E, Pelemans W, Hiele M, et al. Prevalence and causes of anemia in a geriatric hospitalized population. *Gerontology* 1992;38:111–117.

37. Looker CA, Dallman RP, Carroll MS, Gunter WE, Johnso LC. Prevalence of iron deficiency in the United States. *JAMA* 1997;277:973–976.

38. Chiel RL, Schrijver J, Odink J, et al. Long term effects of a vegetarian diet on the nutritional status of the elderly (Dutch nutrition study). *J Am Coll Nutr* 1990;9:600–609.

39. Fleming DJ, et al. Dietary determinants of iron stores in the elderly population in the Framingham Heart Study. *Am J Clin Nutr* 1998;67:722–733.

40. Hillman RS, Finch CA. *Red Cell Manual*. Philadelphia, PA: FA Davis Co; 1985.

41. Balducci L. Epidemiology of anemia in the elderly: information on diagnostic evaluation. *JAGS* 2003;51:S1–9.

42. Brise H. Influence of meals on iron absorption in oral therapy. *Acta Med Scand* 1962;171(suppl 376):39.

43. Fulcher RA, Hyland CM. Effectiveness of once daily oral iron in the elderly. *Age Ageing* 1981;10:44.

44. Reizenstein P, Ljunggren G, Smedby B, et al. Overprescribing iron tablets to elderly people in Sweden. *Br Med J* 1979;2:962.

45. Lipschitz D. Medical and functional consequences of anemia in the elderly. *JAGS* 2003;51(suppl):S10–13.

46. Ahluwalia N, Sun J, Krause D, Mastro A, Handte G. Immune function is impaired in iron deficient, homebound, older women. *Am J Clin Nutr* 2004;79:516–521.

47. Fulop T, Wagner JR, Khalil A, Weber J, Trottier L, Payette H. Relationship between the response to influenza vaccination and the nutritional status of institutionalized elderly subjects. *J Gerontol* 1999;54A:M59–64.

48. Smith D. Anemia in the elderly. *Amer Fam Phys* 2000;62:1565–1572.

49. Elwood PC, Shinton NK, Wilson CID, et al. Haemoglobin, vitamin B_{12} and folate levels in the elderly. *Br J Haematol* 1971;21:557.

50. Craig GM, Elliot C, Hughes KR. Masked vitamin B_{12} and folate deficiency in the elderly. *Br J Nutr* 1985;54:613–619.

51. Ubbink JB. Should all elderly people receive folate supplements? *Drugs Aging* 1998;6:415–420.

52. Ubbink JB, Vermaak WJH, Van der Merwe A, et al. Vitamin requirements for the treatment of hypercysteinemia in humans. *J Nutr* 1994;124:1927–1933.

53. Joosten E, Vandenberg A, Reizler R, et al. Metabolic evidence that deficiencies of vitamin B_{12}, folate and vitamin B_6 occur commonly in elderly people. *Am J Clin Nutr* 1993;58:468–4676.

54. Naurath HJ, Joosten E, Riezler R, et al. Effects of vitamin B_{12}, folate, and vitamin B_6 supplements in elderly with normal serum vitamin concentrations. *Lancet* 1995;346:85–89.

55. Selhub J, Jacques PF, Bostom AG, et al. Association between plasma homocysteine concentrations and extracranial carotid artery stenosis. *N Engl J Med* 1995;332:286–291.

56. Stampfer MJ, Malinow R, Willet WC, et al. A prospective study of plasma homocysteine and risk of myocardial infarction in US physicians. *JAMA* 1992;268:877–881.

57. Nicolas AS, Andrieu S, Nourhashemi F, Rolland Y, Vellas B. Successful aging and nutrition. *Nutr Rev* 2001;59:S88–S91.

58. Rosenberg IH, Bowman BB, Cooper BA, et al. Folate nutrition in the elderly. *Am J Clin Nutr* 1982;36:1060.

59. Brussaard JH, et al. Folate intake and status among adults in the Netherlands. *Eur J Clin Nutr* 1997;51(suppl 3):S46–S50.

60. *Nutrition Canada. Food Consumption Patterns Report.* Ottawa, Ontario, Canada: Department of National Health and Welfare; 1979.

61. Lindenbaum J, Roman MJ. Nutritional anemia in alcoholism. *Am J Clin Nutr* 1980;33:2727.

62. Chanarin I. *The Megaloblastic Anaemias.* 2nd ed. Oxford, England: Blackwell Scientific Publications Ltd; 1979.

63. Stott D, Langhorne P, Hendry A, et al. Prevalence of hematological effects of low serum vitamin B_{12} levels in geriatric medical patients. *Br J Nutr* 1997;78:57–63.

64. Lindenbaum J, Rosenberg IH, Wilson PWF, Stabler SP, Allen RH. Prevalence of cobalamin deficiency in the Framingham elderly population. *Am J Clin Nutr* 1994; 60:2–11.

65. Lindenbaum J, Healton EB, Svage DG, et al. Neuropsychiatric disorders caused by cobalamin deficiency in the absence of anemia or macrocytosis. *N Engl J Med* 1988;318:1720–1728.

66. Russell RM, Baik HW. Clinical implications of vitamin B_{12} deficiency in the elderly. *Nutr Clinical Care* 2001; 4:214–220.

67. Krasinski SD, Russell RM, Samloff IM, et al. Fundic atrophic gastritis in an elderly population. Effect on hemoglobin and several scrum nutritional indicators. *JAGS* 1986;4:806.

68. Chanarin I. Pernicious anemia. Diagnosis should be certain before treatment is begun. *Br Med J* 1992;304: 1584–1585.

69. Murphy PT, Hutchinson RM. Identification and treatment of anemia in older patients. *Drugs Aging* 1994; 4(2):13–127.

70. Joosten E, Ghesquiere B, Linthoudt H, Krekelberghs F, Dejaeger E, Boonen S, et al. Upper and lower gastrointestinal evaluation of elderly inpatients who are iron deficient. *Am J Med* 1999;107:24–29.

CHAPTER 14

Skeletal Aging

Gustavo Duque, MD, PhD and Bruce R. Troen, MD

The integrity of bone is essential, not only to sustain the structure of the human body, but also to host the bone marrow with all of its cellular interactions. Bone strength is not only dependent upon bone mass, which is most often related to bone mineral density, but also upon bone quality, structure, and turnover. Although 60–80% of bone strength is genetically determined,[1,2] many other nutritional and lifestyle factors are determinants of bone health. After birth, human growth determines the increase in bone mass. Bone grows in both length and width, and bone mass is accumulated until the formation of the peak of bone mass (PBM), usually during the third decade of life. This bone mass reflects the amount of bone gained during growth minus that which has been subsequently lost. It now appears that about 60% of final adult bone mass is acquired during the pubertal growth spurt, particularly during the 3- to 4-year period surrounding the time of maximum height velocity, with only about 5% of final bone mass accruing during the decade from age 18 to 28 years. After that time, bone balance is largely negative as a consequence of changes in bone remodeling and hormonal status. The rate at which bone is lost in adults varies from one skeletal site to another and, according to measurement technique, is highly influenced by an assortment of so-called lifestyle factors, including body weight, reproductive hormonal function, habitual physical activity, diet, tobacco and alcohol consumption, illness, and medication (Figure 14–1). The combination of all these multiple factors will determine both the amount of bone mass in the individual and the susceptibility to bone loss in adult life. Although bone loss with advancing age is a universal phenomenon, some individuals undergo more severe bone loss than others due to the balance among these determinants. Specific mechanisms that lead to severe bone loss in some people but not in others are not completely understood. However, considerable interest has been directed toward clarifying the elements that determine peak bone mass at maturity and its subsequent decline.

Osteoporosis is a condition of skeletal fragility that is associated with low bone mass and disruption of the normal bony microarchitecture (bone quality). It appears clinically as fractures that are sustained with little or no trauma. These have been described most frequently for the spine, wrist, and hip. However, osteoporosis is a condition of global fragility, and fractures elsewhere in the skeleton are also common. Osteoporotic fractures are more commonly observed in women. This reflects the fact that women have lower bone mass than men and that there are twice as many older women as men. Nonetheless, while fracture incidence rises substantially as men age, their age-specific incidence of fracture is about half that of women. Osteoporosis may be the consequence of a continuum (or a combination) of factors that include a low PBM, poor nutrition and physical activity, genetic predisposition, and aging *per se*. In this chapter we will attempt to illustrate the interaction between the factors shown in Figure 14–1 and their role in the process of aging bone, as well as the potential approach to prevent osteoporosis and its manifestations.

SKELETAL ORGANIZATION

The skeleton is organized into two compartments, peripheral and axial. The peripheral (cortical) skeleton constitutes 80% of skeletal mass and is composed primarily of compact plates (lamellae) organized around central nutrient canals. The shafts of long bones consist almost entirely of cortical bone that envelopes the central marrow cavity.

The axial, or central, skeleton is composed about 70% (by volume) and about 35% (by weight) of trabecular (cancellous) bone. Trabecular bone is a honeycomb of vertical and horizontal bars (trabeculae), inside which is found bone marrow (Figure 14–2). The metaphyseal ends of long bones also contain trabecular bone,

but they contain no red marrow in the adult. Since marrow elements are the source of osteoclast precursors, and since bone turnover occurs on bone surfaces, the occurrence of high-surface density bone in close proximity to the cellular elements that participate in its turnover results in trabecular bone's responding earlier and more intensely to whole-body changes in bone remodeling rate.

THE PIVOTAL ROLE OF BONE REMODELING

Bone undergoes three fundamental activities: modeling, repair, and remodeling. Modeling refers to the process by which the characteristic shape of a bone is achieved and maintained. Repair is the regenerative response to fracture. Remodeling is a continuous cycle of destruction and renewal of bone that occurs throughout life in humans, primates, and some other mammals.[5] The objectives of the remodeling process are both to replace microdamage and to adapt bone shape and density to patterns of usage. This process is carried out by independent osteons,

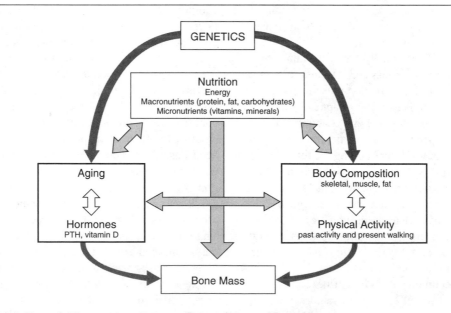

Figure 14–1 Potential Interactions Between Determinants of Bone Mass
Source: Adapted from Ilich et al.[3]

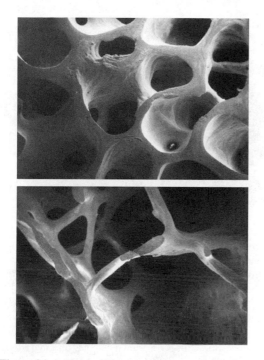

Figure 14–2 Normal Young and Osteoporotic Bone Structure
Trabecular mass is a honeycomb of vertical and horizontal struts (trabeculae), hosting the bone marrow. Due to its proximity to bone marrow, trabecular bone is a very active tissue with multiple cell/cell interactions. In addition, with age, the quality and quantity of the trabeculae decrease and the bone marrow space is increasingly occupied by adipose tissue. From Dempster et al.[4]

sorption front leaves a cavity about 60 μm deep, whose deepest boundary appears as a cement line, a region of poorly organized collagen fibrils, as opposed to the surrounding lamellar bone.

The process of remodeling is dependent upon two types of cells, osteoblasts and osteoclasts. Osteoblasts belong to the fibroblast lineage and are the product of the differentiation of bone marrow mesenchymal stem cells, whereas hematopoietic monocytic precursors differentiate into osteoclasts, which share the characteristics of macrophages in other tissues (Figure 14–3). Coupled to resorption, which is executed by mature osteoclasts, bone formation is triggered when the local release of chemical mediators embedded in the bone matrix attracts preosteoblasts into the resorption cavity.[6] The identity of these mediators is not known with certainty, but bone morphogenic proteins, transforming growth factor-3, and insulin-like growth factors may each play a role. The preosteoblasts mature into osteoblasts and replace the missing bone by secreting new collagen and matrix constituents. Matrix production is initially rapid, with the new osteoid seam approaching 20 μm in thickness when mineral deposition begins. With time, mineralization catches up to matrix deposition, and the new bone becomes fully mineralized. A normal bone-remodeling cycle takes about 2–6 months to reach completion.

Bone formation and bone resorption are tightly coupled; more recently the molecular basis for this linkage has become elucidated (Figure 14–4).[8] Osteoblasts produce both macrophage colony stimulating factor (M-CSF) and membrane bound receptor activator of NFkB ligand (RANKL), which are critical and necessary factors for osteoclastogenesis. Osteoclasts and their precursors express RANK, which is the cognate receptor of RANKL and, upon binding, activates multiple intracellular signaling pathways leading to osteoclast differentiation and activation. A large variety of signals regulates the production of RANKL, including stimulators such as vitamin D, parathyroid hormone, tumor necrosis factor-α, glucocorticoids, prostaglandins, interleukins, insulin-like growth factor-1, and low gravity. Inhibitors of RANKL expression

called bone remodeling units (Figure 14–3), and alterations in remodeling activity constitute the final common pathway through which diverse stimuli, such as dietary or hormonal insufficiency, affect the rate of bone loss.

Normally, 90% of bone surfaces are at rest, covered by a thin layer of inactive lining cells. Remodeling is initiated by hormonal or physical signals that cause marrow-derived precursor cells to cluster on the bone surface, where they fuse into multinucleated osteoclasts, which in turn dig a cavity into the bone. In cortical bone, this cavity appears as a resorption tunnel within a Haversian canal. On trabecular surfaces, it is a scalloped area called a Howship's lacuna. The re-

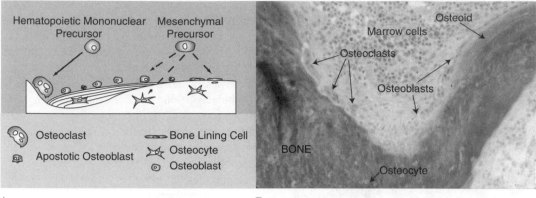

A   B

Figure 14–3A and 14–3B The Cellular Components of Bone Turnover
A) Bone cell formation: After the expression of specific transcription factors, mesenchymal precursors differentiate into osteoblasts. In contrast, osteoclasts differentiate from mononuclear precursors and will act as bone resorbing cells in the bone multicellular unit (BMU). After the completion of bone resorption, osteoclasts die by apoptosis and are replaced by active osteoblasts, which are responsible for the formation of new bone. Finally osteoblasts end as either lining cells, as osteocytes embedded into the osteoid, or die by apoptosis. From Chan & Duque, 2002.[6] B) Basic multicellular unit (BMU—also known as bone metabolic unit): Large multinucleated osteoclasts resorb bone on the left. Osteoblasts cascade into the resorption pit, laying down osteoid (unmineralized bone). The darker gray area in Figure B reflects mineralized bone. From Ott, 2004.[7] Reprinted by permission of Ott, SM, "Osteoporosis and Bone Physiology," http:// courses.washington.edu, 2005.

include estrogen and tumor growth factor-β (TGF-β). Concurrently, osteoblasts secrete osteoprotegerin (OPG), which is a decoy receptor for RANKL and inhibits RANKL-RANK signaling. Therefore, osteoclast differentiation, formation, and activation depend upon the proximity and products of the osteoblast. However, osteoblast differentiation and activation are also significantly modulated by the osteoclast. Both osteoblasts and osteoclasts synthesize and secrete latent TGF-β.[9] Resorption of bone by osteoclasts releases latent TGF-β from the organic matrix, wherein it potently stimulates osteoblastogenesis and concurrently inhibits RANKL expression by osteoblasts.[10] In addition, osteoclasts produce and secrete bone morphogenetic protein-2 (BMP-2),[11] which is a powerful inducer of osteoblast differentiation.[12] Both TGF-β and BMP-2 appear to act directly upon osteoclasts to potentiate RANKL mediated formation and survival.

Furthermore, osteoclasts secrete Mim-1, which is a chemokine that stimulates migration and differentiation of osteoblastic precursor cells.[13,14] Osteoclasts also secrete platelet-derived growth factor (PDGF), which inhibits osteoblast differentiation.[15] These potent secreted molecules and other molecules act in both endocrine and autocrine fashion to exert multiple stimulatory and inhibitory effects upon both osteoclasts and osteoblasts. It appears that the balance between osteoblastogenesis and osteoclastogenesis and between the resultant bone formation and bone resorption are dependent upon threshold levels of these cytokines and the stage of differentiation of both osteoblasts and osteoclasts. This dynamic equilibrium is also modulated by biomechanical stresses associated with weight bearing, exercise, and trauma.[16] Nonetheless, it is clear that osteoblasts are essential mediators of osteoclastogenesis, just as osteoclasts appear to play a major role in osteoblast formation and activity.

If the remodeling cycle were completely efficient, bone would be neither lost nor gained. Each remodeling unit would be associated with

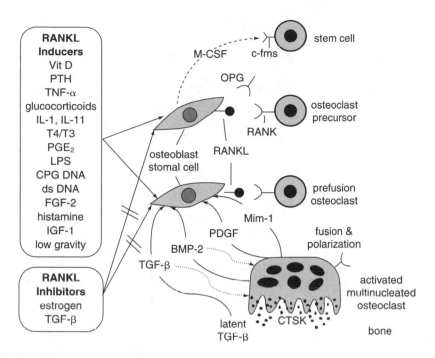

Figure 14–4 Osteoblast–Osteoclast Coupling
Osteoblast production of M-CSF and RANKL plays a critical role in the differentiation and activation of osteoclasts. Inducers and inhibitors of RANKL expression are listed on the left of the figure. M-CSF acts to maintain monocytic stem cell survival, and subsequently RANKL acts to commit the cell toward osteoclast differentiation, fusion, polarization, and activation. TGF-ß, BMP-2, PDFG, and Mim-1 appear to play important roles in the intercellular communication between osteoblasts and osteoclasts. From Troen.[8] Reprinted with permission from Elsevier.

complete replacement of the packet of bone that was initially lost. However, remodeling, like most biological processes, is not entirely efficient. The amount of bone replaced by formation does not always equal the amount previously removed, so that a small bone deficit persists after each cycle. This remodeling imbalance is minuscule for any single normal bone-remodeling event. Unless remodeling dynamics are perturbed, the resulting accumulation of bone deficits may be detected only after many years and would represent a reduction of 0.5%/year after the third decade of life. The concept of remodeling imbalance carries the profound implication that age-related bone loss is a normal, predictable phenomenon and that any increase in the overall rate of bone remodeling will increase the rate of bone loss. Another long-term consequence of remodeling is the acquisition of cement lines. These areas of woven bone are not as strong as the surrounding lamellar bone and thus form a site of least resistance to strain. In fact, examination of fractured bone shows propagation of fracture from one cement line to the next.

After the completion of their function, bone cells in the BMU have different fates (Figure 14-3). Osteoclasts die by apoptosis, or programmed cell death, and are phagocytosed *in situ*. In contrast, osteoblasts can undergo multiple possible fates. They can become lining cells, migrate to a new BMU, become embedded within the osteoid, become osteocytes, or finally die by apoptosis. The predominance of any of these fates will determine the amount of osteoblasts available in the BMU and thus, ultimately, the differentiation and activation of osteoclasts.

IN VIVO ASSESSMENT OF BONE MASS

Accurate, noninvasive measurement of bone mass emerged with the development of photon absorptiometry. Results are given as the mass of bone mineral (grams) contained within a given area (square centimeters) of scanned bone. The resulting value, called bone mineral density (BMD) is therefore an areal density, and not a true volumetric density. Single-photon absorptiometry (SPA) is based on the attenuation of a narrowly focused photon beam by bone. Measurements are accurate, precise, and suited to skeletal regions in which variations in soft tissue composition are minimal, such as the forearm or heel. Estimates of cortical bone mass at these sites correlate reasonably well with whole-body bone mineral, but only poorly reflect the axial skeleton.[17] However, BMD detects only the mineral component of the bone and therefore does not directly reflect the degree of bone turnover and remodeling activity.

This guides us to the concept of the "remodeling space," which refers to the amount of bone tissue which is temporarily "out of service" and that amounts to about 1–1.5% of cortical bone and about 6% of cancellous bone. Despite the limitations due to this underdetection, dual-energy X-ray absorptiometry (DEXA) has emerged as the most useful of the techniques to assess BMD.[18] Subjects lie recumbent while a photomultiplier tube records transmission from an X-ray source located under the scanning table. The lumbar spine is scanned in about 4 minutes with a radiation exposure of less than 5 mrem. DXA measurements in the usual anteroposterior position record the complete mineral content of a vertebra, including the cortical shell and posterior elements, in addition to the vertebral body itself. Moreover, patients with degenerative joint disease of the spine and aortic calcifications may have falsely elevated spine BMD readings. DXA is also routinely used to measure BMD at the proximal femur, which is not subject to these latter artifacts but requires very careful attention to positioning of the leg, particularly for repeated measurements. DEXA software also permits some machines to provide measurements of whole-body and regional skeletal mineral, as well as body composition assessments (lean and adipose tissue). The precision error for DEXA varies from 1–1.5% in young and older subjects, respectively. Although there is a good correlation between the level of bone mineralization measured by DEXA and the risk of fracture, a normal BMD does not exclude the possibility of fractures. Furthermore, treatment with antiresorptive agents can lead to significant reductions in fracture risk with only small improvements in BMD, suggesting that additional factors contribute to bone quality.[19] Between 20% and 40% of bone strength is dependent upon such factors.[20,21] Bone quality also depends upon collagen content, uniformity of mineral distribution, crystallinity, and maintenance of microarchitecture. Consequently the measurement of BMD, though accurate, could be limited in determining a patient's fracture risk. Indeed, it is possible that a significant deterioration in bone microarchitecture can occur before it is detected by DEXA. Therefore, bone microarchitecture seems to be important to understand the mechanisms of bone fragility as well as the action of the drugs used to prevent osteoporotic fractures.

Quantitative computed tomography (QCT) has been used frequently to estimate trabecular bone density at the lumbar spine. The subject lies on a scanning table above a set of materials of standard densities. The operator selects a region of pure trabecular bone for analysis, and the mineral density, given as milligrams per cubic centimeter of bone volume, is calculated. Although this technique can be modified for any skeletal region, most work has involved the lumbar spine, for which commercial software is available. For healthy, nonosteoporotic subjects, the precision error in experienced hands may approach that of DEXA. However, in routine clinical practice such performance is rarely achieved. Radiation exposure, usually 500 to 1000 mrem, is modest but substantially greater than that of DEXA. Modifications of these technologies have become available, including DEXA and CT scanners that are used exclusively on the forearm or leg.

Besides their research applications, these techniques may permit bone density screening of large populations at much lower cost than can be accomplished with DEXA. In addition, several companies are developing methods based on the transmission of ultrasound through bones, such as the heel and patella. As a result of these, measurements correlate well with BMD measurements and could therefore be used as a screening modality to identify those individuals who should undergo comprehensive testing with DEXA.[22] Quantitative ultrasound also provides information on bone mass and structure and has some potential advantages, including cost, portability, and the absence of ionizing radiation.[23] Quantitative ultrasound can distinguish women with and without vertebral fracture over a broad range of ages.[24]

CHANGES IN BONE MASS WITH AGE

Overview

Accumulation of bone during the growth years exactly mirrors linear growth. Bone mass increases linearly until the onset of puberty and then undergoes an intense and rapid increase that is followed by a short interval at the time of maximum height velocity. About 95% of ultimate, "peak" bone mass is acquired by age 18 in girls, perhaps a year or two later in boys.[25–27] Between the ages of 18 and 28 years, small amounts of bone continue to be accrued, but bone acquisition is essentially complete by age 28 years. As measured by noninvasive techniques, bone mass then remains stable until about the third decade of life, when progressive decrease in BMD occurs in both men and women. A woman's loss of estrogen at menopause results in an accelerated rate of loss, particularly from trabecular sites, during the first several years after menopause. Afterward the rates of loss in women and men are fairly similar.

Adolescent Bone Acquisition

The 2- to 3-year period corresponding to the time of peak height velocity represents a brief window of opportunity for laying down bone. Sixty percent of peak bone mass is acquired during this period. Its onset is triggered by pubertal progression, and increases in bone mass are highly correlated to body weight, height, and pubertal stage. In young American women, 90% of total bone mineral content was attained at age 17 and 99% was achieved by age 26. The peak bone density in hip and vertebrae is achieved between ages 17 and 20.[25]

The greatest influence on pubertal bone acquisition is genetics, which appears to account for approximately 75% of the population variance in peak bone mass. The largest single influence of genetics on BMD is bone size, which itself is a polygenic function, reflecting at the very least the activities of the somatotrophic (growth hormone and somatomedin) and gonadotrophic axes. Genetic polymorphisms in the vitamin D receptor have been implicated as being significantly related to bone mass.[28] In addition, a recent study by Peacock et al.[29] reported that chromosomes 14q and 15q harbor genes that affect peak bone mass at the hip of women, suggesting pleiotropic effects of these genes on hip phenotypes. Furthermore, variations in specific genes such as the lipoprotein receptor-related protein 5 (LRP5) and part of the Wnt-frizzled pathway, have been independently identified by linkage in high and low bone mass families.[30] It is highly likely that other genes will also be found to be related to bone mass in the future.

Environmental or lifestyle elements that affect bone acquisition are not completely understood, but substantial evidence suggests that adequacy of dietary calcium (Figure 14–5) and habitual physical activity are very important. Epidemiological data have not been consistent in defining the relationship of dietary calcium to bone acquisition by children. During recent years, several well-conceived placebo-controlled clinical trials have consistently shown larger increases in bone mass by children and adolescents receiving supplemental calcium than were observed in those receiving placebo.[25] In adolescent females, Matkovic et al[31] demonstrated that calcium supplementation and dairy products

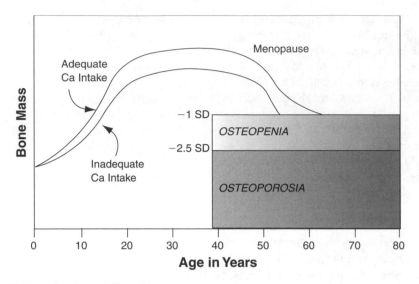

Figure 14–5 Calcium Intake and Bone Mass
Comparison between the curve of bone mass between an adequate and inadequate calcium (Ca) intake. Subjects with inadequate Ca intake show a lower BMD and a higher susceptibility to osteoporosis in later years than those subjects with an adequate Ca intake. From Ilich.[35]

increased bone mineral density of the hip and forearm in adolescent females. Although most of the calcium intervention studies performed in children and adolescents show a positive effect of calcium on bone accretion, follow-up data from some studies in young individuals indicated that 2 years after termination of the calcium intervention, the difference in bone mass between the two treatment groups was no longer significant.[32,33] This could be related to the concept of "bone remodeling transient," which is a temporary alteration in the balance between bone formation and bone resorption.[34] Thus, one possibility is that to achieve permanent skeletal benefit, it is necessary to maintain an increased calcium intake over the long term.

It should be noted that habitual calcium intakes of American girls and women are seriously deficient. According to data from the United States Center for Health Statistics (NHANES), median calcium intake of girls decreases below recommended standards at age 11 and never recovers.[36] Of teenage girls, about 30% consume less than 400 mg of calcium per day, reflecting a serious reduction in milk consumption over the past few decades.

A meta-analysis by Cumming et al.[37] demonstrated that dietary calcium during adolescence is correlated with bone mineral content during the premenopausal years, with a significant prevention of bone loss of about 1% in all measured skeletal sites. Calcium supplementation in healthy older postmenopausal women can also significantly reduce bone loss.[38] This evidence and other reports[39,40] indicate that the adolescent growth spurt represents a window of opportunity for achieving major increases in bone mass and maximizing an individual's chances for achieving full peak bone mass potential. To support this concept, population studies have shown that calcium-rich foods or calcium supplementation increase the peak of bone mass in comparison with nonsupplemented groups.[31] In summary, reaching an adequate PBM will protect the individual to a degree from the "normal" decline in BMD associated with aging and, most importantly, with the abnormalities in bone turnover seen during the perimenopausal years.

ADULT BONE LOSS

The traditional model of age-related bone loss was clearly enunciated by the landmark studies of Garn et al.[41] Using careful measurements of metacarpal cortical thickness from hand radiographs, they described a characteristic trajectory of bone mass change that was similar in men and women and was observed in virtually all ethnic groups: Bone is gained during adolescence, remains stable until about age 50 years, then progressively decreases. This model has been independently validated by numerous laboratories using newer densitometric methods[42-44] and has been modified by the observation that the initial rate of loss at age 50 in women is temporarily more rapid than in men, reflecting the effects of menopausal estrogen loss.

Although the age-related decline in BMD of the radius accurately describes the trajectory of appendicular (limb) cortical bone mass, it was difficult for many years to validate its applicability to other regions of the cortical skeleton, such as the proximal femur, or to the axial or trabecular skeleton. Pioneering studies with postmortem material[45 47] clearly indicated that loss of axial bone occurred earlier than one would predict from noninvasive data. Subsequent analyses of iliac crest biopsy material confirm this view.[48] There is unanimous agreement, using multiple techniques, that trabecular bone is lost with age and that axial density is substantially lower in older subjects than in young people. Uncertainty remains over the timing of onset of axial bone loss.

ONSET OF BONE LOSS

A decline in bone density has been reported to begin after the second,[49] third,[50] fourth,[51] or fifth[52] decade. Measurements of anatomic specimens and results from biopsy studies indicate that axial loss occurs as early as the third decade.[48,53,54] In particular, iliac crest biopsy data suggest that trabecular bone mass declines significantly in women before menopause. Meunier and colleagues showed an age-related loss of trabecular bone that began as early as the third decade in a series of specimens obtained from sudden death accident victims. Marcus et al.[48] examined trabecular bone volume in biopsy specimens taken from active women with normal menstrual function and reported that trabecular bone volume was negatively correlated with age, with an annual predicted loss of 0.7%. The cumulative effect of such loss over a span of 30 years might amount to a deficit of 25% of original trabecular bone volume before menopause is reached. Birkenhager-Frenkel et al.[55] conducted iliac crest biopsies on a large group of healthy men and women and reported a correlation of trabecular bone volume with age for premenopausal women that was the same as that observed by Marcus and colleagues.[48] Trabecular vertebral specimens show the same pattern with age as iliac crest samples. Mosekilde and Mosekilde[56] examined postmortem trabecular samples of the first lumbar vertebra and found an age-related decrease in vertebral bone mass beginning in the third decade.

These changes in bone mineral density are the consequence of changes in both hormones and cells associated with the normal aging process. There are significant changes in the levels of vitamin D due to a reduction in sunlight as well as in vitamin D-rich food intake.[57,58] In addition, the capacity to metabolize vitamin D in the skin is reduced with aging.[59] All these factors determine that serum levels of vitamin D, with a subsequent increase in parathyroid hormone (PTH) levels,[60] will induce an increase in osteoclastic activity, bone resorption, and loss of bone mineral density.

Associated with the hormonal changes, cellular changes in the bone microenvironment will include a predominance of adipogenic differentiation of mesenchymal stem cells with a reduction in the amount of mature osteoblasts as well as a reduction in the life span of active osteoblasts in the BMU. This increase in adipogenesis with reduction in osteoblastogenesis and increased osteoblast/osteocyte apoptosis will have as a consequence a reduction in bone formation and lower mineral content (Figure 14–6). Furthermore,

Ilich et al.[3] have shown that significant changes in nutrient intake or metabolism including protein, magnesium, iron, and vitamin C might have an effect on bone mineral density in elderly women and could induce a more significant deficit in bone mass. The mechanisms to explain the role of each one of these nutrients in bone formation remain unclear, but their deficit is clearly associated with advanced bone loss.

CHANGES IN BONE MASS AT MENOPAUSE

Most studies confirm that trabecular bone loss accelerates at menopause.[50–52,62–67] Gallagher et al.[64] measured spine BMD of almost 400 women and reported that the largest decrease occurred in the first 5 years after menopause. They found a 3.4% annual decline in the second year, a 1.7% decline in the fourth year, and a 0.8% decline in the ninth year. Cann and associates,[66] using QCT to measure spine BMD, found that values for tra-

becular mineral remained stable until menopause, declined rapidly for 5 to 8 years, and then continued to decline more slowly. Firooznia et al[67] showed the same trend. This decline in bone density is the consequence of an increase in osteoclastic activity and bone resorption (Figure 14-6) and could be reverted after the administration of estrogen in experimental models. However, recent evidence obtained from the HERS study has discouraged the use of estrogen supplementation in perimenopausal women due to the risk of estrogen dependent neoplasia and effects on the cardiovascular system. Despite this evidence, further studies are being conducted to assess new dosages and compounds for estrogen supplementation and replacement.

To summarize, trabecular bone loss in women begins before age 50 years and increases at menopause. The weight of evidence supports the conclusion that menopausal loss of bone is curvilinear; that is, most rapid within the first few years (Figure 14–5). The absolute rates of

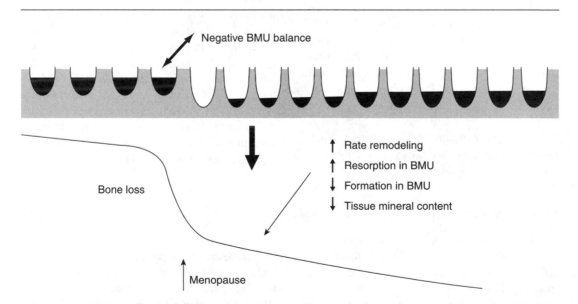

Figure 14–6 Age-Related Bone Loss and Bone Turnover
After the achievement of peak bone mass, progressive bone loss is associated with aging due to a negative BMU balance. After the arrival of menopause in women, there is an increased rate of bone remodeling due to enhanced osteoclastic activity. In both men and women, a significant reduction in the number and activity of osteoblasts in the BMU leads to a reduction in the rate of bone formation and tissue mineral content. From Seeman.[61]

menopausal bone loss are highly variable and appear to follow a normal distribution. In general, a woman whose peak bone density was already low might be predicted to have a low rate of loss, but since her skeleton was already at jeopardy, it would be important to assess her and offer treatment. By contrast, another woman might have rapid bone loss, but starting with an initial bone mass that was greater than 1 standard deviation above age-related norms, she would still have a very low risk of fracture even if she were untreated.

RELATIONSHIP OF LOSS OF BONE MASS TO BONE STRENGTH

Most patients with vertebral, wrist, and hip fractures have low bone mass. However, it is important to understand that bone's strength depends not only on its amount but on its material quality and architecture. A number of so-called qualitative abnormalities have been described in bone from older individuals that render older bone more fragile in comparison to bone of equal BMD in younger individuals. These abnormalities include the lifelong accumulation of cement lines as a consequence of remodeling events (Figure 14–6) and the presence of unremodeled fatigue damage. Other qualitative abnormalities include subtle degrees of undermineralization at critical areas of Haversian systems, loss of trabecular connectivity, and the accumulation of cortical porosity.[68]

Mosekilde and Mosekilde[56] demonstrated the importance of bone quality to vertebral body strength by showing 90% reductions in strength between ages 15 and 87, whereas as density (the amount of mineral present) declined only 50% over this span. In a young person, trabecular bone is characterized by thick vertical plates and columns that are connected by thinner horizontal elements. Maximal strength is provided by the connection of all trabecular elements into a honeycomb-like structure. With age, skeletal fragility is created by both the thinning of trabecular plates and the dropout of complete horizontal elements, with a corresponding increase in intertrabecular spaces.[69]

Another important determinant of bone strength is its geometry. The strength of a bone in compression reflects its mineral density squared times its cross-sectional area. Thus, a larger bone will be stronger than a small bone even if BMD values are equivalent. Recent attention has focused on a measurement called the hip axis length (HAL), seen on bone density printouts as the straight-line distance between the inferior surface of the greater trochanter to the inner surface of the acetabulum. Faulkner et al.[70] have shown that longer HAL is independently predictive of hip fracture. It appears that shorter HAL values are characteristic of Asian women and may contribute to their lower incidence of hip fracture.

MECHANISMS OF BONE MASS REGULATION

As stated above, alteration in remodeling activity is the final common pathway to modulating bone mass in adults. Primary regulators of this process include physical activity, calcium nutriture, and reproductive endocrine status (Figure 14–1). The relationship of these issues to bone acquisition has been discussed above. This section will consider these relationships in adults.

Physical Activity

The estimated loss of bone from its peak value to age 80 years is comparable to the reported 35% to 45% decline in muscle strength over the same period. Since a clear relationship between muscle strength and bone mass has been established, physical activity has gained attention as a strategy for improving bone mass.[47,71–73] The mechanisms by which the skeleton responds to activity remain incompletely understood,[55] but overwhelming evidence indicates that bone mass increases in response to the cyclic administration of mechanical loads.[74–76] Not only is bone density higher in physically active people, but the literature suggests that exercise reduces the rate of age-related bone loss.[77–79] Devine et al.[80] showed that high physical activity associated with calcium consumption reduced the risk of fractures by 17% in 1363 older women (mean age 75±3 years). In contrast, another study by Remes et al.[81] was unable to obtain benefits after 4 years of exercise in men. The explanation for these contradictory gender-related differences remains unclear. Remarkably high BMD values in gymnasts raises the possibility that high-impact activity, such as jumping or high-impact aerobics, may be uniquely potent stimuli for increased bone mass. However, applying such activity to older, frailer individuals may not be practical for safety reasons.

Calcium and Vitamin D Nutriture

The skeleton is the repository for 99.5% of total body calcium and constitutes a source of mineral that can support plasma calcium concentrations at times of need. Despite the evidence supporting the positive effects of dietary calcium on bone, national surveys indicate that calcium intakes in females of all age groups in the United States are consistently lower than current recommendations. The average calcium intake reported in the 1994 USDA Continuing Survey of Food Intakes by Individuals (CSFII) was 657 mg/day in both men and women, which strongly suggests that calcium intake is suboptimal in this population. During the third through fifth decades, robust compensatory mechanisms permit rapid adaptation to even severe dietary restriction. Therefore, it should not be surprising that calcium nutritional state appears to exert less of an influence on changes in bone mass during this period;[82] as a corollary, it is unlikely that calcium supplementation will exert important beneficial effects on bone mass for women in this age group.

After age 60 years, early effects of estrogen deficiency have subsided, whereas the compensatory mechanisms for accommodating dietary deficiencies have become less efficient in both men and women. In elderly subjects diminished absorption of calcium and reduced serum levels of vitamin D result in elevated PTH levels, leading to support of plasma calcium at the expense of aggravated bone loss.[83,84] Duque et al.[57] have

recently shown that, despite the availability of vitamin D supplemented food, 35% of an ambulatory elderly population in Quebec presents with either vitamin D deficiency or insufficiency with a compensatory elevation of PTH levels. Similar findings have been reported in healthy elderly in Argentina.[85] Furthermore, even in significantly sunnier climates, vitamin D deficiency is a significant problem in the elderly population, affecting greater than 30% of elderly veterans.[86] Even with seasonal changes vitamin D inadequacy results in important consequences. Pasco et al[87] demonstrated that the winter decline in vitamin D is accompanied by increases in bone resorption and fractures of both the hip and wrist. At this time, attention to proper calcium nutriture, whether from dietary calcium or from supplementation with calcium/vitamin D, is rational and has been shown to have beneficial effects on bone mass as well as on fracture incidence in elderly men and women.[88,89] In order to compensate for the impact of dietary deficiencies upon bone mineral density, the Institute of Medicine has recommended the following daily intakes:[90]

Age	Calcium	Vitamin D
19–30	1000 mg/day	5 mg/day (200 IU/day)
31–50	1000 mg/day	5 mg/day (200 IU/day)
51–70	1200 mg/day	10 mg/day (400 IU/day)
greater than 70	1200 mg/day	15 mg/day (600 IU/day)

Reproductive Endocrine Status

Formidable evidence supports an important role for gonadal function in the acquisition and maintenance of bone mass. Hypogonadal boys and girls have substantial deficits in both cortical and trabecular bone mineral. Loss of endogenous androgen or estrogen during adult life regularly leads to accelerated loss of bone, an effect that is particularly striking when it occurs at an early age, such as after oophorectomy in a young woman. In women, loss of estrogen has dual effects. Decreased efficiency of intestinal and renal calcium homeostasis increases the level of calcium intake necessary to maintain calcium balance. In addition, estrogen directly affects bone cell function,[91–93] an interaction thought to underlie the accelerated bone loss of early estrogen deficiency. With respect to bone remodeling, estrogen deficiency permits the recruitment of increased numbers of osteoclasts, which individually also seem to resorb bone with greater efficiency. This may lead to perforation of trabeculae, with no scaffold left for initiation of new bone formation. Therefore, entire trabecular elements may be permanently eliminated. Replacement of estrogen at menopause protects bone mass and gives significant protection against fracture. Estrogen deficiency may have an overwhelming influence on bone mass even when adequate attention is given to other important influences on bone health. For example, women athletes who experience interruption of menstrual function lose bone, despite regular exercise at high intensity.

More recently the skeletal role of androgens has been better understood. Local aromatization of androgens to estrogens in large part mediates the androgenic effect upon cancellous bone.[94] Androgens can also act directly via androgen receptors, even in the absence of estrogen receptors. Androgen deficiency in men induces cancellous bone loss similar to estrogen deficiency in postmenopausal women.[95,96] Orchiectomy has been shown to induce changes similar to those seen in postmenopausal women; the rate of bone remodeling is increased, as well as the number of osteoclast progenitors, resulting in enhanced osteoclastogenesis and bone resorption.[97] This imbalance between resorption and formation, together with a delay of osteoclast apoptosis, is responsible for a decrease in trabecular bone volume, thickness, and connectivity. Androgens also increase cortical bone size via stimulation of both longitudinal and radial growth.[97,98] Androgens, like estrogens, have a biphasic effect on endochondral bone formation. At the start of puberty, sex steroids stimulate endochondral bone formation, whereas they induce epiphyseal closure at the end of puberty. In elderly men, testosterone deficiency due to hypogonadism can contribute to osteoporosis.[98] Greater than 40% of men in their 60s and greater than 80% of men in their 80s have total serum testosterone levels below the 5th percentile of healthy young men.[99] A corresponding increase in sex hormone binding globulin results in a significant decline in free bioavailable testosterone.[100] It is now well known that the treatment of androgen deficiency with androgen replacement therapy is beneficial for bone.[98] In contrast, the benefits of replacement therapy in partially androgen-deficient elderly men are not unequivocal, and the overall effects on all target tissues and quality of life and survival need to be further explored.

The unitary model for involutional osteoporosis supports estrogen deficiency as the main cause of perimenopausal type I osteoporosis and the age-related type II osteoporosis in both males and females.[101] There are many perimenopausal hormonal changes in women and increasing evidence of age-related changes in testosterone and estrogen bioavailability in men that influence bone mineral density.[94] Decreasing estradiol levels with age in both men and women are correlated with decreased bone mineral density.[102] Furthermore, decreasing levels of dehydroepiandrosterone (DHEA) and insulin-like growth factor-1 (IGF-1) with age in women are paralleled by decreased bone mineral density,[103] and decreasing levels of DHEA, IGF-1, estradiol, testosterone, and free androgen with age in men are correlated with decreased bone turnover.[104] Constitutive marrow secretion of IL-6 and IL-11 in women also increases with age.[105] OPG in the marrow is markedly lower in older subjects.[106] RANKL expression is significantly higher in bone marrow cells isolated from older postmenopausal women.[107] The changes in the expression and secretion of these hormones and growth factors in the bone microenvironment are consistent with enhanced bone resorption and decreased bone formation via their actions upon both osteoclasts and osteoblasts (Figure 14–7). Additional studies are required in order to more completely assess changes in osteoclast formation with age and changes in hormonal status. Furthermore, the degree of osteoclastogenesis and osteoblastogenesis will likely depend upon whether the bone or specific sample sites exhibit a high turnover or low turnover state.[108] Nevertheless, both aging and declines in bioavailable estradiol and testosterone probably contribute to enhanced osteoclastic bone resorption.

During aging the bone marrow is increasingly occupied by adipose tissue[109,110] (Figure 14–7). Although the exact explanation of the link between aging and bone marrow adipogenesis remains unclear, the expression of a transcription factor (peroxisome proliferator-activated receptor gamma—PPAR), which regulates adipogenesis, is increased in aging bone marrow.[111] Osteoblasts and adipocytes arise from a common mesenchymal progenitor cell.[112] Indeed, bone marrow mesenchymal stem cells will differentiate into adipocytes when PPAR is upregulated.[113] The role of PPAR in bone marrow adipogenesis

and thus in aging bone has been assessed in a model for senile osteoporosis, the Senescence Accelerated Mice (SAM-P/6),[111] where high levels of PPAR correlate with marked bone marrow adiposity associated with low bone mass and a deficit in osteoblastogenesis.[114] Furthermore, this bone marrow adipogenesis has been found to be reversible after treatment with vitamin D in SAM-P/6 mice with a concomitant reduction in PPAR expression.[111] The potential effect that inhibiting adipogenesis may have in gaining bone mass was demonstrated *in vitro* by Akune et al.,[115] who demonstrated that PPAR insufficiency increases bone mass by stimulating osteoblastogenesis from bone marrow progenitors. This is a promising field of research, since adipogenesis is a major finding and a potential explanation for the deficit in bone formation and osteoblastogenesis that are seen in aging bone. In fact, the potential for the transdifferentiation of adipocytes into active osteoblasts could provide a therapeutic approach for senile osteoporosis in the future.

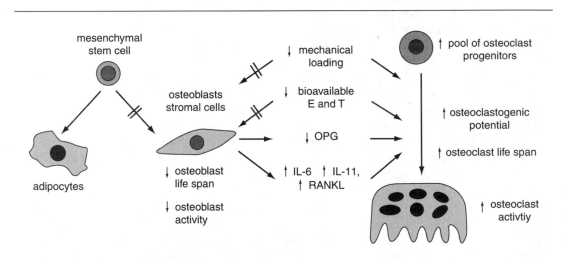

Figure 14–7 Bone Cells and Aging

The balance in mesenchymal stem cell differentiation shifts toward adipocyte differentiation and away from osteoblast differentiation. Decreased levels of bioavailable estradiol and testosterone exert diminished effects upon osteoblasts (depicted by the arrow with the hatches) resulting in decreased osteoblast secretion of OPG and increased expression and secretion of IL-6, IL-11, and RANKL. In turn, the RANKL, IL-6, and IL-11 directly stimulate greater osteoclast formation and activity. The reduced OPG also permits greater binding of RANKL to RANK, which also facilitates increased osteoclastogenesis and resorption. Adapted from Troen.[8] Reprinted with permission from Elsevier.

CONCLUSION

Bone is an active tissue that acts not only as the body support but also as an active metabolic organ with multiple cell/hormone interactions. The maintenance of bone strength should be a major goal during all periods of life but most importantly before the peak bone mass is reached. Preventive measures should include appropriate calcium intake associated with physical activity during the early years of life. By reaching an appropriate level of bone mass in the first decades of life we will be able to face the onset of age-related bone loss with stronger bones.

Furthermore, maintenance of adequate calcium intake and exercise in later decades will enhance the chances of preserving both bone strength and quality of life.

REFERENCES

1. Audi L, Garcia-Ramirez M, Carrascosa A. Genetic determinants of bone mass. *Horm Res* 1999;51:105–123.

2. Peacock M, Turner CH, Econs MJ, Foroud T. Genetics of osteoporosis. *Endocr Rev* 2002;23:303–326.

3. Ilich JZ, Brownbill RA, Tamborini L. Bone and nutrition in elderly women: protein, energy, and calcium as main determinants of bone mineral density. *Eur J Clin Nutr* 2003;57:554–565.

4. Dempster DW, Shane E, Horbert W, Lindsay R. A simple method for correlative light and scanning electron microscopy of human iliac crest bone biopsies: qualitative observations in normal and osteoporotic subjects. *J Bone Miner Res* 1986;1:15–21.

5. Marcus R. Normal and abnormal bone remodeling in man. *Annu Rev Med* 1987;38:129–141.

6. Chan GK, Duque G. Age-related bone loss: old bone, new facts. *Gerontology* 2002;48:62–71.

7. Ott SM in, 2004 pp. Osteoporosis web site maintained by Dr. Susan M. Ott, Associate Professor, Department of Medicine, University of Washington.

8. Troen BR. Molecular mechanisms underlying osteoclast formation and activation. *Exp Gerontol* 2003; 38:605–614.

9. Oursler MJ. Osteoclast synthesis and secretion and activation of latent transforming growth factor beta. *J Bone Miner Res* 1994;9:443–452.

10. Quinn JM, Itoh K, Udagawa N, Hausler K, Yasuda H, Shima N, Mizuno A, Higashio K, Takahashi N, Suda T, Martin TJ, Gillespie MT. Transforming growth factor beta affects osteoclast differentiation via direct and indirect actions. *J Bone Miner Res* 2001;16:1787–1794.

11. Itoh K, Udagawa N, Katagiri T, Iemura S, Ueno N, Yasuda H, Higashio K, Quinn JM, Gillespie MT, Martin TJ, Suda T, Takahashi N. Bone morphogenetic protein 2 stimulates osteoclast differentiation and survival supported by receptor activator of nuclear factor-kappa B ligand. *Endocrinology* 2001;142:3656–3662.

12. Katagiri T, Takahashi N. Regulatory mechanisms of osteoblast and osteoclast differentiation. *Oral Dis* 2002; 8:147–159.

13. Falany ML, Thames AM 3rd, McDonald JM, Blair HC, McKenna MA, Moore RE, Young MK, Williams JP. Osteoclasts secrete the chemotactic cytokine mim-1. *Biochem Biophys Res Commun* 2001;281:180–185.

14. Ponomareva LV, Wang W, Koszewski NJ, Williams JP. Mim-1, an osteoclast secreted chemokine, stimulates differentiation, matrix mineralization and increased vitamin D receptor binding to the VDRE of osteoblastic precursor cells. *J Bone Miner Res* 2002;17: S155.

15. Kubota K, Sakikawa C, Katsumata M, Nakamura T, Wakabayashi K. Platelet-derived growth factor BB secreted from osteoclasts acts as an osteoblastogenesis inhibitory factor. *J Bone Miner Res* 2002;17:257–265.

16. Kurata K, Uemura T, Nemoto A, Tateishi T, Murakami T, Higaki H, Miura H, Iwamoto Y. Mechanical strain effect on bone-resorbing activity and messenger RNA expressions of marker enzymes in isolated osteoclast culture. *J Bone Miner Res* 2001;16:722–730.

17. Mazess RB. The noninvasive measurement of skeletal mass. In: Peck WA, ed. *Bone and Mineral Research Annual*. New York, NY: Elsevier; 1981.

18. Wahner HW. Use of densitometry in management of osteoporosis. In Marcus R, Feldman D, Kelsey J, eds. *Osteoporosis*. San Diego, CA: Academic Press; 1996: 1055–1074.

19. Cummings SR, Karpf DB, Harris F, Genant HK, Ensrud K, LaCroix AZ, Black DM. Improvement in spine bone density and reduction in risk of vertebral fractures during treatment with antiresorptive drugs. *Am J Med* 2002;112:281–289.

20. Moro M, Hecker AT, Bouxsein ML, Myers ER. Failure load of thoracic vertebrae correlates with lumbar bone mineral density measured by DXA. *Calcif Tissue Int* 1995;56:206–209.

21. Weinstein RS. True strength. *J Bone Miner Res* 2000; 15:621–625.

22. Bauer DC, Gluer CC, Genant HK, Stone K. Quantitative ultrasound and vertebral 341 fracture in postmenopausal women. Fracture Intervention Trial Research Group. *J Bone Miner Res* 1995;10:353–358.

23. Stewart A, Reid DM. Quantitative ultrasound in osteoporosis. *Semin Musculoskelet Radiol* 2002;6:229–232.

24. Gluer CC, Eastell R, Reid DM, Felsenberg D, Roux C, Barkmann R, Timm W, Blenk T, Armbrecht G, Stewart A, Clowes J, Thomasius FE, Kolta S. Association of five quantitative ultrasound devices and bone densitometry with osteoporotic vertebral fractures in a population-based sample: the OPUS Study. *J Bone Miner Res* 2004;19:782–793.

25. Bonjour JP, Theintz G, Buchs B, Slosman D, Rizzoli R. Critical years and stages of puberty for spinal and femoral bone mass accumulation during adolescence. *J Clin Endocrinol Metab* 1991;73:555–563.

26. Katzman DK, Bachrach LK, Carter DR, Marcus R. Clinical and anthropometric correlates of bone mineral acquisition in healthy adolescent girls. *J Clin Endocrinol Metab* 1991;73:1332–1339.

27. Bhudhikanok GS, Wang MC, Eckert K, Matkin C, Marcus R, Bachrach LK. Differences in bone mineral in young Asian and Caucasian Americans may reflect differences in bone size. *J Bone Miner Res* 1996;11:1545–1556.

28. Gross C, Eccleshall TR, Feldman D. Vitamin D receptor gene alleles and osteoporosis. In: Bilezikian JP, Raisz LG, Rodan G, eds. *Principles of Bone Biology.* San Diego, CA: Academic Press; 1996:917–934.

29. Peacock M, Koller DL, Hui S, Johnston CC, Foroud T, Econs MJ. Peak bone mineral density at the hip is linked to chromosomes 14q and 15q. *Osteoporos Int* 2004;15:489–496.

30. Baldock PA, Eisman JA. Genetic determinants of bone mass. *Curr Opin Rheumatol* 2004;16:450–456.

31. Matkovic V, Landoll JD, Badenhop-Stevens NE, Ha EY, Crncevic-Orlic Z, Li B, Goel P. Nutrition influences skeletal development from childhood to adulthood: a study of hip, spine, and forearm in adolescent females. *J Nutr* 2004;134:701S–705S.

32. Slemenda CW, Reister TK, Hui SL, Miller JZ, Christian JC, Johnston CC Jr. Influences on skeletal mineralization in children and adolescents: evidence for varying effects of sexual maturation and physical activity. *J Pediatr* 1994;125:201–207.

33. Lee WT, Leung SS, Leung DM, Cheng JC. A follow-up study on the effects of calcium-supplement withdrawal and puberty on bone acquisition of children. *Am J Clin Nutr* 1996;64:71–77.

34. Heaney RP. The bone remodeling transient: interpreting interventions involving bone-related nutrients. *Nutr Rev* 2001;59:327–334.

35. Ilich JZ, Kerstetter JE. Nutrition in bone health revisited: a story beyond calcium. *J Am Coll Nutr* 2000;19:715–737.

36. Eck LH, Hackett-Renner C. Calcium intake in youth: sex, age, and racial differences in NHANES II. *Prev Med* 1992;21:473–482.

37. Cumming RG. Calcium intake and bone mass: a quantitative review of the evidence. *Calcif Tissue Int* 1990;47:194–201.

38. Dawson-Hughes B, Dallal GE, Krall EA, Sadowski L, Sahyoun N, Tannenbaum S. A controlled trial of the effect of calcium supplementation on bone density in postmenopausal women. *N Engl J Med* 1990;323:878–883.

39. Reid IR, Ames RW, Evans MC, Gamble GD, Sharpe SJ. Effect of calcium supplementation on bone loss in postmenopausal women. *N Engl J Med* 1993;328:460–464.

40. Aloia JF, Vaswani A, Yeh JK, Ross PL, Flaster E, Dilmanian FA. Calcium supplementation with and without hormone replacement therapy to prevent postmenopausal bone loss. *Ann Intern Med* 1994;120:97–103.

41. Garn SM, Rohman CG, Nolan PJ. The developmental nature of bone changes during aging. In: Birren JE, ed. *Relations of Development and Aging.* Springfield, IL: Charles C Thomas; 1966.

42. Mazess RB. On aging bone loss. *Clin Orthop* 1982;(165)239–252.

43. Smith DM, Khairi MR, Norton J, Johnston CC Jr. Age and activity effects on rate of bone mineral loss. *J Clin Invest* 1976;58:716–721.

44. Hui SL, Wiske PS, Norton JA, Johnston CC Jr. A prospective study of change in bone mass with age in postmenopausal women. *J Chronic Dis* 1982;35:715–725.

45. Arnold JS, Bartley MH, Tont SA, Jenkins DP. Skeletal changes in aging and disease. *Clin Orthop* 1966;49:17–38.

46. Trotter M, Broman GE, Peterson RR. Densities of bones of white and Negro skeletons. *Am J Orthop* 1960;42A:50–58.

47. Doyle F, Brown J, Lachance C. Relation between bone mass and muscle weight. *Lancet* 1970;1:391–393.

48. Marcus R, Kosek J, Pfefferbaum A, Horning S. Age-related loss of trabecular bone in premenopausal women: a biopsy study. *Calcif Tissue Int* 1983;35:406–409.

49. Riggs BL, Wahner HW, Melton LJ 3rd, Richelson LS, Judd HL, Offord KP. Rates of bone loss in the appendicular and axial skeletons of women. Evidence of substantial vertebral bone loss before menopause. *J Clin Invest* 1986;77:1487–1491.

50. Geusens P, Dequeker J, Verstraeten A, Nijs J. Age-, sex-, and menopause-related changes of vertebral and peripheral bone: population study using dual and single photon absorptiometry and radiogrammetry. *J Nucl Med* 1986;27:1540–1549.

51. Krolner B, Pors Nielsen S. Bone mineral content of the lumbar spine in normal and osteoporotic women: cross-sectional and longitudinal studies. *Clin Sci (Lond)* 1982;62:329–336.

52. Aloia JF, Vaswani A, Ellis K, Yuen K, Cohn SH. A model for involutional bone loss. *J Lab Clin Med* 1985; 106:630–637.

53. Weaver JK, Chalmers J. Cancellous bone: its strength and changes with aging and an evaluation of some methods for measuring its mineral content. *J Bone Joint Surg Am* 1966;48:289–298.

54. Arnold JS. Amount and quality of trabecular bone in osteoporotic vertebral fractures. *Clin Endocrinol Metab* 1973;2:221–238.

55. Birkenhager-Frenkel DH, Courpron P, Hupscher EA, Clermonts E, Coutinho MF, Schmitz PI, Meunier PJ. Age-related changes in cancellous bone structure. A two-dimensional study in the transiliac and iliac crest biopsy sites. *Bone Miner* 1988;4:197–216.

56. Mosekilde L. Iliac crest trabecular bone volume as predictor for vertebral compressive strength, ash density and trabecular bone volume in normal individuals. *Bone* 1988;9:195–199.

57. Vecino C, Gratton M, Rodriguez-Manas L, Kremer R, Duque G. The seasonal variance in serum levels of vitamin D determines a concurrent compensatory response by parathyroid hormone: study in an ambulatory elderly population in Quebec [Submitted]. *J Gerontol Med Sci* 2004.

58. Deplas A, Debiais F, Alcalay M, Bontoux D, Thomas P. Bone density, parathyroid hormone, calcium and vitamin D nutritional status of institutionalized elderly subjects. *J Nutr Health Aging* 2004;8:400–404.

59. Simon J, Leboff M, Wright J, Glowacki J. Fractures in the elderly and vitamin D. *J Nutr Health Aging* 2002, 6:406–412.

60. Lips P. Vitamin D deficiency and secondary hyperparathyroidism in the elderly: consequences for bone loss and fractures and therapeutic implications. *Endocr Rev* 2001;22:477–501.

61. Seeman E. Invited Review: Pathogenesis of osteoporosis. *J Appl Physiol* 2003;95:2142–2151.

62. Buchanan JR, Myers C, Lloyd T, Greer RB 3rd. Early vertebral trabecular bone loss in normal premenopausal women. *J Bone Miner Res* 1988;3:583–587.

63. Hansson T, Roos B. Age changes in the bone mineral of the lumbar spine in normal women. *Calcif Tissue Int* 1986;38:249–251.

64. Gallagher JC, Goldgar D, Moy A. Total bone calcium in normal women: effect of age and menopause status. *J Bone Miner Res* 1987;2:491–496.

65. Nilas L, Gotfredsen A, Hadberg A, Christiansen C. Age-related bone loss in women evaluated by the single and dual photon technique. *Bone Miner* 1988;4:95–103.

66. Cann CE, Genant HK, Kolb FO, Ettinger B. Quantitative computed tomography for prediction of vertebral fracture risk. *Bone* 1985;6:1–7.

67. Firooznia H, Golimbu C, Rafii M, Schwartz MS, Alterman ER. Quantitative computed tomography assessment of spinal trabecular bone. I. Age-related regression in normal men and women. *J Comput Tomogr* 1984;8:91–97.

68. Marcus R. The nature of osteoporosis. In: Marcus R, Feldman D, Kelsey J, eds. *Osteoporosis*. San Diego, CA: Academic Press; 1996:647–659.

69. Parfitt AM. Age-related structural changes in trabecular and cortical bone: cellular mechanisms and biomechanical consequences. *Calcif Tissue Int* 1984:36 (suppl 1):S123–S128.

70. Faulkner KG, Cummings SR, Black D, Palermo L, Gluer CC, Genant HK. Simple measurement of femoral geometry predicts hip fracture: the study of osteoporotic fractures. *J Bone Miner Res* 1993;8:1211–1217.

71. Aloia JF, Cohn SH, Babu T, Abesamis C, Kalici N, Ellis K. Skeletal mass and body composition in marathon runners. *Metabolism* 1978;27:1793–1796.

72. Sinaki M, Offord KP. Physical activity in postmenopausal women: effect on back muscle strength and bone mineral density of the spine. *Arch Phys Med Rehabil* 1988;69:277–280.

73. Sinaki M, McPhee MC, Hodgson SF, Merritt JM, Offord KP. Relationship between bone mineral density of spine and strength of back extensors in healthy postmenopausal women. *Mayo Clin Proc* 1986;61:116–122.

74. Rubin CT, Lanyon LE. Regulation of bone formation by applied dynamic loads. *J Bone Joint Surg Am* 1984;66:397–402.

75. Rubin CT, Lanyon LE. Regulation of bone mass by mechanical strain magnitude. *Calcif Tissue Int* 1985;37:411–417.

76. Carter DR, Fyhrie DP, Whalen RT. Trabecular bone density and loading history: regulation of connective tissue biology by mechanical energy. *J Biomech* 1987;20:785–794.

77. Talmage RV, Stinnett SS, Landwehr JT, Vincent LM, McCartney WH. Age-related loss of bone mineral density in non-athletic and athletic women. *Bone Miner* 1986;1:115–125.

78. Brewer V, Meyer BM, Keele MS, Upton SJ, Hagan RD. Role of exercise in prevention of involutional bone loss. *Med Sci Sports Exerc* 1983:15:445–449.

79. Smith EL Jr, Reddan W, Smith PE. Physical activity and calcium modalities for bone mineral increase in aged women. *Med Sci Sports Exerc* 1981;13:60–64.

80. Devine A, Dhaliwal SS, Dick IM, Bollerslev J, Prince RL. Physical activity and calcium consumption are important determinants of lower limb bone mass in older women. *J Bone Miner Res* 2004;19:1634–1639.

81. Remes T, Vaisanen SB, Mahonen A, Huuskonen J, Kroger H, Jurvelin JS, Penttila IM, Rauramaa R. The

association of bone metabolism with bone mineral density, serum sex hormone concentrations, and regular exercise in middle-aged men. *Bone* 2004;35:439–447.

82. Riggs BL, Wahner HW, Melton LJ 3rd, Richelson LS, Judd HL, O'Fallon WM. Dietary calcium intake and rates of bone loss in women. *J Clin Invest* 1987; 80:979–982.

83. Young G, Marcus R, Minkoff JR, Kim LY, Segre GV. Age-related rise in parathyroid hormone in man: the use of intact and midmolecule antisera to distinguish hormone secretion from retention. *J Bone Miner Res* 1987;2:367–374.

84. Eastell R, Heath HI, Kumar R. Hormonal factors: PTH, vitamin D and calcitonin. In: Riggs BL, Melton, LJ, eds. *Osteoporosis: Etiology, Diagnosis, and Management.* New York, NY: Raven Press; 1988.

85. Oliveri B, Plantalech L, Bagur A, Wittich AC, Rovai G, Pusiol E, Lopez Giovanelli J, Ponce G, Nieva A, Chaperon A, Ladizesky M, Somoza J, Casco C, Zeni S, Parisi MS, Mautalen CA. High prevalence of vitamin D insufficiency in healthy elderly people living at home in Argentina. *Eur J Clin Nutr* 2004;58:337–342.

86. Levis S. Vitamin D deficiency in elderly South Florida veterans. *J Amer Geriatr Soc* 2003;51:S84.

87. Pasco JA, Henry MJ, Kotowicz MA, Sanders KM, Seeman E, Pasco JR, Schneider HG, Nicholson GC. Seasonal periodicity of serum vitamin D and parathyroid hormone, bone resorption, and fractures: the Geelong Osteoporosis Study. *J Bone Miner Res* 2004; 19:752–758.

88. Chapuy MC, Arlot ME, Duboeuf F, Brun J, Crouzet B, Arnaud S, Delmas PD, Meunier PJ. Vitamin D3 and calcium to prevent hip fractures in the elderly women. *N Engl J Med* 1992;327:1637–1642.

89. Trivedi DP, Doll R, Khaw KT. Effect of four monthly oral vitamin D3 (cholecalciferol) supplementation on fractures and mortality in men and women living in the community: randomised double blind controlled trial. *Br Med J* 2003;326:469.

90. Standing Committee on the Scientific Evidence on Dietary Reference Intakes, Food and Nutrition Board. *Dietary Reference Intakes for Calcium, Phosphorus, Magnesium, Vitamin D, and Fluoride,* Washington, DC: Institute of Medicine, National Academy Press; 1997.

91. Eriksen EF, Colvard DS, Berg NJ, Graham ML, Mann KG, Spelsberg TC, Riggs BL. Evidence of estrogen receptors in normal human osteoblast-like cells. *Science* 1988;241:84–86.

92. Komm BS, Terpening CM, Benz DJ, Graeme KA, Gallegos A, Korc M, Greene GL, O'Malley BW, Haussler MR. Estrogen binding, receptor mRNA, and biologic response in osteoblast-like osteosarcoma cells. *Science* 1988;241:81–84.

93. Gray TK, Flynn TC, Gray KM, Nabell LM. 17 beta-estradiol acts directly on the clonal osteoblastic cell line UMR106. *Proc Natl Acad Sci U S A* 1987:84:6267–6271.

94. Riggs BL, Khosla S, Melton LJ 3rd. Sex steroids and the construction and conservation of the adult skeleton. *Endocr Rev* 2002;23:279–302.

95. Vanderschueren D, Bouillon R. Androgens and bone. *Calcif Tissue Int* 1995;56:341–346.

96. Compston JE. Sex steroids and bone. *Physiol Rev* 2001;81:419–447.

97. Vanderschueren D, Vandenput L, Boonen S, Lindberg MK, Bouillon R, Ohlsson C. Androgens and bone. *Endocr Rev* 2004;25:389–425.

98. Olszynski WP, Shawn Davison K, Adachi JD, Brown JP, Cummings SR, Hanley DA, Harris SP, Hodsman AB, Kendler D, McClung MR, Miller PD, Yuen CK. Osteoporosis in men: epidemiology, diagnosis, prevention, and treatment. *Clin Ther* 2004;26:15–28.

99. Comhaire FH. Andropause: hormone replacement therapy in the ageing male. *Eur Urol* 2000;38:655–662.

100. Allan CA, McLachlan RI. Age-related changes in testosterone and the role of replacement therapy in older men. *Clin Endocrinol (Oxf)* 2004;60:653–670.

101. Riggs BL, Khosla S, Melton LJ 3rd. A unitary model for involutional osteoporosis: estrogen deficiency causes both type I and type II osteoporosis in postmenopausal women and contributes to bone loss in aging men. *J Bone Miner Res* 1998;13:763–773.

102. Greendale GA, Edelstein S, Barrett-Connor E. Endogenous sex steroids and bone mineral density in older women and men: the Rancho Bernardo Study. *J Bone Miner Res* 1997;12:1833–1843.

103. Haden ST, Glowacki J, Hurwitz S, Rosen C, LeBoff MS. Effects of age on serum dehydroepiandrosterone sulfate, IGF-I, and IL-6 levels in women. *Calcif Tissue Int* 2000;66:414–418.

104. Fatayerji D, Eastell R. Age-related changes in bone turnover in men. *J Bone Miner Res* 1999;14:1203–1210.

105. Cheleuitte D, Mizuno S, Glowacki J. In vitro secretion of cytokines by human bone marrow: effects of age and estrogen status. *J Clin Endocrinol Metab* 1998;83: 2043–2051.

106. Makhluf HA, Mueller SM, Mizuno S, Glowacki J. Age-related decline in osteoprotegerin expression by human bone marrow cells cultured in three-dimensional collagen sponges. *Biochem Biophys Res Commun* 2000;268: 669–672.

107. Eghbali-Fatourechi G, Khosla S, Boyle WJ, Lacey DL, Riggs BL. Role of RANK ligand (RANKL) in mediating increased bone resorption in early postmenopausal women. *J Bone Miner Res* 2002;17:S128.

108. Kawaguchi H, Manabe N, Miyaura C, Chikuda H, Nakamura K, Kuro-o M. Independent impairment of

osteoblast and osteoclast differentiation in klotho mouse exhibiting low-turnover osteopenia. *J Clin Invest* 1999;104:229–237.

109. Meunier P, Aaron J, Edouard C, Vignon G. Osteoporosis and the replacement of cell populations of the marrow by adipose tissue. A quantitative study of 84 iliac bone biopsies. *Clin Orthop* 1971:80:147–154.

110. Burkhardt R, Kettner G, Bohm W, Schmidmeier M, Schlag R, Frisch B, Mallmann B, Eisenmenger W, Gilg T. Changes in trabecular bone, hematopoiesis and bone marrow vessels in aplastic anemia, primary osteoporosis, and old age: a comparative histomorphometric study. *Bone* 1987;8:157–164.

111. Duque G, Macoritto M, Kremer R. 1,25(OH)2D3 inhibits bone marrow adipogenesis in senescence accelerated mice (SAM-P/6) by decreasing the expression of peroxisome proliferator-activated receptor gamma 2 (PPARgamma2). *Exp Gerontol* 2004;39:333–338.

112. Pittenger MF, Mackay AM, Beck SC, Jaiswal RK, Douglas R, Mosca JD, Moorman MA, Simonetti DW, Craig S, Marshak DR. Multilineage potential of adult human mesenchymal stem cells. *Science* 1999;284: 143–147.

113. Nuttall ME, Gimble JM. Controlling the balance between osteoblastogenesis and adipogenesis and the consequent therapeutic implications. *Curr Opin Pharmacol* 2004;4:290–294.

114. Jilka RL, Weinstein RS, Takahashi K, Parfitt AM, Manolagas SC. Linkage of decreased bone mass with impaired osteoblastogenesis in a murine model of accelerated senescence. *J Clin Invest* 1996;97:1732–1740.

115. Akune T, Ohba S, Kamekura S, Yamaguchi M, Chung UI, Kubota N, Terauchi Y, Harada Y, Azuma Y, Nakamura K, Kadowaki T, Kawaguchi H. PPARgamma insufficiency enhances osteogenesis through osteoblast formation from bone marrow progenitors. *J Clin Invest* 2004;113:846–855.

CHAPTER 15

Endocrine Aspects of Nutrition and Aging

John E. Morley, MB, BCh

Hormones play a major role in the regulation of nutrient intake and utilization within an individual. Conversely, nutritional status can markedly affect circulating hormone levels. Treatment of a number of endocrine disorders (eg, diabetes mellitus and osteoporosis) involves dietary modification.

With advancing age, there are several alterations in circulating hormone levels and hormonal action. Some of these changes are related to the multiple diseases often present in older individuals, while other changes are due to aging *per se*. The loss of functional reserve in many endocrine organs increases the propensity for the elderly to develop deficiency diseases, such as diabetes mellitus, hypothyroidism, and hypogonadism. With advancing age, there is a tendency for endocrine disease to present with atypical or nonspecific symptoms, making diagnosis increasingly difficult. Weight loss is the classic nonspecific presentation of endocrine disease in elderly people.

In this chapter, the interactions of the endocrine system and nutrition are examined, and the impact of aging and its modulation of these interactions are described. More detailed information on the effect of aging on hormones is reported elsewhere.[1,2]

NUTRITIONAL ASPECTS OF DIABETES MELLITUS

Diabetes mellitus occurs in approximately 18% of the population between ages 65 and 75 years.[3] Almost half of the persons with type 2 diabetes mellitus are older than 60 years. The diagnosis is missed in almost half of older patients who have frank diabetes. In many older patients with diagnosed diabetes mellitus, the diabetes is inadequately treated.[4]

In general, older subjects tend to have an impaired glucose tolerance compared with younger subjects; however, recent data suggest that only 10% of the variance in total serum glucose response to an oral glucose load can be attributed to age.[5]

The level of body weight and physical activity appears to have a more important role in the pathogenesis of the hyperglycemia of aging. Recent data have suggested that a failure to suppress the pancreatic hormone amylin in older persons may play a role in the pathogenesis of the hyperglycemia of aging. Table 15–1 lists the major factors thought to play a role in the pathogenesis of the hyperglycemia of aging and the development of type 2 diabetes mellitus. It should be recognized that older persons with type 2

Table 15–1 Major Factors Involved in the Pathogenesis of the Hyperglycemia of Aging and Type 2 Diabetes Mellitus

1. Poor insulin secretion
2. Failure to inhibit hepatic glucose production
3. Insulin receptor and post-receptor defect
4. Obesity
5. Lack of physical activity
6. Failure to suppress amylin
7. Increased leptin

---

diabetes tend to be less overweight than middle-aged diabetics and are more likely to have a significant degree of insulin insufficiency.

Although fasting and postprandial glucose levels increase slightly with age, the basic definition for treatable diabetes mellitus should not change. Treatment should be instituted when any individual has two fasting plasma glucose levels greater than 7.8 mmol/L. Alternatively, 2-hour postprandial values greater than 10.0 mmol/L on two or more occasions would also suggest the need for treatment.

Regardless of the causes of diabetes mellitus in elderly people, there is increasing evidence that reasonable control of glucose will improve the patient's quality of life, as well as possibly decrease morbidity and mortality rates. The major reasons for control of diabetes in elderly people are listed in Table 15–2. The special features of diabetes mellitus in elderly individuals have been the subject of a number of recent reviews.[6–8] At present, it is recommended that the blood glucose be maintained between 5.6 and 11.1 mmol/L for all diabetics older than 70 years.

Treatment of Diabetes Mellitus

The modalities for treatment of diabetes mellitus in elderly subjects are the same as those used in younger subjects: diet, exercise, oral medications, and insulin. In 1674, Sir Thomas Willis advised patients with diabetes mellitus to have gummy and starchy foods. Since then, diabetologists have made a variety of recommenda-

tions about what should constitute the appropriate diet for diabetic patients. The following are the current recommendations of the American Diabetes Association[9] for the dietary management of persons with type 2 diabetes mellitus:

- The approach should be individualized and based on a careful nutrition assessment.
- The number of calories should aim at a weight that both the patient and the health care provider believe is achievable and maintainable.
- Moderate weight loss (5–9 kg) can have important effects, including reducing hyperglycemia, blood pressure level, and lipid levels.
- Protein intake should make up about 10% to 20% of the total caloric intake (0.8 g/kg per day). Protein restriction below this level has no clear benefit and may lead to sarcopenia.
- Fat intake should be limited to 30% of calories, with less than 10% of fat from polyunsaturated fat and 10% to 15% from monounsaturated fats. The use of omega-3 polyunsaturated fats (fish fats) should not be curtailed.
- The rest of the caloric content should obviously be made up of carbohydrate. There is little scientific evidence that simple sugars impair the blood glucose concentration more than complex carbohydrates, and they are therefore no longer proscribed. Some soluble fibers may delay glucose absorption. An ideal diet should contain 20 to 35 g of a mixture of soluble and insoluble fibers. It should be recognized that the modern diabetic diet does not differ from the recommended healthy diet for all Americans. Alcohol should be limited to two or fewer alcoholic beverages per day.

Finally, there are no studies on dietary intervention in ambulatory individuals older than 70 years. A study of elderly nursing home patients suggested that the "diabetic" diet resulted in no better glycemic control than did a regular diet; diabetics receiving "concentrated sweets" in

Table 15–2 Reasons to Control Diabetes Mellitus in Elderly People

Prevention of acute complications
    Diabetic coma
    Hyperosmolar ketoacidotic lactic acidosis
    Complications related to hyperosmolality
Diuresis leading to incontinence and nocturia
    Visual disturbances
    Falls related to above two factors
    Poor outcome following stroke
    Increased pain perception
    Cognitive dysfunction
Complications related to altered function of circulating blood cells
Worsening peripheral vascular disease due to decreased erythrocyte deformability
Increased prevalence of myocardial infarction and stroke due to increased platelet stickiness
Prevention of chronic complications*
Neuropathic complications
Diabetic retinopathy
Diabetic nephropathy
Amputation

*There is some evidence that these complications occur more rapidly in late-onset diabetes.

a nursing home had no deterioration in their glycemic control.[10,11] For these reasons, it is difficult to make a firm recommendation on the ideal diet for the older diabetic. It is important that state surveyors in nursing homes recognize that an order for a "diabetic special diet" represents an order for a regular diet.

Cross-sectional studies have shown that the impaired glucose tolerance of aging is significantly related to the level of physical fitness or activity.[7] Only one prospective trial of the effects of exercise on glucose tolerance has been carried out in men older than 60 years. While glucose levels did not change, both insulin and C peptide levels were lower.[12] In addition, high density lipoprotein cholesterol levels increased, and triglyceride levels decreased. Exercise trials in patients with type 2 diabetes mellitus have failed to show a major advantage of short-term exercise programs over diet alone.[13] However, two trials that lasted 5 months and 11 months did find improvements in glucose tolerance without change in body weight.[14,15] Besides the possible beneficial effects of exercise on glu-

cose tolerance, exercise training may improve cardiovascular fitness, lipid profiles, hypertension, osteopenia, and psychological function in diabetic patients. Risks of exercise in diabetics include hypoglycemia, ketosis, dehydration, myocardial ischemia, arrhythmias, acceleration of proliferative retinopathy, increased proteinuria, and trauma (particularly in patients with neuropathy). The NIH consensus panel concluded that the effect of exercise on metabolic control in non-insulin-dependent diabetes mellitus is often variable and of small magnitude.[16] Pacini and colleagues[17] have demonstrated that physically active older subjects with normal weight have normal insulin-binding capacity, insulin sensitivity, and insulin secretory capacity in response to a glucose stimulus. An individualized 12-week exercise program in elderly African Americans with type 2 diabetes mellitus improved glycemic control and reduced high blood pressures.[18] Studies of long-term exercise programs need to be undertaken before a formal recommendation for an exercise prescription can be given.

The sulfonylurea oral hypoglycemic agents produce their major effect by stimulating insulin release from pancreatic B cells through a different signal recognition system than that by which glucose stimulates insulin release. Chlorpropamide should never be used in subjects older than age 60 years because it produces prolonged hypoglycemia and hyponatremia. The prevalence of hypoglycemia with other sulfonylureas is less than that with chlorpropamide; nevertheless, elderly people are always at increased risk for developing hypoglycemia. The combination of insulin and sulfonylureas has not been proven to be effective. For the majority of older diabetics, Glimepiride, a third-generation sulfonylurea whose actions appear similar to those of the second-generation agents, is an effective choice.

Metformin is a biguanide that enhances insulin action and produces anorexia. It acts, in part, through effects on nitric oxide synthase. It should not be used in persons with a serum creatinine greater than 1.4 g/dL or in those who have severe heart failure or chronic acidosis. In persons older than 80 years, a normal creatinine clearance needs to be demonstrated before it should be used. Its major side effect is lactic acidosis, which occurs extremely rarely if the above prescribing precautions are followed. Older persons need to be monitored for the possibility of excessive weight loss. Metformin may decrease vitamin B_{12} levels.

Thiazolidinediones, eg, Prioglitazone and Rosiglitazone, enhance peripheral insulin action. They work through the activation of PPARγ and do not produce hypoglycemia. They can be used as monotherapy or in combination with other oral antidiabetic agents or insulin. They may produce liver dysfunction and this needs to be monitored.

Acarbose and Miglitol are α-1-glucosidase inhibitors. They delay the absorption of complex carbohydrates, thus smoothing out the glycemic response to a meal. They also release the incretion glucagons, like peptide 1 from the gastrointestinal tract, resulting in enhanced insulin levels in response to the meal.[19] The major side effects are diarrhea, gastrointestinal gas production, and abdominal pus.

Chronic insulin deficiency is similar to starvation in that both conditions are catabolic states that lead to cachexia. The catabolic state of uncontrolled diabetes mellitus is readily reversed by insulin therapy. For this reason, and those listed in Table 15–2, insulin should not be withheld from elderly patients whose glucose levels cannot be reduced below 11.1 mmol/L. At present, human insulin is recommended as the insulin of choice to decrease the formation of anti-insulin antibodies; however, polymerization of human insulin at therapeutic dosage levels does lead to some antibody formation.

Older diabetics may have up to a 20% error when drawing up their insulin into a syringe.[20] For this reason, older diabetics with visual deficiencies should use syringe magnifiers or dose gauges. Some patients also benefit from using needle guides and vial holders. Older diabetic persons with depression have poor outcomes, and depression needs to be vigorously treated in these persons.[21] Much of the diabetic care for older persons is carried out by caregivers; therefore, they should be involved in appropriate diabetic education programs if optimal outcomes are to be obtained.

Micronutrient Status and Diabetes Mellitus

Diabetes mellitus produces a number of effects on vitamin and mineral status of patients.[22] Many of these changes are similar to those seen with aging (Table 15–3). Elderly people often have a decreased zinc intake and are at risk for developing zinc deficiency when illness occurs (Chapter 6). Diabetes mellitus is associated with decreased zinc absorption and hyperzincuria.[23] Zinc deficiency is associated with poor wound healing, poor immune function, immune dysfunction, and anorexia.[24] In addition, zinc is co-secreted from pancreatic islets and enhances insulin binding, suggesting a possible role of zinc in the pathogenesis of some forms of diabetes. Pharmacologic zinc administration has been demonstrated to improve immune function[25] and foot ulcer healing[26] in patients with deficient zinc status.

Table 15–3 Comparison of the Effects of Type 2 Diabetes Mellitus and Aging on Micronutrients

Micronutrient	Changes in Type II Diabetes Mellitus	Changes with Aging
Vitamins		
A	N	N
B_1	N	N
B_6	N or ↓	↓
B_{12}	N or ↓	↓
C	↓	N or ↓
25-hydroxyvitamin D_3	N	↓
E in serum	N	N
E in platelets	↓	↑
Trace elements		
Zinc	N or ↓	↓
Chromium	N	↓
Copper	N or ↓	↑
Manganese	↑	?
Selenium	?	N or ↓

Note: N, Normal; ↑, increased; ↓, decreased.

Source: Adapted with permission from *Journal of American Geriatrics Society* (1987; 35:435–447), Copyright © 1987, American Geriatrics Society.

Chromium has been suggested to have a role in normal glucose homeostasis; however, replacement studies have minimal effect.[27] Deficiency of chromium (Chapter 6) or its biologically active form, glucose tolerance factor, has been implicated in the glucose intolerance of aging.[28] The main sources of glucose tolerance factor include brewer's yeast, liver, and kidney.

In most double-blind studies, chromium supplementation has failed to reverse the hyperglycemia of aging. In one recent small study, the combination of chromium and nicotinamide resulted in a minor diminution of the glucose response to oral glucose, but it did not alter fasting glucose levels.[29] In chromium-deficient areas, such as parts of China, chromium replacement can have more dramatic effects on glucose tolerance.[28]

Copper and ceruloplasmin levels are elevated in type 2 diabetes mellitus. Copper deficiency, induced experimentally, results in elevated total cholesterol levels.[30]

Thiamine is essential for the transport of metabolized glucose from the Embden-Meyerhof pathway into the Krebs cycle. The elevated levels of erythrocyte transketolase activity (an indirect measure of thiamine status) in type 2 diabetes mellitus may be related to the poor availability of intracellular glucose. When malnourished patients receive glucose, they may utilize all of the available thiamine, resulting in Wernicke's syndrome. Conversely, in malnourished patients, thiamine administration may result in hypoglycemia.

Diabetes mellitus may be associated with pernicious anemia. Vitamin B_{12} deficiency should be suspected in any diabetic patient with macrocytic anemia, posterior column neuropathy, or dementia. Recent studies have suggested that low vitamin B_{12} levels, in the absence of macrocytic anemia, may explain the cognitive dysfunction seen in elderly individuals. Low vitamin B_{12} levels are associated with increased levels of methyl malonic acid and homocysteine. Elevated homocysteine levels have been associated with coronary artery disease.

Vitamin C in large doses acts as a reducing agent and can interfere with glucose measurements in both urine and serum.

Diabetes Mellitus in Long-term Care

The management of diabetes mellitus in the long-term care setting is steeped in mythology.[31] It should be realized that hypoglycemic reactions occur infrequently in institutionalized patients, permitting reasonable control of diabetes mellitus in this population.[32] In a study of diabetic patients in a nursing home, it was found that one in five were 20% below average body weight.[32] Weight loss often leads to improved glycemic control in nursing home patients. Awareness of weight loss in this population is important, since it may necessitate a reduction in insulin or oral hypoglycemic dosage. As previously mentioned, neither the American Dietetic Association nor the American Diabetes Association recommend therapeutic diets for diabetic patients in long-term care.

Generally, the management of diabetes mellitus in older patients is the same as that in younger patients. In elderly patients, diabetes mellitus can interact with the normal aging process to produce major changes in micronutrient requirements. In particular, older diabetics are at risk for developing minor degrees of zinc deficiency. When instituting dietary changes in older diabetics, care needs to be taken to avoid producing protein-calorie malnutrition. This is particularly true of patients residing in nursing homes.

THYROID FUNCTION

With advancing age, there is no change in the circulating levels of total thyroxine, tri-iodothyronine, or the free hormone.[1] However, this apparent stability of the circulating thyroid hormones belies the underlying physiologic turmoil that results in the hypothalamic-pituitary-adrenal axis with advancing age. There is a decreased production of thyroid hormones with aging that is counterbalanced by a decreased thyroid hormone degradation. In addition, there is a tendency for diminished feedback of thyroid hormones, leading to a mild increase in thyrotropin (TSH) levels, particularly in women. In older men, there is an increased prevalence of failure for TSH to respond to thyrotropin-releasing hormone (TRH).

In subjects younger than age 60 years, the prevalence of hypothyroidism tends to be 1% or less, whereas in those older than age 60 years, the prevalence rises to 4–7%.[33,34] Between 7% and 12% of patients with hyperthyroidism are older than 60 years.[1] Whereas there are limited changes in circulating thyroid hormones with aging, when illness supervenes, there can be major changes in thyroid hormones that can mimic the changes seen with hypothyroidism.[35] These changes are delineated in Table 15–4. Malnutrition is a particularly common cause of the euthyroid sick syndrome in elderly people.

Atypical presentations of thyroid disease become increasingly common with advancing age. One study estimated that only 10% of older patients with biochemical hypothyroidism were suspected of having thyroid disease on clinical examination.[36] The classic hyperkinetic state, thyromegaly, and eye signs of hyperthyroidism may be replaced by heart failure, apathy, and unexplained weight loss in elderly persons, so-called apathetic hypothyroidism.[37] For these reasons, it is recommended that all patients older than age 60 years who are admitted to the hospital or who have unexplained weight loss, fatigue, depression, dementia, or atrial fibrillation be screened biochemically for thyroid disease.[35]

Nutritional Aspects of Thyroid Disease

The classic nutritional change associated with hyperthyroidism is weight loss. Thyroid hormones produce a marked increase in the basal metabolic rate. The exact mechanism by which thyroid hormones increase the metabolic rate remains controversial.[38] There is an increase in mitochondrial size, number, and surface area, and thyroid hormone stimulates mitochondrial turnover. Thyroid hormone also increases Na^+, K^+-adenosine triphosphatase activity. Pharmacologic concentrations of thyroid hormone produce uncoupling of oxidative metabolism in vitro.

Thyroid hormone results in stimulation of both protein synthesis and degradation. In hyperthyroidism, the predominance of protein degradation leads to loss of muscle mass, muscle weakness, and a negative nitrogen balance. In

Table 15–4 Typical Changes in Thyroid Hormone Levels with Various Diseases

Hormone	Aging	Hyperthyroid	Hypothyroid	Euthyroid Sick
Thyroxine	N	↑	↓	N or ↓
Triiodothyronine	N	↑	N or ↓	↓
Uptake	N	↑	↓	↑
Free thyroxine index	N	↑	↓	N or ↓
TSH				
Normal	N	N	↑	N or ↑
Supersensitive	N	↓	↑	↓ N ↑
Response to TRH	↓	↓	↑	↓

Note: N, Normal; ↑, increased; ↓, decreased.

younger subjects, hyperthyroidism is often associated with hyperphagia, which tends to offset the weight loss to some degree. However, anorexia occurs in up to 30% of older hyperthyroid subjects

Hyperthyroidism is associated with an increase in glucose utilization and a depletion of liver glycogen. While fasting glucose levels are generally normal in hyperthyroidism, glucose intolerance is present in approximately half of these patients.[39] In hypothyroidism, there is decreased glucose absorption from the gastrointestinal tract and a reduction in peripheral glucose utilization. A flat glucose tolerance curve is not unusual in hypothyroidism.

In hyperthyroid subjects, there is an increase in free fatty acid and triglyceride levels and a decrease in cholesterol levels.[38] In hypothyroidism, fat cell lipolysis in response to catecholamine is reduced.[38] Free fatty acid levels are normal or slightly decreased in hypothyroidism.[38] Plasma triglyceride levels are markedly increased secondary to a marked decrease in the triglyceride removal rate.[40] Cholesterol levels are also increased in hypothyroidism; more than 80% of hypothyroid patients have cholesterol levels greater than 250 mg/dL.[41] The increase is mostly in low-density-lipoprotein cholesterol. Cholesterol secretion in the bile is markedly decreased in hypothyroidism.

Osteopenia commonly is present in hyperthyroidism, and the development of hyperthyroidism aggravates normal age-related bone loss. Mild hypercalcemia commonly is seen in hyperthyroidism. Calcium absorption is decreased and calcium excretion is increased in hyperthyroidism. In hypothyroidism, there is a mild decrease in the rate of calcium deposition in bone.

The alterations in vitamin status that occur in thyroid disease are outlined in Table 15–5.[42,43] Decreased dark adaptation occurs occasionally in hyperthyroidism and may be related to diminished vitamin A levels in this disorder. The characteristic yellow color of the skin of hypothyroid patients is due to increased carotene values secondary to decreased conversion of carotene to vitamin A.

Effects of Nutritional Status on Thyroid Hormones

There is increasing evidence that vitamin status may alter thyroid function. Vitamin A deficiency in animals leads to mild increases in circulating thyroid hormones in the presence of normal TSH secretion, suggesting a resetting of the hypothalamic-pituitary axis in response to thyroid hormones.[44] Vitamin A excess lowers circulating total thyroid hormone levels, but not free hormone levels, as the dialyzable function of thyroid hormones increases.[45] In animals, thiamine administration decreases the weight loss seen when pharmacologic amounts of thyroid hormone are administered.[46] Riboflavin deficiency diminishes the hepatic deiodination of thyroxine.[47] Vitamin E may attenuate the effects of

Table 15–5　Effects of Thyroid Diseases on Vitamin Status

Vitamin	Hypothyroid	Hyperthyroid
Vitamin A	↑	↓
Retinol-binding protein	↑	↓
Thiamine		
Erythrocyte transketolase	?	↓
In vitro thiamin pyridinylase (thiammase)	?	None[a]
Riboflavin	?	↑
Pyridoxine		
Xanthurenic acid excretion after tryptophan administration	?	[b]
Vitamin B$_{12}$	↓ or N[c]	↓
Folate	N	?
Vitamin C	N	N
25-Hydroxyvitamin D$_3$	N	N
1, 25-Hydroxvitamin D$_3$	↑	↓
α-Tocopherol (vitamin E)	↑	↓

Note: N, Normal; ↑, increased; ↓, decreased.

a. The decrease in erythrocyte transketolase suggests thiamine deficiency, but the failure of in vitro thiamine augmentation suggests other causes.

b. Suggests pyridoxine deficiency.

c. About 5% to 10% have pernicious anemia.

thyroid hormone on some of its target organs.[48] These findings and others suggest that a careful study of vitamin status in elderly patients with hyperthyroidism is warranted. A recent study also suggested that some protection from thyroid cancer is afforded by vitamins C and E and that there is an inverse association between beta carotene and thyroid cancer.[49]

ADRENAL CORTEX

Aging produces only minor changes in the hypothalamic-pituitary-adrenal axis. There are mild decreases in both cortisol production and clearance rates; as a result, plasma cortisol levels remain unchanged with aging.[1] In addition, with advancing age there is a decreased sensitivity of the anterior pituitary to negative feedback by circulating cortisol.[50] Therefore, with advancing age there is an increased prevalence of failure of dexamethasone to suppress cortisol adequately.

Less than 10% of patients with Addison disease (hypoadrenalism) are older than age 60 years.[51] Nutritional and clinical manifestations are commonly seen in patients with Addison disease. These include weakness, easy fatigability, vomiting, constipation or diarrhea, abdominal pain, salt craving, weight loss, hypoglycemia, hyponatremia, and hyperkalemia. Additional manifestations include hyperpigmentation and postural hypotension.

The clustering of hypertension, hypokalemia, diabetes mellitus, and osteopenia is suggestive of Cushing's syndrome. However, in elderly people all of these conditions occur commonly, and the presence of multiple disease states represents a more likely finding. The classic appearance of patients with Cushing's syndrome is central obesity with thin arms and legs, although weight loss may occur in elderly individuals. The screening test for Cushing's syndrome is the failure of 1 mg of dexamethasone to suppress cortisol levels below 138 mmol/L. In elderly patients, failure of dexamethasone suppression may be secondary to depression, Alzheimer's disease, obesity, or alcoholism.

Whereas Cushing's syndrome is rare in elderly individuals, ectopic corticotropin syndrome (secondary to tumors), such as oat cell carcinoma of the lung, is relatively common. These patients are usually cachectic rather than obese and have severe proximal muscle weakness, hypokalemic alkalosis, mental changes, and hyperpigmentation. Patients with ectopic corticotropin fail the dexamethasone suppression test and have relatively high circulating corticotropin levels.

In elderly people, by far the most common cause of elevated cortisol levels is exogenous cortisol administration. The use of steroids in elderly patients should be limited to situations in which they are absolutely essential, and the steroids should be tapered off as rapidly as possible. Exogenous steroid use is a major cause of osteopenia; patients receiving steroids should receive calcium prophylactically and possibly vitamin D supplementation, as steroids inhibit the conversion of 25-hydroxyvitamin D_3 (25(OH)D_3) to 1,25-dihydroxyvitamin D_3 (1,25(OH)$_2D_3$).

Nutritionally, glucosteroids promote the conversion of protein to carbohydrate (gluconeogenesis). This leads to a negative nitrogen balance, an increase in circulating glucose, and increased liver glycogen. Corticosteroids also reduce hexose transport into the cells, which further increases circulating glucose levels and produces a secondary hyperinsulinemia. Patients receiving corticosteroids who develop frank diabetes mellitus usually require insulin therapy rather than oral hypoglycemic agents.

Cortisol increases DNA synthesis in human adipose cells in vitro. Cortisol promotes hyperphagia and mobilization of free fatty acids. Pharmacologic doses of cortisol elevate triglyceride levels.

Megestrol acetate is a progestagen/glucocorticoid that increases food intake. Because of it, glucocorticoid activity decreases ACTH production, and withdrawal may rarely produce an adrenal crisis. Megestrol also lowers testosterone levels.[52]

Other Adrenal Hormones

Plasma levels and urinary excretion of aldosterone tend to fall with advancing age. Active renin levels also fall with advancing age.[53] These changes increase the propensity of older subjects to develop hyperkalemia secondary to hyporeninemic hypoaldosteronism. This is particularly common in patients with diabetes mellitus and mild renal failure.

In contrast to the relative preservation of cortisol secretory dynamics, dehydroepiandrosterone (DHEA) secretion declines dramatically with advancing age.[54] In animals, DHEA administration prolongs life span, which may be related to its ability to reduce weights.[55] In men, DHEA-sulfate (DHEA-S) has been suggested to be inversely related to death from cardiovascular disease, though this has not been a universal finding.[56] Diminished levels of DHEA and DHEA-S are associated with hypercholesterolemia[57] and hypertension.[58] The mechanism by which DHEA deficiency promotes atherosclerosis is uncertain but may be related to excessive stimulation of lipogenesis by reduced nicotinamide-adenine dinucleotide phosphate (NADPH). Replacement studies with DHEA have been disappointing, though high doses (100 mg) have resulted in reduced body fat and increased muscle mass and strength. A large yearlong study of a 50 mg DHEA dose produced minimal effects in older persons.[59]

WATER METABOLISM

Elderly people are at increased risk for developing disturbances of water metabolism[60] (Chapter 3). Aging is associated with a decline in total body water and intravascular water. Both dehydration and hyponatremia occur with increasing frequency in elderly subjects. Phillips and colleagues[61] have demonstrated that even healthy elderly subjects fail to respond adequately to mild dehydration. In part, this failure to develop an appropriate thirst response may be secondary to an impaired secretion of angiotensin.[62] The mu opioid drinking drive is also severely impaired in older persons. This has led to the concept that elderly people live in a "water desert" and that hospitalized elderly patients need a prescription of at least 1.5 L of fluid intake per day. Most community-dwelling older persons can maintain their hydration status if they drink 4 to 6 glasses of fluid per day.[63]

There is greater arginine vasopressin (antidiuretic hormone) release for a given osmotic stimulus in elderly subjects than in younger subjects.[64] Older subjects also have a decrease in free water clearance in response to argipressin, predominantly related to the age-related fall in glomerular filtration rate.[65] Atrial natriuretic factor (ANF) is released by volume overload and acts on the kidney to increase glomerular filtration rate and induce natriuresis. Recently, ANF levels have been demonstrated to be elevated in elderly individuals.[66] Greater elevations of ANF and brain derived natriuretic factor occur in persons with heart failure.

These hormonal changes explain why hyponatremia occurs commonly in elderly people.[67] Many institutionalized elderly persons have the syndrome of inappropriate secretion of antidiuretic hormone, which may lead to hyponatremia; tube feeding represents another major cause of hyponatremia in institutionalized elderly people.

GROWTH HORMONE AND INSULIN GROWTH FACTORS

There is evidence that growth hormone secretion is impaired with advancing age. A single study of medically impaired elderly subjects found adequate nitrogen retention and free fatty acid increase after growth hormone administration, but impaired urinary hydroxyproline secretion.[68] This highly limited study is the basis for the claim that metabolic responses to growth hormone are impaired in elderly persons.

In contrast to the minor decreases in growth hormone with aging, plasma levels of insulin-like growth factor 1 (IGF-1; somatomedin C) are markedly decreased with advancing age.[69] IGF-1 levels are also decreased by malnutrition. In malnourished, institutionalized elderly patients, the levels of IGF-1 are even lower than those seen in healthy elderly people, suggesting an interaction between nutrition and aging in these individuals.[70]

Rudman[71] and colleagues[72] have suggested that the growth hormone "menopause" that occurs with advancing age may explain a number of the normal changes seen with aging. These include the diminished nitrogen retention, the decrease in lean body mass, the increase in adipose tissue, and some of the osteopenia characteristically associated with aging. Overall, growth hormone replacement studies in older persons have been disappointing. At best, these studies have demonstrated an increase in muscle mass with no increase in strength. Side effects, such as carpal tunnel syndrome, appear to limit the long-term use of growth hormone.[72,73] On the other hand, severely ill older persons who are highly catabolic may benefit from short-term growth hormone treatment.[74] In these patients, growth hormone improved nutrition and function.[75] However, in malnourished severely ill older persons growth hormone was associated with an increased mortality.[76] The muscle isoform of IGF-1 plays an important role in age-related muscle loss.[77]

MALE HYPOGONADISM

With advancing age, sexual dysfunction occurs with increasing frequency. Kinsey and colleagues[78] reported that impotence occurred in 18.6% of 60-year-old men and 75% of 80-year-old men. One in three men over the age of 50 years old who are examined by a physician are impotent.[79] The causes of impotence in older men are multifactorial.[80] The major cause for the increasing prevalence of impotence with advancing age is arteriosclerosis. Medications also have an important role in the pathogenesis of impotence. Nutritionally, it has been found that a small subset of older impotent men have low serum zinc levels and hyperzincuria.[81] Approximately half of these subjects improve after the administration of pharmacologic amounts of zinc.

Hypogonadism occurs with increasing frequency with advancing age. In older men, there is a marked decrease in testosterone and bioavailable testosterone.[82] A longitudinal study demonstrated that testosterone levels decline in all elderly men. Both luteinizing hormone and follicle-stimulating hormone levels tend to increase with advancing age in an attempt to compensate for the decreased levels of testosterone.[83] However, in a number of older individuals, the hypothalamus fails to detect the decrease in testosterone adequately, resulting in the development of hypothalamic hypogonadism.[84]

Testosterone not only plays a role in maintaining normal sexual function (libido and potency) but also has a number of effects that enhance the general well-being of the individual.[85] Testosterone promotes nitrogen retention, maintains muscle mass, protects bone from excessive calcium loss, helps to maintain erythrocyte mass, and produces a general feeling of well-being. Testosterone deficiency appears to play an important role in the development of age-related sarcopenia. Testosterone replacement in older individuals improved muscle strength and libido and decreased serum leptin levels. For these reasons, it is recommended that testosterone replacement therapy be instituted in all subjects with proven hypogonadism, regardless of whether they desire to have sexual intercourse. In patients receiving testosterone, regular rectal examinations need to be conducted to detect prostatic growth.

CALCIUM METABOLISM

Both calcium intake and calcium absorption diminish with advancing ages[1] (Chapter 5). With advancing age, there is a decrease in vitamin D synthesis in the skin[86] and decreased activity of 1-α-hydroxylase in the kidney (Chapter 4). Recent studies have clearly demonstrated that at least a proportion of older individuals have a decrease in $25(OH)D_3$ and its active metabolite, $1,25(OH)_2D_3$.[87] A longitudinal study demonstrated that vitamin D falls with age even in older persons in sunny climates.[88] Lower vitamin D levels are particularly prevalent in institutionalized and housebound elderly people who are rarely exposed to sunlight and who have low calcium intakes. Our longitudinal study in healthy older persons suggests that decreased sunlight exposure is more important than aging *per se* in the pathogenesis of the age-related decline in serum vitamin D levels. Treatment with vitamin D and calcium has been demonstrated to decrease hip fracture in nursing home residents.[89] Vitamin D

also decreases falls and improves function in older persons who are vitamin D deficient.[90]

These changes tend to lead to a decrease in ionized calcium, which, in turn, results in a compensatory increase in parathyroid hormone (PTH) levels.[91] Calcitonin levels may decline slightly with advancing age.[92] As already mentioned, the age-related declines in IGF-1 and testosterone also impinge on calcium metabolism. The changes in calcium metabolism that occur with age are summarized in Figure 15–1.

Seventeen percent of patients with hyperparathyroidism are older than age 60 years.[93] Clinically, hyperparathyroidism is often characterized by vague complaints, including anorexia, weight loss, weakness, abdominal symptoms, cognitive disturbances, polyuria, and dehydration. Diagnosis is made by demonstrating elevated calcium and PTH levels.

Treatment consists of surgical removal of the parathyroid adenoma. In postmenopausal women, estrogen therapy has been shown to lower mild hyperparathyroidism. In the differential diagnosis of hypercalcemia, it should be remembered that megadoses of vitamin A activate cathepsin D, resulting in increased PTH secretion and elevated calcium levels.

A detailed discussion of osteopenia in elderly people is presented elsewhere[86] (Chapter 14). In postmenopausal (type I) osteopenia, clearly estrogen deficiency represents the major problem. The etiologic factors involved in type II osteopenia are multifactorial and include a variety of nutritional factors such as low calcium intake, a high-protein diet that produces hypercalciuria, late-onset lactase deficiency, coffee consumption, alcoholism, lack of physical exercise, and cigarette smoking. Boron supplementation has been demonstrated to reduce the urinary excretion of calcium.[93]

HORMONAL REGULATION OF ENERGY BALANCE

The early phase of aging typically is associated with a positive energy balance and an increase in adiposity, but a decrease in lean body mass.[94] While lean body mass continues to decline in the last phase, often seen beyond age 65 years, negative energy balance often is maintained.[95] Protein-energy malnutrition occurs in this age group at an alarming frequency.[24,96] In elderly people, both energy intake and output typically are reduced, but reduction in intake exceeds the reduced output, leading to the observed loss in energy stores, including lean body mass.

Control of energy intake and output involves complex autonomic, hormonal, and metabolic mechanisms that are only partially understood. It is therefore difficult to identify, with any level of certainty, the age-related dysfunctions responsible for the status of negative energy balance in elderly individuals.

Hormonal Control of Energy Intake

The control mechanism of food intake has central and peripheral components. The primary central structures are in the hypothalamus and include the ventromedial hypothalamus (VMH), lateral hypothalamus (LH), and paraventricular nucleus (PVN).[97] The primary peripheral aspects are thought to include the gastrointestinal tract, liver, and adipose tissue and to involve some key hormones and metabolites.

Whatever effect a peripheral hormone or metabolite has on feeding, its effect will be encoded into the neurotransmitter system in the hypothalamus, and a behavioral feeding response will be elicited subsequent to the specific neurotransmitter signal. Accordingly, discussion of hormone influences on feeding must include the neurotransmitter system (neurohormones), exerting a direct effect in the hypothalamus, and hormones secreted in the periphery.

Neurohormones

Monoamines. Norepinephrine, dopamine, and serotonin all have important roles in determining feeding behavior.[97] Direct injection of norepinephrine into the VMH or PVN will stimulate

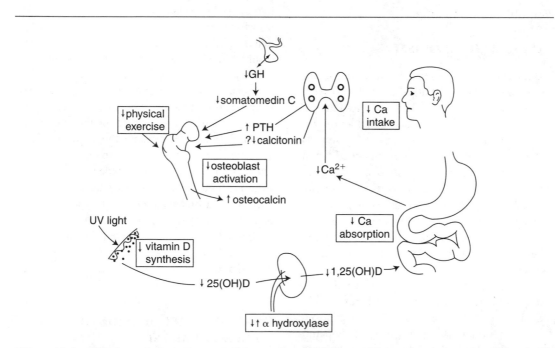

Figure 15–1 Overview of the Effects of Aging on Calcium Metabolism. GH, Growth hormone; PTH, parathyroid hormone
Source: Reprinted with permission from *Journal of American Geriatrics Society* (1988;36: 845–859), Copyright © 1988, American Geriatrics Society.

feeding; its administration into the LH will inhibit feeding. This effect of norepinephrine is mediated through α-adrenergic receptors in the VMH and β-adrenergic receptors in the LH.[97] Brain tissue from aged rats has an impaired capacity for synthesis and regulation of α- and β-adrenergic receptors. This impairment has been demonstrated in the cortex and cerebellum, but it has not been studied in the hypothalamus.

The effects of serotonin on feeding also appear to depend on the type of serotonin receptor, with a decrease in feeding induced by 1_B receptor agonist in the PVN and an increase in feeding with a 1_A receptor agonist.[98] Dopamine neurotransmitters have also been thought to have a role in controlling feeding behavior, but the effects of aging on the serotonin and the dopamine feeding systems have not been studied.

Neuropeptides. Several peptide neurotransmitters have been found in recent years in mammalian brain. These include cholecystokinin (CCK), bombesin, substance P, neurotensin, opioids, neuropeptide Y (NPY), and others.[99] A number of these peptides were shown to decrease feeding after central administration. However, a reduced food intake need not imply a physiologic role for these neuropeptides in modulating feeding behavior, as their effect may be secondary to nonspecific behavioral effects. The administration of either opioid peptides[100] or NPY[101] was reported to stimulate feeding, suggesting a physiologic role for these neuropeptides. Moreover, the opioid antagonist naloxone suppresses food intake.[100] Recently, it was reported that older rats display a much smaller response to opioid agonists and antagonists.[102] However, a human study failed to find an age-related change in the opioid feeding drive.[103] Older rats also have a lower concentration of opioid peptides in the hypothalamus.[100] Aging is thus associated with a decreased opiate-based feeding drive, but the relative importance of the latter in anorexia of aging is not clear. The orexigenic effect of NPY is less age dependent.[104]

Nitric Oxide. Nitric oxide is a gaseous neurotransmitter. It appears to play an important role in increasing food intake. It produces its effects both within the central nervous system and by increasing adaptive relaxation to food in the fundus of the stomach. Available studies suggest that nitric oxide deficiency may play a role in the anorexia of aging.[105]

Peripheral Hormones

Growth Hormone. Administration of growth hormone into experimental animals stimulates food intake and growth of lean, but not adipose, tissue.[106] A similar effect has been reported in humans.[107] It is not clear to what extent small changes in growth hormone activity (within the normal range) influence food intake or whether the reduction in growth hormone activity, which is often observed in elderly subjects (see above), contributes to their anorexia.

Insulin. Daily single injections of insulin stimulate food intake and produce obesity. Moreover, the hyperphagia and obesity that develop after placement of lesions in the ventromedial hypothalamus are contributed to by a vagally mediated insulin hypersecretion induced by the lesions. The stimulatory effect of insulin on food intake is thought to result from its lipolytic effect, which decreases availability of endogenous substrate to the tissues and to specific glucose-sensitive hypothalamic sites. The role of age-associated hyperglycemia (impaired glucose tolerance) in the anorexia of aging is not known.

Glucocorticoids. The stimulatory effect of norepinephrine administered in the PVN of the hypothalamus on food intake is absent in adrenalectomized rats; it is restored with corticosterone.[108] Also, peak hormone concentration in blood is observed before onset of feeding.[109] However, corticosterone administered into nonadrenalectomized rats has little or no effect on food intake.[110] Combined, these data suggest that glucocorticoids have an important "permissive" role in the central control mechanism of feeding. In both animals and humans, glucocorticoid hyperactivity is associated with a redistribution of body energy stores toward increased adiposity and decreased lean body mass.[111] In humans, this is known as Cushing's syndrome, which is rare in elderly persons.

Thyroid Hormone. Thyroid hormone stimulates food intake,[112] but this effect appears to be secondary to a stimulated metabolic rate and a compensatory replenishment of the greater energy losses.

Gonadal Steroids. The gonadal steroid estrogen suppresses food intake in female subjects; its site of action is thought to be in the VMH.[113] Food intake is decreased during days of estrus (high estrogen) and increased during diestrus (low estrogen).[114] Castration of female rats leads to overeating and obesity. Testosterone, on the other hand, increases food intake and lean tissue growth, while decreasing body fat.[115]

Although there is little change in estrogen levels, bioavailable testosterone levels are reduced in the majority of elderly people. These sex hormone changes would be compatible with reduced ingestion with advancing age.

Gastrointestinal Hormones. Peripheral injections of a variety of gastrointestinal hormones and other peptides into rats reduce food intake. These peptides include CCK, bombesin, gastrin-releasing peptide, glucagon, somatostatin, and substance neurotensin.[100] However, the physiologic significance of these hormones in producing normal satiety is not clear. It has been proposed that CCK exerts a weak effect on food intake, amounting to some 10–20% of the total intake at a single meal.[99] Higher than normal serum levels of CCK were observed in elderly men, perhaps contributing to their anorexia.[116,117] Silver and colleagues[118] have reported an increased ability of pharmacologically administered CCK-8 to decrease feeding in older mice compared with younger mice. In older humans CCK is more effective at reducing food intake than in younger persons.[119]

Leptin. Leptin is a protein hormone that is secreted from fat cells.[120] It has been shown to decrease food intake and increase metabolic rate in rodents. It decreases food intake by decreasing nitric oxide synthase activity in the hypothalamus. In humans, leptin levels are strongly related to total adiposity, particularly visceral adiposity. With aging, leptin levels decline in females but increase in males. The increase in males is due to declining testosterone levels that occur with aging. Testosterone replacement therapy in older males causes leptin levels to decline. Elevated leptin levels in older males are related to decreased food intake. Resistance to leptin effects occurs in obese persons related to hypertriglyceridemia.[121]

Hormonal Control of Energy Output

Energy output may be divided into the following components: basal metabolic rate, physical activity, and thermic effect of feeding. A brief discussion of each of these components, their hormonal mediators, and how they interact is necessary to present a complete discussion of the control of hormones on energy balance.

Resting Metabolic Rate

Resting metabolic rate (RMR) accounts for about 1400 to 1600 kcal, constituting about 60–75% of total energy expenditure. It has several major metabolic origins. It is thought to reflect the energy cost of protein and, to a much smaller extent, carbohydrate and fat turnover. It reflects the activity of the sodium pump, the cost of maintaining muscle tone, and the work done by involuntary muscles (heart, respiratory, and gastrointestinal).[120–126] It originates primarily in, and therefore is highly correlated with, lean body mass; men, having a greater lean body mass, have a higher RMR than do women. RMR is governed by thyroid hormones through a mechanism that is not fully understood. The hormone stimulates activity of the sodium pump[127] as well as protein turnover;[128] protein turnover is stimulated through enhancement of protein breakdown via lysosomal proteinases[128] and through stimulation of protein synthesis in conjunction with other anabolic hormones, namely insulin and growth hormone. Triiodothyronine stimulates release of both insulin[129] and growth hormone.[105] Triiodothyronine is also required for sympathetic activation,[130] which can, in turn, stimulate metabolic rate. RMR is reduced in elderly people some 10–20%;[131,132] it is thought that this decline in metabolic rate reflects, by and large, the reduced lean body mass.[131] Females show a lesser decline in RMR than males do. The reduction in BMR is accompanied by a decrease in the rate of protein turnover[133] but with no clear change in activity of the sodium pump in the small number of tissues examined.[134] The metabolic origins for the age-dependent compositional changes have not been clearly identified. Activities of growth hormone and testosterone, which promote lean tissue growth, are reduced with aging. This may contribute to the shift in balance from lean to adipose tissue. A decreased trophic effect of the autonomic nervous system on muscle and a decreased capacity for muscle fiber regeneration have also been suggested.[135]

Physical Activity

Physical activity is an important determinant of energy balance status. Muscle mass is increased and adiposity is decreased with physical training.[94] In elderly people, there is usually a decline in physical activity[94] imposed by age-related conditions such as cardiovascular disease, musculoskeletal disease, osteopenia, and obesity. In addition, there is a decline in physical working capacity (VO$_2$max), amounting to about 10% per decade between ages 25 and 65 years. The latter means that the same physical tasks require a greater physical effort in elderly people. Elderly individuals retain the ability to enjoy the benefit of training,[136] and physical training can correct these age-related changes in physical working capacity by as much as 50%. The level of physical activity is not under hormonal control but is determined by motivational factors.

Thermic Effect of Feeding

The thermic effect of feeding[137,138] represents two components: an obligatory component and an adaptive component. In the obligatory component, heat is a by-product of the metabolic cost of converting the ingested macronutrient into body glycogen, protein, and fat.[139] It amounts to an average of 5–10% of the energy value of the food. It is minimal after fat intake and maximal after protein intake.[139] In the adaptive component, heat is the primary end product. In rodents, this heat is produced exclusively in the brown adipose tissue, where substrate oxidation is uncoupled from phosphorylation.[140] The brown fat has the potential of dissipating a large portion of the caloric intake in rodents, but in humans, the capacity for adaptive thermogenesis is relatively small, apparently because of the small quantity of brown fat in humans. Thermogenic activity of brown adipose tissue is controlled primarily by norepinephrine released from a dense sympathetic innervation of this tissue. Insulin and glucagon, which are released in response to feeding, stimulate thermogenesis of brown adipose tissue in rodents, whereas glucocorticoids inhibit it.

In rodents, the capacity for feeding-induced thermogenesis declines rapidly after sexual maturity is reached. In old rats, there is a 30% decrease in brown adipose tissue mass, a twofold decrease in β-adrenergic receptors (primarily due to receptors of the β$_1$ subtype), and a decrease in the activation of adenylate cyclase. These biochemical abnormalities may contribute to the decreased capacity for feeding-induced thermogenesis in older animals. An analogous reduction in adaptive thermogenesis in humans would contribute to the observed age-related decrease in energy expenditure.

CONCLUSION

Nutrition and the endocrine system are closely integrated. Nutritional status influences glandular activities, while endocrine function can have marked influences on nutrient requirements and status. With advancing age, changes occur in both endocrine and nutritional status.

Several factors enhance development of diabetes mellitus in elderly people, including weight gain, decreased physical activity, and defective mechanisms for insulin secretion and action. Although the efficacy of the American Dietetic Association/American Diabetes Association diet for glucose control in elderly diabetics is not clear, there is no better dietary recommendation for them at the present time. Long-term exercise programs are beneficial to elderly diabetics and should be encouraged.

A hypothyroid state is much more prevalent in elderly people than in young people. In elderly individuals, hypothyroidism is often contributed to by the presence of malnutrition. In the hyperthyroid elderly person, the rise in metabolic rate is not fully compensated for by a corresponding rise in voluntary food intake. Thyroid status can have profound effects on vitamin and calcium requirements, and their proper intake should be monitored in hyperthyroid elderly people.

Aging produces only minor changes in the hypothalamic-pituitary-adrenal axis. Diseases of the adrenal cortex, namely Addison's disease and Cushing's syndrome, are not common in elderly people. However, ectopic corticotropin production, secondary to tumors, is relatively common. Steroid treatment should be used in elderly patients with extreme caution, as it can cause negative nitrogen and calcium balances as well as hyperglycemia and resistance to insulin.

Growth hormone secretion is mildly reduced in the elderly, but IGF-1 is markedly reduced. These may contribute to the diminished nitrogen retention and increased adiposity observed with aging. Another possible contributor to the decline in nitrogen retention in elderly persons is reduced serum testosterone levels. However, the main cause for impotence in elderly men is thought to be arteriosclerosis and not reduced testosterone levels.

In elderly individuals, both energy intake and output are reduced, but reduction in intake often exceeds output. In humans, aging is associated with a greater suppression of feeding by CCK. There is some evidence that leptin may play a role in the alterations in energy metabolism that occur with aging, particularly in males. The smaller energy expenditure observed in elderly people is brought about by a reduced RMR, by reduced physical activity, and possibly by a reduced thermic response to feeding.

REFERENCES

1. Morley JE. Hormones and the aging process. *J Am Geriatr Soc* 2003;51(7 suppl S):S333–S337.
2. Banks WA, Morley JE. Endocrine and metabolic changes in human aging. *J Am Aging Assoc* 2000;23:103–115.
3. Harris MI, Hadden WC, Knowler WC, et al. Prevalence of diabetes and impaired glucose tolerance and plasma glucose levels in U.S. population aged 20–74 years. *Diabetes* 1987;4:523–534.
4. Morley JE. Impaired cognitive function and mental performance in mild dehydration. *Euro J Clin Nutr* 2003; 57(suppl 2):S24–S29.
5. Zavaroni I, Dall'Aglio E, Bruschi F. Effect of age and environmental factors on glucose tolerance and insulin secretion in a worker population. *J Am Geriatr Soc* 1986;34:271–278.
6. Meneilly GS, Tessier D. Diabetes in elderly adults. *J Gerontol Med Sci* 2001;56A:M5–M13.
7. Morley JE, Perry HM III. The management of diabetes mellitus in older individuals. *Drugs* 1991;41:548–565.
8. Morley JE. The metabolic syndrome and aging. *J Gerontol Med Sci* 2004;59A:139–142.
9. American Diabetes Association. Diabetes nutrition recommendations for health care institutions. *Diabetes Care* 2004;27:555–564.
10. Coulston A, Mandelbaum D, Reaven G. Dietary management of nursing, home residents with diabetes: diabetic versus regular diet. *Clin Res* 1988;36:95A.
11. Tariq SH, Karcic E, Thomas DR, Thomson K, Philpot C, Chapel DL, Morley JE. The use of a no-concentrated-sweets diet in the management of type 2 diabetes in nursing homes. *J Am Dietetic Assoc* 2001;101:1463–1466.
12. Seals DR, Hagberg JM, Hurley BF, et al. Effects of endurance training on glucose tolerance and plasma lipid levels in older men and women. *JAMA* 1984;252: 645–649.
13. Krotkiewski M, Lonnroth P, Mandroukas K, et al. The effects of physical training on glucose metabolism in obesity and type 2 (noninsulin-dependent) diabetes mellitus. *Diabetologia* 1985;28:881–890.
14. Saltin B, Lindgarde F, Houston M, et al. Physical training and glucose tolerance in middle-aged men with chemical diabetes. *Diabetes* 1979;28(suppl 1):30–32.
15. Bogardus C, Ravussin E, Robbins DC, et al. Effects of physical training and diet therapy on carbohydrate metabolism in patients with glucose intolerance and noninsulin-dependent diabetes mellitus. *Diabetes* 1984; 33:311–318.
16. Karam JH. Therapeutic dilemmas in type II diabetes mellitus: improving and maintaining B-cell and insulin sensitivity. *West J Med* 1988;148:685–690.
17. Pacini G, Valerio A, Beccaro F, et al. Insulin sensitivity and beta-cell responsivity are not decreased in elderly subjects with normal OGTT. *J Am Geriatr Soc* 1988; 36:317–323.
18. Agurscollins TD, Kumanyika SK, Tenhave TR, Adams Campbell LL. A randomized controlled trial of weight reduction and exercise for diabetes management in older African-American subjects. *Diabetes Care* 1997;20: 1503–1511.

19. Lee A, Patrick P, Wishart J, Horowitz M, Morley JE. The effects of miglitol on glucagon-like peptide-1 secretion and appetite sensations in obese type 2 diabetics. *Diabetes, Obesity & Metab* 2002;4:329–335.

20. Puxty JAM, Hunter DM, Burr WA. Accuracy of insulin injection in elderly patients. *Br Med J* 1983;287: 1762–1763.

21. Rosenthal MJ, Fajardo M, Gilmore S, Morley JE, Naliboff BD. Hospitalization and mortality of diabetes in older adults: a 3-year prospective study. *Diabetes Care* 1998;21:231–235.

22. Mooradian AD, Morley JE. Micronutrient status in diabetes mellitus. *Am J Clin Nutr* 1987;45:877–895.

23. Kinlaw WB, Levine AS, Morley JE, et al. Abnormal zinc metabolism in type II diabetes mellitus. *Am J Med* 1983;75:273–277.

24. Morley JE. Nutritional status of the elderly. *Am J Med* 1986;81:679–695.

25. Niewoehner CB, Allen JI, Boosalis M, et al. The role of zinc supplementation in type II diabetes mellitus. *Am J Med* 1986;81:63–68.

26. Hallbook T, Lanner E. Serum-zinc and wound healing of venous leg ulcers. *Lancet* 1972;2:780–782.

27. Amato P, Morales AJ, Yen SSC. Effects of chromium picolinate supplementation on insulin sensitivity, serum lipids, and body composition in healthy, nonobese, older men and women. *J Gerontol Med Sci* 2000;55A: M260–M263.

28. Anderson RA, Cheng N, Bryden NA, et al. Elevated intakes of supplemental chromium improve glucose and insulin variables in individuals with type 2 diabetes. *Diabetes* 1997;46:1786–1791.

29. Urberg M, Zemel MD. Evidence for synergism between chromium and nicotinic acid in the control of glucose tolerance in elderly humans. *Metabolism* 1987;36:896–899.

30. Klevay LM. Hypercholesterolemia in rats produced by an increase in the ratio of zinc to copper ingested. *Am J Clin Nutr* 1978;26:1060–1065.

31. Sinclair AJ, Allard I. Observations of diabetes care in long-term institutional settings with measures of cognitive function and dependency. *Diabetes Care* 1997;20:778–784.

32. Mooradian AD, Osterweil D, Petrasek D, et al. Diabetes mellitus in elderly nursing home patients: a survey of clinical characteristics and management. *J Am Geriatr Soc* 1988;36:391–396.

33. Robuschi G, Safran M, Braverman LE. Hypothyroidism in the elderly. *Endocr Rev* 1987;8:142–153.

34. Prinz PN, Scanlan JM, Vitaliano PP, Moe KE, Borson S, Toivola B, Merriam GR, Larsen LH, Reed HL. Thyroid hormones: positive relationships with cognition in healthy, euthyroid older men. *J Gerontol Med Sci* 1999;54A:M111–M116.

35. Morley JE, Slag MF, Elson MK, et al. The interpretation of thyroid function tests in hospitalized patients. *JAMA* 1983;249:2377–2379.

36. Lloyd WA, Goldberg IJL. Incidence of hypothyroidism in the elderly. *Br Med J* 1961;2:1256–1258.

37. Martin FI, Deam DR. Hyperthyroidism in elderly hospitalized patients: clinical features and treatment outcomes. *Med J Aust* 1996;164:200–203.

38. Loeb JN. Metabolic changes in hyperthyroidism. In: Ingbar SM, Braverman LE, eds. *Werner's The Thyroid*. Philadelphia, PA: JB Lippincott Co; 1986.

39. Kreines K, Jett M, Knowles HC. Observations in hyperthyroidism of abnormal glucose tolerance and other traits related to diabetes mellitus. *Diabetes* 1965;14:740–744.

40. Nikkala EA, Kekki M. Plasma triglyceride metabolism in thyroid disease. *J Clin Invest* 1972; 51:2103–2111.

41. Watanakunakorn C, Hodges RE, Evans TC. Myxedema. *Arch Intern Med* 1965;116:183–187.

42. Rivlin RS. Vitamin metabolism in hyperthyroidism. In: Ingbar SM, Braverman LE, eds. *Werner's The Thyroid*. Philadelphia, PA: JB Lippincott Co; 1986.

43. Rivlin RS. Vitamin metabolism in hypothyroidism. In: Ingbar SM, Braverman LE, eds. *Werner's The Thyroid* Philadelphia, PA: JB Lippincott Co; 1986.

44. Morley JE, Damassa DA, Gordon J, et al. Thyroid function and vitamin A deficiency. *Life Sci* 1978;22.1901–1906.

45. Morley JE, Melmed S, Reed A, et al. The effect of vitamin A on the hypothalamic-pituitary-thyroid axis. *Am J Physiol* 1980;238:E174–E179.

46. Drill VA. Interrelationships between thyroid function and vitamin metabolism. *Physiol Rev* 1942;23:355–372.

47. Galton VA, Ingbar SM. Effects of vitamin deficiency on the in vitro and in vivo deiodination of thyroxine in the rat. *Endocrinology* 1965;77:169–174.

48. Postelnicu D. Action of an antioxidant substance (alpha tocopherol) on the myocardium of rats treated with thyroxine. *Stud Cercet Endocrinol* 1972;23:175–182.

49. D'Avanzo B, Ron E, LaVecchia C, Francaschi S, Negri E, Zieglar R. Selected micronutrient intake and thyroid carcinoma risk. *Cancer* 1997;79:2186–2192.

50. Oxenburg GF, Pomara N, McIntyre IM. Aging and cortisol resistance to suppression by dexamethasone: a positive correlation. *Psychiatry Res* 1983;10:125–130.

51. Irvine WJ, Barnes EW. Addison's disease, ovarian failure and hypoparathyroidism. *Clin Endocrinol Metab* 1975;4:379–334.

52. Lambert CP, Flynn MG, Sullivan DH, Evans WJ. Effects of megestrol acetate on circulating interleukin-15 and interleukin-18 concentrations in healthy elderly men. *J Gerontol Med Sci* 2004;59A:855–858.

53. Tsundo K, Abe K, Goto T. Effect of age on the renin-angiotensin-aldosterone system in normal subjects: simultaneous measurement of active and inactive renin, renin substrate, and aldosterone in plasma. *J Clin Endocrinol Metab* 1986;62:384–389.

54. Yen SSC. Dehydroepiandrosterone sulfate and longevity: new clues for an old friend. *Proc Nat Acad Sci USA* 2001;98:8167–8169.

55. Pashko LL, Schwartz AG. Effect of food restriction, dehydroepiandrosterone or obesity on the binding of 3H-7,12 dimethylbenz (a) anthracene to mouse skin DNA. *J Gerontol* 1983;38:8–12.

56. Barrett-Connor E, Shaw-XT, Yen SSC. A prospective study of dehydroepiandrosterone sulfate, mortality and cardiovascular disease. *N Engl J Med* 1986;315:1519–1524.

57. Sonka J, Fassati M, Fassati P. Serum lipids and dehydroepiandrosterone excretion in normal subjects. *J Lipid Res* 1968;9:769–772.

58. Nowaczynski W, Fragachon F, Silah J. Further evidence of altered adrenocortical function in hypertension: dehydroepianodrosterol excretion rate. *J Physiol (London)* 1964;56:650–651.

59. Baulieu EE, Thomas G, Legrain S, et al. Dehydroepiandrosterone (DHEA), DHEA sulfate, and aging: contribution of the DHEAge Study to a sociobiomedical issue. *Proc Nat Acad Sci USA* 2000;97:4279–4284.

60. Wilson MMG, Morley JE. Impaired cognitive function and mental performance in mild dehydration. *Eur J Clin Nutr* 2003;57(suppl 2):S24–S29.

61. Phillips PA, Rolls BJ, Ledingham JGG. Reduced thirst after water deprivation in healthy elderly men. *N Engl J Med* 1984;311:753–759.

62. Yamamoto T, Harada H, Fukeiyama J, et al. Impaired arginine-vasopressin secretion associated with hypoangiotensinemia in hypernatremic dehydrated elderly patients. *JAMA* 1988;259:1039–1042.

63. Lindeman RD, Romero LJ, Liang HC, Baumgartner RN, Koehler KM, Garry PJ. Do elderly persons need to be encouraged to drink more fluids? *J Gerontol Med Sci* 2000;55A:M361–M365.

64. Helderman JH. The impact of normal aging on the hypothalamic-neurohypophyseal-renal axis. In: Korenman SG, ed. *Endocrine Aspects of Aging*. New York, NY: Elsevier-North Holland, NY; 1982.

65. Lindeman RD, Lee TD Jr, Yiengst MJ. Influences of age, renal diseases, hypertension, diuretics, and calcium on the antidiuretic responses to suboptimal infusions of vasopressin. *J Lab Clin Med* 1966; 68:206–223.

66. Ohashi M, Fujia N, Nawata H. High plasma concentrations of human atrial natriuretic polypeptide in aged men. *J Clin Endocrinol Metab* 1987; 64:81–85.

67. Miller M, Morley JE, Rubenstein LZ. Hyponatremia in nursing home population. *J Am Geriatr Soc* 1995;43:1410–1413.

68. Manson JMK, Wilmore DW. Positive nitrogen balance with human growth hormone and hypocaloric intravenous feeding. *Surgery* 1986;100:188–197.

69. Florini J, Prim PN, Vitiello MV. Somatomedin-C levels in healthy young and old men: relationship to peak and 24 hours integrated levels of growth hormone. *J Gerontol* 1985;40:2–7.

70. Rudman D, Nagraji HS, Mattson DE. Hyposomatomedinemia in the nursing home patient. *J Am Geriatr Soc* 1986;34:427–430.

71. Rudman D. Growth hormone, body composition and aging. *J Am Geriatr Soc* 1985;33:800–807.

72. Cohn L, Feller AG, Draper MW, Rudman IW, Rudman D. Carpal tunnel syndromes and gynaecomastia during growth hormone treatment of elderly men with low circulating IGF-I concentrations. *Clin Endocrinol* 1993; 39:417–425.

73. Papadakis MA, Grady D, Black D, et al. Growth hormone replacement in healthy older men improves body composition but not functional ability. *Ann Intern Med* 1996;124:708–716.

74. Kaiser FE, Silver AJ, Morley JE. The effect of recombinant human growth hormone on malnourished older individuals. *J Am Geriatr Soc* 1991; 39:235–240.

75. Chu LW, Lam KSL, Tam SCF, Hu WJHC, Hui SL, Chiu A, Chiu KC, Ng P. A randomized controlled trial of low-dose recombinant human growth hormone in the treatment of malnourished elderly medical patients. *J Clin Endocrinol Metab* 2001;86:1913–1920.

76. Takala J, Ruokonen E, Webster NR, et al. Increased mortality associated with growth hormone treatment in critically ill adults. *N Engl J Med* 1999;341:785–792.

77. Musaro A, McCullagh K, Paul A, et al. Localized IGF-1 transgene expression sustains hypertrophy and regeneration in senescent skeletal muscle. *Nature Genetics* 2001;27:195–200.

78. Kinsey AC, Pomeroy WB, Martin CE. *Sexual Behavior in the Human Male*. Philadelphia, PA: WB Saunders Co; 1948.

79. Slag MF, Morley JE, Elson MK, et al. Impotence in medical clinic outpatients. *JAMA* 1983;249:1736–1740.

80. Morley JE. Impotence. *Am J Med* 1986;80:897–905.

81. Billington CJ, Levine AS, Morley JE. Zinc status in impotent patients [abstract]. *Clin Res* 1983;31:714A.

82. Asthana S, Bhasin S, Butler RN, et al. Masculine vitality: pros and cons of testosterone in treating the andropause. *J Gerontol Med Sci* 2004;59A:461–465.

83. Morley JE, Perry HM. Andropause: an old concept in new clothing. *Clin Geriatr Med* 2003;19:507–528.

84. Morley JE, Perry HM. Androgen treatment of male hypogonadism in older males. *J Steroid Biochem Molecul Biol* 2003;85:367–373.

85. Mooradian AD, Morley JE, Korenman SG. Biological actions of androgens. *Endocrinol Rev* 1987; 8:1–28.

86. MacLaughlin J, Holick MF. Aging decreases the capacity of human skin to produce vitamin D3. *J Clin Invest* 1985;76:1536–1538.

87. Armbrecht HJ, Zenser TV, Davis BB. Effect of age on the conversion of 25-hydroxyvitamin D_3 to 1,25-dihydroxy-vitamin D_3 by kidney of rat. *J Clin Invest* 1980;66:1118–1123.

88. Perry HM, Horowitz M, Morley JE, et al. Longitudinal changes in serum 25-hydroxyvitamin D in older people. *Metab Clin Exper* 1999;48:1028–1032.

89. Chapuy MC, Arlot ME, Delmas PD, Meunier PJ. Effect of calcium and cholecalciferol treatment for three years on hip fractures in elderly women. *Brit Med J* 1994;308:1081–1082.

90. Bischoff-Ferrari HA, Dawson-Hughes B, Willet WC, et al. Effect of vitamin D on falls—a meta-analysis. *JAMA* 2004;291:1999–2006.

91. Morley JE, Gorbien MJ, Mooradian AD, et al. UCLA geriatric grand rounds: osteoporosis. *J Am Geriatr Soc* 1988;36:845–859.

92. Somaan NA, Anderson GD, Adam-Mayne ME. Immunoreactive calcitonin in mother, neonate, child and adult. *Am J Obstet Gynecol* 1975;121:622–625.

93. Nielson FH, Hunt CD, Mullen LM, et al. Effect of dietary boron on mineral, estrogen, and testosterone metabolism in postmenopausal women. *FASEB J* 1987;1:394–397.

94. Wilson MMG, Morley JE. Aging and energy balance. *J Appl Physiol* 2003;95:1728–1736.

95. Frisancho AR. New standards of weight and body composition by frame size and height for assessment of nutritional status of adults and the elderly. *Am J Clin Nutr* 1984;40:808–819.

96. Morley JE. Anorexia of aging: physiologic and pathologic. *Am J Clin Nutr* 1997;66:760–773.

97. Leibowitz SF. Neurochemical-neuroendocrine systems in the brain controlling macronutrient intake and metabolism. *Trends Neurosci* 1992;15:491–497.

98. Morley JE, Blundell JE. The neurobiological basis of eating disorders: some formulations. *Biol Psychiatry* 1988;23:53–78.

99. Morley JE. Neuropeptide regulation of appetite and weight. *Endocrinol Rev* 1987;8:256–287.

100. Morley JE, Levine AS, Yim GK, et al. Opioid modulation of appetite. *Neurosci Biobehav Rev* 1983;7:281–305.

101. Morley JE, Levine AS, Gosnell BA, et al. Effect of neuropeptide Y on ingestive behaviors in the rat. *Am J Physiol* 1987;252:R599–R609.

102. Gosnell BA, Levine AS, Morley JE. The effects of aging on opioid modulation of feeding in rats. *Life Sci* 1983;32:2793–2799.

103. MacIntosh CG, Sheehan J, Davani N, et al. Effects of aging on the opioid modulation of feeding in humans. *J Am Geriatr Soc* 2001;49:1518–1524.

104. Morley JE, Hernandez EN, Flood JF. Neuropeptide Y increases food intake in mice. *Am J Physiol* 1987;253:8516–8522.

105. Towle HC. Effects of thyroid hormones on cellular RNA metabolism. In: Oppenheimer JH, Samuels HH, eds. *Molecular Basis of Thyroid Hormone Action*. New York, NY: Academic Press; 1983.

106. York DA, Bray GA. Dependence of hypothalamic obesity on insulin, the pituitary, and the adrenal gland. *Endocrinology* 1972;90:885–894.

107. Bray GA. *The Obese Patient*. Philadelphia, PA: WB Saunders Co; 1976:9. Saunders Monographs on Major Problems in Internal Medicine.

108. Leibowitz SF, Roland CR, Hor L, et al. Noradrenergic feeding elicited via the paraventricular nucleus is dependent upon circulating corticosterone. *Physiol Behav* 1984;32:857–864.

109. Dalman MF. Viewing the ventromedial hypothalamus from the adrenal gland. *Am J Physiol* 1984;246:R1–R12.

110. Freedman MR, Castunguay TW, Stern JS. Effect of adrenalectomy and corticosterone replacement on meal patterns of Zucker rats. *Am J Physiol* 1985;249:R584–R594.

111. Hollifield G. Glucocorticoid-induced obesity: a model and a challenge. *Am J Clin Nutr* 1968;21:1471–1474.

112. Donhoffer SZ, Vonotzky J. The effect of thyroxine on food intake and selection. *Am J Physiol* 1947;150:334–339.

113. Wade GH, Zucker I. Modulation of food intake and locomotor activity in female rats by diencephalic hormone implants. *J Comp Physiol Psychol* 1978;72:328–336.

114. Wade GH, Zucker I. Development of hormonal control over food intake and body weight in female rats. *J Comp Physiol Psychol* 1970;70:213–220.

115. Numez AA, Grundman M. Testosterone affects food intake and body weight of weanling male rats. *Pharmacol Biochem Behav* 1982;16:933–936.

116. Khalil T, Walker JP, Wiener J, et al. Effect of aging on gallbladder contraction and release of cholecystokinin-33 in humans. *Surgery* 1985;98:423–429.

117. Morley JE. Anorexia and weight loss in older persons. *J Gerontol Med Sci* 2003;58A:131–137.

118. Silver AJ, Flood JF, Morley JE. Effect of gastrointestinal peptides on ingestion in young and old mice. *Peptides* 1988;9:221–226.

119. MacIntosh CG, Morley JE, Wishart J, et al. Effect of exogenous cholecystokinin (CCK)-8 on food intake and plasma CCK, leptin, and insulin concentrations in older and young adults: evidence for increased CCK activity as a cause of the anorexia of aging. *J Clin Endocrin Metab* 2001;86:5830–5837.

120. Morley JE, Perry HM, Baumgartner RP, Garry PJ. Leptin, adipose tissue and aging—is there a role for testosterone? *J Gerontol Biol Sci* 1999;54A:B108–B109.

121. Banks WA, Coon AB, Robinson SM, Moinuddin A, Shultz JM, Nakaoke R, Morley JE. Triglycerides induce leptin resistance at the blood-brain barrier. *Diabetes* 2004;53:1253–1260.

122. Garrow J. *Energy Balance and Obesity in Man.* New York, NY: American Elsevier; 1974.

123. Perry HM, Morley JE, Horowitz M, Kaiser FE, Miller DK, Wittert G. Body composition and age in African-American and Caucasian women: relationship to plasma leptin levels. *Metabolism* 1997;46:1399–1405.

124. Keynes RD. The energy cost of active transport. In: Bolis L, Manddrell HP, Schmidt-Nielsen K, eds. *Comparative Physiology: Functional Aspects of Structural Materials.* Amsterdam, Netherlands: North Holland Publishing Co; 1975.

125. Waterlow JC, Garlick PJ, Millward DJ. *Protein Turnover in Mammalian Tissues and in Whole Body.* New York, NY: Elsevier-North Holland; 1978.

126. Newsholme EA. A possible metabolic basis for the control of body weight. *N Engl J Med* 1980;302:400–405.

127. Guernsey DL, Edelman IS. Regulation of thermogenesis by thyroid hormones. In: Oppenheimer JH, Samuels HH, eds. *Molecular Basis of Thyroid, Hormone Action.* New York, NY: Academic Press; 1983.

128. Millward DJ. Human protein requirements: the physiological significance of changes in the rate of whole body protein turnover. In: Garrow JW, Holliday D, eds. *Substrate and Energy Metabolism in Man.* London, England: John Libbey; 1985.

129. Mariash CN, Oppenheimer JH. Thyroid hormone: carbohydrate interaction. In: Oppenheimer JH, Samuels HH, eds. *Molecular Basis of Thyroid Hormone Action.* New York, NY: Academic Press; 1983.

130. Rothwell NJ, Saville ME, Stock MI. Sympathetic and thyroid influences on metabolic rate in fed, fasted, and refed rats. *Am J Physiol* 1982;243:R339–R346.

131. Lipson LG, Bray GA. Energy. In: Chen LH, ed. *Nutritional Aspects of Aging.* Cleveland, OH: CRC Press; 1986.

132. Chernoff R, Lipschitz DA. Nutrition and aging. In: Shils ME, Young VR, eds. *Modern Nutrition in Health and Disease.* 7th ed. Philadelphia, PA: Lea & Febiger; 1988.

133. Young VR. Impact of aging on protein metabolism. In: Armbrecht HJ, Prendergast JM, Coe RM, eds. *Nutritional Intervention in the Aging Process.* New York, NY: Springer-Verlag; 1984.

134. Guernsey DL, Koebbe M, Thomas JE, et al. An altered response in the induction of cell membrane (Na+ K+) ATPase by thyroid hormone is characteristic of senescence in cultured human fibroblasts. *Mech Ageing Dev* 1986;33:283–293.

135. Evans WJ. Exercise and muscle metabolism in the elderly. In: Hutchinson ML, Munro HN, eds. *Nutrition and Aging.* New York, NY: Academic Press; 1986.

136. Singh MAF. Exercise comes of age: rationale and recommendations for a geriatric exercise prescription. *J Gerontol Med Sci* 2002;57A:M262–M282.

137. Glick Z. The thermic effect of a meal. *J Obes Weight Regul* 1987;6:170–178.

138. Rothwell NJ, Stock MJ. Diet-induced thermogenesis: concepts and mechanisms. *J Obes Weight Regul* 1987; 6:162–169.

139. Flatt JP. The biochemistry of energy expenditure. In: Bray GA, ed. *Recent Advances in Obesity Research: Proceedings of the 2nd International Congress on Obesity.* London, England: Newman Publishing; 1978.

140. Himms-Hagen J. Brown adipose tissue metabolism and thermogenesis. *Ann Rev Nutr* 1985;5:69–94.

CHAPTER 16

Pharmacology, Nutrition, and the Elderly: Interactions and Implications

R. Rebecca Couris, PhD, RPh, Kathleen M. Gura, PharmD, BCNSP, FASHP, and Jeffrey Blumberg, PhD, FACN, CNS

Despite the established recognition of the interactions between pharmacology and nutrition, especially in the elderly population, the clinical significance of this relationship remains largely unappreciated. Although much of the early information on this topic had been based on anecdotal reports, current understanding of the interactions among pharmacotherapeutics, nutrition, and aging has been reviewed and compiled such that many adverse outcomes can now be predicted and avoided.[1–11] The adverse consequences of drug-nutrient interactions in elderly people can include nutritional deficiency, drug toxicity, loss of drug efficacy and disease control, and unwanted changes in body weight.

Adverse drug reactions (ADR) are responsible for significant morbidity and mortality among elderly individuals. ADRs are expected to increase as the proportion of individuals over the age of 65 continues to grow over the next few decades. In 2011, the oldest member of the "baby boom generation" will turn 65, ushering in an increase of approximately 22 million individuals over the age of 65 in the decade that follows.[12] Even though they comprise about 13% of the population of the United States today, elderly people consume more than 25% of all prescription drugs, 50% of nonprescription drugs, and experience 39% of the ADR.[13–16] In 1984, the estimated annual expenditure on prescription drugs by the elderly population in the United States was $15 billion, a fourfold greater per capita expenditure on medications compared to younger individuals, making the elderly the largest consumers of legal drugs in the United States.[12] Although the relative contribution of drug-drug interactions and drug-nutrient interactions to this problem among elderly people has not been established, the disproportionately greater exposure to medications, along with age-related physiologic changes in pharmacokinetics and pharmacokinetics, coupled with the presence of multiple disease states and the poor nutritional status, suggests the increased likelihood of medication-related adverse events.

EXTENT AND PATTERNS OF DRUG USE BY THE ELDERLY

The growing numbers of elderly, and the multiple pathologic processes that affect them, inevitably lead to increased use of drugs in old age. Clinicians manage most illnesses in elderly patients with prescription drugs. Moreover, conditions such as memory loss, confusion, and changed sleep patterns are also treated with drug therapy by some physicians. Four of every five individuals over age 65 years are afflicted with chronic conditions such as heart disease, hypertension, arthritis, and diabetes; 35% have three or more of these problems.[17] Many older patients living at home take 3 or more different drugs daily; in institutions the quantity frequently increases to 10 or more different drugs per day.[18] This situation carries with it an increased likelihood of overprescribing practices, including inappropriate or excessive drug use, excessive dosage, and prolonged drug use. Drug interactions are especially likely in geriatric patients who use numerous prescription drugs coupled with self-administered therapies, such as over-the-counter (OTC) and herbal remedies.[19]

ADR events are a common form of preventable iatrogenic injury among older adults in all care settings.[20,21] Gurwitz and colleagues reported that among the 1.6 million United States residents of nursing homes, drug-related injuries are estimated to occur at a rate of 350,000 events per year, and more than half may be preventable.[22] There may be as many as 20,000 fatal or life-threatening ADR events per year among the nursing home population; of these, 80% may be preventable. A subsequent report noted that among 1523 identified ADR events that occurred in elderly patients in the ambulatory setting, 421 (27.6%) were considered preventable.[23] Cardiovascular drugs also were the most frequently implicated (24.5%), followed by diuretics (22.1%), nonopioid analgesics (15.4%), hypoglycemics (10.9%), anticoagulants (10.2%), and opioids (6.7%). Although antibiotics/anti-infectives were the second most common cause of ADR overall, they were associated with only 3.1% of all preventable ADR.

Cardiovascular drugs (eg, digitalis glycosides, diuretics, antiarrhythmics, antihypertensives, and anticoagulants) are the medication class most often prescribed for older patients, followed by psychoactive drugs (eg, neuroleptics and sedative hypnotics) and gastrointestinal drugs (eg, histamine 2 [H_2] blockers and laxatives) (Table 16–1).[18,23–25] More than 60% of the elderly population regularly use nonprescription drugs, especially nonnarcotic analgesics such as acetaminophen, antacids, antihistamines, and nutrient supplements.[26,27] Interestingly, the 10 most common medical conditions reported by elderly people during health interviews include (by rank) arthritis, hearing problems, heart diseases, hypertension, visual handicaps, digestive diseases, chronic sinusitis, mental and nervous disorders, genitourinary tract problems, and circulatory problems.[28] Therefore, despite the patterns of illness among older adults, actual prescribing practices and use of over-the-counter drugs may be different from the incidence of diseases.

The problems associated with trying to provide rational drug treatment for older people can be categorized as extrinsic issues (ie, drug prescription and drug compliance) and intrinsic issues (ie, age-related pharmacokinetic and pharmacodynamic changes).[29] Polypharmacy prescribing patterns provide elderly patients with more drugs than they can reasonably be expected

Table 16–1 Patterns of Drug Use by the Elderly

Therapeutic Class of Drug	Percentage of Prescriptions for Patients ≥65 Years			
	U.K.	Germany	Netherlands	Belgium
Peripheral vasodilators	68	67	68	65
Cardiac drugs	68	59	60	57
Diuretics	60	57	51	54
Antihypertensives	53	64	51	31
Psycholeptics	38	41	26	33
Antirrheumatics	43	37	25	31

to cope with in a practical way. This situation leads to difficulty with compliance and greatly increases the risk of drug-drug and drug-nutrient interactions. In the context of multiple diseases, treatment without drugs is often insufficiently explored, although the risk-benefit ratio is higher in older adults than in young people.

It has been noted that the withdrawal of drug treatment once the initial indication has resolved often requires greater initiative and discipline than the original act of prescribing. "Inherited therapy," when drugs started in middle age are automatically continued, is common among elderly people. Periodic reevaluation of all drugs prescribed on a chronic basis is an essential component of rational drug therapy.[30] There is now evidence that long-term drug treatment with some compounds (eg, hypnotics, diuretics, cardiotonic glycosides, and nonsteroidal anti-inflammatory agents) is not necessary for many patients. Some drug category–specific suggestions to minimize potential ADR in elderly patients are listed in Table 16–2.[31]

Even when prescribed appropriately, poor adherence is a major reason for therapeutic failure. Issues concerning compliance are not unique to elderly people, although they are more vulnerable to problems associated with packaging and labeling, difficult-to-follow regimens, and poor physician-patient communication about drug use. Often the patients themselves may share the blame for ADR due to noncompliance with their drug therapy. Studies have estimated noncompliance rates as high as 59% in the geriatric population.[22] Compliance also decreases when the older patient does not comprehend the importance or the directions for drug therapy. Intentional or unintentional changes in drug therapy by the elderly are frequent. Failing memory or vision may result in the patient dosing too frequently or not frequently enough. Many patients may remember their drugs by appearance rather than by name. If an alternate or generic brand is substituted by the pharmacist, the patient loses these visual cues which could result in medication errors. Transferring medications from their original container to another or combining multiple medications in the same container may lead to use of the wrong medication. Attention must also be directed to the self-medicating practices of the older individual; ubiquitous over-the-counter drugs and putative antiaging remedies

---

Table 16–2 Guidelines for Minimizing Adverse Drug Reactions in the Elderly

Drug Category	Recommendation
Antihypertensives	Select peripherally acting drugs; avoid agents with high lipophilic properties
Antiarrhythmics	Suspect cardiosensitivity
Diuretics	Suspect risk for electrolyte disturbances
Anxiolytics/Sedatives	Avoid long-acting agents with active metabolites
Anticoagulants	Suspect sensitivity to warfarin; monitor INR
Antidepressants/Antipsychotics	Select agents with the least amount of sedative, anticholinergic, and orthostatic hypotension side effects
Analgesics	Monitor use of salicylates and nonsteroidal anti-inflammatory agents; suspect central nervous system sensitivity
Antiulcer agents	Suspect drug interactions and adverse reactions
Hypoglycemic agents	Suspect altered kinetics and increased sensitivity
Antacids	Suspect risk for nutrient deficiencies; monitor for drug-drug interactions
Laxatives	Suspect risk for electrolyte disturbances and nutrient deficiencies

may interfere with other drugs and nutrients. Intrinsic factors of prescribing for the geriatric patient are discussed below.

The underuse of beneficial therapies may considerably dwarf overuse problems in this population. Such underuse problems have been identified in the management of a broad range of chronic conditions in elderly patients, including cardiovascular disease, hypertension, stroke prevention, osteoporosis prevention, pain management, and depression.[22] The rising cost of medications is also a contributing factor to the elderly not complying with their drug therapy. Because seniors are often on a limited income, they may fail to have prescribed medications filled. They may also skip doses attempting to make a prescription last longer or delay having medications refilled when they run out. Saving medications to use at a later time is associated with taking expired drugs. Borrowing or sharing medications can further exacerbate the situation. As would be expected, the more medications the patient takes, the greater the likelihood of noncompliance. Table 16–3 summarizes the factors that contribute to noncompliance with drug therapy in the elderly.

AGE-RELATED PHARMACOKINETIC CHANGES

Aging produces changes in pharmacokinetics (absorption, disposition, excretion) such that any given maintenance dose can lead to a higher steady-state concentration during repeated drug administration (Table 16–4).[32–34] However, before 1990, few geriatric patients participated in the premarketing phases of human studies because most studies of drug kinetics and efficacy were conducted in young and middle-aged patients. In 1997, the United States Food and Drug Administration (FDA) published guidelines encouraging the inclusion of elderly participants in trials of drugs likely to be used to treat diseases prevalent in older patients.[35] This led to improved labeling instructions to help guide therapeutic decisions, such as those on appropriate dosages for geriatric patients, and a "Geriatric Use Subsection" that contained further information specific to use of drugs in elderly patients. However, since many older drugs do not have such information, increased drug monitoring is essential in elderly individuals because the clinical basis for quantitatively predicting changes in pharmacokinetics is not available for all compounds. Lower initial doses are usually indicated in treating elderly patients.

Absorption

Although few studies have evaluated drug absorption in the elderly, there is considerable evidence that advancing age is associated with reduced absorption of many nutrients, such as calcium, folic acid, thiamine, and vitamin B_{12}. With the exception of a few acidic drugs (eg, aspirin), maximal absorption of most drugs and nutrients takes place in the small bowel, so gastric emptying and intestinal transit time have significant impact on the rate and magnitude of the oral absorption of the drugs and certain nutrients. In most instances, age-related physiologic changes in the gastrointestinal (GI) tract that could affect

---

Table 16–3 Factors That Contribute to Noncompliance with Drug Therapy

Borrowing/Sharing Medication	Number of Medications
Cognitive deficits/memory loss	Physical limitations (can't open container, read the label)
Drug cost	Scheduling difficulties
Hoarding medication for future use	Self-medication with OTC/herbals
Improper storage/transferring to another container	Transportation issues
Lack of understanding	Using expired medications

Table 16–4 Physiologic Changes Relevant to Pharmacokinetics in the Elderly

Pharmacokinetic Step		Age-Related Changes*
Absorption	↓	Absorptive surface
	↓	Splanchnic blood flow
	↑	Gastric pH
	↓	Gastrointestinal motility
	↓	Gastric secretion
	↓	Pancreatic trypsin
	↓	Gastric emptying
		Malabsorption
	↑	Blood levels of water-soluble drugs
Distribution	↓	Lean body mass
	↓	Total body water
	↓	Serum albumin
	↑	Body fat
	↑	Serum α-glycoprotein
	↓	Cardiac output
	↓	Cerebral blood flow
	↑/↓	Membrane permeability
	↓	Drug binding
	↓	Blood levels of fat-soluble drugs
Metabolism	↓	Hepatic mass
	↓	Hepatic flood flow
	↑/↓	Enzyme activity/inducibility
Excretion	↓	Renal blood flow
	↓	Glomerular filtration
	↓	Tubular secretion

* ↑, increased; ↓ decreased; ↑/↓, change dependent on specific drug.

drug absorption, such as decreases in gastric emptying, splanchnic blood flow, and intestinal motility, are overcome to a considerable degree by the very large capacity of the system for passive absorption of small-molecular-weight compounds. Drugs absorbed via active transport may be affected by the age-related decline in the efficiency of these mechanisms.[36] The presence of chronic diseases and the interference of foods can further alter drug pharmacokinetics. Other changes may include decreased salivation, decreased gastric acidity, and increased intestinal transit time. Thus, absorption of drugs normally soluble in acid (eg, dipyridamole, itraconazole) could be slowed when gastric pH increases.

However, an increase in intestinal transit time may compensate for this phenomenon.[37]

Distribution

Age-related changes in body composition, such as the increase in adipose tissue and loss of skeletal muscle, can affect drug distribution. These changes are more marked in women than in men. Whereas a significant gain of fat mass, decrease in total body water, and/or a loss of lean mass (sarcopenia) has been noted in healthy individuals over 70, very old subjects lose fat and muscle and this tendency is amplified when malnutrition occurs. Body composition changes may lead to changes in the metabolism of drugs via several mechanisms like changes in the volume of distribution or protein-binding capacity. The volume of distribution (Vd) is the space in which a drug is stored in the body. The Vd for lipophilic drugs (eg, diazepam, lidocaine) and hydrophilic drugs (eg, acetaminophen, digoxin, morphine) can thus be altered in older patients. For example, the elimination half-life of diazepam has been shown to increase in a linear manner with age due to an increased Vd.[38,39]

Plasma protein binding of drugs also alters drug distribution and is affected by age-related declines in serum albumin levels. Decreased protein binding in the presence of lowered albumin levels has been demonstrated for antipyrine, meperidine, phenytoin, propranolol, salicylates, and warfarin.[40,41] Although many drugs exhibit decreased binding (increased free fraction) in elderly subjects, a few show increased binding because of a greater affinity for α_1-acid glycoprotein, which increases with age, than for albumin.[42] It should be noted, however, that in many instances alterations in plasma protein binding seen in the elderly are not age-related, but are due to physiological and pathophysiologic changes or disease states that may occur more frequently in the elderly, thus accounting for altered protein binding. Age-related physiological changes, such as decreased renal function, decreased hepatic function, and decreased cardiac output, generally produce more clinically significant alterations in drug disposition than that seen with alterations in drug plasma protein binding.[43] Hypoalbuminemia is accompanied by a diminished protein-binding capacity, which leads to an increased free concentration of extensively protein-bound drugs. This situation can result in an increase in free drug concentrations and may put patients at risk of developing toxic drug levels, especially for medications with a narrow therapeutic index (digoxin, warfarin, sulfamides, theophylline, and lithium). Although changes in protein binding can be an important factor in determining drug dosage, it is difficult to establish a direct relationship because such changes occur along with concomitant alterations in the Vd and the metabolic clearance of the drug.

Metabolism

The metabolism of orally administered drugs involves various steps that present opportunities for drug-nutrient interactions. Presystemic clearance (first-pass metabolism) occurs primarily in the intestine and the liver, whereas the stomach appears to play only a minor role.[44,45] Phase I biotransformation creates more polar compounds, usually via oxidation, reduction, and hydroxylation reactions, that may either activate or deactivate the drug. Phase II biotransformations are a synthetic process, involving conjugation of the drug or its initial metabolites with glucuronic acid, sulfate, glutathione, glycine or acetate, creating more hydrophilic compounds that can be more readily excreted into bile or urine.[46] Thus, reduced hepatic blood flow can decrease first-pass metabolism and increase the half-life of some medications, eg, phenobarbital and diazepam. It is worth noting that some drugs do not pass through phase I prior to phase II metabolism, eg, lorazepam, undergoes glucuronidation directly by UGT2B7 with its conjugated metabolite then is excreted via the kidney. The enzyme system responsible for the oxidative metabolism of a very wide range of both nutrients and drugs is the cytochrome P450 enzyme super family (CYP), principally located in the endoplasmic reticulum of hepatocytes and enterocytes. CYP is markedly impaired by severe malnutrition.[47]

Hepatic function and perfusion tend to be diminished in older adults.[48] Pharmacokinetic studies suggest that diminished hepatic oxidative (phase I) metabolism reduces the clearance of many drugs in geriatric patients. However, this decline is not universal, due in part to the differential effects of aging on individual CYP 450 isozymes.[32,49] A decrease in the metabolic clearance of drugs such as antipyrine, barbiturates, diazepam, and phenylbutazone, is indicative of reduced oxidative drug-metabolizing enzyme activity in the elderly.[41,50,51] A reduction in biotransformation capacity decreases total drug clearance and results in higher steady-state plasma concentrations during repeated drug administration (Table 16–5). Experimental studies

Table 16–5 Drugs Showing Reduction in Hepatic Biotransformation in the Elderly

Alprazolam	Meperidine HCl
Antipyrine	Midazolam
Carbenoxolone sodium	Norepinephrine
Celecoxib	Nortriptyline HCl
Chlordiazepoxide	Oxazepam
Chlormethiazole	Phenytoin
Clobazam	Piroxicam
Desalkylfurazepam	Propanolol
Desmethyldiazepam	Procainamide
Desipramine	Propranolol
Diltiazem	Quinidine
Imipramine	Quinine
Isoniazid	Theophylline
Indocyanine green	Trazodone
Lidocaine	Triazolam
Lorazepam	Verapamil

Table 16–6 Examples of Medications Showing a Reduction in Renal Excretion in the Elderly

Acetohexamide	Kanamycin
Acetylprocainamide	Levofloxacin
Amikacin	Lisinopril
Ampicillin	Lithium
Atenolol	Methotrexate
Azapropazone	Nadolol
Cefuroxime	Nizatidine
Cephalothin	Ofloxacin
Cephradine	Pancuronium bromide
Chlorpropamide	Penicillin
Ciprofloxacin	Phenobarbital
Cimetidine	Quinapril
Digoxin	Quinidine
Dihydrostreptomycin	Ramipril
Dofetilde	Ranitidine
Doxycycline	Sotalol HCl
Enalapril	Sparfloxacin
Ethambutol	Streptomycin
Famotidine	Sulfamethizole
Gentamicin	Tetracycline
Glyburide	Tobramycin
Imipenem	Vancomycin

indicate drugs metabolized principally via phase II reactions appear to be less influenced by age.[32, 34, 36,38–42, 49–52] However, studies with nonhuman primates indicate that conclusions drawn from the extensive data on hepatic metabolism in rodent models may not be completely relevant to humans.[53–55] For example, the decline in liver size with age in humans does not occur in rats and may account, in part, for the lower drug-metabolizing capacity in older people.[53,56] When evaluating the potential impact of these changes, it should be noted that standard liver function tests do not predict hepatic metabolism because they reflect synthetic, not degradation, function.

Excretion

Most drugs and their metabolites are eliminated via urinary excretion so changes in renal function can affect the drug clearance. Renal blood flow declines linearly with age as does the kidney's ability to acidify, concentrate, and dilute urine. The glomerular filtration rate (GFR) falls approximately 1 mL/min each year after age 40. The reduction of renal function (ie, GFR, tubular secretion, and total renal plasma flow) and the decrease in nephrons and renal mass underlie the slower rate of drug elimination in elderly individuals.[41,57]

Diminished renal function may be the most important single factor responsible for altered drug levels in older people (Table 16–6). Decreased muscle mass with aging is associated with decreased creatinine synthesis, so "normal" blood urea nitrogen (BUN) and creatinine values do not necessarily indicate normal renal function in the elderly. Drug dosages should be adjusted in older patients by taking into account their reduced creatinine clearances, not their serum creatinine levels. Steady-state GFR estimates are readily accomplished with the use of the Cockcroft-Gault equation: $140 - \text{age} \times \text{weight}$ (kg, lean) $/72 \times$ serum creatine (mg/dL) $\times 0.85$ (for women). The presence of obesity may lead to an underestimation of GFR, while in frail geriatric patients, the equation tends to an overestimate of creatinine clearance by as much as 20%, because of the lack of correlation between lean body weight and muscle mass. If such measurements cannot be obtained, nomograms are available that adjust for the expected change related to both age and sex.[58] In addition to the normal decline in renal function with aging, a variety of conditions (eg, congestive heart failure, dehydration, hypotension, and diabetes) can further reduce renal elimination of drugs.[59]

AGE-RELATED PHARMACODYNAMIC CHANGES

Despite the various alterations in pharmacokinetics that occur with different drugs in geriatric patients and the associated changes in drug efficacy with toxicity, there remains a significant residue of altered responsiveness; this can be explained by differences in sensitivity to the drugs.[34] Many factors contribute to the different response to drugs by older people compared to those in young adults. Pharmacodynamic theories suggest that altered pharmacologic effects result from age-related changes in drug receptors, homeostasis, or tissue sensitivity (Q). These components may have different weights, depending on the drug and the individual. Pharmacodynamic explanations are difficult to test in vivo and most studies depend on comparisons of correlations of drug effects versus simultaneously measured plasma drug concentrations, ie, demonstrating different responses between young and old subjects with similar tissue exposures to the drug.

Receptors

Mechanisms for age-related alterations in target tissue sensitivity could include changes in receptor number or affinity, receptor regulation, or translation of binding into a response. Elderly patients are less responsive to β-adrenergic agonists and more responsive to β-adrenergic antagonists as a result of alterations in the cyclic adenosine monophosphate (cAMP) second-messenger system.[60,61] On the other hand, α-adrenergic receptors do not appear to change with age.[62] Age-related changes have also been documented for brain benzodiazepine receptors and several hormone receptors.[63] The pharmacologic effects

of cholinergic agonists increase with age, while those of parasympathetic antagonists produce less response in the heart rates of geriatric patients. The beneficial effects of anticholinergics have been reported to decrease while their ADR become more hazardous to elderly subjects. The progressive depletion of brain dopamine with age enhances the risk of drug-induced extrapyramidal side effects. Baroreceptor sensitivity is responsible for the high incidence of drug-induced orthostatic hypotension.[64] Age-related alterations in receptor-drug interactions are difficult to evaluate because of the influence of confounding factors such as disease, previous drug exposure, and nonreceptor drug-binding sites.

Homeostasis

A reduced homeostatic vitality may be the basis of some examples of increased drug sensitivity among the elderly. The ventilatory response to hypoxic challenge is affected by age, with direct consequences for hypoxic disease states and drug therapy. Older people also tend to show a decreased response to dietary challenges in acid-base balance; eg, ammonium chloride lowers blood pH and prolongs recovery time more markedly in older than in young subjects, despite identical resting steady-state conditions. Older people are also less able to regulate blood glucose levels, pulse rate, blood pressure, and oxygen consumption, but to varying degrees. These variations are great enough to preclude clinically useful generalizations.[65,66]

Tissue Sensitivity

Mechanisms for age-related alterations in target tissue sensitivity often appear to be based on changes in receptor number, affinity, or signal translation. However, many altered drug actions can be ascribed partially to age-related changes in the cardiovascular, endocrine, and central nervous systems. With age, decreases in cellular brain mass, sensory condition time, and cerebral blood flow may contribute to a greater vulnerability to adverse drug effects such as confusion, falls, and urinary incontinence.[63] Changes with age in the cardiovascular system result in a decreased response of the heart to stress and catecholamines and altered sensitivity to the toxic effects of some drugs. Alterations in pancreatic and adrenal hormone levels result in decreased glucose tolerance with age and an increased susceptibility of older patients to drug-induced hypoglycemia.[67] With age, there is a progressive decline in pulmonary function and a greater rigidity of the lung, which may cause an exaggerated respiratory depression after administration of narcotic analgesics. Decreases in thyroid hormone levels can make elderly individuals less sensitive to ß-adrenergic sympathomimetics and more sensitive to digitalis and drug-induced hypothermia.[68] An age-related reduction in the synthesis of hepatic blood-clotting factors may underlie an increased sensitivity to oral anticoagulant drugs. Age- and nutrient-induced declines in immune responsiveness may alter the expected efficacy of antibiotic and antiviral medications. Physiologic losses of vestibular and cochlear hair cells and ganglia make geriatric patients more susceptible to irreversible drug-induced hearing loss.

FOOD CHOICE AND NUTRITIONAL STATUS OF THE ELDERLY

Economic, physical, psychosocial, and pathologic factors may significantly affect elderly people's accessibility to food (Table 16–7). These elements may result from lack of money to purchase food; physical disability; loss of spouse, affecting motivation to cook and eat; isolation from family and community; limited knowledge concerning balanced diets; and existing disease processes. Chronic conditions such as arthritis, impaired hearing and vision, coronary heart disease, and other physical disabilities may affect health such that the ability to carry out food-related activities (eg, shopping and cooking) is significantly affected. Reduced appetite and food intake due to decreases in taste sensitivity, inability to chew, or problems in swallowing make eating more difficult and less pleasurable. Age-related changes in body composition and physiologic function also alter the dietary requirement for some nutrients.

National surveys reveal that substantial numbers of older adults are seriously lacking in adequate intake of some nutrients, including calories, calcium, and vitamin D. In some studies, over half of the respondents fail to meet the recommended level of calorie intake and two-thirds have less than adequate calcium intake. Decreasing energy intake with advancing age has important implications for the diet in terms of protein, vitamins, and minerals. Allowances for these nutrients assume that elderly people actually consume levels of energy that considerably exceed the amounts of food actually consumed. Dietary quality becomes difficult to assure when overall energy intake is low; prudent diets in elderly individuals require a careful selection of nutrient-dense foods. Energy intake decreases more rapidly in the very old because of disabilities that limit physical activity. Many elderly eat few fruits and vegetables, particularly vitamin A– and vitamin C–rich varieties. Despite the widespread use of enriched breads and cereals, low intake of the B-complex vitamins is common in the aged. Many studies demonstrate, however, that elderly people who take advantage of community services providing nutritional support, particularly those in congregate settings, show improved overall dietary intake and nutritional status.

Although the prevalence of nutrient supplementation among elderly people is high, exceed-

Table 16–7 Factors Affecting Food Choices of the Elderly

Primary Factors	Secondary Factors
Poverty	Chronic drug therapy
Social isolation/ depression	Gastrointestinal disorders/ malabsorption
Loss of spouse	Disease/pathologic processes
Physical disability	Alcoholism
Poor dentition	Inadequate knowledge of nutrition

ing 50% in some areas, the use of such supplements often appears irrational and inappropriate to their needs.[69] As with drug regimens, there can be serious problems in compliance with nutritional therapies for chronic disease.[70] The generally poor nutritional status of hospitalized and institutionalized elderly patients has been well documented.[71]

Nutrient Interactions and the Elderly Patient

A drug-nutrient interaction is defined as an alteration of kinetics or dynamics of a drug or a nutritional element or a compromise in nutritional status as a result of the addition of a drug.[72] There are four principal types of drug-nutrient interactions based on the nature and the mechanisms of the interactions: (1) Ex vivo bioinactivation refers to interactions between the drug and the nutrient(s) or dietary formulation through either a biochemical or physical reaction. Examples of this type of interaction involve hydrolysis, oxidation, neutralization, precipitation, and complexation. These reactions usually take place when the interacting agents are in direct physical contact and occur usually before the nutrients or drugs enter the body. (2) Interactions affecting absorption impact drugs and nutrients delivered by mouth or via enteral delivery devices. These interactions cause either an increase or decrease of oral bioavailability of the affected agent. In some cases, the causative agent may modify the function of an enzyme or an active transport mechanism responsible for the biotransformation or transport of the affected drug or nutrient. (3) Interactions affecting systemic/physiologic disposition occur after the drug or the nutrient has been absorbed from the GI tract and has entered the systemic circulation. The mechanisms involve changing the cellular or tissue distribution, systemic metabolism, or transport of the affected agent. In some cases, the interaction between the causative agent and the drug (or nutrient) may involve changing the function of other cofactors (eg, clotting factors) or hormones. (4) Interactions affecting the elimination or clearance of drugs or nutrients may involve enhancing or re-

ducing renal or enterohepatic elimination of a particular agent.

The elderly are at particular risk for drug-nutrient interactions. Several factors may influence these possible interactions, including: (1) the typically higher dietary or nutrient needs of older compared to young people; (2) the systems for detoxification of nutrients can be impaired with age; and (3) the elderly tend to restrict food intake and thus are unable to meet recommended micronutrient intakes.[73] Further, the minimum dietary requirement may be insufficient when a patient is under pathological stresses. Decreased active intestinal transport and an increased propensity for atrophic gastritis may also reduce the absorption of vitamins A, B_1, B_{12}, and folate. Moreover, decreased exposure to sunlight and reduced cutaneous synthesis impair the vitamin D status. When recognized, the negative effects of drug-vitamin interactions can be minimized with adequate vitamin supplementation and modification of the patient's drug regimen.

DRUG EFFECTS ON NUTRITIONAL STATUS

Several classification schemes have been proposed to categorize the ways in which drugs affect nutritional status.[74] Although many of these schemes provide a sense of coherence and organization to the topic, there are difficulties or limitations with each scheme. The reason for this situation is the lack of any comprehensive theory underlying the numerous biochemical and clinical observations that have been reported. For the purpose of this discussion, it is useful to employ the same scheme used to illustrate the interaction between aging and pharmacokinetics (Table 16–8).

Drugs may potentially cause vitamin deficiencies ranging from subclinical status to clinical manifestations. The intensity of the interaction may in many cases be dependent upon the nutritional status of the patient. Patients with borderline micronutrient intakes or those in poor nutritional health appear to be at greater risk of developing symptomatic deficiency states. Other

Table 16–8 Drug-Induced Alterations in Nutrient Kinetics

Drug Category/ Medication	Kinetic Alteration	Mechanism*	Affected Nutrient
Anticoagulants			
Warfarin	metabolism	↓ reductase/carboxylation	vitamin K
Anti-infectives			
Antibiotics (general)	absorption	Δ bacterial flora	vitamins B_1, B_2, B_6, B_{12}, K, biotin
Cephalosporins	metabolism	↓ reductase/carboxylation	vitamin K
Tetracyclines	absorption	chelation	Ca
Neomycin	absorption	mucosal injury	Na, K, Ca, vitamins B_{12}, K
Trimethoprim	metabolism	folate antagonist	folic acid
Isoniazid	metabolism	↓ pyridoxal kinase and ↓ hepatic/renal vitamin D hydroxylation	vitamin B_6 Ca
Anticonvulsants			
Phenobarbital	metabolism	Δ vitamin D metabolites ↑ hepatic microsomal enzymes	vitamin D, Ca, folic acid
Phenytoin	metabolism	Δ vitamin D metabolites ↑ hepatic microsomal enzymes	vitamin D, Ca, folic acid
Antihypertensives			
Vasodilators	metabolism	↓ pyridoxal kinase	vitamin B_6
Loop diuretics	excretion	↑ renal excretion	Na, K, Ca, Cr, Mg, Zn, vitamins B_1, B_6
Thiazide diuretics	excretion	↑ renal excretion	Na, K, Mg, Zn
Triamterene/	excretion	↑ renal excretion	Na, Ca
Hydrochlorothiazide	metabolism	↓ dihydrofolate reductase	folic acid
Antihyperlipidemics			
Cholestyramine	absorption	adsorption to anion	vitamins A, D, E, K, B_{12},
Colestipol		exchange resin	β-carotene Ca, Fe, Zn folic acid
Anti-inflammatory			
Prednisone	metabolism	↓ hepatic/renal vitamin D hydroxylation	vitamin D, Ca
Colchicine	absorption	mucosal injury	vitamin B_{12}
Sulfasalazine	metabolism	dihydrofolate reductase	folic acid
Indomethacin	absorption	mucosal injury	vitamin C, Fe
Sulindac	metabolism	dihydrofolate reductase	folic acid
Aspirin	absorption	mucosal injury	vitamin C, Fe
	excretion	competition for binding sites	folic acid

continues

Table 16–8 continued

Drug Category/ Medication	Kinetic Alteration	Mechanism*	Affected Nutrient
Antineoplastics			
(general)	absorption	mucosal injury	most nutrients
Methotrexate	metabolism	folate antagonist	folic acid
Antiulcer Agents			
H_2 receptor antagonists	absorption	↓ gastric acid secretion	vitamin B_{12}, folic acid, Fe, Zn
Cimetidine			
Famotidine	metabolism	↓ hepatic/renal vitamin D hydroxylation	vitamin D, calcium
Proton Pump Inhibitors	absorption	↓ gastric acid secretion	vitamin B_{12}, folic acid, Fe, Zn
Omeprazole			
Lansoprazole	metabolism	↓ hepatic/renal vitamin D hydroxylation	vitamin D, calcium
Antacids			
Aluminum and magnesium hydroxides	absorption	precipitation and ↓ gastric acid secretion	phosphate, vitamin B_{12}, folic acid, Fe, Zn
Sodium bicarbonate	absorption	↓ gastric acid secretion	vitamin B_{12}, folic acid, Fe, Zn
Laxatives			
Lubricants			
Mineral oil	absorption	solubilization	vitamins A, D, E, K, ß-carotene
Stimulant Cathartics			
Phenolphthalein	absorption	↑ GI motility	K, Ca, vitamin D
Psychotherapeutics			
Tricyclic Antidepressants			
Amitriptyline	metabolism	↓ flavin adenine dinucleotide	vitamin B_2
Neuroleptics			
Chlorpromazine	metabolism	↓ flavin adenine dinucleotide	vitamin B_2

* ↑, increase/induce; ↓, decrease/inhibit; Δ; change.

factors include the type of drug treatment, the dose, and duration of therapy, as well as the age of the patient.[73] For example, individuals on a normal diet rarely become vitamin K deficient. However, malnourished patients (regardless of cause) often have moderate or significant deficiency with prolonged bleeding times.[75] Cohen and colleagues reported that hospitalized patients may become vitamin K deficient within 7 to 10 days after admission, with those at greatest risk being those who were previously malnourished and had received antibiotics for 7 or more days.[76]

Absorption of Nutrients

The best described and most frequent type of drug-nutrient interaction results from drug-induced alteration of nutrient absorption.[77] Drugs cause malabsorption by exerting an effect in the intestinal lumen or by impairing the absorptive ability of the GI mucosa. These effects can be limited and specific for a particular nutrient or they can be general and can affect an entire class of nutrients, such as fat-soluble vitamins or trace minerals. Drugs may decrease nutrient bioavailability by a variety of mechanisms, including adsorption of the nutrient itself or of bile acids, therefore inhibiting the intraluminal phase of fat digestion and absorption. Drugs may form insoluble precipitates or chelate with a nutrient. Drugs may also affect the environment of the GI lumen through changes in pH, motility, or composition of bacterial flora.[78]

Some drugs may damage the intestinal mucosa and destroy the structure of the villi and microvilli, resulting in an inhibition of brush-border enzymes and intestinal transport systems needed for nutrient absorption. The malabsorptive effect of colchicine, neomycin, and p-aminosalicylic acid appears to be the result of such mucosal injury.

Drugs may also interfere with nutrient absorption through secondary mechanisms. Drugs can impair digestion of food directly via initial adverse effects on gastric or intestinal secretion, pancreatic exocrine function, or hepatic bile secretion. Malabsorption of glucose, xylose, and amino acids has been observed when using nonsteroidal anti-inflammatory drugs (indomethacin) and antidiabetic drugs (sulfonylureas).[79] Proton pump inhibitors (eg, omeprazole, lansoprazole) and H_2 antagonists (eg, cimetidine, ranitidine), because of their inhibitory effects on gastric acid productions, reduce the liberation of vitamin B_{12} from its protein-bound state, making it less avail-

able for association with intrinsic factor.[79] Further, in older adults with atrophic gastritis, changes in bacterial flora result in colonies with an increased affinity for vitamin B_{12}, making the nutrient less bioavailable.[80] Chronic effects of hepatotoxic drugs, notably alcohol, include maldigestion with reduced absorption of fats and fat-soluble vitamins.[81] Direct systemic effects of a drug on one nutrient may also have secondary consequences on another nutrient. For example, drugs such as isoniazid[82] and cimetidine,[83] which inhibit the hepatic or renal hydroxylation of vitamin D, and those such as phenytoin[84] and phenobarbital,[85] which promote the catabolism of vitamin D metabolites, produce a functional deficiency of vitamin D with a secondary impairment in calcium absorption.

Alterations in vitamin and mineral absorption can also occur due to chelation or precipitation by a medication. Hypolipidemic drugs of the absorbable and nonabsorbable types may improve lipid status and decrease the risk of coronary artery disease, but pose nutritional hazards.[86] Cholestyramine is a basic anion-exchange resin that binds salts and impairs the absorption of a number of nutrients including β-carotene; vitamins A, B_{12}, D, K; folic acid; and the minerals calcium, iron, and zinc.[87] Clofibrate and colestipol have similar, although less pronounced, effects. Aluminum and magnesium hydroxide-containing antacids may form nonabsorbable phosphate in the gut lumen, resulting in hypophosphatemia along with anorexia and secondary syndromes of hypomagnesemia and osteomalacia.[88] Moreover, antacids, by increasing gastric pH, can negatively impact the bioavailability of riboflavin and folic acid as well as copper and iron, all of which are dependent upon a low pH.[89]

Several classes of OTC drugs may induce adverse nutritional effects. Indeed, drug-induced malnutrition in the elderly may be commonly due to their excessive use of OTC drugs such as antacids, laxatives, and nonnarcotic analgesics.[90] As noted, antacids formulated with aluminum and magnesium hydroxides form nonabsorbable phosphates in the GI lumen and may induce hypophosphatemia[91] with the development of proximal limb muscle weakness, malaise, paresthesias, anorexia, and secondary syndromes of hypomagnesemia, tetany,[92] and osteomalacia.[93] These antacids have also been associated with impaired absorption of riboflavin, copper, and iron. Excessive use of sodium bicarbonate can result in sodium overload and may render the pH of the jejunum sufficiently alkaline to decrease the absorption of folic acid.[94]

Laxative abuse is common among the elderly and has been implicated in cases of malabsorption of vitamin D and calcium. Use of irritant laxatives, such as phenolphthalein and bisacodyl, may damage GI epithelial cells and impair colonic reabsorption, resulting in steatorrhea or protein losing enteropathy, and decrease the absorption of glucose, potassium, calcium, and vitamin D.[95,96] Other stool regimen medications, such as the stool softener, docusate, alter electrolyte transport and induce hypomagnesemia due to GI losses and failure of colonic reabsorption.[97] Orally ingested mineral oil can coat ingested food particles along with the surface of the intestines to form a mechanical barrier to the digestion and absorption of nutrients. Mineral oil also increases gastric motility, which reduces the time required to adequately absorb ingested nutrients.[98] Mineral oil, especially when taken at mealtime or during the postprandial absorptive period, can reduce the absorption of vitamin D.[98] In geriatric patients, the risks of hypokalemia and potassium deficiency with the attendant hazards of cardiac arrhythmias, digitalis toxicity, and hyperglycemia are associated with concurrent use of laxatives and thiazide diuretics.[99] Osteomalacia resulting from excessive laxative use has also been reported.[100]

Anti-inflammatory drugs such as aspirin and indomethacin produce multiple small hemorrhages of the GI mucosa, leading to iron deficiency anemia and decreased absorption of vitamin C.[101] Chronic aspirin therapy is also associated with folic acid deficiency and macrocytic anemia; the greatest risk occurs in patients with a low intake of folic acid.[102] Colchicine has been noted to decrease the absorption of protein, fat, lactose, β-carotene, vitamin B_{12}, sodium, potassium, and bile acids as a result of villous damage.[103]

Physical and chemical interactions between food and drugs may also occur with the use of enteral feeding tubes, which allow easy access for administering drugs to patients unable to swallow. Enteral feeding formulas, however, have been implicated in a number of drug-nutrient interactions. For example, the oral absorption of warfarin, tetracycline, fluoroquinolone antibiotics, and phenytoin are decreased with concomitant enteral feeding.[104–108] Possible mechanisms of action include a decrease in the anticoagulant effect of warfarin caused by increased vitamin K absorption from the enteral formulas or binding of warfarin by a protein component of the enteral formula.[106,107] Drug-nutrient interactions through chelation of divalent and trivalent cations have also been proposed. Enteral feeding formulas and dairy products interact with fluoroquinolones through chelation at the 3-carboxy and 4-oxy functional groups resulting in the formation of nonabsorbable quinolone-cation complexes. Other possible drug interactions with enteral nutrition components have been extensively reviewed.[104,109,110] Esophageal obstruction due to solidification of enteral feed refluxed from the stomach has also been reported in patients also being administered drugs, eg, sucralfate, via the tube.[111]

Drug Effects on Nutrient Transport

There are several mechanisms by which a drug can impact nutrient transport and increase the risk of nutritional deficiencies. For example, a nutrient can be displaced from its plasma protein binding sites by a drug, leading to an increase in its renal excretion. Additionally, a drug may compete with a nutrient such that intracellular utilization of the nutrient is impaired, as when folate stores are depleted in patients receiving therapeutic doses of aspirin.[112]

Metabolism of Nutrients

Drugs may affect nutrient metabolism by inhibiting its essential intermediary metabolism or promoting its catabolism. Drugs with these properties may be used therapeutically, like the "anti-nutrient" actions of coumarin anticoagulants and methotrexate against vitamin K and folate, respectively.[113] In contrast, this action may create an untoward side effect, eg, the antagonism of pyridoxal kinase by isoniazid and hydralazine resulting in depleted pyridoxine stores, reduced γ-aminobutyric acid neurotransmission, and lowered seizure thresholds. Administration of pyridoxine in cases of isoniazid overdose eliminates seizures and metabolic acidosis.[114]

Many drugs induce drug metabolism enzymes, increasing the demand for their vitamin cofactors. Together with chronic drug therapy and marginal nutrient intakes, this interaction can precipitate vitamin deficiencies. Triamterene inhibits dihydrofolate reductase resulting in megalobastosis.[115] Antihyperlipidemic statins, which are HMG-CoA reductase inhibitors, reduce the synthesis and plasma status of ubiquinone (coenzyme Q), a cellular antioxidant.[116]

Patients receiving chronic anticonvulsant therapy are at particular risk of developing metabolic bone disease as a result of these nutrient deficiencies.[117] For example, phenytoin, a microsomal enzyme inducer, stimulates the catabolism of vitamin D to produce an inactive metabolite.[118] Early studies investigating this interaction were confounded because they were conducted in institutionalized patients who were predisposed to other risk factors, such as poor dietary vitamin D intake and/or reduced exposure to sunlight.[117] Further, phenytoin, alone or in combination with phenobarbital, interferes with vitamin K metabolism with a corresponding elevation in serum osteocalcin levels without α-carboxyglutamate (Gla) residues, resulting in metabolic bone disease since osteocalcin containing Gla residues are necessary for normal bone mineralization.[119]

Patients treated with cephalosporin antibiotics may develop a hemorrhagic syndrome due to drug-induced vitamin K deficiency.[120,121] These antibiotics block vitamin K reductase, a reaction necessary to vitamin K activation.[122] They may also block carboxylation of vitamin K–dependent peptides to yield Gla residues required for calcium binding during the conversion of vitamin K–dependent pro-enzymes to their active state. This antagonism inhibits the normal coagulation cascade.[122]

Some drugs have been linked with subnormal serum folate levels due to the weak binding of folate to serum proteins such that this vitamin can be readily displaced by drugs.[123] The mechanism for this interaction has not been fully elucidated, but appears, in part, the result of a decrease in serum binding of methyltetrahydrofolate caused by the drug or one of its metabolites.[124] Folate deficiency secondary to long-term phenytoin therapy is not uncommon; approximately 75% of patients taking anticonvulsants have low serum folic acid status;[125] however, progression to megaloblastic anemia is rare.[126] Importantly, efforts to correct this folate deficiency must be cautious because supplementation with 1 mg/d folic acid can lead to a significant decrease in serum phenytoin concentrations in 15–50% of the patients.[98] Pharmacokinetic analysis of phenytoin suggests that folic acid may increase the affinity of the metabolic enzyme(s) involved in the elimination of the phenytoin without causing overall enzymatic induction.[127] To avoid potential folate deficiency and subsequent fluctuations in serum phenytoin levels, practitioners should routinely supplement all patients with folate when phenytoin therapy is initiated and maintain a schedule of drug monitoring.[128] Aspirin has also been linked with folate deficiency; serum folate levels are low in many patients with rheumatoid arthritis, perhaps as a result of competition for transport binding sites on serum proteins.[73] Methotrexate, a chemotherapeutic agent often used at lower doses to treat psoriasis, rheumatoid arthritis, and Crohn's disease, acts as an antimetabolite, limiting the availability of methyl groups derived from one-carbon metabolism by competitive inhibition of dihydrofolate reductase.[73,129]

Valproic acid (VPA), an antiepileptic agent, has also been associated with folate deficiency, possibly via an alteration in the methionine cycle;[130] this action may also underlie the tetratogenic effect of VPA.[131] VPA may also induce L-carnitine deficiency resulting in a hyperammonemia syndrome but with no other abnormality in the liver function tests. If diagnosed early, the clinical presentation, which includes altered mental status or encephalopathy, can be reversed by L-carnitine supplementation.[132–138]

Intestinal epithelial cells are rich in drug-metabolizing enzymes. CYP 3A4 isoenzyme is present in the small bowel and plays a role in the regulation of oral bioavailability of many drugs. Induction or inhibition of the enzyme in the gut by nutrients may lead to a significant change in oral bioavailability of drugs; the reverse relationship has also been demonstrated. Grapefruit juice represents an example of intestinal CYP 3A4 inhibition.[44,45] Water-soluble vitamin E (α-tocopheryl polyethylene glycol succinate) has been found to increase the oral absorption of cyclosporine, although it is not clear whether this occurs via an effect on intestinal drug metabolizing enzymes or transporters.[139–142] Drug-nutrient interactions that lead to increased drug bioavailability may result in ADR, but can also present useful therapeutic opportunities.

Excretion

Drugs may act to increase the excretion of a nutrient by displacement from plasma protein-binding sites, chelation, or reduction of renal reabsorption. Aspirin competes for folic acid-binding sites on serum proteins and enhances the vitamin's excretion.[143] Long-term administration of penicillamine for rheumatoid arthritis results in chelation of essential minerals such as copper and zinc.[144] Although diuretic therapy effectively decreases the resorption of sodium, it also enhances the renal excretion of calcium, chromium, magnesium, potassium, and zinc.[145] Thiamine deficiency can occur in patients treated with chronic loop diuretic therapy. Patients with congestive heart failure treated with long-term furosemide therapy have been reported to have increased urinary excretion of thiamine leading to frank deficiency over time that may have contributed to poor cardiac performance.[146] Similar findings were reported by Brady et al.[147] who observed laboratory evidence of thiamine deficiency in CHF patients being treated with loop diuretics on a chronic basis.

Drug-Induced Fluid and Electrolyte Imbalance

Several widely used medications can affect electrolyte balance as summarized in Table 16–9. Sodium balance is altered by thiazide diuretics and the neuroleptic carbamazepine.[148,149] Patients treated long term with carbamazepine have been reported to develop a syndrome of inappropriate antidiuretic hormone (SIADH), resulting in hyponatremia and water retention.[149] In SIADH patients, hyponatremia develops due to the enhanced renal conservation of water. Similarly, patients receiving excessive diuretic therapy with fluid loss replaced with excessive water are prone to developing SIADH.[150] Conversely, certain medications can cause hypernatremia as a result of water loss and subsequent dehydration. Hypernatremia, secondary to excessive lactulose therapy for hepatic encephalopathy or constipation, is a common drug-induced cause of this disorder.[151]

Renal wasting of potassium, resulting in hypokalemia, has been associated with thiazide and loop diuretics, corticosteroids, amphotericin B, and antipseudomonal penicillins.[150] Insulin as well as inhaled $\beta2$ agonists such as albuterol can cause a shift of potassium from the extracellular to the intracellular spaces.

Potassium-sparing diuretics (eg, spironolactone), angiotensin converting enzyme inhibitors (eg, enalapril), heparin, and trimethoprim can cause hyperkalemia via different mechanisms of action.[152] Trimethoprim has weak diuretic properties with potassium-sparing activity.[153] Heparin can suppress aldosterone, leading to sodium wasting and potassium retention. Importantly, patients with renal insufficiency or diabetes mellitus appear to be more susceptible to heparin-induced hyperkalemia.[154]

The impact of medications on phosphorus balance is important in patients receiving nutritional support as the synthesis of new cells increases the need for phosphorus. Patients already at risk for refeeding syndrome are particularly susceptible to the effects of drugs known to decrease available phosphorus stores.[155] Antacids and sul-

Table 16–9 Examples of Nutrient-Nutrient Interactions

Nutrient	Interaction
Calcium	High calcium intake interferes with phosphorus absorption
	Interferes with iron absorption
Cysteine	May chelate with copper in parenteral nutrition solutions
Magnesium	High magnesium intake may impair calcium absorption, Decreases phosphorus absorption
Phosphorus	High intake decreases magnesium absorption
Zinc	High zinc intake may impair copper absorption
Vitamin A	Mega doses may interfere with iron, iodine, copper, calcium absorption
	Can also interfere with absorption of ascorbic acid, vitamin K, vitamin E, and vitamin D
Vitamin C	Increases iron absorption
	Impairs copper absorption
	Interferes with cyanocobalamin absorption
Vitamin D	Reduced intake impairs calcium and phosphorus absorption and utilization
Vitamin E	Inhibits the reticulocyte and hemoglobin response to iron

cralfate can alter the absorption of phosphorus from the GI tract by binding to dietary phosphate, thus preventing its absorption. Conversely, patients with renal dysfunction are at risk for development of hyperphosphatemia due to the phosphate content present in the phospholipid emulsifiers formulated into intravenous fat emulsions or clindamycin phosphate injections.[156]

As noted above, isoniazid and cimetidine can inhibit the hepatic and/or renal hydroxylation of vitamin D, leading to impaired calcium absorption.[157,158] Odes et al.[158] found even short-term (30-day) therapy with cimetidine alters vitamin D metabolism and reduces 25-dihydroxyvitamin D status.

Chronic corticosteroid use can cause a net negative calcium balance and increased bone resorption due to suppressed intestinal absorption of calcium in conjunction with increased renal calcium and phosphate excretion and subsequent decrease in renal tubular calcium resorption, resulting in bone osteopenia.[88,159,160] Frequent use of inhaled steroids has also been associated with this response.[161]

Hypomagnesemia as a result of renal wasting can occur in patients treated with loop diuretics, thiazide diuretics, amphotericin B, aminogly-cosides, cisplatin, or cyclosporine. Cisplatin-induced hypomagnesemia is dose- as well as duration-dependent and occurs by reducing magnesium reabsorption in the ascending loop of Henle and the distal tubule.[162,163] Carboplatin, an antineoplastic agent with a chemical structure similar to cisplatin, has been reported to have a lower incidence of hypomagnesemia.[164,165] Renal wasting of magnesium is also common in patients on prolonged courses of high doses of aminoglycosides.[88,166] These drugs can inhibit the proximal tubular transport of magnesium in the kidney, predisposing patients with already low intakes of magnesium to hypomagnesemia.[166] If left untreated, hypomagnesemia can lead to hypocalcemia and induction of transient hypoparathyroidism by reducing parathyroid hormone (PTH) secretion and blunting the PTH response. This situation results in an inhibition of the hypocalcemic feedback loop.[162] Aluminum salts also suppress PTH secretion resulting in hypocalcemia. Treatment for hypocalcemia induced by hypomagnesemia involves correcting the hypomagnesemia first, then managing the magnesium losses. In some cases, calcium supplementation may also be unnecessary.[162]

Trace Elements (Zinc)

Zinc is essential for the function of many enzymes, including dehydrogenases, aldolases, and peptidases and is involved in a variety of other metabolic processes.[167] The formation and activation of zinc-dependent enzymes are regulated by zinc tissue levels.[168] Zinc metalloenzymes are responsible for structural integrity at the cellular level and for the regulation of various aspects of RNA and DNA metabolism.[168] Zinc deficiency limits the activity of these enzymes, resulting in decreased cell replication and tissue growth and repair.

Zinc also interacts with other nutrients. At supplemental doses, zinc may impair copper absorption.[169] Zinc deficiency can also negatively impact vitamin A metabolism by impairing the mobilization of retinol from the liver and altering retinal visual pigment metabolism, thereby contributing to the night blindness associated with zinc deficiency.[170] Zinc deficiency may also result in abnormal dark adaptation and age-related macular degeneration.[171]

Glucose Metabolism

Patients with diabetes mellitus or insulin resistance are susceptible to the effects of medications known to impact glucose metabolism. Thiazide diuretics, corticosteroids, and cyclosporine have all been associated with the induction hyperglycemia in susceptible patients.[172] The long-acting somatostatin analog, octreotide, inhibits insulin secretion and may result in a transient deterioration in glucose tolerance upon initiation of therapy.[173] In most cases, alteration of carbohydrate metabolism does not appear to be a problem. Drugs or foods that have the ability to induce a rapid release of insulin can increase the risk of hypoglycemia, especially if taken with alcohol.[174]

Lipid Metabolism

Drug-induced lipoprotein abnormalities and dyslipidemia are not uncommon. When a drug is used only for a short period, practitioners need to be aware of the effects on their patients' lipoprotein profiles and consider the possibility that an underlying dyslipidemia has been exacerbated. Drugs used chronically may be more problematic because they may be a risk factor for atherosclerosis.[175] Table 16–10 lists medications associated with dyslipidemia.

Orally administered estrogens decrease serum LDL and increase serum HDL in a dose-related manner.[175] Moreover, these agents are known to increase serum triglyceride levels 30–90%.[175] Low-dose estrogens have been proposed to minimize elevations in triglyceride levels without compromising their favorable impact on LDL and HDL levels.[175] Interestingly, topical, intradermal, and intramuscular routes of estrogen administration tend to have a less pronounced effect on lipoproteins, perhaps due to first-pass hepatic metabolism and a smaller impact on hepatic protein synthesis.[175,176]

Like estrogens, anabolic steroids can also cause profound, dose-related effects on lipoprotein metabolism. Reductions in HDL in conjunction with an elevation in LDL levels have been reported in patients using these agents.[175] Because their mechanisms of action have not yet been defined, caution is advised in using these agents in patients prone to dyslipidemia or atherosclerosis.

Food Intake

Impairment of nutritional status due to drug use often results in drug-induced nutritional deficiencies in cases where the medication results in appetite suppression and decreased food intake (Table 16–8). In such instances, these signs and symptoms of nutrient deficiencies are nonspecific and may mimic those of other age-related diseases and conditions. Changes in the ability to taste food, which make eating less enjoyable for many older people, are often blamed on aging (Chapter 7), but disease and the medications can be the real culprits. Aging appears to be associated with some loss in the ability to discriminate aroma, which can impair the appreciation of food. Also, the mouth's ability to feel the

Table 16–10 Medications Associated with Dyslipidemia

Medication	Total Lipids	Total Cholesterol	Triglycerides	Low-Density Lipoprotein	High-Density Lipoprotein	Very-Low-Density Lipoprotein
Abacavir			↑			
Amiodarone		↑	↑			
Amprenavir		↑	↑			
Anabolic steroids				↑	↓	
Beta-blockers			↑			
Calcitriol		↑				
Cholestyramine			↑			
Cyclosporine	↑	↑	↑			
Dexrazoxane			↑	↑		
Didanosine			↑			
Disopramide		↑	↑			
Efavirenz		↑	↑		↑	
Enoxaparin	↑					
Ergocalciferol		↑				
Estrogen			↑			
Fluconazole		↑	↑			
Glucocorticoids	↑	↑	↑	↑	↓	↑
Interferons			↑		↑	↑
Isotretinoin		↑	↑			
Itraconazole			↑			
L-asparaginase			↑			
Miconazole (IV)	↑	↑				
Mycophenolate	↑					
Nelfinavir	↑					
Paclitaxel			↑			
Phenothiazines		↑			↓	
Progestins		↓		↑	↓	↓
Propofol	↑					↑
Retinoids (Vitamin A)			↑	↑	↓	
Risperidone			↑			
Ritonavir		↑	↑			
Testosterone	↑	↑	↑	↑	↓	
Thiazide diuretics	↑	↑	↑	↑		↑
Vitamin E		↑	↑			

Source: Adapted from: Henkin J, Como JA, Oberman A. Secondary dyslipidemia: inadvertent effects of drugs in clinical practice. *JAMA* 1992;267:961–968.

fattiness of foods like butter and ice cream may decline with increasing age. Importantly, some medications affect taste and smell sufficiently that geriatric patients develop ageusia, the inability to taste food and drink or the distortion of normal taste.

Drugs that can affect taste include most antibiotics, chemotherapeutic agents, and antidepressants. Many drugs often create some change in taste, usually a bitter metallic sensation, because of the taste of the drugs themselves. Not all bitter taste sensations are related to the taste of the drug, because some agents may act to block other tastes, such as sweet and salt, which make bitter tastes more prominent.[177]

Several drugs have been noted to alter food intake, primarily through changes in appetite or the senses of taste and smell or through their adverse GI side effects.[178] Drugs may be hyperphagic or hypophagic, but the effects of drugs on appetite are strongly influenced by situational factors.[179] Drugs that affect appetite may do so by either a central or peripheral effect, including loss of appetite, induction of sedation, or evocation of adverse responses when food is ingested (Table 16–11).[180] Appetite suppression via centrally acting mechanisms is found among catecholaminergic (eg, dextroamphetamine), dopaminergic (eg, levodopa), and serotonergic (eg, fenfluramine) drugs as well as endorphin modulators (eg, naloxone).[180] Peripherally acting mechanisms that can indirectly suppress appetite include those agents that inhibit gastric emptying (eg, levodopa) or bulking agents (eg, methylcellulose).

Psychotropic agents, including the phenothiazines and benzodiazepines, improve mood and psychologic function with a consequent increase in food intake in some individuals; however, in elderly patients, whose rate of drug metabolism is slow, these drugs may induce somnolence and disinterest in food. Amitriptyline hydrochloride and related tricyclic antidepressants appear to stimulate appetite, but in elderly subjects they can cause behavioral agitation that interferes with eating.[181]

A secondary response may also occur when an adverse response to food caused by the drug results in a loss of appetite.[180,182] The emetic center in the brain stem can be stimulated by the action of several drugs. Antineoplastic drugs induce nausea, vomiting, and aversion to food.[183] Cardiac glycosides produce anorexia accompanied by nausea; high-dose treatment may result in digitalis cachexia.[184] Several antihypertensive drugs (eg, hydralazine, minoxidil, and diazoxide) are also associated with side effects of anorexia, nausea, vomiting, and diarrhea. Alcohol abuse can cause anorexia, but even elderly social drinkers tend to have lower food intakes than do age-matched nondrinkers. As noted above, some drugs (eg, lithium carbonate) produce an abnormal, unpleasant taste sensation (dysgeusia). A few drugs may also induce an unusual desire for certain foods, such as has been reported by patients taking diuretics who crave salt. Other drugs may induce untoward problems in the mouth that affect food intake, eg, dry mouth (xerostomia) resulting from the anticholinergic action of tricyclic antidepressants and tranquilizers, gingival hyperplasia from phenytoin, oral ulcerations from captopril, and parotid inflammation from guanethidine.

Other ways medications can cause anorexia are through depletion of various nutrients. High doses of aluminum- or magnesium-containing antacids can result in phosphate depletion, leading not only to muscle weakness but also to anorexia.[185] Similarly, loop diuretics can lead to depletion of sodium, potassium, and magnesium that can result in anorexia.[186] Drugs known to deplete folate, such as phenytoin, sulfasalazine, and trimethoprim, can result in anorexia and weight loss.[187,188] Penicillamine, which induces zinc depletion via chelation, can lead to diminished taste acuity and possible decreased food intake.[189]

Belle and Halpern[190] reported that patients taking high-dose niacin therapy for hyperlipidemia experienced GI symptoms that resulted in poor appetite and moderate weight loss. Similar findings were noted by Wilkens et al[191] in a study involving niacin dyslipidemia.

Zinc supplements have been used to treat drug-induced hypogeusia with mixed results, but have been used more successfully managing hypogeusia in patients undergoing dialysis.[192] Dahl and colleagues did not observe a benefit of zinc supplementation in patients with acetazolamide-induced taste disturbances.[193]

FOOD EFFECTS ON DRUG THERAPY

The clinical effects of food on drug absorption and disposition, particularly in geriatric patients and during chronic care, have not been well studied. Nonetheless, food and food com-

Table 16–11 Drug-Induced Alteration of Food Intake

Drugs Producing

Hypophagia	Hyperphagia	Hypogeusia/Dysgeusia
Actinomycin D	Amitriptyline HCl	Amydricaine
Alcohol	Anabolic steroids	Amylocaine HCl
Aluminum hydroxide	Benzodiazepines	Captopril
Amphetamine	Buxclizine HCl	Clofibrate
Cisplatin	Chlorpropamide	d-Penicillamine
Cocaine	Chlortetracycline	Encainide
Dactinomycin	Clemestine	5-Fluorouracil
Diethrlopropion HCl	Cyproeptadine Hcl	Griseofulvin
Digoxin	Dronabinol	Lincomycin
Fenfluramine HCl	Glucocorticoids	Lithium carbonate
Furosemide	Insulin	Methimazole
Griseofulvin	Megestrol acetate	Methylthiouraci
Hydralazine	Phenothiazines	Oxyfedrine
Mazindol	Reseroubel	
Methotrexate	Reserpine	
Methylcellulose	Tolbutamide	
Mineral oil	Tricyclic antidepressants	
Penicillamine		
Phenethylbiguanide		
Phenmetrazine		
Phenmetrazine HCl		
Phenethylbiguanide		
Spironolactone		
Sulfasalazine		
Thiazide diurotics		
Topiramate		

ponents have been shown to interact with drugs in various ways.[194] Food may influence both the absorption and presystemic metabolism of drugs and these effects may be caused by food intake or by different nutrients or additives, food/fluid volume, or polycyclic hydrocarbons present in grilled foods. Whether the changes induced by food are clinically significant depends both on the type of drug and the extent of the change.

Absorption

Food and its constituents can influence drug absorption as a result of physical or chemical in-teractions between the food product and the drug or because of physiologic changes in the GI tract induced by eating or drinking. The net effect of this interaction may be that drug absorption is re-duced, slowed, or increased by food intake (Table 16–12).[195,196]

Food can act to alter the rate of gastric empty-ing and drug dissolution in the stomach. It can also increase the viscosity of the gastric medium, decreasing the rate of drug diffusion to mucosal absorption sites. Food can also act as a simple mechanical barrier, preventing drug access to the mucosal surface. Food components can act as well to complex or chelate drugs. The effect of food on drug absorption may also be dependent

Table 16–12 The Potential Effect of Food on Drug Absorption

Drug Absorption Reduced/Delayed by Food

Acetaminophen	Ethanol	
Amoxicillin	Famciclovir	Penicillamine
Ampicillin	Fursemide	Penicillin
Aspirin	Glipizide	Phenobarbital
Atenolol	Griseofulvin	Phenytoin
Captopril	Hydrochlorothiazide	Propranolol
	Hydralazine	Pseudoephedrine
Carbamazepine	Indinavir	Quinidine
Cefaclor	Isoniazid	Rifampicin
Cephalexin	Ketoconazole	Sucralfate
Chlorothiazide	Levodopa	Sulfadiazine
Cimetidine	Lincomycin	Sulfasoxazole
Ciprofloxacin	Lithium	Tetracycline
Diazepam	Loratidine	Theophylline
Didanosine	Metronidazole	Thiamine
Diclofenac	Metoprolol	Thioridazine
Digoxin		
Dirthromycin	**Nafcillin**	**Valproic acid**
Doxycycline	Nitrofurantoin	Zafirlukast
Erythromycin stearate		

Drug Absorption Increased by Food

Atovaquone	Famotidine	Metoprolol
Carbamazepine	Ganciclovir	Nelfinavir
Chlorothiazide	Griseofulvin	Nitrofurantoin
Cefuroxime	Hydralazine	Phenytoin
Clofazimine	Hydrochlorothiazide	Propranolol
Diazepam	Itraconazole	Prophyphene
Dicoumarol	Lithium	Riboflavin
Lithium	Lovastatin	Ritonavir
Propranolol	Methylphenidate	Squinavir
Erythromycin estolate		
Erythromycin ethyl succinate		

on the drug formulation with enteric-coated tablets most affected by foods, and drugs in solution are least affected.[197]

Several food-related effects on GI function that also affect drug absorption and may augment age-related changes include alteration in gastric emptying time; intestinal motility; splanchnic blood flow; and alteration in the secretion of bile, gastric acid, and digestive enzymes.[198] The β-blockers propranolol and metoprolol are better absorbed after meals because of food-related increases in splanchnic blood flow and reduced first-pass metabolism in the intestinal mucosa or liver.[199]

Drug Absorption Increased by Food

When the effect of food on drug absorption is related to interactions between the food and the drug in the GI tract, then the timing of drug intake in relation to mealtime is of practical importance. Acetaminophen absorption, for example, is five times more rapid after fasting than after consumption of a high-carbohydrate meal containing large amounts of pectin.[200] Foods can also interfere with the mucosal transfer of drugs absorbed by active transport. Drugs such as levodopa and methyldopa with structures similar to amino acids are absorbed by the transport mechanism for amino acids.[201] Competition for transport between the drug and amino acids from protein in the diet diminish drug uptake and appear partly responsible for the "on-off" phenomenon of levodopa in patients with Parkinson's disease.[202] In geriatric patients, particularly those having difficulty with mastication or who have had gastric surgery, long-term cimetidine administration, coupled with high fiber intake, may lead to the formation of phytobezoars.[203]

The effects of changes in gastric emptying time on drug absorption are dependent on the water solubility of the drug; drugs with very low solubility are better absorbed when they remain longer in the stomach, as they will do after large, hot or high-fat meals.[204] For drugs that are weak bases, eg, amitriptyline hydrochloride, diazepam, and pentazocine, gastric emptying rate is critical because absorption occurs in the less acidic intestine. The gastric emptying time is approximately 50 minutes in young, healthy volunteers but greater than 120 minutes in subjects over age 77 years.[205] Food-induced decreases in gastric clearance can cause more of drugs such as digoxin, levodopa, and penicillin to be metabolized in the stomach and less of the unchanged drug to be available for absorption, resulting in an erratic therapeutic response.[40] Changes in gastric emptying affect mainly drugs that are rapidly absorbed or that have a short biologic half-life.

Distribution

Nutritional influences on drug distribution appear to be limited to the large reduction of plasma albumin seen in poorly nourished geriatric patients. However, even in well-nourished and healthy elderly, albumin concentrations have been found to be lower than those in young adults.[206] Therefore, for extensively protein-bound drugs, such as diazepam and warfarin, a reduced binding capacity in old age results in an increase in the drugs' free fractions, so lower ranges of therapeutic and toxic plasma concentrations should be anticipated.[207] Dietary fats may modify drug distribution; free fatty acids compete for anionic binding sites on plasma albumin, increasing the pharmacologic activity of displaced drugs.

Metabolism

Diet and nutritional status may have a marked effect on the way drugs are metabolized, although studies in this area have rarely been conducted with elderly subjects.[208] Because the rate of drug metabolism tends to decrease with age, this type of interaction is likely to be more marked in older adults.[209] In studies conducted on healthy young men given antipyrine or theophylline during sequential feeding of high-carbohydrate, high-fat, or high-protein diets, the rate of drug elimination was slowest when the high-carbohydrate, diet was fed and fastest during the high-protein period.[210,211] The high-fat diet produced a small decrease in the rate of antipyrine loss but did not alter theophylline pharmacokinetics. Reduced drug clearance has been demonstrated in lactovegetarians, whose diets are characterized by a low-protein intake.[212] Balanced-protein diets produce an acid urine, whereas low-protein diets usually result in an alkaline urine. Many older adults shift toward dietary patterns with lower protein, a change with implications for drug elimination and half-life.[213–215]

Subjects who switch between saturated and polyunsaturated dietary fats show a concurrent alteration in plasma lipids but no change in CYP 450-mediated drug metabolism.[216] In cases of mild or moderate undernutrition, particularly in adults, the rate of drug metabolism has been found to be either normal or slightly increased.[208] Only in severely malnourished adults with nutritional edema is drug metabolism impaired, with significant increases in plasma half-life of the drug.[217]

Natural nonnutrient components of the diet may exert a profound influence on the rate of drug metabolism, and these effects may occur rapidly after food ingestion. For example, alterations of intestinal microflora produced by changes in the dietary level or source of protein or fiber may influence intestinal drug metabolism. Cruciferous vegetables of the Brassica family, such as broccoli, Brussels sprouts, cabbage, and cauliflower, contain indols capable of inducing aryl hydrocarbon hydroxylase activity as well as the conjugation of phenacetin and acetaminophen.[218–220] Flavones occurring in citrus and other fruits and polycyclic aromatic hydrocarbons generated during charcoal broiling stimulate hepatic microsomal drug metabolism.[221,222]

Grapefruit juice can inhibit the presystemic metabolism of drugs metabolized by CYP 3A4 in the small intestine, including carbamazepine, cyclosporine, terfenadine, several dihydropyridines (eg, felodipine, nifedipine, and nisoldipine), and short-acting benzodiazepines like triazolam.[223–227] The impact of this interaction may result in serious ADR such as hypotension and tachycardia by dihydropyridines and increased sedation by benzodiazepines. On the other hand, there is potential to employ the inhibition of CYP 450 by grapefruit juice therapeutically to increase the bioavailability of poorly absorbed agents like cyclosporine and rapidly metabolized HIV protease inhibitors like saquinavir.[228,229] However, it has not been established whether the elderly are as susceptible as younger people to this type of induction and inhibition of hepatic and intestinal enzymes. Nonetheless, grapefruit juice has been removed from some institutional formularies to minimize the potential risk of this interaction. It is important to note that the grapefruit juice–drug interaction studies have utilized double-strength frozen concentrates (diluting frozen concentrates with water as 1:1 rather than 1:2 or more) that does not represent the way most consumers prepare this beverage; thus, the actual magnitude of this drug-nutrient interaction may be overestimated.

Excretion

Renal elimination of drugs involves glomerular filtration, active tubular secretion, and passive tubular excretion. Drugs or their metabolites that are primarily filtered and excreted by the kidney may be affected by nutritional status, eg, dietary protein increases renal blood flow, glomerular filtration rate (GFR), and renal tubular function.[230] Severe protein energy malnutrition is associated with decreased GFR and renal blood flow.[231] Refeeding an undernourished patient can increase the systemic clearance of some drugs, necessitating a dosage adjustment to maintain efficacy;[150] eg, the Vd of theophylline decreases and the elimination rate gradually increases in malnourished patients given a dextrose-based parenteral nutrition solution for more than a couple days.[232] The protein component of enteral or parenteral nutrition, however, appears to be the major macronutrient enhancing systemic clearance of effected drugs in patents transitioned from an unfed to fed state.

IMPACT OF MACRONUTRIENTS ON DRUG THERAPY

Carbohydrates

Some suggest that carbohydrates have little impact on drug metabolism,[233,234] while others, such as Kappas et al,[235] report that the oxidative metabolism of model drugs such as antipyrine and theophylline decreases with carbohydrate-supplemented diets and increases with protein-enriched diets. Although many liquid medications are manufactured in sugar syrup, little research has been done on its effect on disposition and action. Animal studies by Sonawane et al[236] suggest that dietary carbohydrates and fat may significantly influence the hepatic drug-metabolizing enzymes via alterations in the phospholipid composition of endoplasmic reticulum or by limiting the supply of cofactors necessary for optimal functioning of CYP and UGT.

Dietary fiber as well as other bulk-forming compounds may interfere with the GI absorption of medications.[237] The bioavailability of digoxin is reduced significantly when given with a fiber-rich meal, with almost half of the dose sequestered in or bound to the fiber.[238,239] Similar effects have been reported with lithium salts and lovastatin.[240,241] Stewart reported that several patients with recurrent major depression that had been successfully treated with tricyclic antidepressants became refractory to treatment after beginning a high-fiber diet.[242] Nutrient absorption can also be negatively impacted in the presence of a high-fiber diet. Zinc absorption in the intestine is reduced by the binding to dietary fiber constituents like phytate.[243]

Protein

Following a high-protein meal, the bioavailability of drugs that undergo an extensive first-pass effect, eg, propranolol, metoprolol, and lidocaine, can be markedly enhanced due to increases in hepatic blood flow. High-extraction drugs can then rapidly pass through the liver, allowing higher drug concentrations in the systemic circulation.[244-246]

A decrease in dietary protein depresses creatinine clearance and renal plasma flow.[247] Dietary protein also affects the renal tubular transport of certain compounds, although the mechanism by which this occurs has not been elucidated. Studies of allopurinol and its active metabolite, oxypurinol, suggest that the dietary manipulation of protein intake can significantly alter clearance. For example, Berlinger et al.[248] provided subjects a low- or high-protein diet for 14 days as well as a single daily 600 mg oral dose of allopurinol; compared with baseline values, renal function was decreased by the low-protein diet and increased by the high-protein diet. Creatinine clearance increased by 30% in the high-protein diet when compared to the low-protein diet. This was consistent with the renal clearance of allopurinol, which mirrors creatinine clearance. The area under the curve (AUC) for allopurinol was approximately 45% greater during protein restriction than during the high-protein diet. Since the renal clearance of allopurinol represents only a small fraction of its total body clearance, the increase in allopurinol AUC may actually reflect a

decrease in the xanthine oxidase-dependent metabolism of allopurinol to oxypurinol that occurs during protein restriction. This contrasts with the very pronounced effect of protein restriction on the renal clearance of oxypurinol, which was reduced by 66% compared to the high-protein diet; both the AUC and half-life of oxypurinol were three times greater in the high-protein diet. In protein restriction, the decrease in the renal clearance of oxypurinol was twice as large as the change in creatinine clearance, suggesting that the mechanism of the interaction also involved a change in tubular function associated with protein restriction. Oxypurinol, a weak acid structurally similar to uric acid, is reabsorbed by the uric acid system in the renal tubules. In subjects fed a high-protein diet, reabsorption is inhibited. However, in protein restriction, oxypurinol undergoes extensive tubular reabsorption resulting in decreased renal clearance and elevated serum levels.

Dietary Fat

Lipids are an essential part of cell membrane structure and are involved in many of the normal enzymatic activities located within the cell membrane.[233] Diets that are deficient in fat or essential fatty acids decrease the activity of the enzyme systems responsible for the metabolism of nutrients.[249] Plasma free fatty acid levels become elevated after consumption of a high-fat meal, increasing the potential to become bound to plasma albumin and subsequently displace albumin-bound drugs, increasing the risk of drug toxicity.[233]

EFFECT OF NUTRIENT SUPPLEMENTS ON DRUG THERAPY

Vitamin Supplementation/Hypervitaminosis

Nutrient supplements are required by those on chronic drug regimens when a risk of progressive nutrient depletion exists as well as when a nutrient deficiency induced by the drug is present (Table 16–13).[27] Appropriate levels of vitamin

Table 16–13 Examples of Vitamin-Drug Interactions

Nutrient	Medication	Interaction
Ascorbic acid (Vitamin C)	coumarin anticoagulants	shortens prothrombin time, may antagonize warfarin response
	gentamicin	acidifies urine, decreases efficacy of gentamicin
	iron salts	increases iron absorption
	oral contraceptives	intermittent use may cause contraceptive failure
	tricyclic antidepressants	high dose (>2 g/d) may reduce therapeutic response
Folic acid	phenytoin	reduces phenytoin bioavailability, may antagonize anticonvulsant action
Niacin	pyrimethamine	reduces pyrimethamine efficacy
	adrenergic blockers	enhances vasodilation, may cause orthostatic hypotension
	aspirin	decreases flushing seen with niacin use
	HMG-CoA reductase inhibitors ("statins")	increases risk of myopathy/rhabodmyolysis with concurrent use
	isoniazid	increases niacin requirement
Pyridoxine (Vitamin B$_6$)	barbiturates	reduces barbiturate response
	levodopa	reduces levodopa response
	phenytoin	high doses reduce phenytoin levels, may impair therapeutic effect
Vitamin A	aluminum hydroxide	reduces vitamin A absorption
	coumarin anticoagulants	high doses of vitamin A may enhance anticoagulant response, increase risk of bleeding
	isotretinoin	competes with vitamin A
	oral contraceptives	increases serum vitamin A levels
Vitamin D	digoxin	vitamin D may cause hypercalcemia, leading to arrhythmias
Vitamin E	coumarin anticoagulants	potentiates anticoagulant response
	vitamin A	increases serum vitamin A levels
	iron salts	inhibits reticulocyte and hemoglobin response to iron therapy
Vitamin K	coumarin anticoagulants	antagonizes anticoagulant response

supplementation have been proposed for specific drug therapies.[6] It is not unusual that drug-related depletion of nutrients in geriatric patients is complicated by dietary inadequacy or disease states that induce nutrient deficiencies. Despite such well-justified therapeutic needs for nutrient supplementation, it is important to recognize the extensive nature of self-prescribed supplement use among older adults. The estimated prevalence of nutrient supplementation in the elderly ranges from 30–70%.[69] In one survey of middle-class elderly individuals who had no known medical illnesses and who were not taking prescription medications, the prevalence of nutrient supplement use was 60%.[250] Although several of the factors discussed above suggest that there may be valid reasons to recommend nutrient supplementation for older adults, current trends indicate that their supplementation regimens are not always appropriate; self-selected supplements are not based on the individual's actual needs.

"Megavitamin therapy" (employing doses greater than 10 times the Recommended Dietary Allowance) has been advocated in the treatment of various disease states including schizophrenia, cancer, and the common cold.[251,252] Although vitamins typically possess low toxicity and a wide therapeutic margin, adverse reactions can occur with excessively high doses.[253] Micronutrient supplementation alone or as part of a fad diet can potentiate or exacerbate nutrient-nutrient interactions (Table 16–14).

Megadoses of vitamin E potentiate the action of the anticoagulant warfarin and produce a hemorrhagic syndrome by further depressing the levels of vitamin K–dependent coagulation factors.[254] Vitamin D supplements can induce hy-

percalcemia and precipitate cardiac arrhythmias in patients receiving digitalis.[255] The administration of supplemental calcium can cause a recurrence of atrial fibrillation in patients maintained on verapamil.[256]

High doses of vitamin C may acidify the urine and alter drug pharmacokinetics because acidic drugs are more readily absorbed and basic drugs are more rapidly excreted from acidic urine.[257] Large doses of vitamin C may also inhibit the anticoagulant response of warfarin.[258] High-dose niacin supplements produce postural hypotension via their additive vasodilating effect with sympathetic antagonists like clonidine hydrochloride.[256] An increase in seizure frequency and a corresponding decrease in serum phenytoin levels have been reported in epileptic patients receiving high-dose folic acid supplements.[259]

Drug metabolizing enzyme systems have been shown to be highly dependent on vitamin C status. Houston et al[260] found healthy individuals

Table 16–14 Chronic Drug Therapy and Nutrient Supplementation

Drug	Supplement
Acitretin	Folic acid
Antacids	Folic acid
Aspirin	Folic acid, iron, vitamin C
Chlortetracycline	Calcium, vitamin C, vitamin B_2
Cholestyramine resin	Vitamins A, D, E, K, folic acid, calcium
Cimetidine	Vitamin B_{12}
Colestipol	Vitamins A, D, E, K, folic acid, calcium
Estrogens/progestin	Vitamin B_6, folic acid
Hydralazine HCl	Vitamin B_6
Isoniazid	Vitamin B_6
Levodopa	Vitamin B_6
Penicillamine	Vitamin B_6
Pentamidine	Folic acid
Phenothiazines	Vitamin B_2
Phenytoin	Folic acid, vitamin D, vitamin K, calcium
Primidone	Vitamin D, folic acid
Proton pump inhibitors	Vitamin B_{12}
Pyrimethamine	Folic acid
Rifampin	Vitamin B_6, niacin, vitamin D
Sulfasalazine	Folic acid
Tetracycline	Calcium, vitamin B_2, vitamin C
Triamterene	Folic acid

receiving supplemental ascorbic acid had a substantial increase in antipyrine clearance, and Beatie et al[261] reported that vitamin C deficiency was partly responsible for impaired drug clearance in patients with liver disease. A rebound scurvy has been reported in individuals abruptly stopping high-dose vitamin C supplementation, so tapered doses rather than immediate cessation of treatment are recommended. High doses of ascorbic acid may also impair vitamin B_{12} status when taken at mealtime.[262,263] Auer et al[264] reported hematuria and calcium oxalate dihydrate crystal formation in a 25-year-old male 8 days after ingesting 4 g/d vitamin C with signs resolving 5 days after discontinuing supplementation. Very high doses of vitamin B_6, from 2–5 g/d, when administered for only a few months can induce sensory neuropathies.[265]

Vitamin K–rich foods (eg, green leafy vegetables, cabbage, broccoli), when intake is irregular, can alter response to anticoagulants such as warfarin. Warfarin creates a partial deficiency of the active form of vitamin K involved in the posttranslational modification factors (II, VII, IX, X, and protein C and S).[266] When ingested in high amounts, vitamin K–rich foods may be associated with anticoagulant failure, resulting in the need for higher doses. Conversely, when patients stable on warfarin therapy suddenly decrease their intake of vitamin K–rich foods, there is a risk for bleeding. Other sources of vitamin K associated with warfarin resistance include intravenous fat emulsions prepared from soybean or safflower oils.[267] Frequent monitoring of the International Normalized Ratio (INR) and warfarin dosage adjustments are imperative in these patients.

Effect of Dietary Manipulation on Drug Kinetics

Several dietary factors can alter the rate of drug metabolism and both food and fluids can alter the rate and extent of drug absorption. These alterations in response may occur as a result of influences on gastric pH, gastric emptying time, intestinal motility, mesenteric and hepatic portal blood flow, or biliary flow.[268] Direct physico-

chemical interactions with dietary components can also alter the absorption of susceptible agents.[269,270] Interactions such as the binding of the medication with metal ions, solubilization of the drug in dietary fat, or adsorption of the drug to insoluble dietary components may occur.[244]

Dietary changes of macronutrient composition and proportion can alter the expression and activity of hepatic drug-metabolizing enzymes, although the clinical impact of the effect can be minimal.[271–273] As noted above, the rate of drug metabolism can be accelerated by drugs themselves or by a variety of dietary factors, such as protein supplementation or inclusion of cruciferous vegetables or charcoal-broiled meats in the diet.[274] Charcoal-broiled beef induces the metabolism of antipyrine and theophylline, reducing their half-lives by 20%, apparently due to its high content of polycyclic aromatic hydrocarbons, which are potent inducers of CYP 1A2.[275,276] Conversely, low-protein, high-carbohydrate diets and various vitamin and mineral deficiencies can reduce levels of drug-metabolizing enzymes such that serum drug concentrations decline more slowly, resulting in increased drug potency.[274]

In general, when orally administered medications are taken with meals, the rate rather than the extent of GI absorption is delayed. Food affects drug absorption by enhancing gastric blood flow in conjunction with delayed gastric emptying. Food can increase, decrease, or have no effect on the absolute systemic availability of a medication.[277] Concomitant food ingestion reduces the absorption of drugs such as ampicillin penicillin, and isoniazid.[278] Conversely, food may actually enhance the absorption of other medications, including diazepam, lithium, carbamazepine, and griseofulvin (Table 16–12).

The composition of a meal may alter splanchnic blood flow. Blood flow can be doubled by a high-protein liquid meal and slightly reduced by a liquid glucose meal.[279] The significance of this effect on splanchnic flow is important for those medications with high hepatic extraction.[244] Food will slow the rate of gastric emptying and may thus result in a delay in drug absorption from the GI tract. Changes in gastric emptying are not only related to the physicochemical properties of the drug, but also on the type of meal itself. Hot meals, highly viscous solutions, or meals rich in fat can delay emptying.[244,280,281]

Meals commonly enhance the presystemic clearance of lipophilic basic drugs, such as amitriptyline and propranolol, but rarely alter the clearance of lipophilic acids, such as penicillin and salicylic acid.[245] Alternately, food may reduce the presystemic clearance of some lipophilic basic drugs via transient, complex effects on splanchnic-hepatic blood flow. Further, repeated intake of specific nutrients (eg, protein) and food contaminants (eg, benzopyrene) can enhance presystemic drug clearance by enzyme induction. As described above, competition between levodopa and the neutral amino acids in a high-protein meal for transport through the blood-brain barrier may be partly responsible for the "on-off" phenomenon in therapy for Parkinson's disease;[282] thus, reducing protein intake may improve the efficacy of levodopa.

EFFECT OF HERBAL SUPPLEMENTS ON DRUG THERAPY

Herbal remedies have been employed in traditional Arabian, Ayurvedic, Chinese, and other medicines purposes for centuries. Herbal therapies have been defined as the use of crude drugs of plant origin and are utilized to promote health and treat both acute and chronic diseases.[283] Herbal products are categorized in the United States as dietary supplements according to the Dietary Supplement and Health Education Act (DSHEA) of 1994.[284–288]

Although interactions between herbal products and drugs are based on the same pharmacokinetic and pharmacodynamic relationships discussed above, relatively little information is available in this arena.

Herbs can affect drug absorption, eg, aloe leaf (*Aloe vera*) and senna (*Senna alexandrina*) exert a laxative effect that may decrease intestinal transit time and alter drug bioavailability. The greatest impact of this interaction would be seen with drugs having a narrow therapeutic index such as

digoxin and warfarin.[289] St. John's wort (*Hypericum perforatum*) has been reported to induce the P-glycoprotein intestinal transporter and thus could have an impact of drug substrates for this protein, such as digoxin.[290,291]

Herbal supplements can influence drug distribution by competing with and displacing a drug from its plasma protein binding site and affect its Vd; eg, aescin, a constituent of horse chestnut seed (*Aesculus hippocastanum*), appears to interfere with warfarin through this mechanism.[288,292]

Like drug-nutrient interactions affecting metabolism, drug-herb interactions may be mediated via an effect on CYP 450 isozymes. St. John's wort, indicated for mild to moderate depression, can induce CYP 3A4[290,293–295] and increase the metabolism of digoxin,[296,297] theophylline,[298] protease inhibitors,[299] cyclosporin,[300,301] corticosteroids,[294,295] amitriptyline,[302] warfarin,[294,295] and oral contraceptives.[295] St. John's wort acts as a selective serotonin reuptake inhibitor (SSRI),[303] so concurrent use with other SSRI agents is generally contraindicated.[304,305] A discretionary clinical approach suggests a 3-week wash-out period between the use of these therapies.[306]

Ginkgo biloba has been indicated in the treatment of Alzheimer's disease and dementia[307,308] and for improving peripheral circulation,[309] but possesses anti-platelet activity and inhibits platelet aggregation.[309,310] Episodes of subdural hematoma,[311] subarachnoid hemorrhage,[312] and spontaneous hyphema[313] have been reported in patients taking ginkgo alone. A potential contraindication may exist for gingko in patients taking drugs and nutrients known to affect platelet activity such as aspirin, vitamin E, and garlic supplements. Ginkgo also inhibits warfarin metabolism and can increase the risk of bleeding disorders when these agents are used concurrently.[310]

Asian (*Panax ginseng*) and American (*Panax quinquefolius*) ginseng are claimed to increase energy, enhance immune function, improve cognitive ability, and promote a sense of overall well-being.[298] Ginseng induces the CYP 2C9 isozyme and can decrease the INR with concomitant use of warfarin.[314] Ginseng may act in an additive or synergistic fashion with insulin or hypoglycemic agents to reduce blood glucose levels and hemoglobin A1c levels in type 2 diabetes, so careful glucose monitoring is required.[315–317]

Garlic (*Allium sativum*) has been promoted as an herbal remedy for lowering serum cholesterol and blood pressure and reducing the risk for cardiovascular disease.[288] However, garlic inhibits platelet aggregation by interfering with thromboxane synthesis and has been associated with postoperative bleeding and altered INR during anticoagulant therapy.[318–322]

Kava kava (*Piper methysticum*), indicated as an anxiolytic agent, appears to act as a dopamine antagonist and, therefore, may reduce the efficacy of levodopa in the treatment of Parkinson's disease.[323,324] Kava kava exhibits an agonist ligand effect in the benzodiazepine γ-aminobutyric acid (GABA) receptor complex and potentiates the sedative effects of drugs like alprazolam.[325]

Licorice (*Glycyrrhiza glabra*) contains glycyrrhizin, an inhibitor of 11 β-hydroxysteroid dehydrogenase in humans, and can reduce the catabolism of corticosteroids and increase their plasma concentrations.[326,327] Licorice may also exacerbate hypokalemia and potentiate the toxicity of cardiac glycosides such as digoxin.[328,329] When used in high doses over long durations, licorice may cause pseudoaldosteronism presenting as sodium and water retention, hypokalemia, hypertension, heart failure, and cardiac arrest.[328,329]

Cat's Claw (*Uncaria tomentosa*), used for GI and immune disorders; chamomile, an herbal tea related to ragweed and also used for GI complaints; and Echinacea (*Echinacea angustifolia, Echinacea pallida*), another relative of ragweed used to treat the common cold and influenza, all appear to inhibit CYP 3A4, an action which could increase serum levels of drugs metabolized by this isoenzyme, including cyclosporine and protease inhibitors.[288,330]

Investigating and predicting drug-herbal interactions can be confounded by the presence of inadvertent or intentional adulteration of the plant material or extract with other bioactive ingredients or drugs, including belladonna alkaloids, digitalis, rauwolfia, indomethacin, phenylbutazone, corticosteroids, benzodiazepine, and warfarin. Some herbal products have also been found to be contaminated with arsenic, cadmium, lead, or mercury; insecticides, herbicides, fungicides, and other pesticides; and microbial toxins like aflatoxins and bacterial endotoxins.[283,288,327]

IMPLICATIONS FOR AGING

The long list of identified drug-nutrient interactions does not implicate the production of a clinically significant ADR whenever these two components are present, ie, the drug prescription and low or supplemental intake of a nutrient. However, both the nutrition- and drug-related risk factors for untoward interactions are greatest in the elderly because of the concomitant presence of age-associated conditions.[331] The nutrient intakes of most older people fail to meet recommended allowances, so they present with suboptimal nutritional status at the outset of drug therapy. Elderly patients are often prescribed multiple drugs requiring frequent administration over long periods of time. Age-associated diseases, changes in body composition, and changes in physiologic function contribute to substantial alterations in drug pharmacokinetics and pharmacodynamics. Therefore, it is important to recognize the multifactorial diet-drug-age-disease interrelationships in determining the benefits and risks of any specific therapeutic intervention.[332] (Table 16–15)

The medical treatment of geriatric patients often tends to include practices that do not fully consider the risk factors that contribute to drug-nutrient interactions. Physician advice to older patients to take medication with foods to decrease GI side effects and enhance compliance may increase the chance of adverse interactions. Drug-nutrient interactions may also occur as a result of the common practice of passing drugs down nasogastric tubes used for enteral feeding. This practice can induce blockage of the tube or reduce bioavailability because of physical incompatibility between the enteral formula and the drug. As discussed above, drug metabolism and efficacy may also be affected simply by

Table 16–15 Risk Factors for Drug-Induced Nutrient Deficiency in the Elderly

Drug-Associated Factors	*Nutrition-Associated Factors*
Dose	Nutritional quality of diet
Duration	Initial nutritional status
Frequency	Use of nutrient supplements
Polypharmacy	Temporal relation between meals and medication administration

Age-Associated Factors	*Pathologic Factors*
Gastrointestinal changes	Cardiovascular disease
Hepatic changes	Gastrointestinal malabsorption
Renal changes	Liver disease
Body composition changes	Renal disease
Homeostatic changes	
Receptor-mediated changes	
Tissue sensitivity changes	

changing the diet (eg, the protein content) or the timing between meals and drug administration. These situations reveal the importance of close and frequent communication among physicians, dietitians, and pharmacists on the health care team. The widespread use of nutrient supplements among older adults may adversely or beneficially influence the therapeutic outcome of drug treatment. Relatively frequent and careful evaluation through drug monitoring and nutritional assessment becomes critical in the geriatric patient.

CONCLUSION

The human diet is highly heterogeneous in its composition, method of preparation, quantity, and time of consumption. Consequently, drug kinetics as a result of diet varies widely in subjects based on age, gender, culture, and economic status. Even within the same individual, seasonal variations will occur that impact dietary habits and, thus, drug-related effects. Although each factor may play a small role by itself, a much larger synergistic effect could occur when combined with other environmental factors as well as genetic factors.

Nutritional deficiencies have been strongly linked to increased susceptibility to disease and behavioral changes. Drug-induced vitamin and mineral deficiencies can lead to a host of symptoms, including anorexia, bone pain, confusion, and malaise, that mimic what are frequently considered as signs of old age. Prolonged nutrient deficiencies can also result in conditions such as anemia, laryngitis and bronchitis, carpal tunnel syndrome, and postoperative confusion. The interactions between drugs and diet have implications for general health as well as drug safety and efficacy. Unless the health care team is aware of drug-nutrient relationships, problems experienced by the geriatric patient may be wrongfully attributed to existing disease(s) or even simply to age. Application of existing knowledge about the relationships among pharmacology, nutrition, and aging can directly contribute to minimizing the iatrogenic impact of drug-nutrient interactions.

Carefully controlled clinical trials as well as hospital- and community-based epidemiologic studies are needed to identify further the risk factors associated with drug-nutrient interactions in geriatric patients. In some cases, the effects of age on drug disposition and action are of less importance than the effects of inappropriate concurrent drug and meal intakes, unscheduled changes in dietary regimens, or ill-considered polypharmacy regimens. There is a need to develop methods of communication to transfer this information to geriatric patients and to their caregivers, including physicians, nurses, pharmacists, dietitians, and home care personnel. Means of communication between caregivers and education programs within geriatric institutions must be developed further so that the potential adverse consequences of changes in diet or drug therapies are recognized before they occur. Although more research is necessary to identify and characterize the mechanisms and symptoms of drug-nutrient interactions in the geriatric patient, much can be done now through education and communication to recognize the risks and avoid their adverse consequences.

REFERENCES

1. Powers DE, Moore AG. *Food-Medication Interactions.* Tempe, AZ: F-M I Publishing; 1983.

2. Roe DA, ed. *Drugs and Nutrition in the Geriatric Patient.* New York, NY: Churchill Livingstone Inc; 1984.

3. Roe DA, Campbell TC, eds. *Drugs and Nutrients: The Interactive Effects.* New York, NY: Marcel Dekker; 1984.

4. Basu TK. *Drug-Nutrient Interactions.* Deckenham, England: Croom Helm; 1988.

5. Roe DA. *Drug-Induced Nutritional Deficiencies.* Westport, CT: Avi Publishing; 1985.

6. Roe DA. *Handbook: Interactions of Selected Drugs and Nutrients in Patients.* Chicago, IL: American Dietetic Association; 1982.

7. Roe DA. *Drug and Drug Interactions.* New York, NY: Van Nostrand Reinhold; 1989.

8. Blumberg JB. Drug-nutrient interrelationships. In: Calkins E, Davis P, Ford A, eds. *The Practice of Geriatrics.* Philadelphia, PA: WB Saunders Co; 1986.

9. Blumberg J. Clinical significance of drug-nutrient interactions. *Trans Pharmacol Sci* 1986;7:33–35.

10. Hershey LA. Avoiding adverse drug reactions in the elderly. *Mt Sinai J Med* 1988;55:244–250.

11. Roe DA. Medications and nutrition in the elderly. *Primary Care: Clinics in Office Practice* 1994;21:135–147.

12. Schmucker DL, Vessel ES. Are the elderly underrepresented in clinical drug trials? *Clin Pharmacol* 1999; 39(11):1103–1108.

13. Young FE. Clinical evaluation of medicine used by the elderly. *Clin Pharmacol Ther* 1987;42:666–669.

14. Skolnick AA. FDA sets geriatric drug use labeling deadlines. *JAMA.1997;*278(16):1302.

15. Stoehr GP, Ganguli M, Seaberg EC, et al. Over-the-counter medication use in an older rural community: the MoVIES Project. *J Am Geriatr Soc* 1997;45:158–165.

16. Diehl M, Lago D, Ahern F, et al. Examination of priorities for therapeutic drug utilization review. *J Geriatr Drug Therapy* 1991;6:65–85.

17. Kovar MG. Health of the elderly and use of health services. *Public Health Rep* 1977;92:9–19.

18. Chen LH, Liu S, Cook-Newell ME, et al. Survey of drug use by the elderly and possible impact of drugs on nutritional status. *Drug Nutrient Interact* 1985;3:73–86.

19. Darnell JC, Murray MD, Martz BL, Weinberger M. Medication use by ambulatory elderly. An in-home survey. *J Am Geriatr Soc* 1986;34:1–4.

20. Gurwitz JH, Field TS, Harrold LR, et al. Incidence and preventability of adverse drug reactions among older persons I. the ambulatory setting. *JAMA* 2003;289:1107–16.

21. Rothschild JM, Bates DW, Leape LL. Preventable medical injuries in older patients. *Arch Intern Med* 1991; 114:956–966.

22. Gurwitz JH. Improving the quality of medication use in elderly patients: a not-so-simple prescription. *Arch Intern Med* 2002;162:1670–1672.

23. Cusak B, Denham MJ, Kelly JG, et al., eds. *Clinical Pharmacology and Drug Treatment in the Elderly.* Edinburgh, Scotland: Churchill Livingstone; 1984.

24. Shapiro S, Avery KT, Carpenter RD. Drug utilization by a non-institutionalized ambulatory elderly population. *Gerodontics* 1986;2:99–102.

25. IMS International Audit of Prescribing in General European Practice, 1981.

26. Rikans LE. Drugs and nutrition in old age. *Life Sci* 1986; 39:1027–1036.

27. Lamy PP. Nonprescription drugs and the elderly. *Am Fam Physician* 1989;39:175–179.

28. Lofholm P. Self-medication by the elderly. In: Kayne KC, ed. *Drugs and the Elderly.* Los Angeles, CA: University of Southern California Press; 1979.

29. Swift CG. Prescribing in old age. *Br Med J* 1988;296: 913–915.

30. Lamy P. The elderly and drug interactions. *J Am Geriatr Soc* 1986;34:586–592.

31. Anon. Long-term care of elderly patients: chronic disease co-morbidity and other considerations. *Consult Pharm* 1995;10:583–593.

32. Greenblatt DJ, Sellers EM, Shader RI. Drug disposition in old age. *N Engl J Med* 1982;306:1081–1088.

33. Schmucker DL. Drug disposition in the elderly: a review of the critical factors. *J Am Geriatr Soc* 1984;32: 144–149.

34. Blumberg JB. A discussion of drug metabolism and actions in the aged. *Drug Nutrient Interact* 1985;4:99–106.

35. Skolnick AA. FDA sets geriatric drug use labeling deadlines. *JAMA* 1997;278(16):1302.

36. Robertson D. Drug handling in old age. In: Brocklehurst JC, ed. *Geriatric Pharmacology and Therapeutics*. Oxford, England: Blackwell Scientific Publications Ltd; 1984.

37. Noble RE. Drug therapy in the elderly. *Metabolism: Clinical & Experimental* 2003; 52(10 suppl 2): 27–30.

38. Klotz U, Avant GR, Hoyumpa A, et al. The effects of age and liver disease on the disposition and elimination of diazepam in adult man. *J Clin Invest* 1975;55:347–359.

39. Greenblatt DJ, Allen MD, Harmatz JS. Diazepam disposition determinants. *Clin Pharmacol Ther* 1980;27:301–312.

40. Lamy PP. Nutrition, drugs, and the elderly. *Clin Nutr (Phila)* 1983;2:9–14.

41. Cohen JL. Pharmacokinetic changes in aging. *Am J Med* 1986;80:31–38.

42. Wallace SM, Verbeeck RK. Plasma protein binding of drugs in the elderly. *Clin Pharmacokinet* 1987;12:41–72.

43. Grandison MK, Boudinot FD. Age-related changes in protein binding of drugs: implications for therapy. *Clin Pharmackinet* 2000;38(3):271–290.

44. Rendic S, DiCarlo FJ. Human cytochrome P450 enzymes: a status report summarizing their reactions, substrates, inducers, and inhibitors. *Drug Metab Rev* 1997; 29:413–580.

45. Lown KS, Bailey DG, Fontana RJ, et al. Grapefruit juice increases felodipine oral availability in humans by decreasing intestinal CYP 3A protein expression. *J Clin Invest* 1997; 99:2545–2553.

46. Guengerich FR. Influence of nutrients and other dietary materials on cytochrome P450 enzymes. *Am J Clin Nutr* 1995;61:651S–658S.

47. Krishaswamy K. Effects of malnutrition on drug metabolism and toxicity in humans. In: Hathcock JN, ed. *Nutritional Toxicology*, Volume II. New York, NY: Academic Press Inc. 1987.

48. Sato K, Kawamura T, Wakusawa R. Hepatic blood flow and function in elderly patients undergoing laparoscopic cholecystectomy. *Anesthesia & Analgesia* 2000;90(5): 1198–1202.

49. Kamataki T, Maeda K, Shimada M, et al. Age-related alteration in the activities of drug-metabolizing enzymes and contents of sex-specific forms of cytochrome P-450 in liver microsomes from male and female rats. *J Pharmacol Exp Ther* 1985;233:222–228.

50. Greenblatt DJ, Allen MD, Harmatz JS, et al. The effects of age and liver disease on the disposition and elimination of diazepam in adult man. *J Clin Invest* 1975;55: 347–359.

51. Crooks J, O'Malley K, Stevenson IH. Pharmacokinetics in the elderly. *Clin Pharmacokinet* 1976;1:280–285.

52. Vestal RE, Woods JA, Branch RA, et al. Studies of drug disposition in the elderly using model compounds. In: Kitani K, ed. *Liver and Aging*. Amsterdam: Elsevier-North Holland; 1978.

53. Kitani K. Hepatic drug metabolism in the elderly. *Hepatology* 1986;6:316–319.

54. Sutter MA, Gibson G, Williamson LS, et al. Comparison of the hepatic mixed function oxidase systems of young, adult and old non-human primates (*Macaca nemiestrina*). *Biochem Pharmacol* 1985;34:2983 2987.

55. Maloney AG, Schmucker DL, Vessey DS, et al. The effects of aging on the hepatic microsomal mixed-function oxidase system of male and female monkeys. *Hepatology* 1986;6:282–287.

56. Kitani K. The role of the liver in the pharmacokinetic and pharmacodynamic alterations in the elderly. In: Waddington JL, O'Malley K, eds. *Therapeutics in the Elderly*. Amsterdam: Elsevier Scientific Publishers BV; 1985.

57. Davies DF, Shock NW. Age changes in glomerular filtration rate, effective renal plasma flow, and tubular excretory capacity in adult males. *J Clin Invest* 1950;29: 496–507.

58. Rowe JW, Andres R, Tobin JD, et al. Age-adjusted standards for creatinine clearance. *Ann Intern Med* 1976;84: 567 569.

59. Chan GL, Matzke GR. Effects of renal insufficiency on the pharmacokinetics and pharmacodynamics of opioid analgesics. *Drug Intell Clin Pharm* 1987;21:773–783.

60. Roth GS. Hormone receptor changes during adulthood and senescence: significance for aging research. *Fed Proc* 1979;38:1910–1914.

61. Feldman RD, Limbird RE, Nadeau J, et al. Alterations in leukocyte beta-receptor affinity with aging: a potential explanation for altered beta-adrenergic sensitivity in the elderly. *N Engl J Med* 1984;310:815–819.

62. Scott PJ, Reid JL. The effect of age on the response of human isolated arteries to noradrenaline. *Br J Clin Pharmacol* 1982;13:237–239.

63. Lamy PP. Age-associated pharmacodynamic changes. *Methods Find Exp Clin Pharmacol* 1987;9:153–159.

64. Gribbin B, Pickering TG, Sleight P, et al. Effect of age and high blood pressure on baroreflex sensitivity in man. *Cir Res* 1971;29:424–431.

65. Kohn RR. Human aging and disease. *J Chronic Dis* 1983;16:5–21.

66. Vestal RE. Drug use in the elderly: a review of problems and special considerations. *Drugs* 1978;16:358–382.

67. Lamy PP. *Prescribing for the Elderly* Littleton, MA: PSG Publishing Co Inc; 1980.

68. Orlander P, Johnson DG. Endocrinologic problems in the aged. *Otolaryngol Clin North Am* 1982;15:439–449.

69. Hartz SC, Blumberg JB. Use of vitamin and mineral supplements by the elderly. *Clin Nutr (Phila)* 1986;5: 130–136.

70. Glanz K. Compliance with dietary regimens. *Prev Med* 1980;9:787–791.

71. Colucci RA, Bell SJ, Blackburn GL. Nutritional problems of institutionalized and free-living elderly. *Compr Ther* 1987;13:20–28.

72. Chan L-N. Redefining drug-nutrient interactions. *Nutr Clin Pract* 2000;15:249–252.

73. Alonso-Aperte E, Varela-Moreiras G. Drugs-nutrient interactions: a potential problem during adolescence. *Eur J Clin Nutr* 2000;54:S69–S74.

74. Roe DA. Concurrent interactions of drugs with nutrients. In: Linder MC, ed. *Nutritional Biochemistry and Metabolism with Clinical Applications.* New York, NY: Elsevier Science Publishing Co Inc.; 1985.

75. Streiff RR. Anemia and nutritional deficiency in the acutely ill hospitalized patients. *Medical Clin North Am* 1993; 77:911–918.

76. Scott D, et al. The development of hypothrombinemia following antibiotic therapy in malnourished patients with low serum vitamin K levels. *Br Haematol* 1988; 68: 63–66.

77. Roe DA. Nutrient and drug interactions. *Nutr Rev* 1984; 42:141–154.

78. Roe DA. Pathological changes associated with drug-induced malnutrition. In: Sidransky H, ed. *Nutritional Pathology.* New York, NY: Marcel Dekker Inc; 1985.

79. Streeter AM, Goldston KJ, Bathur FA, et al. Cimetidine and malabsorption of cobalamine. *Dig Dis Sci* 1982;27: 13–16.

80. Kassarjian Z, Russell RM. Hypochlorhydria: a factor in nutrition. *Annu Rev Nutr* 1989;9:271–285.

81. Leiber CS. Alcohol, protein nutrition and liver injury. In: Winick M, ed. *Nutrition and Drugs.* New York, NY: John Wiley & Sons; 1983.

82. Brodie MJ, Boobis AR, Hillyard CJ, et al. Effect of isoniazid on vitamin D metabolism and hepatic monooxygenase activity. *Clin Pharmacol Ther* 1981;30:363–367.

83. Bengoa JM, Bolt MJG, Rosenberg IH. Hepatic vitamin D-25-hydroxylase inhibition by cimetidine and isoniazid. *J Clin Med* 1984;104:546–552.

84. Robbro OT, Christiansen C, Lund M. Development of anticonvulsant osteomalacia in epileptic patients on phenytoin treatment. *Acta Neurol Scand* 1974;50: 527–532.

85. Hahn TJ, Birge SJ, Sharp CR, et al. Phenobarbital-induced alterations in vitamin D metabolism. *J Clin Invest* 1972;51:741–748.

86. Miettinen TA. Effects of hypolipidemic drugs on bile acid in man. *Adv Lipid Res* 1981;18:65–97.

87. West RJ, Lloyd JK. The effect of cholestyramine on intestinal absorption. *Gut* 1975;16:93–98.

88. Gura KM, Couris RR. Drug-induced bone disease. *U.S. Pharmacist* 2002; 27:HS43-57.

89. Walan A. Strom M. Metabolic consequences of reduced gastric acidity. *Scandinavian J Gastroenterology* 1985; 111(suppl):24–30.

90. Roe DA. Adverse nutritional effects of OTC drug use in the elderly. In: Roe DA, ed. *Drugs and Nutrition in the Geriatric Patient.* New York, NY: Churchill-Livingstone Inc; 1984.

91. Lotz M, Zisman E, Bartter C. Evidence for phosphorus depletion syndrome in man. *N Engl J Med* 1968;278: 409–415.

92. Rud RK, Singer FR. Magnesium deficiency and excess. *Annu Rev Med* 1981;32:245–259.

93. Insogna KL, Bordley DR, Caro JF, et al. Osteomalacia and weakness from excessive antacids. *JAMA* 1980; 244: 2544–2546.

94. Benn A, Swan CJH, Cooke WT, et al. Effect of intraluminal pH on the absorption of pteroylmonoglutamic acid. *Br Med J* 1971;16:148–150.

95. Tolstoi LG. Nutritional problems related to stimulant laxative abuse. *Hospital Pharmacy* 1988;23:564–573.

96. Becker GI. The case against mineral oil. *Am J Digestive Dis* 1953;19:344–347.

97. Schindler AM. Isolated neonatal hypomagnesaemia associated with maternal overuse of stool softener (letter). *Lancet* 1984; 2:822.

98. Clark JH, Russell GJ, Fitzgerald JF, et al. Serum beta-carotene, retinol, and alpha-tocopherol levels during mineral oil therapy for constipation. *Am J Dis Child* 1987;141:1210–1212.

99. Roe DA. Drug interference with the assessment of nutritional status. *J Clin Lab Med* 1981;1:647–664.

100. Frame B, Guiang HL, Frost HN, et al. Osteomalacia induced by laxative (phenolphthalein) ingestion. *Arch Intern Med* 1971;128:794–796.

101. Leonards JH, Levy G. Gastrointestinal blood loss during prolonged aspirin administration. *N Engl J Med* 1973;289:1020.

102. Gouf KR, McCarthy C, Read AE, et al. Folic acid deficiency in rheumatoid arthritis. *Br Med J* 1964;1: 212–216.

103. Race TF, Paes IC, Faloon WW. Intestinal malabsorption induced by oral colchicine: comparison with neomycin and cathartic agents. *Am J Med Sci* 1970;259:32–41.

104. Singh BN. Effects of food on clinical pharmacokinetics. *Clin Pharmacokinet* 1999;37:213–255.

105. Mueller BA, Brierton DG, Abel SR, Bowman L. Effect of enteral feeding with Ensure on oral bioavailabilities

of ofloxacin and ciprofloxacin. *Antimicrob Agents Chemother* 1994; 38(9).2101–2105.

106. Howard PA, Hannaman KN. Warfarin resistance linked to enteral nutrition products. *J Am Diet Assoc* 1985; 713–715.

107. Penrod LE, Allen JB, Cabacungan LR. Warfarin resistance and enteral feedings: 2 case reports and a supporting in vitro study. *Arch Phys Med Rehabil* 2001; 82:1270–1273.

108. An Yeung SCS, Ensom MHH. Phenytoin and enteral feedings: does evidence support an interaction? *Ann Pharmacother* 2000;34:896–905.

109. Chan L-N. Drug-nutrient interactions in transplant recipients. *JPEN* 2001;25:132–141.

110. Wright DH, Pietz SL. Konstantinides FN, Rotschafer JC. Decreased in vitro fluroquinolone concentrations after admixture with an enteral feeding formulation. *JPEN* 2000;24:42–48.

111. Garcia-Luna P, Garcia E, Pereira JL, et al. Esophageal obstruction by solidification of the enteral feed: a complication. *Intensive Care Med* 1997;23:790–792.

112. Branda RF, Nelson NL. Inhibition of 5-methyltetrahydrolic acid transport by amphipathic drugs. *Drug-Nutrient Interact* 1981;1:45–53.

113. Roe AD. Drug effects on nutrient absorption, transport, and metabolism. *Drug Nutrient Interactions* 1985; 4(1–2):117–135.

114. Romero JA. Kuczler FJ Jr. Isoniazid overdose: recognition and management. *Am Fam Physician* 1998; 57(4): 749–752.

115. Corcino J, Waxman S, Herbert V. Mechanism of triamterene-induced megalobastosis. *Ann Intern Med* 1970;73:419.

116. Palomaki A, Malminiemi K, Solakivi T, Malminiemi O. Ubiquinone supplementation during lovastatin treatment: effect on LDL oxidation ex vivo. *J Lipid Res* 1998; 39(7):1430–1437.

117. Williams C, Netzloff M, Folkerts L, et al. Vitamin D metabolism and anticonvulsant therapy: effect of sunshine on incidence of osteomalacia. *South Med J* 1984; 77:834–836.

118. Hahn TJ, Avioli LV. Anticonvulsant-drug-induced mineral disorders. In: Roe DA, Campbell TC, eds. *Drugs and Nutrients: The Interactive Effects.* New York, NY: Marcel Dekker Inc; 1984.

119. Keith DA, Gundbeg CM, Japour A, et al. Vitamin K-dependent protein and anticonvulsant medication. *Clin Pharm Therap* 1983;34:529–532.

120. Jones Sr, Kimbrough RC. Moxalactam and hemorrhage. *Ann Intern Med* 1983;99:126.

121. Reddy J, Bailey RR. Vitamin K deficiency developing in patients with renal failure, treated with cephalosporin antibiotics. *N Z Med J* 1980;92:378–379.

122. Editorial. New example of vitamin K-drug interaction. *Nutr Rev* 1984;42:161–163.

123. Lambie DG, Johnson RH. Drugs and folate metabolism. *Drugs* 185;30:145–155.

124. Labadarios D. The effect of chronic drug administration on folate status and drug toxicity. In: Parks DV, Ioannides C, Walker R, eds. *Food, Nutrition and Chemical Toxicity.* London: Smith-Gordon; 1993.

125. Mallek HM, Nakamoto T. Dilantin and folic acid status. Clinical implications for the periodontist. *J Periodontol* 1981;52(5):255–259.

126. Rivey MP, Schottelius DD, Berg MJ. Phenytoin-folic acid: a review. *Drug Intell Clin Pharm* 1984;18(4): 292–301.

127. Seligmann H, Potasman I, Weller B, Schwartz M, Prokocimer M. Phenytoin-folic acid interaction: a lesson to be learned. *Clin Neuropharmacol* 1999;22(5): 268–272.

128. Lewis DP, Van Dyke DC, Wilhite LA, et al. Phenytoin-folic acid interaction. *Ann Pharmacother* 1995;29: 726–735.

129. Selhub J, Seyoum E, Pomfret EA, Zeisel SH. Effects of choline deficiency and methotrexate treatment upon liver folate content and distribution. *Cancer Res* 1991; 51:16–21.

130. Wegner C, Nau H. Alteration of embryonic folate metabolism by valproic acid during organogenesis: implications for mechanism of teratogenesis. *Neurology* 1992;42(suppl 5):17–24.

131. Ubed N, Alonso E, Martin-Rodriguez JC, et al. Valproic induced developmental modifications may be partially prevented by coadministration of folinic acid and S-adenosylmethionine. *Int J Dev Biol* 1996; (suppl 1): 291S–292S.

132. Ohtani Y, Endo F, Matsuda I. Carnitine deficiency with hyperammonemia associated with valproic acid therapy. *J Pediatr* 1982;101:782–785.

133. Zaccara G, Paganini M, Campostrini R, et al. Hyperammonemia and valproate-induced alterations of the state of consciousness. A report of 8 cases. *Eur Neurol* 1984;23:104–112.

134. Thurston JH, Hauhart RE. Amelioration of adverse effects of valproic acid on ketogenesis and liver coenzyme. A metabolism by cotreatment with pantothenate and carnitine in developing mice: possible clinical significance. *Pediatr Res* 1992;31:419–423.

135. Sugiomoto T, Nishida N, Murakami K, et al. Valproate-induced hepatotoxicity: protective effect of L-carnitine supplementation. *Jpn J Psychiatry Neurol* 1990;44: 387–387.

136. Bohles H, Sewell AZ, Wenzel D. The effect of carnitine supplementation in valproate-induced hyperammonemia. *Acta Paediatr* 1996;85:446–449.

137. Beversdorf D, Allen C, Nordgren R. Valproate-induced encephalopathy treated with carnitine in an adult [letter]. *J Neurol Neurosurg Psychiatry* 1996;61:211.

138. Triggs WJ, Gilmore RL, Millington DS, et al. Valproate-associated carnitine deficiency and malignant cerebral edema in the absence of hepatic failure. *Int J Clin Pharmacol Ther* 1997;35:353–356.

139. Sokol RJ, Johnson KE, Karrer FM, et al. Improvement of cyclosporine absorption in children after liver transplantation by means of water-soluble vitamin E. *Lancet* 1991;338:212–215.

140. Boudreaux JP, Hayes DH, Mizrahi S, et al. Use of water-soluble vitamin E to enhance cyclosporine absorption in children after liver transplant. *Tranplant Proc* 1993;25:1875.

141. Pan S, Lopez RR, Sher LS, et al. Enhanced oral cyclosporine absorption with water-soluble vitamin E after liver transplantation. *Pharmacotherapy* 1996;16:59–65.

142. Chang T, Benet LZ, Hebert MF. The effect of water-soluble vitamin E on cyclosporine pharmacokinetics in healthy volunteers. *Clin Pharmacol Ther* 1996;59:297–303.

143. Lawrence VA, Lowenstein JE, Eichner ER. Aspirin and folate binding: in vivo and in vitro studies of serum binding and urinary excretion of endogenous folate. *J Lab Clin Med* 1984;103:944–948.

144. Day AT, Golding JR, Lee PN, et al. Penicillamine in rheumatoid disease: a long term study. *Br Med J* 1974;1:180–183.

145. Wester PO. Zinc curing diuretic treatment. *Lancet* 1975;1:578.

146. Seligman H, Halkin H, Rauchefleisch S, et al. Thiamin deficiency in patients with congestive heart failure receiving long-term furosemide therapy: a pilot study. *Am J Med* 1991;91:151–155.

147. Brady JA, Rock CL, Horneffer MR. Thiamin status, diuretic medications, and the management of congestive heart failure. *J Am Diet Assoc* 1995;95:541–544.

148. Sonnenblick M, Friedlander Y, Rosin AJ. Diuretic-induced severe hyponatremia. Review and analysis of 129 reported patients. *Chest* 1993;103:601–606.

149. Lahr MB, Hyponatremia during carbamazepine therapy. *Clin Pharmacol Ther* 1985;37:693–696.

150. Brown RO, Dickerson RN. Drug-nutrient interactions. *Am J Managed Care* 1999;5(3):345–352.

151. Nelson DC, McGrew WR, Hoyumpa AM. Hypernatremia and lactulose therapy. *JAMA* 1983;249:1295–1298.

152. Tolstoi LG . Drug-induced hyperkalemia. *Hosp Pharm* 1996;31:221–228.

153. Velazquez H, Perazella MA, Wright FR, Ellison DH. Renal mechanism of trimethoprim-induced hyperkalemia. *Ann Intern Med* 1993;119:296–301.

154. Oster JR, Singer I, Fishman LM. Heparin-induced aldosterone suppression and hyperkalemia. *Am J Med* 1995;98:575–586.

155. Brown GR, Greenwood JK. Drug- and nutrition-induced hypophosphatemia: mechanisms and relevance in the critically ill. *Ann Pharmacother* 1994;28:626–632.

156. Malluche HH. Monier-Faugere MC. Understanding and managing hyperphosphatemia in patients with chronic renal disease. *Clin Nephrology* 1999;52(5):267–277.

157. Williams SE, Wardman AG, Taylor GA, et al. Long term study of the effect of rifampicin and isoniazid on vitamin D metabolism. *Tubercule* 1985;66:49–54.

158. Odes HS, Fraser GM, Krugliak P, et al. Effect of cimetidine on hepatic vitamin D metabolism in humans. *Digestion* 1990;20:251–262.

159. Roe DA. Nutrient and drug interactions. *Nutr Rev* 1984;42:141–154.

160. LoCascio V, Bonucci E, Imbinbo B, et al. Bone loss in response to long term glucocorticoid therapy. *Bone Miner* 1990;8:39–51.

161. Israel E, Banerjee TR, Fitzmaurice GM, et al. Effects of inhaled glucocorticoids on bone density in premenopausal women. *N Engl J Med* 2001;345:941–947.

162. al-Ghamdi SM, Cameron EC, Sutton RA. Magnesium deficiency: pathophysiologic and clinical overview. *Am J Kidney Dis* 1994;24:737–752.

163. Lajer H, Gaugaard G. Cisplatin and hypomagnesemia. *Cancer Treat Rev* 1999;25:47–58.

164. Leyvaz S, Ohnuma T, Lassus M, et al. Phase 1 study of carboplatin in patients with advanced cancer, intermittent intravenous bolus and 24-hour infusion. *J Clin Oncol* 1985;3:1385–1392.

165. Ferra C, Berlanga JJ, Gallardo D, et al. Mitoxantreone, etoposide, carboplatinum and Ara-C combination therapy in refractory and relapsed acute leukemia. *Leukemia Lymphoma* 2000;39:583–590.

166. Shetty AK, Rogers NI, Mannick EE, Aviles DH, Syndrome of hypokalemic metabolic alkalosis and hypomagnesemia associated with gentamicin therapy: case reports. *Clin Peds* 2000;39:529–533.

167. Arlette JP. Zinc and the skin. *Ped Clin N Amer* 1983;30:583–596.

168. Prasad AS. Clinical, biochemical and pharmacological role of zinc. *Ann Rev Pharmacol Toxicol* 1979;2:393–426.

169. Prasad AS, Brewer GJ, Schoomaker EB, et al. Hypocupremia induced by zinc therapy in adults. *JAMA* 1978;240:2166–2168.

170. Solomons NW. Zinc and copper in human nutrition: *Nutrition in the 1980's: Constraints On Our Knowledge.* New York, NY: Alan R. Liss Inc; 1981.

171. Ugarte M, Osborne NN. Zinc in the retina. *Prog Neurobio* 2001;64:219–249.

172. Pandit MK, Burke J, Gustafson AB, et al. Drug-induced disorders of glucose tolerance. *Ann Intern Med* 1993;118:529–539.

173. Plewe G, Beyer J, Krause U, et al. Long-acting and selective suppression of growth hormone secretion b somatostatin analogue SMS 201-995 in acromegaly. *Lancet* 1984;2:782–784.

174. Mills GA, Horn JR. Beta-blockers and glucose control. *Drug Intell Clin Pharm* 1985;19:246–251.

175. Henkin J, Como JA, Oberman A. Secondary dyslipidemia: inadvertent effects of drugs in clinical practice. *JAMA* 1992;267:961–968.

176. Baker VL. Alternatives to oral estrogen replacement. Transdermal patches, percutaneous gels, vaginal creams and rings, implants, other methods of delivery. *Ob Gynecol Clin N America* 1994;21(2):271–297.

177. McDonough RP, Cooper JW Jr. Drug-related problems in older adults. *J Am Pharm Assoc* 2002;42(5 Suppl 1):S32–33.

178. Pawan GLS. Drugs and appetite. *Proc Nutr Soc* 1974; 33:239–244.

179. Syiel JN, Liddle GW, Lacey WW. Studies of the mechanism of cyproheptadine-induced weight gain in human subjects. *Metabolism* 1970:19:192–200.

180. Welling PG. Effects of food on drug absorption. *Annu Rev Nutr* 1996;16:383–415.

181. Paybel PS, Mueller PS, DeLa Vergne PM. Amitriptyline weight gain and carbohydrate craving: a side effect. *Br J Psychiatry* 1973;123:501 507.

182. Willoughby JMT. Drug induced abnormalities of taste sensation. *Adverse Drug Reaction Bull* 1983;100: 368–371.

183. Morrison SD. Origins of anorexia in neoplastic disease. *Am J Clin Nutr* 1978;31:1104–1107.

184. Banks T, Ali N. Digitalis cachexia. *N Engl J Med* 1974; 290:746.

185. Herzog P. Holtermuller KH. Antacid therapy—changes in mineral metabolism. *Scandinavian J Gastroenterol* 1982;75(suppl):56–62.

186. Kinzie BJ. Management of the syndrome of inappropriate secretion of antidiuretic hormone. *Clinical Pharmacy* 1987;6(8):625–633.

187. Keenan WF Jr. Macrocytosis as an indicator of human disease. *J Amer Board Fam Pract* 1989;2(4):252–256.

188. Dreizen S, McCredie KB, Keating MJ, Andersson BS. Nutritional deficiencies in patients receiving cancer chemotherapy. *Postgrad Med* 1990;87(1):163–167, 170.

189. Knudsen L, Weismann K. Taste dysfunction and changes in zinc and copper metabolism during penicillamine therapy for generalized scleroderma. *Acta Med Scand* 1978;204(1–2):75–79.

190. Belle M, Halpern MM. Oral nicotinic acid for hyperlipidemia with emphasis on side effects. *Am J Cardiol* 1985;2:449–452.

191. Wilkins RW, Bearman JE, Boyle E, et al. Coronary Research Drug Project Group: Clofibrate and niacin in coronary heart disease. *JAMA* 1975;231:360–381.

192. Heyneman CA. Zinc deficiency and taste disorders. *Ann Pharmacother* 1996;30:186–187.

193. Dahl H, Norskov K, Peitersen E, et al. Zinc therapy of acetazolamide-induced side effects. *Acta Opthalmol* 1984;62:739–745.

194. Roe DA. Food, formula and drug effects on the disposition of nutrients. *World Rev Nutr Diet* 1984;43:80–94.

195. Toothaker RD, Welling PG. The effect of food on drug bioavailability. *Annu Rev Pharmacol Toxicol* 1980;20: 173–199.

196. Welling P. Nutrient effects on drug metabolism and action in the elderly. *Drug-Nutrient Interact* 1985;4: 183–193.

197. Rosenberg HA, Bates TR. The influence of food on nitrofurantoin bioavailability. *Clin Pharmacol Ther* 1976; 20:227–232.

198. Gibaldi M. *Biopharmaceutics and Clinical Pharmacokinetics.* Philadelphia, PA: Lea & Febiger; 1977.

199. McLean AJ, Isbister C, Bobik A, et al. Reduction of first-pass hepatic clearance of propranolol by food. *Clin Pharmacol Ther* 1981;30:31–34.

200. Lamy PP. *Prescribing for the Elderly.* Littleton, MA: PSG Publishing Co Inc; 1980.

201. Gillespie NG, Mena I, Cotzias GS, et al. Diets affecting treatment of parkinsonism with levodopa. *J Am Diet Assoc* 1973;62:525–532.

202. Nutt JG, Woodward WR, Hammerstad JP, et al. The "on-off" phenomenon in Parkinson's disease: relation to levodopa absorption and transport. *N Engl J Med* 1984;310:483–488.

203. Nichols TW. Phytobezoar formation: a new complication of cimetidine therapy. *Ann Intern Med* 1981;95: 70–73.

204. Welling PG. Influence of food and diet on gastrointestinal drug absorption: a review. *J Pharmacokinet Biopharm* 1977;5:291–315.

205. Evans MA, Triggs EJ, Cheung M. Gastric emptying in the elderly: implications for drug therapy. *J Am Geriatr Soc* 1981;29:201–207.

206. McLennan EJ, Martin P, Mason BJ. Protein intake and serum albumin levels in the elderly. *Gerontology* 1977; 27:360–367.

207. Richey DP, Bender AD. Pharmacokinetic consequences of aging. *Annu Rev Pharmacol Toxicol* 1977;17:49–65.

208. McDannell RE, McLean AEM. Role of nutrition status in drug metabolism and toxicity. In: Sidransky H, ed. *Nutritional Pathology.* New York, NY: Marcel Dekker Inc; 1985.

209. O'Malley K, Crooks J, Duke E, et al. Effect of age and sex on human drug metabolism. *Br Med J* 1971;3: 607–609.

210. Conney AH, Pantuck EJ, Juntzman R, et al. Nutrition and the chemical biotransformation in man. *Clin Pharmacol Ther* 1977;22:707–716.

211. Alvares AP, Anderson KE, Conney AH, et al. Interactions between nutritional factors and drug biotransformations in man. *Proc Natl Acad Sci USA* 1976; 73:2501–2504.

212. Mucklow JC, Caraher MT, Henderson DB, et al. Relationship between individual dietary constituents and antipyrine metabolism in Indo-Pakistani immigrants to Britain. *Br J Clin Pharmacol* 1982;13:481–486.

213. Vendrely B, Chauveau P, Barthe N, et al. Nutrition in hemodialysis patients previously on a supplemented very low protein diet. *Kidney International* 2003;63(4): 1491–1498.

214. Pijls LT, de Vries H, van Eijk JT, Donker AJ. Protein restriction, glomerular filtration rate and albuminuria in patients with type 2 diabetes mellitus: a randomized trial. *Eur J Clin Nutr* 2002;56(12):1200–1207.

215. Maiorca R, Brunori G, Viola BF, et al. Diet or dialysis in the elderly? The DODE study: a prospective randomized multicenter trial. *J Nephrology* 2000;13(4): 267–270.

216. Anderson KE, Conney AH, Kappas A. Nutrition and oxidative drug metabolism in man: relative influence of dietary lipids, carbohydrate and protein. *Clin Pharmacol Ther* 1979;26:493–501.

217. Krishnaswamy K, Naidu AN. Microsomal enzymes and malnutrition as determined by plasma half-life of antipyrine. *Br Med J* 1977;1:538–542.

218. Pantuck EJ, Pantuck CB, Garland WA, et al. Stimulatory effect of Brussels sprouts and cabbage on human drug metabolism. *Clin Pharmacol Ther* 1979;25:88–95.

219. Williams D, Hill DP, Davis JA, et al. The influence of food on the absorption and metabolism of foods: an update. *Eur J Metab Pharmacokinet* 1996;21:201–211.

220. Kall M, Vang O, Clausen J. Effects of dietary broccoli on human drug metabolizing activity. *Cancer Letters* 1997;114:169–170.

221. Lasker JM, Wuang MT, Conney AH. In vivo activation of zoxazolamine metabolism by flavone. *Science* 1982; 216:1419–1421.

222. Slaughter DL, Edwards DJ. Recent advances, the cytochrome P450 enzymes. *Ann Pharmacother* 1995;29: 619–624.

223. Edwards DJ, Bernier SM. Naringin and naringenin are not the primary CYP3A inhibitors in grapefruit juice. *Life Sci* 1996;59:1025–1030.

224. Anon. Grapefruit juice interactions with drugs. *Med Letter Drug Ther* 1995;37:73–74.

225. Josefesson M, Zackrisson AL, Ahlner J. Effect of grapefruit on the pharmacokinetics of amlodipine in health volunteers. *Eur J Clin Pharm* 1996;51:189–193.

226. Rau SE, Bend JR, Arnold Mo, et al. Grapefruit juice-terfenadine single-dose interaction: magnitude, mechanism and relevance. *Clin Pharmacol Ther* 1997;61: 1–9.

227. Hukkinen SK, Varke A, Olkkaol KT, et al. Plasma concentrations of triazolam are increased by concomitant ingestion of grapefruit juice. *Clin Pharmacol Ther* 1995;58:127–131.

228. Min DI, Hu YM, Perry PJ, et al. Effect of grapefruit juice on cyclosporine pharmacokinetics in renal transplant patients. *Transplantation* 1996;62:123–125.

229. VanCleef GF, Fisher EJ, Polk RE. Drug interaction potential with inhibitors of HIV protease. *Pharmacotherapy* 1997;17:774–778.

230. Park GD, Spector R, Kitt TM. Effect of dietary protein on renal tubular clearance of drugs in humans. *Clin Pharmacokinetic* 1989;17(6):441–451.

231. Alleyne GAO. The effect of severe protein calorie malnutrition on renal function of Jamaican children. *Pediatrics* 1967;400–411.

232. Cuddy PG, Bealer JF, Lyman EL, Pemberton B. Theophylline disposition following parenteral feeding of malnourished patients. *Ann Pharmacother* 1993;28: 836–837.

233. Williams L, David JA, Lowenthal DT. The influence of food on the absorption and metabolism of drugs. *Med Clin N Amer* 1993;77:815–829.

234. Welling P. Nutrient effects on drug metabolism and action in the elderly. *Drug-Nutrient Interactions* 1985; 4:173–207.

235. Kappas A, Anderson KE, Conney AH, et al. Influence of dietary protein and carbohydrate on antipyrine and theophylline metabolism in man. *Clin Pharmacol Ther* 1976;20:643–653.

236. Sonawane BR, Coates PN, Yaffe SJ, et al. Influence of dietary carbohydrates (alpha-saccharides) on hepatic drug metabolism in male rats. *Drug Nutr Interact* 1983; 2:7–16.

237. D'Arcy PF. Nutrient-drug interactions. *Adverse Drug React Toxicol Rev* 1995;14:233–254.

238. Floyd RA, Greenberg WM, Caldwell C. In vitro interaction between digoxin and bran. 12th Annual ASHP Midyear Clinical Meeting, Atlanta, Georgia, Dec. 6, 1977.

239. Reissell P, Manninen V. Effect of administration of activated charcoal and fibre on absorption, excretion and steady state blood levels of digoxin and digitoxin. Evidence for intestinal secretion of the glycosides. *Acta Med Scan* 1982; 668(suppl):88–89.

240. Beach RS, Mantero-Atienza E, Fordyce-Baum MK. Dietary supplementation in HIV infection. *FASEB J* 1988;2:A1435.

241. Richter WO, Jacob BG, Schwandt P. Interaction between fibre and lovastatin. *Lancet* 1991;338:706.

242. Stewart DE. High-fiber diet and serum tricyclic antidepressant levels. *J Clin Psychopharmacol* 1992;12: 438–440.

243. Champagne ET. Low gastric hydrochloric acid secretion and mineral bioavailability. *Advances in Experimental Medicine & Biology* 1989;249:173–184.

244. Vessell ES. Complex effects of diet on drug disposition. *Clin Pharm Ther* 1984;36:285–296.

245. Melander A, Danielson K, Schersten B, Wahlin E. Enhancement of the bioavailability of propranolol and metoprolol by food. *Clin Pharmacol Ther* 1977; 22(1):108–112.

246. Elvin AT, Cole D, Peper JA, et al. Effect of food on lidocaine kinetics: mechanism of food-related alteration in high intrinsic clearance drug elimination. *Clin Pharmacol Ther* 1981;30:455–460.

247. Anderson KE. Influences on diet and nutrition on clinical pharmacokinetics. *Clin Pharmacokinetics* 1988; 14:325–346.

248. Berlinger WG, Park GD, Spector R. The effect of dietary protein on the clearance of allopurinol and oxypurinol. *N Engl J Med* 1985;313:771–776.

249. Guengerich FB. Effects of nutritive factors on metabolic processes involving bioactivation and detoxification of chemicals. *Ann Rev Nutr* 1984;4:207–231.

250. Garry PJ, Goodwin JS, Hunt MA, et al. Nutritional status in a healthy elderly population: dietary and supplemental intakes. *Am J Clin Nutr* 1982;36:319–331.

251. Ban TA. Pharmacotherapy of schizophrenia with special reference to megavitamin therapy. *Canad J Psychiat Nurs* 1973;14:6–9.

252. Dipalma JR. Vitamin toxicity. *Am Fam Physic* 1978; 18:106–109.

253. Anon. On the toxicity of water-soluble vitamins. *Nutr Revs* 1984;42:265–267.

254. Anon. Megavitamin E supplementation and vitamin K-dependent carboxylation. *Nutr Revs* 1983;41:268–270.

255. Krishnaswamy K. Drug metabolism and pharmacokinetics in malnutrition. *Trans Pharmacol Sci* 1983;4: 295–297.

256. Garvadian-Ruffalo SM. Alterations in drug effects secondary to vitamin supplementation. *Intern Med* 1984; 5:129–137.

257. Levy G, Leonards JR. Urine pH and salicylate therapy. *JAMA* 1971;217:81.

258. Rosenthal G. Interaction of ascorbic acid with warfarin. *JAMA* 1971;215:1671–1672.

259. Rall TN, Schleifer LS. Drugs effective in the therapy of the epilepsies. In: Gilman AG, Goodman LS, Gilman A, eds. *The Pharmacological Basis of Therapeutics*. New York, NY: Macmillan Publishing Co; 1980.

260. Houston JB. Effect of vitamin C supplement on antipyrine disposition in man. *Br J Clin Pharmacol* 1977; 4(2):236–239.

261. Beattie AD, Sherlock S. Ascorbic acid deficiency in liver disease. *Gut* 1976;17:571–575.

262. Herbert VD. Megavitamin therapy. *J Amer Pharmaceut Assoc* 1977;17(12):764–766.

263. Herbert V, Jacob E. Destruction of vitamin B_{12} by ascorbic acid. *JAMA* 1974;230:241–242.

264. Auer BK, Auer D, Rodgers AL. Relative hyperoxaluria, crystalluria and haematuria after megadose ingestion of vitamin C. *Eur J Clin Invest* 1998;28:695–700.

265. Schaumburg H, Kaplan J, Winderbank A, et al. Sensory neuropathy from pyridoxine abuse. *N Engl J Med* 1983; 309:445–448.

266. Stirling Y. Warfarin-induced changes in procoagulant and anticoagulant proteins. *Blood Coagulation & Fibrinolysis* 1995;6(5):361–373.

267. Lutomski DM, Palascak JE, Bower RH. Warfarin resistance associated with intravenous lipid administration. *JPEN* 1987;11:316–318.

268. Evans AM. Influence of dietary components on the gastrointestinal metabolism and transport of drugs. *Therapeutic Drug Monitoring* 2000;22:131–136.

269. Charman WN, Porter CJH, Mithani S, et al. Physicochemical and physiological mechanism for the effects of food on drug absorption: the role of lipids and pH. *J Pharm Sci* 1997;86:269–282.

270. Fleisher D, Li C, Zhou Y, et al. Drug, meal and formulation interactions influencing drug absorption after oral administration. Clin Implications. *Clin Pharmacokinet* 1999; 36:233–254.

271. Ioannides C. Effect of diet and nutrition on the expression of cytochrome P450. *Xenobiotica* 1999; 29:109–54.

272. Anderson KE. Influences of diet and nutrition on clinical pharmacokinetics. *Clin Pharmacokinet* 1988;14: 325–346.

273. Walter-Sack I, Klotz U. Influence of diet and nutritional status on drug metabolism. *Clin Pharmacokinet* 1996; 31:47–64.

274. Kappas A, et al. Influence of dietary protein and carbohydrate on antipyrine and theophylline metabolism in man. *Clin Pharmacol Ther* 1976;20:643–53.

275. Kappas A, et al. Effect of charcoal broiled beef on antipyrine and theophylline metabolism. *Clin Pharmacol Ther* 1978;23:445–450.

276. Conney AH. Pharmacological implications of microsomal enzyme induction. *Pharmacol Rev* 1967;19: 317–366.

277. Welling PG, Lyons LL, Craig WA, Trochta GA. Influence of diet and fluid on bioavailability of theophylline. *Clin Phamacol Ther* 1975;17:475–480.

278. Mayhew SL, Christensen ML. Pharmacokinetic alterations in malnutrition and obesity. *Hosp Pharm* 1993; 28:836–837.

279. Schwartz JG, McMahan CA, Green GM. Phillips WT. Gastric emptying in Mexican Americans compared to non-Hispanic whites. *Dig Dis & Sciences* 1995;40(3): 624–630.

280. Davenport HW. *Physiology of the Digestive Tract*. Chicago, IL: Chicago Year Book Publishers; 1961.

281. Marcus CS, Lengemann FW. Absorption of 45Ca and 85Sr from solid and liquid food at various levels of the alimentary tract of the rat. *J Nutr* 1962;77:155–160.

282. Nutt JG, Woodward WR, Hammerstad JP, Carter JH, Anderson JL. The "on-off" phenomenon in Parkinson's disease. Relation to levodopa absorption and transport. *N Engl J Med* 1984;310(8):483–488.

283. DeSmet PAGM. Herbal remedies. *N Engl J Med* 2002; 347(25):2046–2056.

284. Dietary Supplement Health and Education Act of 1994. http://Thomas/loc.gov/cgi-bin/query/d?c103: 6:./temp~c103705qih:e13550 (accessed 2000 Sep 20).

285. Gugliotta G. Health concerns grow over herbal aids. http://washingtonpost.com/wp-dn/articles/a32685-2000mar17.html (accessed 2000 Sep 20).

286. American Society of Health-System Pharmacists. Snapshot of medication use in the US. www.ashp.org/public/public_relations/snapshot.pdf (accessed 2001 Feb 3).

287. Food and Drug Administration. Regulations on statements made for dietary supplements concerning the effect of the product on the structure or function of the body; final rule. *Fed Reg* 2000;65:1000–1005.

288. Jellin JM, Gregory P, Batz F, et al, eds. Pharmacist's letter/prescriber's letter natural medicines comprehensive database. www.naturaldatabase.com (accessed 2001 Feb 3).

289. Smith M. Drug interactions with natural health products/dietary supplements: a survival guide. Paper presented at: Complementary and Alternative Medicine: Implications for Clinical Practice and State-of-the-Science Symposia; March 12, 2000; Boston, MA.

290. Durr D, Stieger B, Kullak-Ublick GA et al. St. John's wort induces intestinal P-glycoprotein/MDRI and intestinal and hepatic CYP3A4. *Clin Pharmacol Ther* 2000;68:598–604.

291. Yu DK. The contribution of P-glycoprotein to pharmacokinetic drug-drug interactions. *J Clin Pharmacol* 1999;39:1203–1211.

292. Rothkopf M, Vogel G, Lang W, et al. Animal experiments on the question of the renal tolerance of the horse chestnut saponin aescin. *Arzneimittelforschung* 1977; 27:598–605.

293. Roby CA, Anderson GD, Kantor E, et al. St. John's wort: effect on CYP3A4 activity. *Clin Pharmacol Ther* 2000; 67:451–457.

294. Food and Drug Administration. Risk of drug interactions with St. John's wort and indinavir and other drugs. www.fda.gov/cder/drug/advisory/stjwort.htm (accessed 2000 Oct 31).

295. Yue Q-Y, Berquist C, Gerden B. Safety of St. John's Wort (hypericum perforatum). *Lancet* 2000;355:576–577.

296. Cheng TO. St. John's wort interactions with digoxin. *Arch Intern Med* 2000;160:2548.

297. John A, Brockmoller J, Bauer S, et al. Pharmacokinetic interaction of digoxin with an herbal extract from St. John's wort (hypericum perforatum). *Clin Pharmacol Ther* 1999;66:338–345.

298. Nebel A, Schneider BJ, Baker RK, et al. Potential metabolic interactions between St. John's wort and theophylline. *Ann Pharmacother* 1999;33:502.

299. Piscitelli SC, Burstein AH, Chaitt D, et al. Indinavir concentrations and St. John's wort. *Lancet* 2000;355: 547–548.

300. Breidenbach Y, Hoffman MW, Becher T, et al. Drug interaction of St. John's wort with cyclosporine. *Lancet* 2000;355:1912.

301. Ruschitzka F, Meier PJ, Turina M, et al. Acute heart transplant refection due to Saint John's wort. *Lancet* 2000;355:548–549.

302. Roots I, Johne A, Schmider I, et al. Interaction of a herbal extract from St. John's wort with amitriptyline and its metabolites. *Clin Pharmacol Ther* 2000;67:159.

303. Henney J. Risk of interactions with St. John's wort. *JAMA* 2000;283:13.

304. Greeson JM, Sanford B, Monti DA. St. John's wort (hypericum perforatum): a review of the current pharmacologic toxicological, and clinical literature. *Psychopharmacology (Berl)* 2001;153:402–414.

305. Gordon JB. SSRI's and St. John's wort: possible toxicity [letter]. *Am Fam Phys* 1998;57:950, 953.

306. Blumental M, Goldberg A, Brinckmann J, eds. *Herbal Medicine: Expanded Commission E Monographs*. Austin, TX: American Botanical Council; 2000.

307. LeBars PL, Katz MM, Berman N, et al. A placebo-controlled, double-blind, randomized trial of an extract of Gingko biloba for dementia. *JAMA* 1997;278: 1327–1332.

308. Sastre J, Millan A, de la Asuncion G, et al. A Gingko biloba extract (Egb761) prevents mitochondrial aging by protecting against oxidative stress. *Free Rad Biol Med* 1998;24:298–304.

309. Diamond BJ, Shiflett SC, Feiwel N, et al. Gingko biloba extract: mechanisms and clinical indications. *Ach Phys Med Rehabil* 2000;81:668–678.

310. Chung KF, Dent G, McCusker M, et al. Effect of a ginkgolide mixture (BN 52063) in antagonizing skin

and platelet responses to platelet activating factor in man. *Lancet* 1987;1:248–251.

311. Rowin J, Lewis SL. Spontaneous bilateral subdural hematomas associated with chronic Gingko biloba ingestion. *Neurology* 1996;46:1775–1776

312. Vale S. Subarachnoid haemorrhage associated with Gingko biloba. *Lancet* 1998;352:36.

313. Rosenblatt M, Mindel J. Spontaneous hyphema associated with ingestion of gingko biloba extract. *N Eng J Med* 1997;336:1108.

314. Janetzky K, Morreale AP. Probable interaction between warfarin and ginseng. *Am J Health-Syst Pharm* 1997; 54:692–693.

315. Sotaniemi EA, Haapakoski E, Rautio A. Ginseng therapy in non-insulin-dependant diabetic patients. *Diabetes Care* 1995;18:1373–1375.

316. Vuksan V, Sievenpiper JL, Koo VY, et al. American ginseng (Panax quinquefolius L) reduces postprandial glycemia in non-diabetic subjects and subjects with type 2 diabetes mellitus. *Arch Intern Med* 2000;160: 1009–1013

317. Vuksan V, Stavro MP, Sievenpiper JL, et al. Similar postprandial glycemic reductions in escalation of dose and administration time of American ginseng in type 2 diabetes. *Diabetes Care* 2000;23:1221–1226.

318. Rose KD, Croissant PD, Parliament CF, et al. Spontaneous spinal epidural hematoma with associated platelet dysfunction from excessive garlic ingestion: a case report. *Neurosurgery* 1990;26:880–882.

319. Legnani C, Frascaro M, Guazzaloca G, et al. Effects of a dried garlic preparation on fibrinolysis and platelet aggregation in healthy subjects. *Arzneimittelforschung* 1993;43:119–122.

320. Burnham BE. Garlic as a possible risk for postoperative bleeding. [letter]. *Plast Reconstr Surg* 1995;95:213.

321. German K, Kumar U, Blackford HN. Garlic and the risk of TURP bleeding. *Br J Urol* 1995;76:518.

322. Sunter WH. Warfarin and garlic. *Pharm J* 1991;246: 772.

323. Pittler MH, Ernst E. Efficacy of kava extract for treating anxiety: systematic review and meta-analysis. *J Clin Psychopharmacol* 2000;20:84–89.

324. Scheloscky L, Raffauf C, Kendroska K, et al. Kava and dopamine antagonism. *J Neurol Neurosurg Psychiatry* 1995;58:639–640.

325. Almeida JC, Grimsley EW. Coma from the health food store: interactions between kava and alprazolam. *Ann Intern Med* 1996;125:940–941.

326. Jonas WB, Levin JS, eds. Idem. The safety of herbal products. In: *Essentials of Complementary and Alternative Medicine*. Philadelphia, PA: Lippincott Williams and Wilkins; 1999:108–147

327. Farese RV Jr, Biglieri EG, Shackelton CHL, Irony I, Gomez-Fontes R. Licorice-induced hypermineral corticoidism. *N Engl J Med* 1991;325(17):1223–1227.

328. Wash LK, Bernard JD. Licorice-induced pseudoaldosteronism. *Am J Hosp Pharm* 1975;32(1):73–74.

329. Bannister B, Ginsburg R, Shneerson J. Cardiac arrest due to licorice-induced hypokalaemia. *Br Med J* 1977; 9(17):738–9.

330. Michalets EL. Update: clinically significant cytochrome P-450 drug interactions. *Pharmacotherapy* 1998;18:84–112.

331. Roe DA. Drug-nutrient interactions in the elderly. *Geriatrics* 1986;41:57–74.

332. Lamy PP. Effects of diet and nutrition on drug therapy. *J Am Geriatr Soc* 1982;30:S99.

CHAPTER 17

The Geriatric Exercise Prescription: Nutritional Implications

Maria A. Fiatarone Singh, MD

At all ages, physical activity and exercise capacity play an important role in health promotion and disease prevention. Nowhere is this dual role more evident than in the care of geriatric patients. It is in this cohort that genetic susceptibility, lifestyle choices, accumulated burden of disease, accidents, and iatrogenic misfortunes intersect to weave an intricate tapestry that represents both current health status as well as prognosis for the coming years. In the following discussion, the potent ability of physical activity and exercise patterns to influence this pathway at all levels beyond genetic susceptibility defines its importance.[1] Physical fitness levels in old age have been shown to be directly related to functional limitations, as well as indirectly related through diseases associated with inactivity.[2-7] Thus, health care practitioners in all disciplines will be better able to serve their elderly clientele if they understand the theoretical basis for, and the practical implementation of, an exercise prescription for this population.

IMPORTANCE OF EXERCISE IN GERIATRICS AND GERIATRIC NUTRITION

Physical activity exerts benefit at multiple levels, including amelioration of the biological changes of aging; prevention or delay in the development of risk factors for chronic diseases

such as ischemic heart disease, stroke, diabetes, and osteoarthritis; primary prevention of some of the most common chronic diseases in the elderly; treatment for disabling geriatric syndromes not well addressed by standard medical practice; and adjunctive treatment for established disease (Table 17–1).

In addition, the pharmacotherapy offered for chronic disease may carry with it a burden of side effects, including often-unrecognized nutritional consequences in the elderly patient. In these situations (Table 17–2), a novel combination of exercise and standard care may shift the risk/benefit ratio of treatment significantly. For example, some common yet unheeded side effects of long-term corticosteroid treatment for chronic obstructive pulmonary disease or inflammatory arthritis are severe osteopenia and osteoporotic fractures, proximal myopathy, and wasting. Progressive resistance training has been shown in both animals and humans to reverse losses of both muscle and bone mass associated with corticosteroid therapy alone.[8,9] Loss of lean tissue secondary to hypocaloric dieting, low-protein diets in chronic renal failure, or disuse accompanying bed rest or decreased mobility with any acute or chronic illness may all be similarly attenuated by an appropriate prescription of resistive exercises in these situations.[10,11]

Many diseases and medications are associated with anorexia and weight loss. It is often

Table 17–1 Benefits of Exercise in the Elderly

Minimizing Physiologic Changes of Aging	Decreasing Risk Factors for Chronic Disease	Preventing or Delaying Onset of Chronic Diseases	Providing Adjunctive Treatment for Established Diseases	Preventing and/or Treating Common Geriatric Syndromes
Atrophy of tendons and ligaments	Glucose intolerance	Breast cancer	Chronic obstructive pulmonary disease	Anorexia/nutrient deficiencies
Decreased aerobic and glycolytic enzyme capacity	Hyperinsulinemia and insulin resistance	Colon cancer	Congestive heart failure	Constipation
Decreased bone mass and fracture threshold	Hyperlipidemia	Coronary artery disease	Coronary artery disease	Functional decline
Decreased capillary density	Hypertension	Endometrial cancer	Depression	Gait and balance disorders/falls
Decreased glycogen storage, insulin sensitivity, glucose tolerance	Inflammatory cytokinemia (CRP, IL-6, etc.)	Hypertension	Diabetes mellitus	Incontinence
Decreased maximal aerobic capacity and cardiovascular efficiency	Obesity, visceral obesity	Osteoporosis	Hypertension	Insomnia / Low back pain
Decreased muscle mass and strength		Stroke	Inflammatory arthritis	Low self-efficacy
Decreased tissue elasticity, joint flexibility		Type 2 diabetes mellitus	Obesity	Low self-esteem
Endothelial cell dysfunction			Osteoarthritis	Social isolation, loneliness, low morale
Immunosenescence			Parkinson's disease	Weakness, fatigue, low exercise tolerance
Increased fat mass			Peripheral vascular disease	
Increased visceral adiposity			Stroke	
			Varicose veins	

Table 17–2 Counteracting Adverse Consequences of Chronic Disease Treatment with Exercise

Disease Treatment	Adverse Consequence	Effective Exercise Modalities
Anorexia secondary to drug therapy (digoxin, serotonin reuptake inhibitors, theophylline, multiple-drug regimens)	Weight loss, sarcopenia	Progressive resistance exercise*
Corticosteroid treatment for chronic pulmonary disease or inflammatory arthritis	Myopathy, osteopenia, osteoporotic fracture	Progressive resistance exercise Progressive resistance exercise and endurance exercise
Hypocaloric dieting for obesity	Loss of lean body mass (muscle and bone)	Progressive resistance exercise
Low-protein diet for chronic renal failure or liver failure	Weight loss, sarcopenia	Progressive resistance exercise*
Postural hypotension secondary to drug therapy (diuretics, anti-hypertensives, Parkinsonian drugs, antidepressants)	Postural symptoms, falls, fractures	Endurance exercise
Slowed gastrointestinal motility secondary to anticholinergics, narcotics, calcium channel blockers, iron therapy	Constipation, fecal impaction, reduced food intake	Progressive resistance exercise and endurance training*
Thyroid replacement for hypothyroidism	Osteopenia	Progressive resistance exercise and endurance exercise
Treatment with beta blockers or alpha-methyldopa for hypertension or heart disease	Depression	Progressive resistance training or endurance training*

*For these conditions, the benefit of exercise remains to be tested in controlled trials in patients receiving the indicated treatment. For example, exercise has been shown to speed gastrointestinal transit time and theoretically would counteract the constipating effect of listed medications.

difficult to treat such patients with nutritional interventions alone because their energy requirements are markedly blunted by both low muscle mass, and thereby basal metabolic rate, and restricted energy expenditure in physical activity. Attempts at nutritional supplementation with additional energy are often not successful in these situations, whereas individuals who begin an exercise regimen along with supplementation have been shown to be able to augment their total energy intake significantly.[12] This combination of multinutrient supplemen-

tation and anabolic exercise also improved adaptations to resistance training, including greater strength gain, muscle hypertrophy, and insulin-like growth factor-1 expression in skeletal muscle in these frail elders.[13] In addition to stimulating appetite, initiation of resistance training has been shown to augment nitrogen retention in older adults.[14,15] Such an adaptation may be especially important for older adults in catabolic situations such as recovery from surgery or trauma, catabolic illnesses, hepatic diseases, and low protein intake.[10,11]

Overall, the concept should be to implement, whenever possible, a multidisciplinary approach to the management of medical and nutritional disorders in the elderly, recognizing the vital interdependence of the elements of nutritional requirements, energy expenditure in physical activity, body composition, and the health and medication profile in geriatric practice.

PHYSIOLOGIC CHANGES OF AGING THAT AFFECT EXERCISE CAPACITY

The important physiologic alterations in the elderly that affect exercise capacity are listed in Table 17–3. Although these changes affect peak athletic performance, they do not prevent physiologic adaptation to an appropriate exercise stimulus, even in individuals of very advanced age. The ability of exercise training to moderate or even reverse some of these changes suggests that a proportion of what we know as "aging" is not inevitable biologic progression but is attributable to disuse of organ systems over time.[7] Unquestionably, certain age-related phenomena would persist despite athletic training, such as the decline in maximal heart rate or perhaps motor neuron death.[16] However, the impact of such "unavoidable" physiologic aging is primarily limited to performance in athletic competitions and will cause little disability in daily functional activities for the otherwise healthy older adult.

Table 17–3 Physiologic Changes of Aging That Impair Exercise Capacity

Physiologic Change	Habitual Exercise Minimizes Change
Decreased glucose transport and glycogen storage capacity in skeletal muscle	Yes
Decreased capillary density in skeletal muscle	Yes
Decreased ligament and tendon strength	Yes
Decreased maximal aerobic capacity	Yes
Decreased maximal heart rate	No
Decreased maximal muscle strength	Yes
Decreased muscle endurance	Yes
Decreased muscle mass	Yes
Decreased muscle power	Yes
Decreased nerve conduction velocity	Yes
Decreased skeletal oxidative muscle and glycolytic enzyme capacity in skeletal muscle	Yes
Decreased pulmonary flow rates	No
Decreased stroke volume	Yes
Decreased tissue elasticity and joint range of motion	Yes
Degeneration of cartilage	Yes*
Increased fat mass and percent body fat	Yes
Increased heart rate and blood pressure response to submaximal exercise	Yes
Loss of motor neurons and motor units	Unknown
Prolonged neural reaction time	Yes

*Although exercise-related injuries may result in chronic damage and degeneration of cartilage, habitual weight-bearing exercise without injury is protective to cartilage viability.

NUTRITIONAL DISORDERS IN THE ELDERLY AND THEIR IMPACT ON EXERCISE CAPACITY

Physiologic aging and chronic diseases are not the only factors that limit functional capacity in the elderly. If nutritional deficiencies exist as well, the potential for clinically overt consequences for functional capacity is even greater (Table 17–4). Protein-calorie malnutrition, alone or in combination with catabolic diseases, will lead to loss of lean body mass. Loss of muscle mass, from undernutrition, aging, or other causes (sarcopenia), may result in weakness, gait and balance disorders, falls and fractures, functional decline, and insulin insensitivity and is thus one of the most important sequelae of malnutrition in the elderly.[17–19]

Micronutrient status is also important for physical function. Skeletal muscle expresses receptors for 1,25 dihydroxyvitamin D, which appear to be necessary for the rapid intracellular reuptake of calcium into the sarcoplasmic reticulum in the relaxation phase of myofilament contraction.[20,21] Muscle that cannot fully relax in this way cannot subsequently produce maximal force during the contractile phase, and this cycle results in clinical muscle weakness, particularly of the proximal muscles of the lower extremities. The proximal myopathy of osteomalacia is also associated with pain and atrophy in the affected muscle groups but is reversible with vitamin D repletion. High-risk individuals for this condition include homebound or institutionalized elders; veiled women; those chronically receiving corticosteroids, dilantin, or phenytoin; those living in countries where dairy products are not fortified with vitamin D; or individuals abstaining from dairy products even when these are fortified due to lactose intolerance or other reasons.

Other nutritional deficiencies that impair muscle contractile activity and result in clinical weakness include deficiencies of the minerals calcium, magnesium, and potassium. Thus, patients administered long-term or high-dose diuretic therapy are at highest risk. Furosemide will cause losses of all three minerals; thiazide-type diuretics will spare calcium but not the other two.

Table 17–4 Nutritional Deficiencies That Impair Exercise Tolerance

Deficiency	Physiologic Consequence	Primary Exercise Capacity Affected
B_{12}	Central and peripheral nervous system dysfunction	Muscle strength and power
Calcium	Muscle contractile dysfunction, cardiac conduction disturbance	Aerobic capacity; muscle strength, power, and endurance
Carbohydrate	Reduced glycogen storage	Aerobic capacity; musculoskeletal endurance
Energy	Sarcopenia, osteopenia	Aerobic capacity; muscle strength, power, and endurance
Iron	Decreased oxygen carrying capacity	Aerobic capacity
Magnesium	Muscle contractile dysfunction, cardiac conduction disturbance	Aerobic capacity; muscle strength, power, and endurance
Potassium	Muscle contractile dysfunction, cardiac conduction disturbance	Aerobic capacity; muscle strength, power, and endurance
Protein	Sarcopenia, osteopenia	Aerobic capacity; muscle strength, power
Thiamin	Nerve conduction impairment, myopathy, cardiac dysfunction	Aerobic capacity; muscle strength, power, and endurance
Vitamin D	Muscle contractile dysfunction and atrophy	Aerobic capacity; muscle strength, power, and endurance

Magnesium replacement is usually not offered even when potassium is replaced, and it should be remembered that intracellular stores of potassium cannot be repleted in the face of inadequate magnesium. Because serum levels of these minerals remain normal even when tissue stores are quite low, they are an insensitive index of deficiency states and should not be relied upon to determine the need for supplementation. Patients with no other definable cause for muscle weakness and fatigue who have risk factors for these mineral losses should be considered candidates for replacement or alternative drug therapy. Sometimes in the elderly, fatigue may be a more prominent complaint than actual muscle weakness in these conditions, so a thorough history and a high index of suspicion are essential to early diagnosis and treatment.

OPTIMIZING BODY COMPOSITION WITH EXERCISE IN OLDER ADULTS

One of the most direct pathways from physical activity to health status involves the modulation of body composition by habitual exercise patterns. The typical patterns of change in body compartments seen in "usual aging" include decreased muscle and bone mass and increased total and central fat mass. The extent to which these changes occur in an individual depend upon a combination of genetic, lifestyle, and disease-related factors that are all interrelated. All of these nutritional and body composition changes may negatively impact metabolic, cardiovascular, and musculoskeletal function, even in the absence of overt disease. Therefore, it is important to anticipate them and optimize lifestyle choices and other treatments that can counteract the negative effects of aging and/or disease on body composition.

Exercise is able to partially offset all of the adverse body composition changes associated with aging. For example, a stabilization or increase in bone mass in pre- and postmenopausal women and older men is achievable by either resistive, weight-bearing aerobic exercise, or high-impact loading (studied only in premenopausal women to

date).[22–27] Such effects on bone density (differences of 1–2% per year associated with exercise) may be important for both prevention and treatment of osteoporosis and related fractures and disability, and should complement the provision of adequate calcium, vitamin D, protein, and energy, which are also required for adequate bone health. Even if exercise alone is an insufficient stimulus to maintain bone density at youthful levels, the combination of exercise effects on bone strength, muscle mass, muscle strength, and balance should lower the risk of injurious falls substantially in physically active individuals.[28–39] However, randomized controlled trials of any exercise modality with osteoporotic fracture itself as a primary outcome remain to be conducted.

Obesity is one of the most important nutritional problems in older adults, as prevalence estimates for overweight/obesity exceed 50% in many Western nations and are linked to increased rates of insulin resistance, hypertension, type 2 diabetes, atherosclerosis, depression, osteoarthritis, sleep apnea, and functional impairment with aging.[40–43] Decreases in both total adipose tissue accumulation and its abdominal (visceral) deposition are achievable by both aerobic[44–46] and resistive training,[11,47,48] with significant changes in total body fat usually only in conjunction with an energy-restricted diet.[49,50] Preferential visceral fat mobilization is often seen in response to exercise and dietary interventions,[51–55] which means that small amounts of total body weight or fat mass (5%) may be associated with substantial changes in visceral fat (20% or more), with important metabolic implications for the prevention or treatment of the insulin resistance syndrome.[28,56] Such prevention of excess adiposity is both protective and therapeutic for many common chronic diseases, offering significant risk reduction in the case of osteoarthritis; cardiovascular disease; gall bladder disease; type 2 diabetes; breast, colon, and endometrial cancer; hypertension; stroke; and vascular impotence, for example.[57–62] Although generalized obesity is associated with excess mortality, cardiovascular disease, osteoarthritis, mobility impairment, and disability, it is predominantly excess visceral fat that is associated with the derangements of dyslipidemia, elevated fibrinogen, hyperinsulinemia, glucose intolerance or diabetes, vascular insulin resistance, hypertension, and cardiovascular disease.

An increase in muscle mass, in contrast to changes in fat and bone, is only achievable to a significant degree with progressive resistance training or generalized weight gain from extra energy and protein consumption[63-67] and has a potential role in prevention for diabetes,[68-71] functional dependency,[17,18,72,73] and falls and fractures,[74-79] as well as being important in the treatment of chronic diseases and disabilities[80] that are accompanied by disuse, catabolism, and sarcopenia.[56,81,82] For some diseases, like type 2 diabetes mellitus, there are potential advantages to both minimizing fat tissue as well as maximizing muscle tissue, since these compartments have opposite and likely independent effects on insulin resistance in elderly individuals.[56] This use of a specific exercise modality (weight lifting) to combat a near-universal condition of older adults (sarcopenia) is one of the most important applications of exercise science to clinical medicine and gerontology in recent years. The remarkable reversibility of the syndrome of muscle atrophy and weakness with such a targeted exercise prescription, even among those over the age of 90 years with advanced disability, attests to the importance of assessment and treatment of remediable conditions and maintenance of preventive health strategies at all ages.

ASSESSING THE ELDERLY PATIENT FOR EXERCISE CAPACITY AND NEEDS

With rare exceptions in the United States, the majority of elderly patients in any geriatric clinical setting will not have optimized their physical fitness level and physical activity habits when they present to their health care professional. Therefore, it is critical to assess the current fitness deficits in order to set appropriate goals and develop a rational and feasible exercise prescription for each individual. The stages necessary for the adequate assessment and recommendation of exercise modalities for the elderly are outlined in Table 17–5.

The first step is to take a current exercise history, much as one would gather dietary intake information before administering any nutritional counseling. The patient should be questioned about previous involvement in sport, recreational, and competitive activities, and information about any remote or chronic exercise-related injuries should be gathered. Current household, work-related, and recreational activities should be solicited and quantified in terms of days per week, weeks per year, average length of each session or activity, and how long this pattern has been followed. In addition, specific questions about distances walked per week (in miles or blocks) and number of flights of stairs climbed per week will provide useful information on which to build the prescription, as well as an

---

Table 17–5 Stages of the Exercise Prescription

1. Assess exercise needs/goals on the basis of history and physical and individual preferences.
2. Identify behavioral readiness to change; provide appropriate counseling for current stage.
3. Identify potential risk factors for exercise-related adverse events.
4. Prioritize physical activity needs in relation to risks.
5. Prescribe the specific exercise modality and dose desired.
6. Provide or refer for specific training, equipment advice, facility options, and safety precautions.
7. Set up behavioral program for adoption, adherence, and relapse prevention.
8. Monitor compliance, benefits, and adverse events over time.
9. Modify exercise prescription as health status/goals/behavioral stage changes.

index of current capacity. Scales such as the Harvard Alumni Questionnaire can be used to score this information in standardized formats, which have been linked to chronic disease outcomes and longevity itself.[83] More recently developed questionnaires such as the Physical Activity Scale for the Elderly (PASE) include activities other than sport (housework, gardening, volunteer work, etc.) that may contribute more to overall physical activity levels in the elderly than exercise itself.[84] Questions about the need for human or mechanical assistance with activities of daily living and household tasks will also point out where the greatest deficits in physiologic capacity lie. Individuals should also be asked about their preferred modes of exercise, specific dislikes or fears, preferences for lone or group activity, and potential limitations to increased activity levels imposed by spousal care, transportation, finances, and so forth.

The physical exam will augment the above exercise history by highlighting physiologic deficits amenable to an exercise prescription. Although formal exercise testing, including maximal oxygen consumption, strength and power tests, range of motion and flexibility, and balance, would be ideal before the offering of advice, time, equipment, and expertise for such testing are outside the realm of possibility for most health care practitioners who are not exercise physiologists or physical therapists. A simplified observational approach in the clinical setting will, however, guide the examiner quite adequately in conjunction with the history of health conditions and functional status.

First, ask the patient to sit in a straight-backed chair with the arms folded across the chest and the feet on the floor. Ask the patient to stand up as quickly as possible without using the arms to assist, and observe the result closely. If the patient takes more than 1 to 2 seconds to stand or cannot do so without using his or her arms to assist, lower extremity power (hip and knee extensors) is compromised, and strengthening is indicated. If the patient complains of pain in the knees with this maneuver, quadriceps strengthening will be able to improve function and mobility and reduce pain. If the individual stands up quickly but appears unsteady and wavering in the upright position, balance or postural hypotension may be a problem. Test the balance further at this point while the patient is in the standing position by asking him or her to stand for 15 seconds in each of the following positions: feet together, one foot halfway in front of the other (semi tandem stand), with the heel of one foot directly in front of the toe of the other (tandem stand), on one leg only, and finally on one leg with the eyes closed. Most elderly people, even in the absence of disease, will not be able to hold the final two postures for 15 seconds without practice, but very early failures in this sequence indicate the need for specific balance training. Next, ask the patient to walk around a circular hallway or path that you have previously measured the distance of for 6 minutes without stopping, trying to cover as much distance as possible. Walk behind the patient and offer encouragement continuously while timing and observing closely for symptoms of dizziness, gait instability, claudication, angina, shortness of breath or wheezing, muscle weakness, joint pain, or overall fatigue. Patients with reduced aerobic capacity from any cause will walk only a few hundred feet to a thousand feet during this test, whereas fit adults may cover 3 to 4 times that distance.[85] This 6-minute walk test has the advantage of being more tolerable than a treadmill test for frail elders, providing a quantitative outcome that can be remeasured over time as an index of improvement. This test is able to point out the specific physical symptoms that are most limiting for the patient, is possible to complete even for those using ambulatory assistive devices or wheelchairs, and requires only a stopwatch to perform. In addition, the 6-minute walk test has been now seen to provide an index of overall exercise capacity that is related to functional independence in older adults. Some of the factors contributing to the distance walked on this test in addition to aerobic capacity are muscle mass, muscle strength, balance, obesity, arthritis pain, depressive symptoms, and cognitive status, attesting to the multifactorial nature of exercise and functional capacity in older adults.[86]

The combination of history and physical tests outlined above will provide the necessary information to prioritize the components of the exercise prescription shown in Table 17–6. In general, if major deficits in strength and balance are identified, along with a history of mobility difficulties, functional decline, and falls, for example, resistance training and balance training should be undertaken before attempts to increase aerobic capacity. For completely sedentary adults and novices at regular exercise, suggesting only one type of new physical activity at a time will enhance compliance. Giving back the capacity to lift one's body weight out of a chair and remain upright should always precede endurance activities such as walking to maximize function safely.

Simply identifying the appropriate exercise goals is not sufficient, however. It is equally important to identify what stage of behavioral change the person is in currently if the counseling is to have any effect. In the transtheoretical model of behavior, individuals advance through stages of precontemplation, contemplation, action, regular activity, and maintenance with regard to any behavioral choice. Offering a "precontemplator" an incentive such as a free membership to a gym will be unlikely to induce exercise adoption, whereas the same incentive given to someone who has advanced to contemplation or action stages may be just the motivation needed to start a regular new habit of physical activity. Once someone is in a regular pattern, behavioral incentives such as positive reinforcement, record keeping, external reminders of the desired behavior, goal setting, and relapse prevention all work to keep the behavior continuous. Maintenance is a phase indicating at least 6 months of continuous adherence to the new behavior, whether it is exercise, dietary change, smoking cessation, or other lifestyle habits, and evidence indicates that recidivism is quite low if you can get patients to this point.[8] Most failures in any new behavior occur long before the 6-month interval has passed, so it makes sense to put in place rigorous behavioral programs in this critical initial period. These may take the form of supervised classes, logs to send in, rewards, telephone calls, financial incentives, or group support mechanisms.

To help patients advance through the behavioral stages or prevent relapse, it is important to identify the specific barriers to changing or maintaining the behavior in that individual. Many of the most often cited barriers to appropriate physical activity in the older adult are listed in Table 17–7. Some of these barriers are at a societal level (expectations, grandparent roles), others involve local regulations or geographical features, and others are personal (fear of injury, boredom, time constraints). In all cases, it is important not to assume that all old people are alike or function with similar reasoning as regards exercise participation. For some, offering exercise in a group setting may relieve fears and provide social support; for others, embarrassment over disabilities or skill level may make exercising at home a much more appealing option. Creativity in exercise planning is a key factor. If transportation is a major barrier, then exercise classes at a meal site where elderly vans are already in service can efficiently overcome this barrier. Perceived lack of time is a barrier frequently cited even by nursing home residents when asked why they do not exercise. It is helpful to go through a daily schedule, pointing out times when watching television or other sedentary activities can be combined with flexibility, resistive, or even stationary aerobic exercise or when stairs can be substituted for elevators and escalators, for example. Balance exercises, such as standing on one leg, can be practiced whenever one is standing in line at a bank or supermarket. Breaking down the exercise prescription into such small pieces throughout the day will encourage the integration of a more active lifestyle into the daily routine most effectively for long-term adherence.

Some elderly patients will have medical problems that place them at higher risk for exercise-related adverse events. Examples include visual impairment, balance disorders, osteoarthritis of the shoulder or weight-bearing joints, low thresholds for ischemia or bronchospasm, peripheral vascular disease, and peripheral neuropathy. In

Table 17–6 Exercise Recommendations for Older Adults

Modality	Resistance Training	Cardiovascular Endurance Training	Flexibility Training	Balance Training
Dose				
Frequency	2–3 days/wk	3–5 days/wk	2–7 days/wk	1–7 days/wk
Volume	1–3 sets of 8–12 repetitions, 6–10 major muscle groups	20–60 minutes	4 repetitions, 30 s/stretch, 6–10 major muscle groups	1–2 sets of 4–10 different exercises, including static and dynamic postures*
Intensity	15–18 on Borg Scale (70–80% 1 RM), 10 s/repetition	11–14 on Borg Scale (50–80% maximal heart rate reserve)	Stretch to maximal pain-free distance and hold	Progressive difficulty as tolerated**
Requirements	Slow speed Good form No breath holding Increase weight progressively	Low-impact activity Weight bearing if possible	Nonballistic movements	Safe environment or monitoring Gradual increase in difficulty

*Examples of balance-enhancing activities include t'ai chi movements, standing yoga postures, tandem standing and walking, standing on one leg, stepping over objects, climbing up and down steps, turning, and standing on heels and toes.

**Intensity is increased by decreasing the base of support (e.g., progressing from standing on two feet while holding onto the back of a chair to standing on one foot with no hand support); by decreasing other sensory input (e.g., closing eyes or standing on a foam pillow); or by perturbing the center of mass (e.g., holding a heavy object out to one side while maintaining balance, standing on one leg while lifting other leg out behind body, or leaning forward as far as possible without falling or moving feet).

Table 17–7 Barriers to Appropriate Physical Activity in the Elderly

- Acute and chronic medical problems and disabilities
- Caregiving role for sick spouse or family member
- Lack of interest
- Exaggerated perception of risk/fear of injury
- Financial limitations
- Geographical constraints and environmental design features
- Institutional/residential policies
- Lack of advocacy by family and health care community
- Lack of appropriately designed exercise equipment
- Lack of health care professional/caregiver/family education about exercise
- Perceived lack of time
- Psychological issues (depression, dementia, bereavement, self-efficacy, fear of falling, low self-esteem, social isolation)
- Reduced appreciation of benefit
- Societal norms/expectations of sedentariness
- Transportation difficulties

general, problems can be avoided by providing monitoring if needed, exercising in adequate lighting, strengthening muscles around arthritic joints before weight-bearing exercise, and keeping intensity levels below those that produce cardiopulmonary symptoms. If the risk of ischemia is very high with aerobic exercise, then prescribing resistance exercises may offer similar benefits in terms of health and functioning with far less potential to provoke cardiac symptoms. If an older runner who likes competition is getting into difficulty with knee and ankle injuries, substituting a lower impact yet intense activity such as race walking can provide all of the physical and psychological benefits desired without the risk of musculoskeletal trauma. In all cases, it is important to balance the pleasurable components of exercise for the individual with the health-maintaining aspects important to the practitioner, or the prescription is likely to be unheeded in the long term.

Exercise prescriptions sometimes fail because they are too vague to be useful. The exercise prescription should be thought of like a medication; the patient needs to know the indication, type, dose, frequency, potential side effects, alternatives, and interactions with other nutritional or pharmaceutical preparations that he or she is already taking. The recommendations in Table

17–6 are consistent with the most recent guidelines of the American College of Sports Medicine for healthy and older adults[9,10] and represent dose ranges of exercise that have been shown to have benefit in terms of disease prevention and treatment as well as maintenance of cardiovascular and musculoskeletal fitness. Higher intensities or greater amounts of exercise may be undertaken for competitive purposes or in highly athletic individuals but are not required for general health in the elderly and are associated with greater risk of injury and higher dropout rates. Thus, a total of about 3 to 4 hours per week is sufficient to meet the requirements for all four modes of exercise, which is feasible for most individuals of retirement age.

Most geriatric patients will require more training than can be provided by the average health care professional without special exercise knowledge. Therefore, a referral to a qualified fitness instructor or physical therapist is often needed, along with explicit graphic instructions or videotapes. Such materials provide both knowledge and motivation for the novice exerciser, and having them on hand in the waiting room or office setting reinforces the power of the prescription and emphasizes the commitment of the practitioner to healthy lifestyle principles. Set up the behavioral program at the same time that the prescription is generated by giving the client an exercise calendar or diary to fill out each week, motivational tokens, and a plan for feedback on his or her progress at frequent intervals. If relapse is likely because of intercurrent illness, caregiving responsibilities, travel, or other identified problems, address these concerns early, and outline plans to anticipate and avoid such pitfalls. Ask about the compliance with the exercise prescription at every health care visit, as well as perceived benefits and adverse events that have occurred. Repeating the physical function testing that was used to generate the initial prescription can be very motivating because the patient can be given direct feedback on the specific physical benefits attributable to his or her new physical activity pattern. As functional status improves, modify the exercise goals to emphasize new areas of fitness once the routine of regular physical activity has been firmly established. Shaping behavior in small increments is more likely to be successful than overwhelming an adult who has been sedentary for 50 years with an overly ambitious plan of physical activity.

MEDICAL SCREENING FOR THE EXERCISE PRESCRIPTION

Many sets of recommendations have been created in an attempt to make exercise as safe as possible for adults, especially those at risk for cardiovascular events.[11] Indeed, exercise carries with it the possibility of complications and adverse events; the most important of which are outlined in Table 17–8. The most feared events are the cardiovascular ones, although they are relatively rare even in cardiac rehabilitation settings, whereas the most common occurrences are minor musculoskeletal injuries. Most such injuries can be prevented by paying attention to proper technique, slowly progressing in intensity as tolerated, avoiding ambulatory activities until strength and balance are adequate to support the body weight safely, and abstaining from exercise during acute illness, extremes of temperature or humidity, or the appearance of new, unidentified medical symptoms.

A broader use and definition of medical screening for exercise for the geriatric patient is suggested. Rather than asking yourself, "Is this patient safe to exercise?" you might pose the question, "Is this patient safe to be sedentary?" It is important to keep in mind that sedentariness is the lethal condition and that habitual exercise protects against many major chronic diseases, as well as being indicated in their treatment. In this broader concept of screening, therefore, the practitioner should be alert to the presence of sedentariness itself as a risk factor for disease and disability, to chronic diseases that are amenable to physical activity, to readiness to change behavior, and finally to exacerbation of chronic diseases that should be brought to the attention of a physician, regardless of whether an exercise prescription is about to be given. In general, hypertension, angina, diabetes, pulmonary disease, obesity, neurologic disease, and arthritis are indications for exercise as long as they are in control, rather than contraindications to more activity.

Some specific areas of concern in the older adult include cardiopulmonary status, musculoskeletal integrity, mental status, podiatric problems, and vision. It is important to know an individual's pattern of angina or shortness of breath and the level of exertion that produces it. Any change in chronic patterns warrants referral to a medical practitioner. For most cardiopulmonary symptoms, activity should be stopped at their onset. The notable exception to this is claudication; evidence indicates that walking a little further once the pain begins is the most effective way to extend the time to claudication and improve pain-free walking distances. Cardiac stress testing should be done for standard medical indications in consultation with the patient's physician, and not simply because an asymptomatic older adult wants to begin a moderate exercise regimen. Requiring such testing before any exercise could be undertaken would pose an enormous psychological and financial disincentive to physical activity and would be likely to result in positive tests in many asymptomatic individuals, which would then require further medical testing

Table 17–8 The Risks of Exercise in the Elderly

Musculoskeletal	Cardiovascular	Metabolic
Falls	Arrhythmia	Dehydration
Foot ulceration or laceration	Cardiac failure	Electrolyte imbalance
Fracture, osteoporotic or traumatic	Hypertension	Energy imbalance
	Hypotension	Heat stroke
Hemorrhoids	Ischemia	Hyperglycemia
Hernia	Pulmonary embolism	Hypoglycemia
Joint or bursa inflammation, exacerbation of arthritis	Retinal hemorrhage or detachment, lens detachment	Hypothermia
		Seizures
Ligament or tendon strain or rupture	Ruptured aneurysm	
Muscle soreness or tear	Syncope or postural symptoms	

such as thallium stress testing or angiography to resolve.

For patients with pulmonary disease, symptoms at rest and with exertion should be elicited, as well as determination of the need for supplemental oxygen during exercise. Plan the use of inhalers if needed for 15 to 30 minutes before exercise to allow maximum effect, and keep them on hand during all sessions. During febrile episodes or acute flares of disease, exercise should be avoided because the risk of cardiac arrhythmias and pulmonary edema is high during this time in the elderly. Some patients may not tolerate aerobic activity at all but are able to perform resistance, balance, and flexibility exercises, which are much less consumptive of oxygen, without any difficulty. It is important to remember that the catabolic effects of chronic pulmonary disease, often accompanied by anorexia, malnutrition, and corticosteroid treatment, produce severe losses of lean tissue (muscle and bone). Such losses cannot be counteracted by cardiovascular endurance training alone but require the adaptive response to resistive exercise to reverse this wasting process. Therefore, patients with the most severe lung disease who are least likely to be able tolerate aerobic activities in fact are more likely to benefit in terms of body composition and function from weight-lifting exercise.

Identification of depression, anxiety, or insomnia on screening is important because these conditions all benefit from both resistive and aerobic exercise. Severe withdrawal or lethargy may require additional treatment and make an unsupervised exercise prescription unlikely to succeed. Cognitive impairment is not a contraindication to exercise, but may necessitate close supervision, group exercise, and safety precautions. Often a nonimpaired spouse or home care worker can be helpful as a walking partner or exercise trainer for those living at home. In an institutional setting, demented patients can successfully participate in all kinds of exercise with adequate staff-to-patient ratios. Aggressive or disruptive behavior, poor safety awareness and judgment, or uncontrolled alcohol intake should be screened for because these will dictate the feasibility of group or isolated activity.

Many exercise-related injuries are related to the foot and ankle, although most injuries of this type are preventable with proper foot care, shoes, socks, orthotics, assistive devices, and avoidance of high-impact activities. Look for ulcers, fungal infections, peripheral neuropathy, infections, edema, ischemic changes, skin rashes or breakdown, calluses, bunions, ingrown or long toenails, and painful points on the ankle, heel, and foot. Those patients with peripheral vascular disease or neuropathy should be particularly careful about sudden increases in weight-bearing activities. If ulcers develop on the foot or ankle and ambulation is restricted temporarily, advise the patient to substitute seated weight-lifting exercises to prevent disuse atrophy from occurring during this period of reduced activity. It is wise to have a family member check the feet, particularly in diabetics who may also have visual impairment that prevents them from seeing early problems as they develop. Shoes with the lowest comfortable heel and nonslip soles are important, particularly in those with balance impairment at risk for falls.

Visual problems are common in the geriatric patient, and optimal lighting, exercise in the daylight hours, and use of corrective lenses at all times will minimize safety problems. Those with active or newly treated proliferative retinopathy, retinal detachment, or cataract surgery should not perform any exercise that raises the blood pressure or lift weights until cleared by their ophthalmologist. Substitution of stationary bikes, rowers, and steppers for other aerobic activities allows even completely blind individuals to exercise vigorously without supervision, and these patients should not therefore be automatically denied an exercise prescription because many such alternatives are now available.

USE OF EXERCISE IN THE PREVENTION AND TREATMENT OF COMMON GERIATRIC SYNDROMES

The exercise prescription for general health addresses the four major components of fitness: strength, endurance, flexibility, and balance (Table 17–6). Therefore, the idea is to gradually get individuals to incorporate most or all of these modalities into their weekly routine, regardless of their specific medical history. Most chronic diseases and their associated disabilities in fact benefit from both resistance training and aerobic training at the dosages indicated in the table, so there is no need to develop a specific exercise prescription for every medical condition that someone has. This is particularly important for individuals who cannot participate in one mode of exercise at all. For example, the depressed,

obese elderly woman with severe degenerative disease of the knees who cannot ambulate without severe pain will benefit in terms of mood, arthritis pain, mobility, and weight loss from resistive exercises, which can be performed without standing.

In addition to isolated diseases, there are many multifactorial syndromes with which geriatric patients commonly present and for which standard medical treatment often has little to offer. For these syndromes, exercise may be very therapeutic and have far fewer side effects than attempts at pharmacological management. Some of the most commonly encountered scenarios and suggested approaches to exercise management are listed in Table 17–9.

PRACTICAL IMPLEMENTATION OF EXERCISE PROGRAMS IN THE CLINICAL SETTING

Ideally, the exercise prescription should be integrated with all other components of the individual's care plan, since it will affect functional capacity, health status, nutritional requirements, psychological status, and other lifestyle changes that may be addressed by other members of the health care team. Physicians should be aware of any new exercise prescription that may affect medication requirements or cause exacerbation of underlying conditions. Many individuals will start an exercise regimen when they are advised to lose weight, so the incorporation of nutritional recommendations with activity suggestions is critical to the success of such attempts. Often, patients will have questions about what to eat when exercising or the need for special drinks, supplements, or protein sources. Guidelines for commonly encountered exercise-nutrition interactions are outlined in Table 17–10. In general, food sources are preferable to packaged supplements because they encourage greater dietary diversity, and education regarding the often overstated advertising claims for many of these expensive products should be given to patients who might better spend their money on good athletic shoes or home exercise equipment.

Include discussions of physical activity patterns in team conferences and planning meetings.

Table 17–9 Choice of Exercise for Common Geriatric Syndromes

Syndrome	Therapeutic Exercise Recommendation
Anorexia	Endurance or resistance training before meals
Constipation	Endurance or resistance exercise
Depression, anxiety, low self-efficacy	Individual or group exercises, including endurance, resistive, and calisthenic activities as preferred
Fatigue	Endurance training in the morning hours; increase duration and intensity as tolerated
Functional dependency	Walking, stair climbing for endurance; resistance training of upper and lower extremities
Incontinence (stress)	Pelvic muscle strengthening (Kegel exercises); mobility improvement with endurance, balance, and resistance training as needed
Insomnia	Endurance or resistance exercise in midafternoon (4–6 hours before bedtime)
Low back pain, spinal stenosis	Resistance training to strengthen the back extensor muscles, rectus abdominus, and hip and knee extensor muscle groups
Recurrent falls, gait and balance disorders	Lower extremity resistance training for hip, knee, and ankle; balance training, t'ai chi, yoga, ballet; walking in safe or supported environment; training in use of ambulatory device as needed
Weakness	Moderate to high-intensity resistance training for all major muscle groups

Make available easily completed forms for patient assessment in terms of exercise history, physical performance, exercise prescription, and activity logs. Add to the health library references on major exercise techniques and videotapes that can be viewed in the waiting room or even bor-

Table 17–10 Nutritional Recommendations for the Physically Active Older Adult

1. Encourage extra water intake (500–1000 mL) on exercise days, especially in those on diuretics or very low sodium diets, during high ambient temperatures or humid conditions, and after recovery from dehydrating illnesses or fevers; sport drink formulations are unnecessary for fluid replacement under normal conditions and in noncompetitive athletes.
2. If a goal is fat/weight loss, combine exercise with a balanced hypocaloric diet, and supplement with multivitamin at RDA levels.
3. If goal is weight maintenance, counsel on increased energy intake (with normal ratios of fat/carbohydrate/protein) as food rather than supplements; encourage dietary diversity to fulfill energy requirements and supply micronutrient needs.
4. If goal is weight gain, add nutrient- and energy-dense food snacks between meals and after exercise sessions.
5. There is no need to supplement protein beyond 1.0 to 1.2 g/kg/per day, which can be achieved with diverse dietary sources rather than amino acid or protein supplements.
6. In diabetics, time exercise sessions for the postprandial peaks in blood glucose (1.5 to 2 hours after a meal); keep high carbohydrate and concentrated sugar snacks available during exercise sessions for brittle or insulin-dependent diabetics; advise against exercise after prolonged fasting or skipping meals.
7. Increase dietary or pharmacological sources of potassium and magnesium if levels are marginal or low, particularly in high-risk coronary artery disease or arrhythmia-prone patients on diuretics or digoxin.

rowed from the library for home use. Consider replacing several chairs in the waiting room or lobby with stationary exercise equipment along with tables of educational materials to read. Make sure that stairways are accessible and well lighted, have sturdy handrails, and are marked clearly to encourage use. Provide incentives for exercise adherence in the form of reduced fees, free exercise equipment, lottery tickets, or whatever is meaningful to the clientele in a particular setting. Practice good exercise habits yourself, as your prescription will carry a lot more credibility if your patient sees you following it yourself in the workplace. Most environments can be creatively modified to encourage rather than restrict activity and this is as true of the doctor's or nutritionist's office as it is of the nursing home. Many small spaces in such settings can be converted to "mini-gyms" with little capital investment and may be the seed from which much larger programs develop.

CONCLUSION

Physical fitness is not merely a medical prescription or treatment; it is a right of individuals, both fit and frail, and thus caregivers, family members, and volunteers are responsible for providing education, opportunity, and access in this domain to the eldest members of our communities. Health care practices and policies for the elderly should be enlarged to promote fitness, activity, and independence to the fullest extent possible for each individual as an important component of overall quality of life.

REFERENCES

1. Fiatarone Singh M. Exercise comes of age: Rationale and recommendations for a geriatric exercise prescription. *J Gerontol: Med Sci* 2002;57(A):M262-M282.

2. Chandler J, Hadley E. Exercise to improve physiologic and functional performance in old age. *Clin Geriatric Med* 1996;12(4):761–784.

3. Huang Y, Macera C, Blair S, Brill P, Kohl H, Kronenfeld J. Physical fitness, physical activity, and functional limitation in adults aged 40 and older. *Med Sci Sports Exerc* 1998;30(9):1430–1435.

4. Kempen GI, van Heuvelen MJ, van Sonderen E, van den Brink RH, Kooijman AC, Ormel J. The relationship of functional limitations to disability and the moderating effects of psychological attributes in community-dwelling older persons. *Social Science & Medicine* 1999;48(9):1161–1172.

5. Miller M, Rejeski W, Reboussin B, Ten Have T, Ettinger W. Physical activity, functional limitations, and disability in older adults. *JAGS* 2000;48:1264–1272.

6. Stuck A, Walthert J, Nikolaus T, Bula C, Hohmann C, Beck J. Risk factors for functional status decline in community-living elderly people: a systematic literature review. *Social Science & Medicine* 1999;48:445–469.

7. Bortz WM. Redefining human aging. *J Am Geriatr Soc* 1989;37(11):1092–1096.

8. Braith R, Mills R, Welsch M, Keller J, Pollock M. Resistance exercise training restores bone mineral density in heart transplant recipients. *J Am Coll Cardiol* 1996;28(6):1471–1477.

9. Braith R, Welsch M, Mills R, Keller J, Pollock M. Resistance exercise prevents glucocorticoid-induced myopathy in heart transplant recipients. *Med Sci Sports Exerc* 1998;30(483–489).

10. Castaneda C, Gordon P, Uhlin K, et al. Resistance training to counteract the catabolism of a low protein diet in chronic renal insufficiency: A randomized controlled trial. *Ann Intern Med* 2001;135: 965–976.

11. Ballor DL, Harvey-Berino JR, Ades PA, Cryan J, Calles-Escandon J. Contrasting effects of resistance and aerobic training on body composition and metabolism after diet-induced weight loss. Metabolism: *Clinical & Experimental* 1996;45(2):179–183.

12. Fiatarone MA, O'Neill EF, Ryan ND, et al. Exercise training and nutritional supplementation for physical frailty in very elderly people. *New Engl J Med* 1994;330:1769–1775.

13. Fiatarone Singh M, Ding W, Manfredi T, et al. Insulin-like growth factor I in skeletal muscle after weight-lifting exercise in frail elders. *Am J Physiol (Endo and Metab)* 1999;277:E136–E143.

14. Campbell WW, Crim MC, Young VR, Evans WJ. Increased energy requirements and changes in body composition with resistance training in older adults. *Am J Clin Nutr* 1994;60(2):167–175.

15. Campbell W, Crim M, Dallal G, Young V, Evans W. Increased protein requirements in the elderly: new data and retrospective reassessments. *Am J Clin Nutr* 1994;60:501–509.

16. Rogers MA, Hagberg JM, Martin WH III, Ehsani AA, Holloszy JO. Decline in VO2 max with aging master athletes and sedentary men. *J Appl Physiol* 1990;68(5):2195–2199.

17. Chumlea W, Guo S, Glaser R, Vellas B. Sarcopenia, function and health. *Nutr Health Aging* 1997;1(1):7–12.

18. Evans W, Campbell W. Sarcopenia and age-related changes in body composition and functional capacity. *J Nutrition* 1993;123:465–468.

19. Morley JE. Anorexia, sarcopenia, and aging. *Nutrition* 2001;17(7-8):660–663.

20. Boland R. Role of vitamin D in skeletal muscle function. Endo Rev 1986;7:434-448.

21. Jeejeebhoy KN. Muscle function and nutrition. *Gut* 1986;27(Suppl 1):25-39.

22. Wolff I, Croonenborg J, Kemper H, Kostense P, Twisk J. The effect of exercise training programs on bone mass: A meta-analysis of published controlled trials in pre- and postmenopausal women. *Osteoporosis Int* 1999;9:1–12.

23. Kelley G, Kelley D, Kristi S, Tran Z. Resistance training and bone mineral density in women: A meta-analysis of controlled trials. *Am J of Phys Med Rehab* 2001;80(1): 65–77.

24. Kelley G. Aerobic exercise and lumbar spine bone mineral density in postmenopausal women: a meta-analysis. *JAGS* 1998;46(2):143–152.

25. Bassey E, Rothwell M, Littlewood J, Pye D. Pre- and postmenopausal women have different bone density responses to the same high-impact exercise. *J Bone Mineral Res* 1998;13:1805 1813.

26. Bassey E, Ramsdale S. Increase in femoral bone density in young women following high-impact exercise. *Osteoporosis Int* 1994;4(2):72–75.

27. Bassey E, Ramsdale S. Weight-bearing exercise and ground reaction forces: A 12-month randomized controlled trial of effects on bone mineral density in healthy postmenopausal women. *Bone* 1995;16:469–476.

28. Menkes A, Mazel R, Redmond R, et al. Strength training increases regional bone mineral density and bone remodeling in middle-aged and older men. *J Appl Physiol* 1993;74:2478-2484.

29. Notelovitz M, Martin D, Tesar R, et al. Estrogen and variable-resistance weight training increase bone mineral in surgically menopausal women. *J Bone Mineral Res* 1991;6(6):583–590.

30. Snow C, Shaw J, Winters K, Witzke K. Long-term exercise using weighted vests prevents hip bone loss in postmenopausal women. *J Gerontol* (Med Sci) 2000;55A(9): M489–M491.

31. Nelson M, Fiatarone M, Morganti C, Trice I, Greenberg R, Evans W. Effects of high-intensity strength training on multiple risk factors for osteoporotic fractures. *JAMA* 1994;272:1909–1914.

32. Aloia J, Cohn S, Ostuni J, Cane R, Ellis K. Prevention of involutional bone loss by exercise. *Ann Intern Med* 1978;89:356–358.

33. Aloia J, Vaswani A, Yeh J, Cohn S. Premenopausal bone mass is related to physical activity. *Arch Intern Med* 1988;148:121–123.

34. Dalsky G, Stocke K, Ehsani A, Slatopolsky E, Lee W, Birge S. Weight-bearing exercise training and lumbar bone mineral content in postmenopausal women. *Ann Intern Med* 1988;108:824–828.

35. Kenny A, Prestwood K, Marcello K, Raisz L. Determinants of bone density in healthy older men with low testosterone levels. *J Gerontol* (Med Sci) 2000; 55A(9):M492–M497.

36. Kohrt WM, Snead DB, Slatopolsky E, Birge SJ, Jr. Additive effects of weight-bearing exercise and estrogen on bone mineral density in older women. *J Bone Mineral Res* 1995;10(9):1303–1311.

37. Krall EA, Dawson-Hughes B. Walking is related to bone density and rates of bone loss. *Am J Med* 1994;96:20–26.

38. Wallace M, Cumming R. Systematic review of randomized trials of the effect of exercise on bone mass in pre- and postmenopausal women. *Calcif Tissue Int* 2000;67: 10–18.

39. Kelley G. Exercise and regional bone mineral density in postmenopausal women: a meta-analytic review of randomized trials. *Am J Phys Med Rehabil* 1998;77(1): 76–87.

40. Despres J-P, Lemieux I, Prud'homme D. Treatment of obesity: need to focus on high risk abdominally obese patients. *Br Med J* 2001;322(7288):716–720.

41. Faith MS, Matz PE, Jorge MA. Obesity-depression associations in the population. *J Psychosomatic Res* 2002; 53(4):935–942.

42. Jadelis K, Miller M, Ettinger W, Messier S. Strength, balance, and the modifying effects of obesity and knee pain: Results from the Observational Arthritis Study in Seniors (OASIS). *JAGS* 2001;49:884–891.

43. Jensen GL, Friedmann JM. Obesity is associated with functional decline in community-dwelling rural older persons. *JAGS* 2002;50(5):918–923.

44. Kohrt WM, Obert KA, Holloszy JO. Exercise training improves fat distribution patterns in 60- to 70-year-old men and women. *J Gerontol* 1992;47(4):M99–105.

45. Despres J, Bouchard C, Savard R, Tremblay A, Marcotte M, Theriault G. The effect of a 20-week endurance training program on adipose-tissue morphology and lipolysis in men and women. *Metabolism* 1984;33:235–239.

46. Dengel DR, Hagberg JM, Coon PJ, Drinkwater DT, Goldberg AP. Comparable effects of diet and exercise on body composition and lipoproteins in older men. *Medicine & Science in Sports & Exercise* 1994;26(11): 1307–1315.

47. Schwartz RS, Shuman WP, Larson V, et al. The effect of intensive endurance exercise training on body fat distribution in young and older men. *Metabolism: Clinical & Experimental.* 1991;40(5):545–551.

48. Treuth M, Hunter G, Szabo T, Weinsier R, Goran M, Berland L. Reduction in intra-abdominal adipose tissue

after strength training in older women. *J Appl Physiol* 1995;78(4):1425–1431.

49. Grundy SM, Blackburn G, Higgins M, Lauer R, Perri MG, Ryan D. Physical activity in the prevention and treatment of obesity and its comorbidities: evidence report of independent panel to assess the role of physical activity in the treatment of obesity and its comorbidities. *Medicine & Science in Sports & Exercise* 1999;31(11): 1493–1500.

50. Fiatarone Singh M. Combined exercise and dietary intervention to optimize body composition in aging. *Ann of the New York Acad Sci* 1998;854:378–393.

51. Horber FF, Kohler SA, Lippuner K, Jaeger P. Effect of regular physical training on age-associated alteration of body composition in men. *Eur J Clin Invest* 1996; 26(4):279-285.

52. Thomas E, Brynes A, McCarthy J, et al. Preferential loss of visceral fat following aerobic exercise, measured by magnetic resonance imaging. *Lipids* 2000;35(7): 769–776.

53. Ross R, Dagnone D, Jones P, et al. Reduction in obesity and related comorbid conditions after diet-induced weight loss or exercise-induced weight loss in men. A randomized, controlled trial. *Ann Intern Med* 2000;133: 92–103.

54. Smith S, Zachwieja J. Visceral adipose tissue: a critical review of intervention strategies. *Int J Obes Relat Metab Disord* 1999;23(4):329–335.

55. Mourier A, Gautier J, DeKerviler E, et al. Mobilization of visceral adipose tissue related to the improvement in insulin sensitivity in response to physical training in NIDDM. Effects of branched-chain amino acid supplements. *Diabetes Care* 1997;20:385–391.

56. Despres J-P. Body fat distribution, exercise and nutrition: Implications for prevention of atherogenic dyslipidemia, coronary heart disease, and non-insulin dependent diabetes mellitus. In: Lamb D, Murray R, eds. *Perspectives in Exercise Science and Sports Medicine: Exercise, Nutrition and Weight Control* Vol 11. Carmel, CA: Cooper Publishing Group; 1998:107–150.

57. Folsom A, Kay S, Sellers T. Body fat distribution and 5-year risk of death in older women. *JAMA* 1993;269: 483–487.

58. Shephard RJ. Physical activity and reduction of health risks: how far are the benefits independent of fat loss? *J Sports Med Physical Fitness* 1994;34(1):91–98.

59. Visser M, Langlois J, Guralnik J, et al. High body fat-ness, but not low fat-free mass, predicts disability in older men and women: the Cardiovascular Health Study. *Am J Clin Nutr* 1998;68:584–590.

60. USDA/USDHHS. *Nutrition and Your Health: Dietary Guidelines for Americans.* Washington, D.C.: U.S. Department of Agriculture and the U.S. Department of Health and Human Services; 1990.

61. Koop C. *The Surgeon General's Report on Nutrition and Health:* U.S. Department of Health and Human Services; 1988. DHHS Publ. No. 88-50210.

62. U.S. Dept of Health and Human Services. *Physical activity and health: A report of the Surgeon General.* Atlanta: US Dept of Health and Human Services, Centers for Disease Control and Prevention, National Center for Chronic Disease Prevention and Health Promotion; 1996.

63. Charette S, McEvoy L, Pyka G, et al. Muscle hypertrophy response to resistance training in older women. *J Appl Physiol* 1991;70(5):1912–1916.

64. Pu C, Johnson M, Forman D, et al. Randomized trial of progressive resistance training to counteract the myopathy of chronic heart failure. *J Appl Physiol* 2001;90: 2341–2350.

65. McCartney N, Hicks A, Martin J, Webber C. Long-term resistance training in the elderly: effects on dynamic strength, exercise capacity, muscle, and bone. *J Gerontology* 1995;50A(2):B97–B104.

66. Morganti CM, Nelson ME, Fiatarone MA, et al. Strength improvements with 1 yr of progressive resistance training in older women. *Med Sci Sports Exerc* 1995;27(6): 906–912.

67. Fiatarone M, Evans W. The etiology and reversibility of muscle dysfunction in the elderly. *J Gerontology* 1993; 48:77–83.

68. Fluckey JD, Hickey MS, Brambrink JK, Hart KK, Alexander K, Craig BW. Effects of resistance exercise on glucose tolerance in normal and glucose-intolerant subjects. *J Applied Physiol* 1994;77(3):1087–1092.

69. Zachwieja JJ, Toffolo G, Cobelli C, Bier DM, Yarasheski KE. Resistance exercise and growth hormone administration in older men: effects on insulin sensitivity and secretion during a stable-label intravenous glucose tolerance test. *Metabolism: Clinical & Experimental* 1996;45(2):254–260.

70. Ishii T, Yamakita T, Sato T, Tanaka S, Fujii S. Resistance training improves insulin sensitivity in NIDDM subjects without altering maximal oxygen uptake. *Diabetes Care* 1998;21(8):1353–1355.

71. Tuomilehto J, Lindstrom J, Eriksson J, et al. Prevention of type 2 diabetes mellitus by changes in lifestyle among subjects with impaired glucose tolerance. *N Engl J Med* 2001;344:1343–1350.

72. Evans WJ. Exercise, nutrition and aging. *J Nutr* 1992; 122:796–801.

73. Hopp JF. Effects of age and resistance training on skeletal muscle: A review. *Physical Therapy* 1993;73(6): 361–373.

74. Rantanen T, Avela J. Leg extension power and walking speed in very old people living independently. *J Gerontol* 1997;52A(4):M225–M231.

75. Skelton DA, Grieg CA, Davies JM, Young A. Strength, power and related functional ability of healthy people aged 65-89 years. *Age Ageing* 1994;23:371–377.

76. King MB, Tinetti ME. Falls in community-dwelling older persons. *JAGS* 1995;43:1146–1154.

77. Lauritzen JB, McNair PA, Lund B. Risk factors for hip fractures. A review. *Danish Medical Bulletin* 1993;40(4): 479–485.

78. Lord SR, Ward JA, Williams P. Exercise effect on dynamic stability in older women: A randomized controlled trial. *Arch Phys Med Rehabil* 1996;77:232–236.

79. Lord SR, Lloyd DG, Nirui M, Raymond J, Williams P, Stewart RA. The effect of exercise on gait patterns in older women: A randomized controlled trial. *J Gerontol* 1996;51A(2):M64–M70.

80. Fiatarone MA, Evans WJ. Exercise in the oldest old. *Top Geriatr Rehab* 1990;5:63–77.

81. Ballor D, Keesey R. A meta-analysis of the factors affecting exercise-induced changes in body mass, fat mass, and fat-free mass in males and females. *Int J Obesity* 1991;15:717–726.

82. Dengel DR, Hagberg JM, Coon PJ, Drinkwater DT, Goldberg AP. Effects of weight loss by diet alone or combined with aerobic exercise on body composition in older obese men. *Metabolism: Clinical & Experimental* 1994;43(7):867–871.

83. Paffenbarger R, Hyde R, Wing A, Hsieh C-C. Physical activity and longevity of college alumni. *N Engl J Med* 1986;315:399–401.

84. Washburn R, Smith K, Jetter A, Janney C. The physical activity scale for the elderly (PASE): development and evaluation. *J Clin Epidemiol* 1993;46(2):153–162.

85. Cahalin L, Mathier M, Semigram M, Dec W, DiSalvo T. The six-minute walk test predicts peak oxygen uptake and survival in patients with advanced heart failure. *Chest* 1996;110:325–332.

86. Bean JF, Kiely DK, Herman S, et al. The relationship between leg power and physical performance in mobility-limited older people. *JAGS* 2002;50(3):461–467.

CHAPTER 18

Nutritional Assessment of the Elderly

Carol O. Mitchell-Eady, PhD, RD and Ronni Chernoff, PhD, RD

One of the more challenging aspects of providing nutrition to elderly individuals is the determination of their nutritional status. Aging has an effect on many of the anthropometric, biochemical, and hematologic parameters commonly used to assess nutritional status in younger adults. Adding to the difficulty of evaluating the results of these measures is the fact that people age at individual rates, thus contributing to the heterogeneity of the older group. To make a considered judgment about the need for nutritional interventions or the possibility of nutritional depletion that may have an impact on health, it is necessary to conduct a thorough, multifaceted nutritional assessment that examines many aspects of the individual to present the most complete picture possible. To evaluate the individual adequately, a thorough nutritional assessment should be made, including appraisal of physical appearance; oral health; social and environmental situation; potential physical and psychologic disabilities; medical and drug history; performance of anthropometric measurements; evaluation of biochemical, hematologic, and immune function; functional competence; and a comprehensive dietary history.

Conducting a comprehensive nutritional assessment is an important component of providing quality health care to elderly people; malnutrition may contribute to the depletion of reserve capacity or the ability to respond rapidly and appropriately to a physiologic insult. Malnutrition may be unrecognized in elderly subjects because many of the changes that are seen with inadequate nutrition are often associated with changes that occur with aging. Severely malnourished individuals are easier to identify than those who are mildly or moderately malnourished because the latter will not manifest overt signs of malnutrition. Many health care professionals are not attuned to the important role that nutrition plays in the maintenance of health throughout life; therefore, subclinical or marginal nutritional deficits may go unnoticed and undocumented.[1]

CLINICAL ASSESSMENT

Physical Assessment

Malnutrition is the consequence of chronically inadequate intake of essential nutrients.[2] Replenishment of normal tissue requires protein, energy, vitamins, and minerals in amounts adequate to replace old cells with new ones. These elements are needed to repair damaged cells and tissues and to make substrate for protein compounds such as antigens, hormones, and enzymes. For many anabolic processes, vitamins and minerals serve as cofactors in metabolic cycles that drive these physiologic mechanisms. When chronic malnutrition of one or more essential nutrients exists, there may be physical manifestations that are associated with the primary functions of the deficient nutrients.[2] It is very important to look at the individual being assessed; a great deal can be ascertained about nutritional status by carefully assessing the state of hair, skin, nails, musculature, eyes, mucosa, and other physical attributes. Basic physical examination techniques needed for a nutrition-focused physical assessment have been described, and the need for formal training and practice in assessment techniques has been stressed.[3] Many of the consequences of specific nutrient deficiencies are listed in Table 18–1.

Another clinical manifestation associated with nutritional deficiencies in elderly people is fluid imbalance. Overhydration that contributes to edema is probably less of a nutritional problem than is dehydration. Presentation of dehydration in elderly individuals is described in Table 18–2. Dehydration is often caused by inadequate ingestion of free fluids and is a potentially precarious state for older people[4] (Chapter 3). Total body water is decreased with changes in body composition. These changes occur with aging: alterations in thirst, osmoreceptor and baroreceptor sensitivities, and impairment of renal capacity to conserve water or to concentrate urine efficiently.[5] Assessment of actual fluid needs is often difficult. Intake and output records may be inaccurate or difficult to collect. Pinching the skin on the back of the hand or on the sternum may be a good physical indicator of hydration status; well-hydrated tissue will resume its normal position immediately on release of the skin pinch. It must be kept in mind that the use of skin turgor to assess fluid status lacks precision and more in-depth evaluation of fluid balance may be needed.[6]

Recommendations for fluid requirements for the elderly of 1 mL/kcal intake have been given by the National Academy of Sciences Food and Nutrition Board.[7] Chernoff, however, recommends 30 mL/kg of body weight with a 1500 mL/day minimum.[8] More recently, Chidester and Spangler found 1500 to 2000 mL of fluid to be necessary for proper hydration of long-term care residents[9] (Chapter 3). Factors that may contribute to risk of dehydration in elderly subjects[10] are listed in Table 18–3.

Many nutritional deficiencies are manifested in the oral cavity; therefore, an oral examination should be included in an assessment of nutritional status[11] (Chapter 8). The condition of an individual's mouth (number and looseness of teeth; presence of caries or plaque; presence of, or need for, dentures and how well they fit; condition of periodontal tissues and tongue; presence of lesions; and condition of the lips and skin around the mouth) can be evaluated easily without invasive procedures. Individuals who have difficulty in chewing because of loose teeth, poorly fitting dentures, or oral lesions have a tendency to eat soft foods, which are usually high in fat and refined carbohydrate and low in most essential nutrients. This may contribute to weight loss in the frail elderly.[12] It is valuable to assess the individual's ability to chew, swallow, and self-feed while evaluating the condition of the teeth, tongue, gums, and oral mucosa. Poor oral status may be both the etiology and manifestation of poor nutrition; therefore, assessment of oral health must always be included as part of the nutritional assessment.[13]

Physical Disabilities

Nutritional status may be affected as a result of physical changes that impede the ability of some older adults to perform normal functions of daily life. For example, eating behavior is influenced by many factors, including taste and smell changes and the ability to feed oneself. These alterations may not be correctable, but they may be overcome if they are first recognized as contributing to nutritional intake problems. Some of these changes occur slowly, and the individual adapts to them with little effort; others occur as the result of acute illness, and the individual may require an intervention to accommodate these changes.

One change that occurs with aging, although at different rates among elderly people, is an alteration in taste and smell sensitivity. Diminished taste and smell acuity contribute to decreased enjoyment of food.[14] Bland, tasteless, odorless food will not be very appetizing and will not be eaten. Loss of certain taste sensations, particularly sweet

Table 18–1 Clinical Signs of Nutritional Deficiencies

Nutrient	Clinical Deficiency Symptoms
Vitamin A	*Eyes* —Bitot's spots; conjunctival and corneal xerosis (dryness); keratomalacia *Skin* —follicular hyperkeratosis; xerosis *Hair* —coiled, keratinized
Vitamin D	*Bone*—bowlegs; beading of ribs; pain; epiphyseal deformities
Vitamin E	Possible anemia
Vitamin K	*Skin*—subcutaneous hemorrhage; ecchymoses (bruises easily)
Thiamine (vitamin B$_1$)	*Neurologic*—mental confusion; irritability; sensory losses; weakness, paresthesias; anorexia *Eyes*—ophthalmoplegia *Cardiac* —tachycardia; cardiomegaly; congestive heart failure *Other*—constipation; sudden death
Niacin (vitamin B$_2$)	*Skin*—nasolabial seborrhea; fissuring eyelid corners; angular fissures around mouth; papillary atrophy; pellagrous dermatitis *Neurologic*—mental confusion *Other*—diarrhea
Riboflavin	*Skin*—nasolabial seborrhea; fissuring and redness around eyes and mouth; magenta tongue, genital dermatosis *Eyes*—corneal vascularization
Pyridoxine	*Skin*—nasolabial seborrhea; glossitis
Vitamin B$_0$	*Neurologic*—paresthesias; peripheral neuropathy *Other*—anemia
Folic acid	*Skin*—glossitis; hyperpigmentation of tongue; pallor *Neurologic*—depression *Other*—diarrhea; anemia
Pantothenic acid	*Other*—headache; fatigue, apathy; nausea; sleep disturbances
Ascorbic acid (vitamin C)	*Skin*—petechiae, purpura; swollen, bleeding gums *Other*—bone pain; dental caries; depression; anorexia; delayed wound healing
Vitamin B$_{12}$	*Skin*—glossitis; skin hyperpigmentation; pallor *Neurologic*—ataxia; optic neuritis; paresthesias; mental disorders *Other*—anemia; anorexia; diarrhea
Biotin	*Skin*—pluckable, sparse hair; pallor; seborrheic dermatitis *Neurologic*—depression *Other*—anemia; fatigue
Iron	*Skin*—pallor; angular fissures; glossitis; spoon nails; pale conjunctiva *Other*—enlarged spleen
Zinc	*Skin*—seborrheic dermatitis; poor wound healing *Eyes*—photophobia *Other*—dysgeusia
Iodine	*Other*—large, swollen tongue; goiter
Protein	*Skin*—dull, dry, easily pluckable hair; "flaky paint" dermatitis; edema
Protein/energy	*Skin*—loss of subcutaneous fat; dull, dry, easily pluckable hair; decubitus ulcers; muscle wasting

Table 18–2 Presentation of Dehydration in the Elderly

- Mucosal xerosis
- Swollen tongue
- Sunken eyeballs
- Elevated body temperature
- Decreased urine output
- Constipation
- Nausea and vomiting
- Decreased blood pressure
- Mental confusion
- Acute renal failure
- Altered drug effects
- Electrolyte disturbances

---

and salt, may contribute to stronger sour or bitter taste sensations.[15] (Chapter 7) The magnitude and etiology of taste sensation changes that occur remain somewhat controversial,[16–18] due in part to the accuracy and validity of the methodologies used in studying the senses of taste and smell; however, improved oral hygiene may help enhance taste sensations.[19] Unless an individual is deficient in zinc, vitamin A, or the B vitamins, supplementing the diet with these nutrients will not correct loss of taste.

Table 18–3 Risk Factors for Dehydration in the Elderly

- Anorexia
- Laxative abuse
- Diuretic abuse
- Disability
- Confinement to chair or bed
- Depression
- Cognitive dysfunction
- Confusion
- Central nervous system impairment
- Diarrhea, vomiting, hemorrhage
- Incontinence
- Unconsciousness
- Dependence on tube or parenteral feeding
- Inability to feed self
- Presence of four or more chronic conditions
- Use of four or more medications
- Presence of chronic infections

Olfactory dysfunction is prevalent in elderly individuals, which results in their inability to identify exactly what is being consumed.[20] Decreased olfactory perception in the elderly has been shown to be associated with lower interest in food-related activities, lower preference for many healthful foods, and higher intake of sweets.[21] Other sensory losses may affect nutrition, although in less direct ways. Loss of vision and hearing will contribute to social isolation and changes in eating behaviors. A decrease in visual acuity will limit shopping and cooking activities. Loss of hearing will also tend to restrict social activities.[22]

Physical disabilities that affect nutritional status in elderly people are related to chronic illnesses or problems with motor or cognitive function.[23,24] Chronic illness can affect appetite and alter nutrient needs, and eventually may lead to tube or parenteral feeding dependency. (Chapter 19) Multiple chronic illnesses can lead to polypharmacy, which may have an impact on absorption, metabolism, and requirements for specific nutrients. (Chapter 16) Assessing the types and doses of various prescription and over-the-counter medications is an essential component of a thorough nutritional assessment.

Functional Assessment

Many of the nutrition-related problems noted thus far may result in some form of functional impairment, which can further affect nutritional status. The benefit of including an assessment of functional status as part of a complete nutritional assessment has been documented in many recent publications.[25–28] Sullivan et al.[29] demonstrated, for a population of institutionalized elderly, that impaired functional status and nutritional status strongly predicted infectious complications. The effect of loss of function in the elderly on their ability to perform activities related to food or nutrition such as shopping, meal preparation, and self-feeding has also been documented.[30–32] A commonly used measure of independence is the ability to perform functional tasks necessary for daily living. These activities of daily living

(ADLs)[33] include basic self-care functions, including self-feeding (Table 18–4). Instrumental activities of daily living (IADLs)[34] are the more involved skills needed to function in the community, including such activities as driving, shopping, paying bills, and preparing food (Table 18–5). Other assessment tools that identify functional impairment as well as nutrition skills are available.[35]

Motor skills that enable elderly individuals to remain independent are important factors in the maintenance of health and nutrition status. The ability to move around unencumbered by walkers or wheelchairs is important for getting out of

---

Table 18–4 Activities of Daily Living

Toileting
1. Cares for self; no incontinence
2. Needs to be reminded, or needs help with cleanliness; accidents rare
3. Soiling or wetting at least once a week
4. No control of bladder or bowels

Feeding
1. Eats without assistance
2. Eats with minor assistance or with help in cleanliness
3. Feeds self with assistance and is messy
4. Requires extensive assistance with feeding
5. Relies on being fed

Dressing
1. Is independent in dressing and selecting clothing
2. Dresses and undresses with minor assistance
3. Requires moderate assistance with dressing and undressing
4. Needs major assistance in dressing but is helpful
5. Completely unable to dress or undress oneself

Grooming
1. Always neatly dressed and well groomed
2. Grooming adequate; may need minor assistance
3. Requires assistance in grooming
4. Needs grooming care but is able to maintain groomed state
5. Resists grooming

Ambulation
1. Totally independent
2. Ambulates in limited geographical area
3. Ambulates with assistance (needs cane, wheelchair, walker, railing)
4. Sits unsupported in chair or wheelchair but needs help with motion
5. Bedridden

Bathing
1. Bathes self independently
2. Bathes self with help getting into bath or shower
3. Washes hands and face but needs help with bathing
4. Can be bathed with cooperation
5. Does not bathe and is combative with those trying to help

Source: Adapted with permission from M.P. Lawton, The functional assessment of elderly people. *Journal of American Geriatrics Society,* Vol.19, p. 4465, © 1971, Williams & Wilkins.

Table 18–5 Instrumental Activities of Daily Living

Ability to use telephone
1. Uses telephone without help
2. Uses telephone only with familiar telephone numbers
3. Answers phone but does not initiate calls
4. Does not use telephone at all

Shopping
1. Shops independently for all needs
2. Shops independently for minor purchases
3. Needs accompaniment on shopping trip
4. Completely unable to shop

Food preparation
1. Plans, prepares, and serves adequate meals independently
2. Prepares adequate meals if foods are provided
3. Heats and serves prepared meals *or* prepares meals that are not adequate
4. Needs to have meals prepared and served

Housekeeping
1. Maintains house alone or with occasional help with heavy work
2. Performs light daily housework
3. Performs light daily tasks incompletely
4. Needs help with all home maintenance tasks
5. Does not participate in any housekeeping tasks

Laundry
1. Does personal laundry completely
2. Launders small items independently
3. All laundry must be done by others

Mode of transportation
1. Travels independently on public transportation or drives car
2. Arranges own travel by taxi but does not use public transportation
3. Travels on public transportation with assistance
4. Travels by private transport with assistance
5. Does not travel at all

Responsibility for own medications
1. Is totally independent in managing medications
2. Takes own medications if prepared in advance
3. Is not capable of dispensing or managing medications

Ability to handle finances
1. Manages financial matters independently
2. Manages day-to-day finances but needs help with more complex tasks
3. Incapable of handling money

Source: Adapted with permission from M.P. Lawton, The functional assessment of elderly people, *Journal of American Geriatrics Society,* Vol. 19, p. 4465, © 1971, Williams & Wilkins.

---

the house as opposed to being homebound. Fine motor skills are necessary for the preparation and consumption of food. Assessing an individual's ability to self-feed should be an essential component of a nutritional evaluation of individuals who have been institutionalized or have had a debilitating illness such as a stroke. These skills can all be evaluated by a functional assessment.

Cognitive and Psychological Function

The effect of alterations in nutritional status in relation to the etiology and treatment of cognitive impairment is hard to establish, but more evidence is becoming available to suggest there may indeed be a relationship.[36] Nutrition-related risk factors may include inadequacy of essential nutrients, particularly vitamin B_{12}, B_6, folate, and the antioxidants vitamin C, vitamin E, and β-carotene. Recent studies suggest that individuals with cognitive impairment are at risk for nutrition-related problems.[37,38] It is well recognized that weight loss occurs in patients with senile dementia, such as Alzheimer's disease, but it is difficult to define the etiology of the weight loss.[39,40] Poor memory, loss of feeding skills, hyperactive behavior, anorexia associated with polypharmacy, and depression may contribute to poor dietary intake. Depression occurs commonly in institutionalized people and is recognized as a treatable cause of weight loss.[41] Changes in cognitive or psychological function must be elicited from family members or caregivers and should be considered as possible etiologies in a chronically malnourished elderly patient.

Socioeconomic Factors

Exploring the environment in which elderly people live is important to gaining an understanding of their nutrition and health status. Financial resources, living situation, degree of independence, level of education, and social support systems are all factors that may influence nutritional intake. Many elderly people live on a fixed income, which limits their purchasing power when the cost of living increases. Of course, there is also a large population of older people who have financial resources to meet their needs. The ability to purchase fruits and vegetables in season and fresh meats may be limited, and this limitation may contribute to reliance on high-calorie foods that are not nutritionally dense, such as those high in carbohydrates and fats. Dietary supplements (eg, vitamin and mineral preparations), however, are used by some older individuals who probably do not require nutritional supplementation.[42]

Financial resources are a factor that determines living arrangements. Individuals who have adequate incomes may still live in their own homes. Many alternatives to housing are available for those who cannot afford to live alone or who need support in their activities of daily living, including group or foster homes, congregate living situations, retirement homes, and minimum to skilled care facilities. For elderly individuals who choose to live at home or alone, there are congregate meal programs, home meal programs, and home health aides (Chapter 20). Access to these services has been shown to contribute to a more successful maintenance of health status and a more rapid recovery from an episodic illness.[43] Several studies indicate that elderly people who live alone or in institutions have dietary intakes below recommended levels.[44,45]

Educational level is linked to both income and nutritional status. Several studies have indicated that level (years) of education is associated with the dietary intake of several nutrients, such as protein, iron, calcium, and several of the B vitamins.[44,46,47]

Health and nutritional status have also been linked with accessibility of social support systems. There appears to be a relationship between health status and social and community support systems, such as senior citizens' centers, churches, and other community groups.[48] This type of extended support system contributes to a sense of extended family and belonging to a caring group.

Examination of as many of these factors as possible in a nutritional assessment will contribute to a clearer picture of an individual's functional ability, lifestyle, and health problems that may interfere with adequate nutritional intake. A clinical assessment will add another dimension to the commonly used tools of nutritional assessment: anthropometric measurements; biochemical, hematological, and immune evaluations; and dietary histories.

ANTHROPOMETRIC ASSESSMENT

The major physiologic effect of malnutrition, either undernutrition or overnutrition, is a detrimental alteration of body composition. Protein-energy malnutrition (PEM) is first evidenced by loss of lean body mass and fat tissue. If the loss of available energy reserve (undernutrition) is severe enough, it can result in a significantly increased incidence of morbidity or mortality. Obesity (overnutrition) is characterized by an abnormal increase in body fat tissue, contributing to an increased risk for many chronic diseases.

Anthropometry is the technique by which the severity and composition of these morphologic changes can be evaluated. It also provides a method of monitoring the appropriateness of nutritional therapy. The anthropometric measurements most commonly used for assessing nutritional status are height, body weight, circumferences, and skinfold thicknesses.[49] For various reasons, the usefulness of these measures as predictors of nutritional status in the elderly is questionable. Major benefits of anthropometry over other nutritional assessment procedures are the ease with which the measurements can be accomplished, their relatively low cost, and their noninvasive nature, all of which make anthropometry particularly desirable for use in an aged population. However, the ability to obtain adequate and reproducible data is dependent on being able to obtain accurate measurements, and many elderly individuals have physical impairments that make this difficult and often impossible. Another significant limitation of anthropometry is the lack of appropriate standards with which to compare results; standards are derived from measurements compiled on younger adults and do not adjust for age-related physiologic changes.

Well-known physiologic changes in stature and body composition that occur with normal aging must be considered when using anthropo-metric measurements to assess nutritional status in older adults.[50] A progressive decrease in height with age is well documented and has been attributed to changes in the integrity of the vertebral column, with postural changes due to generalized osteoporosis.[51–53] An average decrease in height of 1.2 cm/20 years postmaturity for whites and blacks of both sexes has been reported;[54,55] other cross-sectional studies have estimated the rate of loss in stature to be between 0.5 and 1.5 cm per decade.[52,56–58] Another longitudinal study observed a decrease in stature of 0.5 cm/year in white, healthy, middle-class, elderly men and women.[59]

Weight and body composition have also been shown to change with age[60–65] (Figure 18–1). Weight tends to increase until the early 40s in men and the early 50s in women, to hold relatively steady for the next 15 to 20 years, and to decrease thereafter.[61,63–65] A decrease in lean body mass is characteristic of aging, regardless of energy intake.[62] Along with the loss of protein mass, there is an increase in the proportion of body weight as adipose tissue. There is approximately a 10% increase in total body fat in an elderly subject above what a young adult carried. This increase in fat is not always visually evident because of the higher proportion of fat deposited around internal organs, particularly in women.[62] Subcutaneous fat on the extremities decreases with age, while fat tends to increase on the trunk.[66–68] This shift in body composition can complicate the interpretation of skinfold and circumference measurement data as predictors of total body fat.[69]

A major objective of anthropometry in nutritional assessment is to establish an individual's protein-energy reserve compared with normal ranges.[70] This presents a perplexing problem when one is using anthropometric measures to assess nutritional status in elderly subjects because of the lack of appropriate standards with which to compare the obtained data.[69] Therefore, extreme care must be used when interpreting results of anthropometric measures; anthropometry must be used in conjunction with clinical, laboratory, dietary, and psychosocial data.

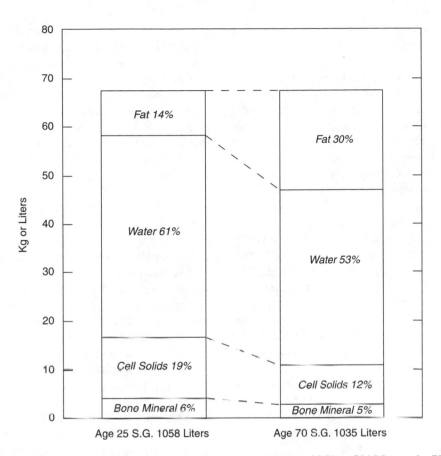

Figure 18–1 A Comparison of Body Composition Compartments in a 25-Year-Old Man and a 70-Year-Old Man
Source: Reprinted with permission from N.W. Shock, *Biological Aspects of Aging,* pp. 59–78, © 1962, Columbia University Press.

Weight for Height

Almost all of the currently used indicators of appropriate body weight, as well as other measures of lean body mass, require knowledge of the individual's height. Accurate measurements of stature are particularly difficult to obtain from most aged subjects because the physical changes that occur with aging make it difficult or even impossible for many elderly people to stand erect. Chronic diseases, such as arthritis, osteoporosis, and Parkinson-like disorders, which affect the neuromuscular systems, contribute to this problem. Individuals who have severe kyphosis (curvature of the spine) and bowing of

the legs present major problems in obtaining accurate measures of height.[49]

Additional problems are related to the fact that these same diseases may result in an actual decrease in height due to a compression of the vertebral disc space.[53] Since height is used as a constant reference point in many weight/height-related measurements, it is difficult to know whether to use actual height as "best measured" or maximal height of the individual as a young adult.[71]

To measure stature in elderly subjects who are able to stand unaided in an erect position, the following standardized procedure, as described in the *Anthropometric Standardization Reference*

Manual[72] and adapted for elderly subjects[73] is recommended:

1. The subject should be measured without shoes and in little or light clothing to allow viewing of the position of the body.
2. He or she should stand on a flat surface; at a right angle to the vertical board of a stadiometer.
3. The subject should stand up straight, with heels close together, legs as straight as possible, arms at the sides, and shoulders relaxed.
4. The head should be in the Frankfort horizontal plane: that is, the line of vision should be perpendicular to the body. The headboard is then lowered onto the crown of the head.
5. The subject should then take a deep breath; the stature measurement is recorded to the nearest 0.1 cm or $\frac{1}{8}$ in at maximal inspiration.
6. A repeated measurement should be taken to ensure reliability and should agree within 1 cm or $\frac{1}{2}$ in of the first measurement.
7. The degree of kyphosis or bowing of the legs should be noted.
8. A sliding bar attached to a beam balance may also be used to measure height; however, this device is generally less accurate.[69]

Because of the problems described, alternative methods for estimating stature in the elderly have been investigated.[74,75] Arm span is highly correlated with stature when an individual reaches his or her maximal height, before age-associated changes occur in the vertebral column.[50,76] Studies indicate that racial differences between American blacks and whites occur in the relationship between arm span and stature.[54] Arm span includes both arms and the breadth of the shoulders and is measured with the subject's arms outstretched maximally. Problems similar to those encountered in measuring stature due to kyphosis, osteoporosis, and arthritis can prevent the use of arm span measurement in this group. As a result, total arm length (TAL) has been evaluated as an alternative

measure.[74] TAL is measured from the tip of the acromial process of the scapula to the end of the styloid process of the ulna. This study[74] indicates that although height decreases with age, arm measurements do not change to the same degree. Therefore, it seems likely that TAL could be a useful value for the development of anthropometric standards for the elderly; however, arm length varies among individuals of the same height, so additional validation and further studies are required to determine the reliability and interpretation of this measurement before its routine clinical use can be advocated.[74]

For those elderly individuals who cannot stand erect, recumbent anthropometric techniques have been developed that can be used to estimate stature from knee height measurements;[75] weight can be estimated by using recumbent measurements of arm and calf circumferences, subscapular skinfold thickness, and knee height.[77] The clinical application of these and other recumbent measures, along with detailed descriptions of the measuring techniques, have been reported elsewhere.[73] For elderly individuals who have severe neuromuscular deformities, the best measurement of height may be obtained by measurement of individual body segments. Segment lengths should be measured between specific bony landmarks and as vertical distances between a flat surface and a bony landmark, but they should not be measured from joint creases[78] (Figure 18–2).

Weight

Body weight is one of the simplest and most routinely collected anthropometric indices used to monitor individuals[79] and is used as a rough estimate of body energy stores. Body weight is a composite measure of total body size, reflecting everything inside the personal envelope,[80] but it provides no information relating to body composition. Absolute weight may stay constant over time, but the proportions of lean muscle mass and fat may change, as seen in many elderly individuals.[55]

To increase the reliability and reproducibility of repeated measures, standardized procedures

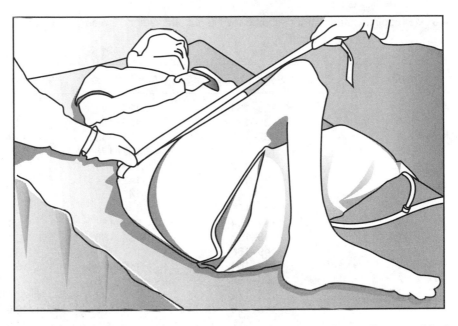

Figure 18–2 An Example of Segmental Measurements in an Elderly, Cachectic, Contracted Patient
Measurement points are from one bony prominence to another bony landmark.

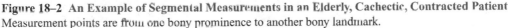

should be followed.[81] Subjects should always be weighed in the same type of clothing, preferably in a lightweight gown or underclothing. Because of diurnal variations in weight, it is best to weigh at the same time of day, before eating and after voiding. These conditions should be recorded each time to help to understand extreme variations in the measurement. For ambulatory persons who can stand unaided, an upright beam scale with movable weights is the most accurate and reliable. One with a wide base and a hand support is best because most elderly individuals are unsteady and need this support to position themselves before accurate measurements can be taken. Subjects should stand with their feet over the center of the platform. Measurements should be recorded to the nearest 0.1 kg or 1/4 lb. A chair scale may be needed for persons who are unable to stand unaided. For the nonambulatory, bedfast patient, it is necessary to use a bed scale; recumbent measures developed to estimate weight can be used.[77] Each scale should be calibrated periodically against a set of standard weights.

As with most nutritional assessment parameters, it is useful to be able to compare a given weight of an individual with that of an ideal weight for a healthy subject of the same sex, age, and stature. This presents a problem, however, since there are no universally accepted standards available for evaluation of weight in very old persons.[49] The Metropolitan Life Insurance Company height and weight tables for 1959[82] and 1983[83] are commonly used standards (Table 18–6). These tables represent weights associated with the lowest mortality rate for persons of various height and body frames. These data were compiled to represent persons up to age 59 years; however, the 1983 tables have been shown to be appropriate for older individuals.[84] Body frame is determined by measuring elbow breadth as described by Frisancho and Flegel.[85] A recent study comparing several reported methods of determining frame size showed that elbow breadth was not the most acceptable measure on the basis of assumptions inherent in use of frame size determinations.[86] No data exist on the reliability of determining frame size in very old people.

Table 18–6 Metropolitan Life Insurance Company Height and Weight Tables, 1983

Height		Men		
Feet	Inches	Small Frame	Medium Frame	Large Frame
5	2	128–134	131–141	138–150
5	3	130–136	133–143	140–153
5	4	132–138	135–145	142–156
5	5	134–140	137–148	144–160
5	6	136–142	139–151	146–164
5	7	138–145	142–154	149–168
5	8	140–148	145–157	152–172
5	9	142–151	148–160	155–176
5	10	144–154	151–163	158–180
5	11	146–157	154–166	161–184
6	0	149–160	157–170	164–188
6	1	152–164	160–174	168–192
6	2	155–168	164–178	172–197
6	3	158–172	167–182	176–202
6	4	162–176	171–187	181–207

Height		Women		
Feet	Inches	Small Frame	Medium Frame	Large Frame
4	10	102–111	109–121	118–131
4	11	103–113	111–123	120–134
5	0	104–115	113–126	122–137
5	1	106–118	115–129	124–140
5	2	108–121	118–132	128–143
5	3	111–124	121–135	131–147
5	4	114–127	124–138	134–151
5	5	117–130	127–141	137–155
5	6	120–133	130–144	140–159
5	7	123–136	133–147	143–163
5	8	126–139	136–150	146–167
5	9	129–142	139–153	149–170
5	10	132–145	142–156	152–173
5	11	135–148	145–159	155–176
6	0	138–151	148–162	158–179

Note: Weights at ages 25 to 59 years based on lowest mortality. Weight in pounds according to frame (in indoor clothing weighing 5 lb, shoes with 1-in heels).

Source: Reprinted with permission from *Statistical Bulletin* Vol. 62, p. 2, Copyright © 1983, Metropolitan Life Insurance Company.

The National Center for Health Statistics has published reference data that include weights for older subjects up to age 74 years[87] (Table 18–7). These data make it possible to locate the 5th- through 95th-percentile values for weight of an elderly person of any given height. The 50th percentile value is probably a reasonable standard for most active elderly patients. It has

Table 18–7 Average Weights for U.S. Men and Women, 1971–1974

Sex and Height	Weight (lb)			
	35–44 Y	45–54 Y	55–64 Y	65–74 Y
Men				
62 in	143	147	143	143
63 in	148	152	147	147
64 in	153	156	153	151
65 in	158	160	158	156
66 in	163	164	163	160
67 in	169	169	168	164
68 in	174	173	173	169
69 in	179	177	178	173
70 in	184	182	183	177
71 in	190	187	189	182
72 in	194	191	193	186
73 in	200	196	197	190
74 in	205	200	203	194
Women				
57 in	125	129	132	130
58 in	129	133	136	134
59 in	133	136	140	137
60 in	137	140	143	140
61 in	141	143	147	144
62 in	144	147	150	147
63 in	148	150	153	151
64 in	152	154	157	154
65 in	156	158	160	158
66 in	159	161	164	161
67 in	163	165	167	165
68 in	167	168	171	169

Note: Weights at ages 25 to 59 years based on lowest mortality. Weight in pounds according to frame (in indoor clothing weighing 5 lb, shoes with 1-in heels). Estimated values from regression equations of weight on height for specified age groups. Examined persons were measured without shoes; clothing weight ranged from 0.20 to 0.62 lb, which was not deducted from weights shown.

Source: Adapted from Weight by Height and Age for Adults 18–74 Years: United States, 1971–1974, Office of Health Research, Statistics and Technology, National Center for Health Statistics, U.S. Department of Health and Human Services.

been recommended that the 5th-percentile value be the acceptable standard for completely inactive patients.[88]

Limited data on average or reference weight are available on persons over age 74 years. Master and Lasser[89] published average height-weight tables for persons aged 64 years and older (Table 18–8). Limitations associated with these data are that only a limited number of subjects were included in the groups age 85 years and older and that the subjects were predominantly white men and women and may not be representative of most elderly populations.[49] More recently, data are available from the National Health and Nutrition Examination Survey (NHANES) III, which contains data collected over the period from 1988 to 1991 (phase 1) on a sample of 600 elderly individuals 60 years of

Table 18–8 Average Height-Weight Table for Persons Aged 65 Years and Older

Men

Weight (lb)

Ht. (in)	65–69 Y	70–74 Y	75–79 Y	80–84 Y	85–89 Y	90–94 Y
61	128–156	125–153	123–151			
62	130–158	127–155	125–153	122–148		
63	131–161	129–157	127–155	122–150	120–146	
64	134–164	131–161	129–157	124–152	122–148	
65	136–166	134–164	130–160	137–155	125–153	117–143
66	139–169	137–167	133–163	130–158	128–156	120–146
67	140–172	140–170	136–166	132–162	130–160	122–150
68	143–175	142–174	139–169	135–165	133–163	126–154
69	147–179	146–178	142–174	139–169	137–167	130–158
70	150–184	148–182	146–178	143–175	140–172	134–164
71	155–189	152–186	149–183	148–180	144–176	139–169
72	159–195	156–190	154–188	153–187	148–182	
73	164–200	160–196	158–192			

Women

Weight (lb)

Ht. (in)	65–69 Y	70–74 Y	75–79 Y	80–84 Y	85–89 Y	90–94 Y
59	121–147	114–146	112–136	100–122	99–121	
60	122–148	116–142	113–1.39	1 06–130	102–124	
61	123–151	118–144	115–144	1 09–133	104–128	
62	125–153	121–147	118–144	112–136	108–132	107–131
63	127–155	123–151	121–147	115–141	112–136	107–131
64	130–158	126–154	123–151	119–145	115–141	108–132
65	132–162	130–158	126–154	122–150	120–146	112–136
66	136–166	132–162	128–157	126–154	124–152	116–142
67	140–170	136–166	131–161	130–158	128–156	
68	143–175	140–170				
69	148–180	144–176				

Source: Reprinted with permission from A.M. Master et a!. *Journal of the American Medical Association,* Vol. 172, p. 659. Copyright © 1960, American Medical Association. Reprinted by permission of the American Medical Association.

age and older, with no upper age limits. Included in this survey were equal numbers of whites, blacks, and Hispanics.[90] Concerns have been expressed regarding the use of these data as reference standards due to the limited sample size.[91] More reliable data will be available when results of the entire NHANES III data is published. This data will represent approximately 5300 people ages 60 years and older. There are limitations associated with the use of each of the different standards. All of the standards should be considered, and the one most representative of the population being evaluated should be selected. It is important that the standards selected be recorded and used consistently by all members of the health care team, according to frame (in indoor clothing weighing 3 lb, shoes with 1-in heels).

A more clinically useful and predictive factor than relative body weight is the evaluation of changes in weight over a given period of time;[92] therefore, a careful history of previous weight gain or loss should be obtained. For a very old individual or an acutely ill, elderly patient, one must usually seek the help of a close family member or care provider to ascertain this information. Extreme differences in either weight gain or loss over very short durations are most probably related to shifts in fluid balance rather than to alterations in nutritional status.[92] Recommendations for evaluating the significance of weight change over time have been published.[70] Similar recommendations specifically for evaluating the anorexia of aging were made at a conference on nutrition in the elderly.[93]

Body Mass Index

Body mass index (BMI), calculated by dividing the individual's weight in kilograms by the square of the height in meters, is being used with more frequency to evaluate nutritional status in the elderly. The BMI has been shown to be a good estimate of body fat. Low levels of BMI are associated with decreases in functional abilities and increased mortality in the elderly.[94] The Nutrition Screening Initiative (NSI) included the use of BMI and stated that elderly individuals with a BMI of greater than 27 or less than 24 may be at increased risk for poor nutritional status.[95] Nomograms for calculating BMI are widely available, as well as tables for the direct conversion of height and weight into BMI.[26,96,97] The reliability of the use of BMI in the elderly has been questioned because of concerns related to changes in height and body composition in the elderly. There is some evidence that BMI in elderly individuals may not be as predictive of health outcomes as has been promoted.[98]

Skinfold and Circumference Measures

Body weight is one indication of available energy stores; however, it is desirable to evaluate the composition of these stores and the severity of loss of lean muscle tissue versus adipose tissue. Depletion of lean muscle mass is more critical because of the role that protein plays in body function. The loss of lean muscle with aging has been referred to as sarcopenia.[99,100] More recently, the term *sarcopenia* is being used to designate abnormal losses of lean muscle; losses greater than what can be accounted for as a mere function of the aging process.[101]

At present, the most clinically applicable procedure for evaluating the degree of muscle loss and adipose mass depletion is anthropometry, particularly skinfold and circumference measurements. These techniques have particular limitations in elderly subjects, due in part to the previously mentioned physical alterations in body composition associated with aging. In addition to the changes in lean muscle tissue and adipose tissue, other factors exist that make these measures more difficult to interpret in elderly subjects. With aging, there are changes in elasticity, hydration, and compressibility of the skin and in subcutaneous adipose and connective tissues that can alter the relationship of skinfold thickness measurements to body composition.[102] These changes may also affect both the accuracy and precision of the skinfold measurements.

Additional problems relating to measuring technique become apparent when working with elderly subjects who have loose skin on the arms and upper body. Therefore, it is imperative that standardized techniques be used[83] and that any major abnormalities in skin and fat distribution be noted.

Skinfold Measures

Skinfold measurements are relatively simple to obtain, are less affected by hydration status than is weight, and are independent of height. Skinfold measurements have been shown to correlate with body fat measured by more sophisticated techniques.[103-107] Formulas have been developed for predicting total body fat from one skinfold[108] and from multiple skinfold measurements.[103] Data from a large study of elderly subjects indicated that skinfold measurements on the trunk may be more reliable predictors of body fat in men, whereas skinfold measurements on the extremities seem to be more accurate in women.[104] In elderly people, the use of multiple skinfold measurements should add to the reliability of the predicted value of body fat. Numerous equations have been developed to determine body composition from skinfold measurements, all of which use various combinations of measurements from different sites.[109]

Although there is no universal agreement about whether to use right-side or left-side body measures, it is very important that the same side of the body always be used for both skinfold and circumference measurements of a given subject. The most commonly used anatomic sites for skinfold measurements are triceps, biceps, subscapular, and suprailiac. The following methods for identifying these sites and performing the measurements are taken from the *Anthropometric Standardization Reference Manual.*[110]

Triceps skinfold is measured at a point midway between the lateral projection of the acromial process of the scapula and the inferior margin of the olecranon. This point is determined by using a tape measure, with the subject's elbow flexed to 90°. The midpoint is marked on the lateral side of the arm. Subjects are measured while standing, if possible; if not, they should be propped upright in a chair or bed. The skinfold is measured with the arm hanging loosely and comfortably at the subject's side. The triceps skinfold is picked up with the left thumb and index finger, approximately 1 cm proximal to the marked level, and the calipers are applied to the skinfold at the marked level. The skinfold should be held for the duration of the measurement. The measurement site must be in the midline posteriorly when the palm is directed anteriorly.

Biceps skinfold is measured by lifting the skin on the anterior aspect of the upper arm, directly above the center of the cubital fossa at the same level as the triceps skinfold. The crest of the fold should run parallel to the long axis of the arm. The subject stands, facing the measurer, with the arm relaxed at the side and the palm directed anteriorly.

Subscapular skinfold is measured by lifting the skin 1 cm under the inferior angle of the scapula with the shoulder and arm relaxed at the side of the body. To locate the site, the measurer palpates the scapula, running the fingers inferiorly and laterally along its vertebral border until the inferior angle is identified. For obese or elderly subjects, gentle placement of the subject's arm behind the back aids in identifying the site. The skinfold thickness is recorded to the nearest 0.1 cm.

Suprailiac skinfold is measured in the midaxillary line immediately superior to the iliac crest. The skinfold is grasped just posterior (about 2 cm) to the midaxillary line, following the natural cleavage lines of the skin. The crest of the fold should be horizontal. The caliper jaws are applied about 1 cm from the fingers holding the skinfold, and the thickness is recorded to the nearest 0.1 cm.

Equations for calculating total body fat and fat-free mass from the sum of the four skinfold measurements are given in Table 18–9. The most widely used data for evaluating skinfold and circumference measurements in elderly subjects are those from a cross-sectional sampling of American subjects aged 25 to 74 years from the NHANES I and II.[87] These data are presented in Tables 18–10 and 18–11. Available percentile norms for upper arm anthropometry in white men and women aged 60 to 89 years are presented in Table 18–12.[111]

Circumference Measurements

Circumferences are measurements that record the size of cross-sectional and circumferential dimensions of the body. They can be used alone, in combination with skinfold measurements, or in combination with other circumferences to help evaluate nutritional status. Specific techniques for measuring circumferences have been described.[112] These measurements require the use of a tape measure, which should be flexible but nonstretchable and should have markings on only

Table 18–9 Calculation of Fat and Fat-Free Mass

1. Determine the patient's age and weight in kilograms.
2. Measure the following skinfolds in millimeters: biceps, triceps, subscapular, suprailiac.
3. Compute Σ by adding four skinfold values.
4. Compute the logarithm of Σ.
5. Apply one of the following age- and sex-adjusted equations to calculate body density *(D)* (in g/mL):

   Equations for men:
   Age Range (y)
   17–19 $D = 1.1620 - 0.0630 \times (\log \Sigma)$
   20–29 $D = 1.1631 - 0.0632 \times (\log \Sigma)$
   30–39 $D = 1.1422 - 0.0544 \times (\log \Sigma)$
   40–49 $D = 1.1620 - 0.0700 \times (\log \Sigma)$
   50+ $D = 1.1715 - 0.0779 \times (\log \Sigma)$

   Equations for women:
   Age Range (y)
   17–19 $D = 1.1549 - 0.0678 \times (\log \Sigma)$
   20–29 $D = 1.1599 - 0.0717, \times (\log \Sigma)$
   30–39 $D = 1.1423 - 0.0632 \times (\log \Sigma)$
   40–49 $D = 1.1333 - 0.0612 \times (\log \Sigma)$
   50+ $D = 1.1339 - 0.0645 \times (\log \Sigma)$

6. Fat mass is then calculated as: Fat mass (kg) = body weight (kg) $\times [(4.95/D) - 4.5]$
7. Fat-free mass is then calculated as: Fat-free mass (kg) = body weight (kg) − fat mass (kg)

Source: Reprinted with permission from J.V. Dumin and J. Womersley, Body fat assessed from total body density and its estimation from skinfold thickness, in *British Journal of Nutrition,* Vol. 32, p. 77, Copyright © 1974, Cambridge University Press.

one side, in either metric or English units. Circumferences should be recorded with the zero end of the tape held in the left hand above the remaining part of the tape, which is held by the right hand.

The tape should be maintained in a horizontal position, touching the skin and following the contours of the limb but not compressing underlying tissue. The tension applied to the tape by the evaluator affects the validity and reliability of the measurement. The mid-upper arm circumference is measured at the midpoint between the acromial process of the scapula and olecranon.

Table 18–10 Average Triceps Skinfold Thickness in Adults

| Age (y) | Average Thickness (mm) | |
	Men	Women
35–44	12	23
45–54	11	25
55–64	11	25
65–74	11	23

Source: Reprinted from 1971–1975 National Health Survey, *Vital and Health Statistics Series No. 219*, U.S. Department of Health and Human Services, Public Health Service, 1981.

Table 18–11 Average Mid-Upper Arm Muscle Circumference in Adults

| Age (y) | Average Circumference (cm) | |
	Men	Women
45–54	28.2	22.7
55–64	27.8	22.8
65–74	26.8	22.8

Source: American Society for Clinical Nutrition, *Journa Clinical Nutrition*, Vol. 34, p. 2530, Copyright © 1981.

Table 18–12 Percentile Norms for Measurements of Upper Arm Anthropometry

Triceps Skinfold Thickness

Sex, Age (Y) Group	Sample	Mean	Percentile						
			5th	10th	25th	50th	75th	90th	95th
			MM						
Women									
60–89	496	25.2	12.5	14.4	18.5	24.0	30.8	38.1	43.6
60–69	146	27.2 ±~0.2*	13.0	14.7	20.7	26.2	33.0	40.3	47.2
70–79	239	25.1 ± .3	13.0	15.0	18.0	23.7	31.0	38.3	41.5
80–89	111	23.3 ±9.7'	10.9	12.9	16.7	21.8	27.5	34.6	43.4
Men									
60–89	250	22.5	5.7	7.6	11.5	20.4	31.8	42.1	45.8
60–69	86	21.9 ±13.6	4.9	6.9	10.8	18.0	31.9	45.1	49.3
70–79	115	23.5 ±13.3	6.3	7.9	12.0	22.0	32.7	41.8	45.4
80–89	49	2?.6 ±11.0	5.8	8.0	11.5	21.0, 29.6		37.5	40.5

Mid–Upper Arm Circumference

Sex, Age (Y) Group	Sample	Mean	Percentile						
			5th	10th	25th	50th	75th	90th	95th
			MM						
Women									
60–89	496	30 0	23.3	25.1	27.0	29.7	32.7	35.9	38.1
60–69	146	31 1 ±4.8	23.5	25.6	27.7	30.6	33.7	37.5	'39.9
70–79	239	30.0 ±4.1	23.5	25.5	27.1	29.5	32.5	35.5	37.8
80–89	111	28.8 ±4.6	22.5	23.5	26.0	28.8	31.6	34.5	36.4
Men									
60–89	250	30.4	24.9	26.6	28.7	30.4	32.2	34.6	36.3
60–69	86	30.5 ±3.0	25.1	27.3	29.0	30.5	32.4	34.2	35.7
70–79	115	30.7 ±3.1	25.3	26.8	29.0	30.7	32.4	34.6	36.6
80–89	49	29.6 ±3.5	23.4	24.9	27.6	29.6	31.5	35.3	36.5

Mid–Upper Arm Muscle Circumference

Sex, Age (Y)			Percentile						
Group	Sample	Mean	5th	10th	25th	50th	75th	90th	95th
			MM						
Women									
60–89	496	22.0	16.7	17.7	19.8	21.9	24.3	26.9	28.3
60–69	146	22.6 ±3.6	17.8	18.4	20.2	22.3	24.6	27.5	29.2
70–79	239	22.1 ±3.5	16.7	17.8	19.8	21.9	24.2	26.7	28.2
80–89	111	21.4 ±4.1	15.2	16.7	19.1	21.3	24.2	26.7	27.5
Men									
60–89	250	23.3	16.6	18.1	20.5	23.4	26.2	28.4	29.7
60–69	86	23.7 ±4.4	16.1	18.0	20.5	23.7	26.7	28.9	31.7
70–79	115	23.3 ±4.1	17.0	18.2	20.4	23.4	26.3	28.4	28.7
80–89	49	22.8 ±3.3	16.6	18.2	20.7	22.8	24.9	27.3	28.6

Mid–Upper Arm Muscle Area

Sex, Age (Y)			Percentile						
Group	Sample	Mean	5th	10th	25th	50th	75th	90th	95th
			MM						
Women									
60–89	496	39.9	22.2	25.0	31.1	38.0	47.1	57.7	63.8
60–69	146	41.6 ±13.5	25.1	27.0	32.6	39.6	48.3	60.3	67.6
70–79	239	39.8 ±12.7	22.1	25.1	31.2	38.0	46.7	56.6	63.2
80–89	111	37.9 ±13.3	18.4	22.3	29.0	36.1	46.5	56.8	60.2
Men									
60–89	250	44.6	22.0	26.2	33.5	43.6	54.4	64.1	70.4
60–69	86	46.0 ±16.5	20.7	25.8	33.4	44.8	56.8	66.7	79.7
70–79	115	44.6 ±14.6	23.0	26.4	33.3	43.7	54.8	64.3	65.7
80–89	49	42.3 ±11.8	21.9	26.5	34.2	41.5	49.4	59.1	64.9

*Mean ±standard deviation.

Source: Adapted from G. Falciglia. Upper Arm Anthropometric Norms in Elderly White Subjects. Copyright The American Dietetic Association. Adapted by permission from The American Dietetic Association, Vol. 85, p. 1296, © 1985.

This location is the same as that marked for the triceps and biceps skinfolds. The measurement is made with the elbow extended and the arm relaxed and hanging just away from the side of the trunk, with the palm facing the thigh.

The mid-upper arm circumference (MAC), in conjunction with the triceps skinfold (TSF) measurement, can be used to calculate the arm-muscle circumference (AMC) and the arm-muscle area (AMA), both of which are estimates of the amount of muscle or lean tissue in the body. Formulas that can be used for these calculations are as follows:

$$AMC \text{ (cm)} = MAC \text{ (cm)} - (3.14 \times TSF \text{ (mm)})$$

$$AMA \text{ (cm}^2) = AMC^2/12.56$$

Reference standards are given in Tables 18–10 and 18–11.

The use of calf circumference has been recommended as a more sensitive measure of the loss of total body muscle mass in the elderly than arm circumference and midarm muscle area.[113] The World Health Organization has recommended that calf circumference be included as a measure of nutritional status in the elderly.[91] Calf circumference is included as one of the anthropometric measures, in addition to MAC, BMI, and history of weight loss, in a Mini Nutritional Assessment form recently developed for assessing nutritional status as part of the geriatric evaluation.[114]

Another measure of lean body mass (LBM) is the creatinine height index (CHI), which has been used to assess nutritional status in the elderly.[115] Creatinine is formed irreversibly from the metabolism of creatine and creatine phosphate found primarily in muscle tissue. The daily production of creatinine is related to the total LBM content of the body and has been shown to be remarkably consistent from day to day.[116] The CHI has been adopted for evaluation of LBM in young, healthy adults and in hospitalized patients who may be protein-energy malnourished.

Several problems are associated with this measurement as a clinical tool in elderly individuals. The measurement requires an accurately timed, 24-hour urine collection, which is very difficult (and often impossible) to obtain from elderly patients. In addition, creatinine excretion must be related to an individual's measured height, which sometimes is difficult to obtain in elderly subjects, as discussed previously. Another problem relates to the fact that LBM decreases with age, and with this decrease there will be a decrease in creatinine excretion unrelated to nutritional status. Many elderly individuals have compromised renal function; if this is the case, urinary creatinine excretion may not be a reliable measure.[117]

The usefulness of the CHI as a tool with which to predict PEM in an elderly population has been evaluated.[69] This research indicated that CHI was a more accurate predictor of PEM in elderly men than in elderly women. In a recent study to determine whether aging alters the usefulness of creatinine excretion as an index of LBM or muscle mass in healthy men and women,[118] total LBM was determined by total-body potassium counting, and cross-sectional areas of upper arm and thigh muscle were determined by magnetic resonance imaging. This study indicated that creatine excretion is useful for evaluating body composition in both young and old subjects.

BIOCHEMICAL MEASURES

A number of biochemical measures are available for use in the assessment of nutritional status. They can be categorized into two groups on the basis of the diagnostic ability of the results.[116] The first group relies on nonspecific indices of nutritional status, and the second group uses nutrient-specific indices of nutritional status. The first group includes determinations of the plasma proteins, which are usually easier to obtain than the nutrient-specific analyses that can detect subclinical micronutrient deficiencies.

As with anthropometric measures, problems exist with the use of biochemical indices in the assessment of elderly people. Factors other than nutrient intake are known to influence biochemical marker levels in the body.

General state of health, past and present history of diseases, and use and abuse of alcohol, tobacco, medications, and over-the-counter drugs can produce alterations in biochemical data. These factors are of particular concern in elderly individuals. There is also a lack of age-adjusted reference data for appropriate interpretation of available results.

Protein Assessment

Several biochemical measurements are available that reflect dietary protein intake as well as body protein stores. Among these, analyses of serum albumin, transferrin, and total iron-binding capacity (TIBC) are the most readily available and least expensive. Transport proteins with more rapid turnover (eg, prealbumin and retinol-binding protein) may be more sensitive to changes in protein nutriture, but tests for these are less readily available. The level of circulating serum albumin is the most consistently used measure of visceral protein status because of its high reliability as a prognostic marker of PEM.

Albumin is the major visceral protein produced by the liver, and its synthesis is dependent on an adequate supply of protein and, to a lesser degree, total energy intake.[119] It has been used extensively as a marker of the degree of PEM, has been shown to correlate positively with post-surgical outcome,[120] and has been reported to be a good prognostic indicator of hospital survival in elderly patients.[121] Albumin has also been found to be a strong predictor of clinical outcomes of hospitalized elderly nursing home residents.[122]

Serum albumin levels appear to be only minimally affected by aging.[123,124] However, some studies indicate a slight reduction in the rate of albumin synthesis in aged subjects.[125] A recent study found hypoalbuminemia to be associated with several sociodemographic, lifestyle, and disease-related factors in community-dwelling older persons.[126] Others have reported lower serum albumin levels in the elderly to be associated with losses in muscle mass.[127] Functional

impairment and disability have also been associated with low serum albumin in the elderly.[123,128]

In the past, hypoalbuminemia has been shown to be a reliable predictor of protein malnutrition in elderly people.[69,129] In a study evaluating several nutritional indices for their predictive ability of mortality in elderly hospitalized patients, a serum albumin level of less than 3 g/dL was found to be the best single predictor of mortality; it has been suggested that this value could provide early identification of elderly people who are at increased risk of death.[121] Another more recent study evaluating predictors of early non-elective hospital readmissions in nutritionally compromised Medicare patients found low albumin levels along with any amount of weight loss to be the most predictive of readmissions.[130]

Even though decreased albumin levels are almost always present in malnourished individuals, caution, along with astute clinical judgment, must be exercised in their interpretation. Many of the concurrent diseases that are common in elderly people are known to alter plasma protein concentrations. Therefore, depressed serum albumin levels due to diminished production in liver diseases, and excess losses as a consequence of renal or gastrointestinal disease or protein-losing enteropathy, must be ruled out before this measure can be used as a reliable indicator of nutritional status. Albumin is an acute phase reactant, so a patient experiencing any inflammatory disease process may have a depressed serum albumin independent of nutritional status.[131] Also, immobilization will contribute a state of negative nitrogen balance, which will compromise albumin levels.

Additionally, plasma albumin concentrations are directly influenced by hydration status. Any situation that results in a decrease in plasma volume will cause an artificially high serum albumin level unrelated to protein intake or albumin synthesis. Depressed levels of serum albumin are seen when plasma volume is expanded, as would occur in a patient with congestive heart failure or renal disease. Albumin values in these individuals might appear to be deceptively low and unrelated to nutritional status. Very old and acutely ill elderly patients are often confined to bed for extended periods of time, and this can contribute to depressed albumin levels.[132]

After the clinical findings described previously are taken into account, a serum albumin level of less than 3.5 g/dL is suggestive of chronic PEM and warrants further evaluation. Albumin's relatively long half-life (approximately 14 to 20 days) explains its slow response to nutritional therapy. A refeeding period of at least 2 weeks is usually required before consistent improvement in serum albumin levels can be noted. Aggressive refeeding in a severely malnourished elderly patient often will result in a further decrease in serum albumin level before an increase is seen. This phenomenon is attributed to the redistribution of extracellular and intracellular fluids.

Another major visceral protein often used for monitoring nutrition status is serum transferrin. It is usually considered a more sensitive marker of protein nutriture than albumin because its half-life is approximately 9 days. However, its usefulness in an aged population is complicated by the fact that there is a strong negative correlation between circulating transferrin and tissue iron stores.[133,134] With advancing age, tissue iron stores increase, and as a result, serum transferrin levels are reduced.[135,136] Thus, some healthy elderly individuals may have transferrin values in the range commonly associated with nutritional deficiency.[137] This fact should always be considered before assuming that reductions in transferrin levels are due to protein malnutrition. Conversely, in individuals who have decreased iron stores, serum transferrin may be within the normal range, even in the presence of PEM.[137]

Often direct measures of serum transferrin are not available, necessitating the estimation of transferrin from TIBC.[136] This is usually accomplished by using the following formula:

$$[TIBC\ (mg/dL) \times 0.8] - 43$$

This may not be the best formula to use in all circumstances, however, and it has been suggested that each laboratory run its own regression analysis to determine a laboratory-specific formula for the estimation of transferrin levels from TIBC.[117]

Thyroxine-binding pre-albumin (PA) and retinol-binding protein (RBP) are two serum proteins synthesized in the liver that have very rapid turnover rates and small body pool sizes; they are therefore sensitive to any changes affecting their synthesis and catabolism.[138] Because of these properties, they may be excellent indicators of subclinical malnutrition and may aid in the long-term management and monitoring of high-risk elderly patients.[139]

RBP is a glycoprotein with a half-life of approximately 12 hours; it is involved in the transport of retinol from the liver to peripheral tissues. Its synthesis is responsive to the need for retinol transport; therefore, circulating serum levels may reflect vitamin A status, not just protein nutriture. In addition, inflated levels of RBP can be seen in patients with renal failure, and the levels may be depressed in patients with liver disease. RBP circulates while bound to PA as a PA-RBP complex. PA has a half-life of 2 days and is responsible for the transport of thyroxine. Its synthesis is not dependent on vitamin A status. The concentration of PA-RBP complex is decreased in the presence of protein-energy metabolism, responds positively to nutritional therapy, and has been shown to be useful as a prognostic indicator of nutritional status.[140–143]

In recent years, C-reactive protein (CRP) has been explored as a possible indicator of nutritional status. Increased CRP serum concentrations are seen in obesity, smoking, infection, and coronary heart disease. The role of CRP as a predictor of asymptomatic heart disease appears to have more reliability than do lipid levels, particularly low density lipoproteins.[144] CRP is normally present in low concentrations, but when inflammation occurs and there is an increase in circulating interleukin-6, CRP concentrations can increase as much as 1000-fold.[145] It has been demonstrated that Ω-3 and Ω-6 fatty acids have anti-inflammatory effects and can, therefore, lower serum levels of CRP. Vitamin E has been shown to have a similar effect. More recently, it has been demonstrated that weight loss can also result in a significant reduction in CRP levels.[146] Although CRP has been suggested as a marker of nutritional status[147] that is affected by dietary intake, it does not appear to be accurate or reliable.

However, albumin, RBP, PA, and CRP are acute-phase reactants and therefore are directly affected by infections and inflammatory states.[148] PA is considered a negative acute-phase reactant because levels decrease after acute stress. This decrease is due to an interruption of hepatic synthesis rather than to increased catabolism or urinary excretion[149] and is influenced by hormonal changes rather than lack of available nutritional substrate. Discretion should be used before ascribing any change in these proteins to nutritional circumstances if either of these conditions exists. There are no data to indicate that any of these markers are altered in elderly people. However, more research is needed to determine the effect of aging on the synthesis and catabolism of these visceral proteins.

Cholesterol

There is some evidence, corroborated by serum protein levels, that serum cholesterol levels in elderly people are associated with poor health status.[150] Cholesterol levels as a disease predictor is different in older adults than it is in younger adults. There is a decreased association between serum cholesterol and coronary heart disease with advancing age,[151–155] and a link between serum cholesterol and mortality has been demonstrated.[156,157] This suggests that further investigation of biochemical measures and nutritional status of the elderly should be pursued.

IMMUNOLOGIC MEASURES

The association between nutritional status and immunocompetence is complex and multifactorial.[158–161] However, one of the strong associations noted is that PEM is accompanied by a reduction in host defense, demonstrated by anergy measured by delayed cutaneous hypersensitivity and lymphocytopenia. Immunologic dysfunction is associated with infections, cancer, and autoimmune diseases and may be a serious problem in elderly adults.

The immune system does not function as efficiently in older individuals as it does in younger individuals. The cell-mediated immune system is related to the T-cell system, which is responsible for the delayed cutaneous hypersensitivity response; responses to certain autoimmune diseases; responses to some bacteria, viruses, and fungi; and responses to cancers. An absolute decrease in the number of T cells with a relative increase in the number of T suppressor cells has been described in elderly subjects.[137,162] One explanation is a progressive decline in thymic function and the production of thymic hormone with advanced age. These factors contribute to the increase in immature lymphocytes and the related decrease in helper/inducer T lymphocytes.[163] These and other changes that occur in immune function are very similar to the changes that are often seen with PEM.[163,164]

The most commonly used assay for immunocompetence is antigen-recall skin testing. The ability to demonstrate a response to recall antigens diminishes with age.[165,166] This same effect has been demonstrated in PEM.[159,165,166] The similarity of the effects of the aging process and those of PEM on immune function makes the usefulness of routine immunologic testing in elderly subjects difficult to interpret. A relationship between anergy and mortality in a nursing home population has been shown,[167] and there appears to be evidence that restoration of some immune function in malnourished elderly patients can be induced by nutritional repletion.[162] The contribution of measures of immune function to the assessment of nutritional status in elderly people is difficult to isolate and therefore must be evaluated within the context of all the previously identified parameters.

HEMATOLOGIC MEASURES

Epidemiologic evidence indicates that anemia is fairly common among elderly subjects.[168,169] (Chapter 13) Whether the anemia is related to the aging process or to nutritional factors is difficult to determine. There is a strong similarity between the alterations in hematologic function seen with advancing age and those seen with PEM. In a study that examined multiple indicators of nutritional status in malnourished, elderly subjects, refeeding corrected most nutritional indicators (weight, serum albumin level, vitamin and mineral levels) but did not correct immunologic and hematologic indices (eg, hemoglobin level).[137]

Hematologic indices such as hematocrit, hemoglobin level, and total lymphocyte count are often available in the medical record since they are routinely obtained on admission to the hospital; they should be followed and changes noted. In a free-living or long-term care environment where complete blood counts are not obtained on a regular basis, it is probably more valuable to follow other nutritional indicators that will provide more reliable nutritional data, such as weight, serum albumin level, and dietary intake.

DIETARY ASSESSMENT

Dietary assessment of elderly subjects should provide insight into both present and past nutrient consumption habits. Finding the methods that can best accomplish this task is complicated by the physical and psychological impairments often seen in this group. While quantitative methods often may be impossible, a qualitative assessment can be used to reveal those individuals who are at risk for nutrient deficiencies. These methods should be able to identify those who are having problems consuming an adequate diet, those who limit their intake to one or two foods or categories of food, those who follow unusual dietary patterns, or those who exclude an important food or food group.[170] Methods available for collecting dietary intake data include diet histories with food frequency checks, food records kept over a specific time period, and 24-hour dietary recalls. All of these methods rely on the cooperation of the elderly subject and the knowledge and skills of the interviewer. Many hospitalized and institutionalized elderly patients are not competent enough to provide accurate self-reported dietary intake information. When this is encountered, the use of a surrogate source is advocated; surrogates include the spouse, child, or close relative or friend of the patient. For a very old individual, it may be difficult to find a person who can provide data adequate to reflect an accurate description of eating habits. In a review of the use of surrogate measures of dietary intake in elderly subjects, it was concluded that surrogate dietary data may introduce misclassification in analytic investigations but may be useful in descriptive studies.[171]

Dietary histories elicit information regarding what subjects generally eat and are based on food frequency checklists. Checklists should be constructed so that food intake over time can be estimated and should minimize the variation of day-to-day intake. Additional data should be gathered concerning food likes and dislikes; socioeconomic factors, such as transportation availability, cooking facilities, and income status; information on health-related special dietary requirements; and use of alcohol and over-the-counter drugs.

In a review by Hankin,[172] the following recommendations were made regarding the development of a diet history questionnaire for studies of older persons:

1. The questionnaire should include items that are representative of the population's usual diet to permit valid associations with biochemical and clinical findings. Both regional and ethnic foods should be included.

2. The questionnaire should provide both qualitative and quantitative information on the usual intake of foods, nutrients, and other dietary components. This can best be accomplished through the use of visual prompts: food models, common household measuring equipment, or actual photographs of serving sizes of different foods.

3. The questionnaire should be objective. Food items and groups should be clearly defined, the range of serving sizes speci-

fied, and the method of recording frequencies clearly presented. This will help to reduce variations among interviewers and will increase clarity and comprehension among the older subjects.

4. The validity of the questionnaire must be determined as accurately as possible.

5. The reproducibility of the questionnaire should be assessed by pretesting on a random sample of the study population on two different occasions and assessing agreement of the two sets of data. This will also help identify potential problems that may occur in the administration of the instrument.

A simplified diet history questionnaire may be adequate for use in an elderly population because the diets of these individuals are usually less varied than those of younger subjects. This is a result of the physiologic, sociologic, and economic changes that are often encountered in this group.[172] Dietary history and food frequency questionnaires, if administered properly, are very time consuming and require a well-trained, experienced professional interviewer. The subjectivity involved in describing a usual eating pattern makes this method vulnerable to memory lapses and psychological tendencies to exaggerate or minimize self-described behavior.[173]

Another method often used to assess the nutrient intake of free-living elderly persons is the self-written dietary food record. A 7-day record is considered to be of an optimal length to obtain a more representative sample of usual intake. The food record technique places most of the responsibility on the subject and is therefore less time consuming for the interviewer. However, this method can be used reliably only for individuals who are well motivated and who can read and write. Level of education is often a factor in determining who will complete a 7-day record;[174] the length of the food record is often a factor relating to compliance. The accuracy of record keeping has been shown to decline before the end of 7 days;[174] therefore, for an older person a 3 day

record may be adequate, but it should include one weekend day. Physical abnormalities, such as arthritis or uncontrollable tremors as a result of neurological damage, may make it very difficult for some elderly people to write. Alterations in eating patterns are often noted by individuals who record their intakes.

The 24-hour recall is used more often than any other technique for assessing dietary intake and the subsequent nutrient status of free-living as well as institutionalized or hospitalized elderly people. The reliability of this method has been questioned for use in this group.[175] Factors that may interfere with the reliability of the method relate to dependence on memory; short-term memory is one of the first physiologic functions to show changes with advancing age. An alternative to these methods is visual observation. This method has been validated as a means of assessing dietary consumption among older adults with cognitive deficits in long-term care settings.[176]

SCREENING VERSUS ASSESSMENT

A thorough, comprehensive nutrition assessment is the approach of choice in determining the nutritional status of an individual and in promoting appropriate therapeutic interventions when necessary. During the past years, there has been much discussion about nutritional screening for elderly adults, and screening has been incorporated into many community and institution-based programs. A screening tool should be easy to administer, easy to score, reliable, and valid. One such instrument is the **DETERMINE Your Nutritional Health** checklist, developed by the Nutritional Screening Initiative (NSI), a collaborative effort of the American Dietetic Association, the American Academy of Family Physicians, and the National Council on the Aging.[177] This one-page instrument poses 10 questions designed to identify eating, economic, and lifestyle behaviors that may contribute to the development of nutritional problems. This tool does not evaluate nutritional status, but it does help to alert service providers and individuals to potentially correctable habits that are associated with poor nutritional status. The **DETERMINE** checklist has been widely used and validated.[178–180]

Another widely used screening tool is the Mini-Nutritional Assessment (MNA).[181] This tool has been validated in the older population for integration into geriatric assessment programs.[182] The MNA has been compared against the Subjective Global Assessment (SGA) and was found to be a more appropriate assessment tool for identifying malnourished elderly patients.[183] The MNA comprises simple measurements and a brief questionnaire. Components include:

1. Anthropometric assessment (weight, height, and weight loss)
2. General assessment (lifestyle, medication, and mobility)
3. Dietary assessment (number of meals, food and fluid intake, autonomy of eating)
4. Self-assessment (self-perception of health and nutrition)

Assessment scores are calculated and compared with malnutrition indicator scores. This will place the patient into one of three groups. The three groups are well-nourished, at risk of malnutrition, or malnourished. From this, the need for specific intervention or appropriate referrals can be determined. Copies of the MNA tool and other information related to this tool are available from Nestec Ltd (Nestle Research Center)/Clintec Nutrition Company and on the Web at www.mna.com (Chapter 21).

Screening should not be confused with assessment but can be very helpful when it is properly used.

CONCLUSION

Assessing nutritional status in elderly individuals is a challenging task for nutrition professionals because of the age- and disease-related alterations of parameters commonly used to evaluate nutritional condition. To assess nutritional status properly, a multifaceted evaluation of the individual is necessary to develop a comprehensive picture of nutritional state. A thorough evaluation should include a physical assessment, including an examination of skin, hair, nails, eyes, oral mucosa, and musculature; fluid balance; physical disability; sensory losses; medical, cognitive, and psychological problems; and socioeconomic conditions. Measures of body composition, such as anthropometric measures including height, weight, skinfold thicknesses, and muscle circumferences, can be used to estimate protein and energy stores. Biochemical, immunologic, and hematological assessments contribute to a more comprehensive evaluation of nutritional status and provide some valuable biomarkers by which to track changes in nutritional status over time. A dietary history will contribute to a more complete profile of an individual's nutritional state and may serve to identify potential nutritional problems that are not obvious to the observer.

An evaluation of nutritional status will help to detect individuals who are at risk for malnutrition before the overt presentation of such a condition. Malnutrition may interfere with the successful treatment of acute medical conditions, with the ability of an individual to recover from an insult or injury, or with an adequate response by the immune system to fight infection. Nutrition assessment will help to identify patients who may benefit from successful nutritional intervention before heroic measures are needed to restore nutritional integrity.

REFERENCES

1. Buzina R, Bates CJ, van der Beek J, et al. Workshop on functional significance of mild-to-moderate malnutrition. *Am J Clin Nutr* 1989;50:172–176.

2. McLaren OS. Clinical manifestations of human vitamin and mineral disorders: a resume. In: Shils ME, Olson JA, Shike M, Ross CA, eds. *Modern Nutrition in Health and Disease.* 9th ed. Philadelphia, PA: Lea & Febiger; 1999.

3. Mackle T, Touger-Decker R, O'Sullivan Maillet J. Registered dietitians' use of physical assessment parameters in professional practice. *J Am Dietet Assoc* 2003;103:1632–1638.

4. Lavizzo-Mourey R, Johnson J, Stolley P. Risk factors for dehydration among elderly nursing home residents. *J Am Geriatr Soc* 1988;36:213–218.

5. Rowe J. Renal system. In: Rowe JW, Besdine RW, eds. *Health and Disease in Old Age*. Boston, MA: Little, Brown & Co; 1982.

6. Larson K. Fluid balance in the elderly: assessment and intervention—important role in the community health and home care nursing. *Geriatr Nurs* 2003;24:306–309.

7. Food and Nutrition Board. *Recommended Dietary Allowances*. 10th ed. Washington, DC: National Academy Press; 1989.

8. Chernoff R. Meeting the nutritional needs of the elderly in the institutional setting. *Nutr Revs* 1994;52:132–136.

9. Chidester JC, Spangler AA. Fluid intake in the institutionalized elderly. *J Am Dietet Assoc* 1997;97:123–128.

10. Chernoff R. Thirst and fluid requirements. *Nutr Revs* 1994;52:132–136.

11. Knapp A. Nutrition and oral health in the elderly. *Dent Clin North Am* 1989;33:109–125.

12. Sullivan DH, Martin W, Flaxman N, Hagen M. Oral health problems and involuntary weight loss in a population of frail elderly. *J Am Geriatr Soc* 1993;41:725–731.

13. Position of the American Dietetic Association: oral health and nutrition. *J Am Dietet Assoc* 2003;103: 615–625.

14. Jurdi-Haldeman D, Napier AK. Perceived relationships between taste and smell acuity and food intake in the elderly. *Top Clin Nutr* 1988;3(4):4–8.

15. Rosenberg IH, Russell RM, Bowman BB. Aging and the digestive system. In: Munro HN, Danford DE, eds. *Nutrition, Aging, and the Elderly*. New York, NY: Plenum Publishing Corp; 1989.

16. Mattes R. The chemical senses and nutrition in aging: challenging and old assumptions. *J Am Dietet Assoc* 2003;102:192–196.

17. Miller IJ. Human taste bud density across adult age groups. *J Gerontol* 1988;43:B26–B30.

18. Chauhan J, Hawrysh ZJ, Gee M, et al. Age-related olfactory and taste changes and interrelationships between change and nutrition. *J Am Dietet Assoc* 1987;87: 1543–1550.

19. Langan MJ, Yearick ES. The effects of improved oral hygiene in taste perception and nutrition of the elderly. *J Gerontol* 1976;31:413–418.

20. Doty RL, Shaman P, Applebaum SL, Rosenberg L. Smell identification ability: change with age. *Science* 1984 Dec 21;226(4681):1441–1443.

21. Duffy VB, Backstrand JR, Ferris AM. Olfactory dysfunction and related nutritional risk in free-living, elderly women. *J Am Dietet Assoc* 1995;95:879–884.

22. Chernoff R. Aging and nutrition. *Nutr Today* 1987; 22(2):4–11.

23. Chernoff R. Nutrition and chronic conditions. *Top Geriatr Rehabil* 1989;5(1):69–78.

24. Kohrs MB, Czajka-Narins DM, Nordstrom IW. Factors affecting nutritional status of the elderly. In: Munro HN, Danford DE, eds. *Nutrition, Aging, and the Elderly*. New York, NY: Plenum Publishing Corp; 1989.

25. Sullivan DH, Patch GA, Walls RC, Lipschitz DA. Impact of nutrition status on morbidity and mortality in a select population of geriatric rehabilitation patients. *Am J Clin Nutr* 1990;51:749–758.

26. Dwyer JT, Gallo JJ, Reichel W. Assessing nutritional status in elderly patients. *Am Fam Physician* 1993;47: 613–620.

27. Guigoz Y, Vellas B, Garry P. Assessing the nutritional status of the elderly: the mini nutritional assessment as part of the geriatric evaluation. *Nutr Rev* 1996;54: S59–S65.

28. Posner BM, Jette A, Smigelski C, Miller D, Mitchell P. Nutritional risk in New England elders. *J Gerontol* 1994;49:MI23–M132.

29. Sullivan DH, Martin WE, Flaxman N, Hagen JE. Oral health problems and involuntary weight loss in a population of frail elderly. *J Am Geriatr Soc* 1993;41: 725–731.

30. Dargent-Molina P, Hays M, Breart G. Sensory impairments and physical disability in aged women living at home. *Int J Epidemiol* 1996;25:621–629.

31. Ostwald SK, Snowdon DA, Keenan NL, et al. Manual dexterity as a correlate of dependency in the elderly. *J Am Geriatr Soc* 1989;37:963–969.

32. Siebens H, Trupa E, Siebens A, et al. Correlates and consequences of eating dependency in institutionalized elderly. *J Am Geriatr Soc* 1986;34:192–198.

33. Katz S, Ford AB, Moskowitz RW, et al. Studies of illness in the aged: the index of ADL; a standardized measure of biological and psychosocial function. *JAMA* 1963;185:914–919.

34. Lawton MP, Brody EM. Assessment of elderly people: self-maintaining and instrumental activities of daily living. *Gerontologist* 1969;9:179–186.

35. Fleming KC, Evans JM, Weber DC, Chutka DS. Practical functional assessment of elderly persons: a primary-care approach. *Mayo Clin Proc* 1995;70: 890–910.

36. Gonzalez-Gross, Marcos A, Pietrzk K. Nutrition and cognitive impairment in the elderly. *Brit J Nutr* 2001; 86:313–321.

37. Faxen-Irving G, Basun H, Cederholm T. Nutritional and cognitive relationships and long-term mortality in patients with various dementia disorders. *J Am Geriatr Soc* 2005;34:136–141.

38. Lee L, Kang SA, Lee HO, Lee B-H, Park JS, Kim J-H, Jung IK, Park YJ, Lee JE. Relationships between dietary

intake and cognitive function level in Korean elderly people. *Public Health* 2001;115:133–138.

39. Franklin CA, Karkeck J. Weight loss and senile dementia in an institutionalized elderly population. *J Am Diet Assoc* 1989;89:790–792.

40. Wright BA. Weight loss and weight gain in a nursing home: a prospective study. *Geriatr Nurs* 1993;14:156–159.

41. Morley JE. Death by starvation: a modern American problem? [editorial]. *J Am Geriatr Soc* 1989;37:184–185.

42. Gray GE, Paganini-Hill A, Ross RK. Dietary intake and nutrient supplement use in a southern California retirement community. *Am J Clin Nutr* 1983;38:122–128.

43. Adams TL, Chernoff R, McCabe BM, et al. *The Effect of Home-Delivered Meals on Length of Hospitalization for Elderly Patients.* 1991. Unpublished master's thesis.

44. O'Hanlon P, Kohrs MB, Hilderbrand E, et al. Socioeconomic factors and dietary intake of elderly Missourians. *J Am Diet Assoc* 1983;82:646–653.

45. Baker H, Frank O, Thind IS, et al. Vitamin profiles in elderly persons living at home or in nursing homes, versus profile in healthy young subjects. *J Am Geriatr Soc* 1979;27:444–450.

46. Singer JD, Granahan P, Goodrich NN, et al. Diet and iron status, a study of relationships: United States 1974. *Vital Health Stat* 1982;229(11).

47. McGandy RB, Russell RM, Hartz SC, et al. Nutritional status survey of healthy noninstitutionalized elderly: energy and nutrient intakes from three day records and nutrient supplements. *Nutr Res* 1986;6:785–798.

48. Mcintosh WA, Shifflet PA. Influence of social support systems on dietary intake of the elderly. *J Nutr Elderly* 1984;4:5.

49. Blackburn GL, Bistrian BR, Maini BS. Nutritional and metabolic assessment of the hospitalized patient. *J Parenter Enter Nutr* 1977;1:11–22.

50. Mitchell CO, Lipschitz DA. Detection of protein calorie malnutrition in the elderly. *Am J Clin Nutr* 1982;35:398–406.

51. Rossman J. The anatomy of aging. In: Rossman J, ed. *Clinical Geriatrics.* Philadelphia, PA: JB Lippincott Co; 1979.

52. Dequeker JV, Baeyens JP, Classens J. The significance of stature as a clinical measurement of aging. *J Am Geriatr Soc* 1969;17:169–179.

53. Miall WE, Ashcroft MT, Lovell HG, et al. A longitudinal study of the decline of adult height with age in two Welsh communities. *Hum Biol* 1967;39:445–454.

54. Trotter M, Bleser G. The effect of aging on stature. *Am J Phys Anthropol* 1951;9:311–324.

55. McPherson JR, Lancaster DR, Carroll JC. Stature changes with aging in black Americans. *J Gerontol* 1978;33:2–25.

56. Young CM, Blondin J, Tensuan R, et al. Body composition studies of "older" women, thirty to seventy years of age. *Ann NY Acad Sci* 1963;110:598–607.

57. Norris AH, Lundy T, Shock NW. Trends in selected indices of body composition in men between the ages 30 and 80 years. *Ann NY Acad Sci* 1963;110:623–639.

58. Hertzog KP, Garn SM, Hempy HO. Partitioning the effects of secular trend and aging on adult stature. *Am J Phys Anthropol* 1969;31:111–116.

59. Chumlea WC, Garry PJ, Hunt WC, et al. Serial changes in stature and weight in a healthy elderly population. *Hum Biol* 1988;60:918–925.

60. Abraham S, Lowenstein FW, Johnson CL. *Preliminary Findings of the First Health and Nutrition Examination Survey, United States, 1971–2: Dietary Intake and Biochemical Findings.* Washington, DC: US Government Printing Office; 1974. National Center for Health Statistics; US Department of Health, Education, and Welfare publication HRA 74-1219-21.

61. Elahi VK, Elahi P, Andres R. A longitudinal study of nutritional intake in men. *J Gerontol* 1983;38:162–180.

62. Forbes GB. The adult decline in lean body mass. *Hum Biol* 1976;48:161–166.

63. Garth S, Young R. Concurrent fat loss and fat gain. *Am J Phys Anthropol* 1956;14:497–504.

64. Hejda S. Skinfold in old and long-lived individuals. *Gerontology* 1963;8:201–297.

65. Stoudt HW, Damon A, McFarland R, et al. Weight, height and selected body dimensions of adults, United States, 1960–1962. *Vital Health Stat* 1963;35(11).

66. Enzi G, Gasparo M, Biondetti PR, et al. Subcutaneous and visceral fat distribution according to sex, age, and overweight, evaluated by computed tomography. *Am J Clin Nutr* 1987;45:7–13.

67. Borkan GA, Hults DE, Gerzof SG, et al. Comparison of body composition in middle-aged and elderly males using computed tomography. *Am J Phys Anthropol* 1985;66:289–295.

68. Baumgartner RN, Heymsfield SB, Roche AF, et al. Quantification of abdominal composition by computed tomography. *Am J Clin Nutr* 1989;50:221–226.

69. Mitchell CO, Lipschitz DA. The effect of age and sex on the routinely employed measurements used to assess the nutritional status of hospitalized patients. *Am J Clin Nutr* 1982;36:340–349.

70. Heymsfield SB, Tighe A, Wang Z-M. Nutritional assessment by anthropometric and biochemical methods. In: Shils ME, Olson JA, Shike M, eds. *Modern Nutrition in Health and Disease.* 8th ed. Philadelphia, PA: Lea & Febiger; 1994.

71. Lipschitz DA, Mitchell CO. Nutritional assessment of the elderly: special considerations. In: Wright RA, Heymsfield S, eds. *Nutritional Assessment.* Boston, MA: Blackwell Scientific Publications Inc; 1984.

72. Gordon CC, Chumlea WC, Roche AF. Stature, recumbent length, and weight. In: Lohman TG, Roche AF, Martorell R, eds. *Anthropometric Standardization Reference Manual*. Champaign, IL: Human Kinetics Publishers Inc; 1988.

73. Chumlea WC, Roche AF, Mukherjee D. *Nutritional Assessment in the Elderly Through Anthropometry*. 2nd ed. Columbus, OH: Ross Laboratories; 1987.

74. Mitchell CO, Lipschitz DA. Arm length measurement as an alternative to height in nutritional assessment of the elderly. *J Parenter Enter Nutr* 1982;6:226–229.

75. Chumlea WC, Roche AF, Steinbaugh ML. Estimating stature from knee height for persons 60 to 90 years of age. *J Am Geriatr Soc* 1985;33:116–120.

76. Harris JA, Jackson CM, Patterson DG, et al. *The Measurement of Man*. Minneapolis, MN: University of Minnesota Press; 1930.

77. Chumlea WC, Guo S, Roche AF, et al. Prediction of body weight for the non-ambulatory elderly from anthropometry. *J Am Dietet Assoc* 1984;88:564–568.

78. Martin AD, Carter JEL, Hendy KC, et al. Segment lengths. In: Lohman TG, Roche AF, Martorell R, eds. *Anthropometric Standardization Reference Manual*. Champaign, IL: Human Kinetics Publishers Inc; 1988.

79. Dwyer JT, Coleman A, Krall L, et al. Changes in relative weight among institutionalized elderly adults. *J Gerontol* 1987;42:246–251.

80. Roche AF. Anthropometric variables: effectiveness and limitations. In: *Assessing the Nutritional Status of the Elderly: State of the Art. Report of the Third Ross Roundtable on Medical Issues*. Columbus, OH: Ross Laboratories; 1982.

81. Sullivan DH, Patch GA, Baden AL, et al. An approach to assessing the reliability of anthropometries in elderly patients. *J Am Geriatr Soc* 1989;37:607–613.

82. Metropolitan Life Insurance Company. New weight standards for men and women. *Stat Bull Metrop Insur Co* 1959;40:1–4.

83. Metropolitan Life Insurance Company. Metropolitan height and weight tables. *Stat Bull Metrop Insur Co* 1989;64:2–9.

84. Russell RM. Evaluating the nutritional status of the elderly. *Clin Nutr* 1983;2:4–8.

85. Frisancho AR, Flegel PN. Elbow breadth as a measure of frame size for U.S. males and females. *Am J Clin Nutr* 1983;73:311–314.

86. Novascone MA, Smith EP. Frame size estimation: a comparative analysis of methods based on height, wrist circumference, and elbow breadth. *J Am Diet Assoc* 1989;89:964–966.

87. Frisancho AR. New standards of weight and body composition by frame size and height for assessment of nutritional status of adults and the elderly. *Am J Clin Nutr* 1984;40:808–819.

88. Clark NG. Nutritional support of elderly patients, II: proposed answers. *Clin Consult* 1982;2:5–9.

89. Master AM, Lasser RP. Tables of average weight and height of Americans aged 65 to 94 years: relationship of weight and height to survival. *JAMA* 1960;172:661.

90. Burt VL, Harris T. The third National Health and Nutrition Examination Survey: contributing data on aging and health. *Gerontologist* 1994;34:486–490.

91. de Oms M, Habicht JP. Anthropometric reference data for international use: recommendations from a World Health Organization Expert Committee. *Am J Clin Nutr* 1996;64:650–658.

92. Chernoff R, Mitchell CO, Lipschitz DA. Assessment of the nutritional status of the geriatric patient. *Geriatr Med Today* 1984;3:129–141.

93. Mooradian AD. Nutrition modulation of life span and gene expression. *Ann Intern Med* 1988;109:890–904.

94. Galanos AN, Peiper CF, Cornoni-Huntley JC, Bales CW, Fillenbaum GG. Nutrition and function: is there a relationship between body mass index and the functional capabilities of community-dwelling elderly? *J Am Geriatr Soc* 1994;42:368–377

95. *Nutrition Interventions Manual for Professionals Caring for Older Americans.*. Washington, DC: Nutrition Screening Initiative; 1992.

96. Obesity in America: an overview. In: Bray GA, ed. *Obesity In America*. Washington, DC: US Department of Health, Education, and Welfare; 1980.

97. Thommas AE, McKay DA, Cutlip MD. A nomograph method for assessing body weight. *Am J Clin Nutr* 1976;29:302–304.

98. Potter JF, Schafer DF, Bohi RL. In-hospital mortality as a function of body mass index: an age-dependent variable. *J Gerontol* 1988;43:M59–M63.

99. Rosenberg IH. Summary comments. *Am J Clin Nutr* 1989;50:1231–1233.

100. Evans WJ. What is sarcopenia? *J Gerontol* 1995;50A: 5–10.

101. Chumlea WC, Guo SS, Glaser RM, Vellas BJ. Sarcopenia, function and health. *Nutr Health Aging* 1997; 1:7–12.

102. Chumlea WC, Baumgartner RN. Status of anthropometry and body composition data in elderly subjects. *Am J Clin Nutr* 1989;50:1158–1166.

103. Dumin JV, Womersley S. Body fat assessed from total body density and its estimation from skinfold thickness: measurements of 481 men and women aged from 16 to 72 years. *Br J Nutr* 1974;32:77–79.

104. Steen B, Bruce A, Isaksson B, et al. Body composition in 70-year-old males and females in Gothenburg, Sweden: a population study. *Acta Med Scand Suppl* 1977;611:87–112.

105. Wilmore JH, Behnke AR. Predictability of lean body weight through anthropometric assessment in college men. *J Appl Physiol* 1968;25:349–355.

106. Watson PE, Watson JD, Batt RD. Total body water volumes for adult males and females estimated from simple anthropometric measurements. *Am J Clin Nutr* 1980;33:27–39.

107. Latin RW, Johnson SC, Ruhling RO. An anthropometric estimation of body composition of older men. *J Gerontol* 1987;42:24–28.

108 Butterworth CE, Blackburn GL. Hospital malnutrition and how to assess the nutritional status of a patient. *Nutr Today* 1975;10:8–18.

109. Fox EA, Boylan ML, Johnson L. Clinically applicable methods for body fat determination. *Top Clin Nutr* 1987;2:1–9.

110. Harrison GG, Buskirk ER, Carter JEL, et al. Skinfold thickness and measurement technique. In: Lohman TG, Roche AF, Martorell R, eds. *Anthropometric Standardization Reference Manual.* Champaign, IL: Human Kinetics Publishers Inc; 1988.

111. Falciglia G, O'Connor J, Gedling E. Upper arm anthropometric norms in elderly white subjects. *J Am Diet Assoc* 1988;88:569–574.

112. Callaway CW, Chumlea WC, Bouchard C, et al. Circumferences. In: Lohman TG, Roche AF, Martorell R, eds. *Anthropometric Standardization Reference Manual.* Champaign, IL: Human Kinetics Publishers Inc; 1988.

113. Chumlea WC, Guo SS, Vellas B, Guigoz Y. Assessing body composition and sarcopenia with anthropometry. Proceedings: CERI Symposium, Nutrition et personnes agees au-dela des apports recommandes. 1997: 161–169. Paris, France.

114. Guigoz Y, Bruno V, Garry PJ. Assessing the nutritional status of the elderly: the mini nutritional assessment as part of the geriatric evaluation. *Nutr Rev* 1996;54: S59–S65.

115. Mitchell CO, Lipschitz DA. Creatinine height index in the elderly. In: *Assessing the Nutritional Status of the Elderly: State of the Art. Report of the Third Ross Roundtable on Medical Issues.* Columbus, OH: Ross Laboratories; 1982.

116. Bloch L, Schoenheimer R, Rittenberg D. Rate of formation and disappearance of body creatinine in normal animals. *J Biol Chem* 1941;138:155–161.

117. Morrow FD. Assessment of nutritional status in the elderly: application and interpretation of nutritional biochemistries. *Clin Nutr* 1986;5:112–120.

118. Welle S, Thornton C, Totterman S, Gilbert F. Utility of creatinine excretion in body-composition studies of healthy men and women older than 60 y. *Am J Clin Nutr* 1996;63:151–156.

119. Mobarhan S. The role of albumin in nutritional support. *J Am Coll Nutr* 1988;7:445–452.

120. Mullen JL, Buzby GP, Waldman MT, et al. Prediction of operative morbidity and mortality by preoperative nutritional assessment. *Surg Forum* 1979;30:80–82.

121. Agarwal N, Acevedo F, Leighton LS, et al. Predictive ability of various nutritional variables for mortality in elderly people. *Am J Clin Nutr* 1988;48:1173–1178.

122. Ferguson RP, O'Connor P, Crabtree B, Batchelor A, Mitchell J, Coppola D. Serum albumin and prealbumin as predictors of clinical outcomes of hospitalized elderly nursing home residents. *J Am Geriatr Soc* 1993; 41:545–549.

123. Salive ME, Cornoni-Huntley J, Phillips CL, et al. Serum albumin in older persons: relationship with age and health status. *J Clin Epidemiol* 1992;45:213–221.

124. Campion EW, deLabry La, Glynn RJ. The effect of age on serum albumin in healthy males: report from the normative aging study. *J Gerontol* 1988;43:MI8–M20.

125. Munro HN. Nutrition and ageing. *Br Med J* 1981;37: 83–88.

126. Reuben DB, Moore AA, Damesyn M, Keeler E, Harrison GG, Greendale GA. Correlates of hypoalbuminemia in community-dwelling older persons. *Am J Clin Nutr* 1994;66:38–45.

127. Baumgartner RN, Doehler KM, Romero L, Garry PJ. Serum albumin is associated with skeletal muscle in elderly men and women. *Am J Clin Nutr* 1996;64: 552–558.

128. Corti MC, Guralnik JM, Salive ME, Sorkin JD. Serum albumin level and physical disability as predictors of mortality in older persons. *JAMA* 1994;272:1036–1042.

129. Finucane P, Rudra T, Hsu R, et al. Markers of the nutritional status in acutely ill elderly patients. *Gerontology* 1988;34:304.

130. Friedmann JM, Jensen GL, Smiciklas-Wright H, McCamish MA. Predicting early nonelective hospital readmission in nutritionally compromised older adults. *Am J Clin Nutr* 1997;65:1714–1720.

131. Sullivan DH. What do the serum proteins tell us about our elderly patients? *J Gerontol:MED SCI* 2001; 56A(2):M71–M74.

132. Eisenberg S. Postural changes in plasma volume in hypoalbuminemia. *Arch Intern Med* 1963;112:544–549.

133. Lipschitz DA, Cook JD, Finch CA. The clinical evaluation of serum ferritin as an index of iron stores. *N Engl J Med* 1974;290:1213–1216.

134. Bothwell TH, Charlton R, Cook J, et al. *Iron Metabolism in Man.* Oxford, England: Blackwell Scientific Publishers Ltd; 1979:295–297.

135. Lipschitz DA, Mitchell CO, Thompson C. The anemia of senescence. *Am J Hematol* 1981;11:47–54.

136. Awad MO, Barford AV, Grindulis KA, et al. Factors affecting the serum iron-binding capacity in the elderly. *Gerontology* 1982;28:125–131.

137. Lipschitz DA, Mitchell CO. The correctability of nutritional, immune, and hematopoietic manifestations of protein-caloric malnutrition in the elderly. *J Am Coll Nutr* 1982;1:16–23.

138. Winkler MF, Gerrior SA, Pomp A, et al. Use of retinol-binding protein and prealbumin as indicators of the response to nutrition therapy. *J Am Diet Assoc* 1989;89:684–687.

139. Prendergast JM. Nutritional evaluation of the institutionalized elderly. In: Armbrecht HJ, Prendergast JM, Coe RM, eds. *Nutritional Intervention in the Aging Process* New York, NY: Springer-Verlag; 1984.

140. Kergoat MJ, Leclerc BS, Pettit-Clerc C, et al. Discriminant biochemical markers for evaluating the nutritional status of elderly patients in long-term care. *Am J Clin Nutr* 1987;46:849–861.

141. Ingenbleek Y, DeVisscher M, DeNayer P. Measurements of prealbumin as an index of protein-calorie malnutrition. *Lancet* 1972;2:106–108.

142. Carpentier YA, Barthel J, Bruyns I. Plasma protein concentration in nutritional assessment. *Proc Nutr Soc* 1982;41:405–417.

143. Bourry J, Milano G, Caldani C, et al. Assessment of nutritional proteins during the parenteral nutrition of cancer patients. *Ann Clin Lab Sci* 1982;12:158–162.

144. Ridker PM, Rifai N, Rose L, et al. Comparison of C-reactive protein and low-density lipoprotein cholesterol levels in the prediction of first cardiovascular events. *N Engl J Med* 2002;347:1557–1565.

145. Liepa GU, Basu II. C-reactive proteins and chronic disease: what role does nutrition play? *Nutr Clin Pract* 2003;18:227–233.

146. Dietrich M, Jialal I. The effect of weight loss on a stable biomarker of inflammation, C-reactive protein. *Nutr Revs* 2005;63(1):22–28.

147. Seltzer MH, Bastidos JA, Cooper DM, et al. Instant nutritional assessment. *J Parenter Enteral Nutr* 1979;3:157–159.

148. Fuhrman MP, Charney P, Mueller C. Hepatic proteins and nutrition assessment. *J Am Diet Assoc* 2004;104:1258–1264.

149. Ramsden D, Prince H, Burr A, et al. The interrelationship of thyroid hormones, vitamin A and their binding proteins following acute stress. *Clin Endocrinol (Oxf)* 1978;8:109–122.

150. Goichot B, Schlienger J-L, Gruenenberger F, et al. Low cholesterol concentrations in free-living elderly subjects: relations with dietary intake and nutritional intake. *Am J Clin Nutr* 1995;62:547–553.

151. Kaiser FE. Cholesterol, heart disease, and the older adult. *Clin Appl Nutr* 1992;2(1):35–43.

152. Harris T, Cook EF, Kannel WB, et al. Proportional hazards analysis of risk factors for coronary heart disease in individuals aged 65 or older. *J Am Geriatr Soc* 1988;36:1023–1028.

153. Benfante R, Reed D. Is elevated serum cholesterol a risk factor for coronary heart disease in the elderly? *JAMA* 1990;263:393–396.

154. Corti M-C, Guralnick JM, Salive ME, et al. HDL cholesterol predicts coronary heart disease mortality in older persons. *JAMA* 1995;274:539–544.

155. Wilson PWF, Anderson KM, Harris T, et al. Determinants of change in total cholesterol and HDL-C with age: the Framingham Study. *J Gerontol Med Sci* 1994;49:M252–M257.

156. Rozzini R, Sabatini T, Franzoni S, Trabucchi M. Cholesterol and mortality in elderly patients. *J Am Geriatr Soc* 2004;52:469–470.

157. Rudman D, Mattson DE, Nagraj HS, et al. Prognostic significance of serum cholesterol in nursing home men. *J Parenter Enter Nutr* 1988;12:155–158.

158. Cunningham-Rundles S. Effects of nutritional status on immunological function. *Am J Clin Nutr* 1982;35:1202–1210.

159. Bistrian BR, Blackburn GL, Scrimshaw N, et al. Cellular immunity in semi-starved states in hospitalized adults. *Am J Clin Nutr* 1975;28:1148–1155.

160. Meakins JL, Pietsch JB, Bubenick O, et al. Delayed hypersensitivity: indicator of acquired failure of host defenses in sepsis and trauma. *Surgery* 1977;82:349–355.

161. Chandra RK, Scrimshaw NS. Immunocompetence in nutritional assessment. *Am J Clin Nutr* 1980;33:2691–2697.

162. Thompson JS, Robbins J, Cooper JK. Nutrition and immune function in the geriatric population. *Clin Geriatr Med* 1987;3:309–317.

163. Katz AE. Immunity and aging. *Otolaryngol Clin North Am* 1982;15:287–291.

164. Delafuente JC, Meuleman JR, Nelson RC. Anergy testing in nursing home residents. *J Am Geriatr Soc* 1988;36:733–735.

165. Chandra RK. Serum thymic hormone activity in protein energy malnutrition. *Clin Exp Immunol* 1979;38:228.

166. Stiehm ER. Humoral immunity in malnutrition. *Fed Proc* 1980;39:3093.

167. Cohn JR, Hohl CA, Bucklby CE III. The relationship between cutaneous cellular immune responsiveness and mortality in a nursing home population. *J Am Geriatr Soc* 1983;3:808–809.

168. Lipschitz DA. Nutrition, aging, and the immunohematopoietic system. *Clin Geriatr Med* 1987;3:319–328.

169. Lipschitz DA. Nutrition and the aging hematopoietic system. In: Hutchinson ML, Munro HN, eds. *Nutrition and Aging.* New York, NY: Academic Press; 1986.

170. Caliendo MA. Validity of the 24-hour recall to determine dietary status of elderly in an extended care facility. *J Nutr Elderly* 1981;1:57–66.

171. Samet JM. Surrogate measures of dietary intake. *Am J Clin Nutr* 1989;50:1139–1144.

172. Hankin JH. Development of a diet history questionnaire for studies of older persons. *Am J Clin Nutr* 1989;50: 1121–1127.

173. Mahalko JR, Johnson LK, Ballagher SK, et al. Comparison of dietary histories and seven-day food records in a nutritional assessment of older adults. *Am J Clin Nutr* 1985;42:542–553.

174. Gersovitz M, Madden JP, Smiciklas-Wright H. Validity of the 24-hr dietary recall and seven-day record for group comparisons. *J Am Diet Assoc* 1978;73:48–55.

175. Bowman BB, Rosenberg IH. Assessment of the nutritional status of the elderly. *Am J Clin Nutr* 1982;35: 1142–1144.

176. Shatenstein B, Claveau D, Ferland G. Visual observation is a valid means of assessing dietary consumption among older adults with cognitive deficits in long-term care settings. *J Am Diet Assoc* 2002;102:250–252.

177. *Report of Nutrition Screening I: Toward a Common View.* Washington DC: Nutrition Screening Initiative; 1991.

178. Posner BM, Jette AM, Smith MA, et al. Nutrition and health risks in the elderly: the Nutrition Screening Initiative. *Am J Public Health* 1993;83:972–978.

179. *Nutrition Screening Initiative Project: Status Report.* Hillsborough County, FL: Senior Citizens Nutrition Program, Nutrition Screening Initiative Project; 1994.

180. *Delaware Nutrition Screening Program.* New Castle, DE: Delaware Health and Social Services, Division of Aging; 1993.

181. Guigoz Y, Vellas B, Garry P. Mini nutritional assessment: a practical assessment tool for grading the nutritional state of elderly patients. *Facts and Research in Gerontology.* 1994;(supp 2):15–59.

182. Vellas B, Guigoz Y, Baumgartner R, Garry PJ, Lauque S, Albarede JL. Relationship between nutritional markers and the mini-nutritional assessment in 155 older persons. *J Am Geriatr Soc* 2000;48:1300–1309.

183. Barone L, Milosavljevic M, Gazibarich B. Assessing the older person: is the MNA a more appropriate nutritional assessment tool than the SGA? *J Nutr Health Aging* 2003;7:13–17.

CHAPTER 19

Nutritional Support for the Older Adult

Ronni Chernoff, PhD, RD

Nutrition is essential to sustain life and health and plays a key role in the recovery from acute and chronic illnesses. For those who are not healthy, have chronic conditions or episodes of acute illness, suffer trauma, or undergo surgeries or other invasive medical procedures, providing nutritional therapies that are timely and appropriate for the patient and the patient's condition is essential to maximize recovery and rehabilitation potential.

Since older adults consume the greatest percentage of health care resources[1,2] and occupy many acute and chronic care beds, it becomes essential that the provision of nutritional therapies, particularly as enteral or parenteral infusions, is done with special consideration to the unique needs of elderly individuals. Many of these specific needs have been addressed in the examination of macronutrient and micronutrient requirements (Chapters 2–6 and in the discussion of nutritional assessment in Chapter 18). However, it is important to review these particular requirements with consideration of the benefits and limitations of nutritional support methodologies. Appropriate selection of nutritional interventions may be key to successful nutritional rehabilitation, correction of nutritional deficits, restoration of nutritional reserves, and avoidance of difficult ethical dilemmas.

INDICATIONS FOR NUTRITIONAL SUPPORT

Gradual loss of weight is a common occurrence among elderly individuals, although the etiology of the weight loss may be undetermined. Involuntary weight loss may occur with a variety of acute and chronic illnesses, such as cancer,[3] sepsis, diabetes, renal disease, and dementia;[4] however, weight loss in elderly subjects may not have an obvious cause.[5–9] Anorexia or diminished nutrient intake usually is associated with the loss of weight. Morley and colleagues[10] describe this syndrome as the "anorexia of aging" and have suggested that the diminished nutrient intake is a consequence of decreased metabolic rate and reduced energy output. Inadequate food intake due to compromised socioeconomic circumstances, depression or dementia, and functional dependency may also contribute to slow, chronic weight loss. Aging may also affect endocrine factors that are involved in appetite control such as cholecystokinin, leptin, cytokines, and testosterone, which may contribute to a decrease in appetite.[11]

Sometimes weight is maintained because of lack of activity and reduced requirements for energy, but chronic malnutrition may occur because of a deficit of essential nutrients other than energy. Maintenance of weight is only part of the picture; although the etiology is not clear, it appears that inactivity (being bed or chair bound) may lead to a chronic loss of lean body mass. This may result in a depletion of all body protein stores leading to muscle wasting, weakness, unsteady gait, compromised immune function,[12] poor wound healing, inefficient gastrointestinal function, and other consequences.[13,14]

Depletion of additional nutrient stores, particularly tissue stores of water-soluble vitamins, may not be apparent until a physiologic insult such as an illness, an accident, a trauma, or emotional stress occurs. When an individual who is chronically undernourished encounters physical stress, his or her physical condition may deteriorate rapidly, and unexpected complications may occur. Repletion of nutrient stores and restoration of nutritional and reserve capacity may require aggressive nutritional intervention, enteral or parenteral support.

Protein-energy malnutrition is often secondary to a primary disease process such as cancer, a chronic cardiac condition, chronic pulmonary disease, renal or hepatic disease, or a gastrointestinal disorder.[15] Many studies indicate that protein-energy malnutrition is prevalent among elderly hospitalized patients[16–22] and institutionalized individuals.[23–25] Many consequences of undernutrition may contribute to delayed recovery or rehabilitation, which, in older adults, may complicate an already complex health status.

One of the profound consequences of protein-energy malnutrition in elderly individuals is impairment of immune function.[12] Immune responses are affected by age (Chapter 18), independent of nutritional status; however, compromised nutritional status contributes to an additional depression of the immune system.[24] This situation may prove life-threatening in seriously ill individuals because of the increased risk of infection and a decreased ability to mobilize host defenses.

If protein-energy malnutrition is suspected in seriously ill patients, it is important that practitioners use clinical judgment to set therapeutic priorities and to select and initiate nutritional interventions. Major medical problems take priority over nutritional deficits and must be corrected before nutritional intervention is considered. Priorities include the management of infection; the control of blood pressure; and the restoration of metabolic, fluid, and electrolyte balances. It is important to monitor fluid and electrolyte equilibration during the acute phase of an illness, or at the time of admission to an acute care facility, to establish the validity of certain nutritional markers. Nutritional indicators may appear to change after fluid and electrolyte therapy is instituted because of serum dilution or rehydration effects. True serum values are necessary for an accurate assessment of nutritional condition and the need for nutritional support intervention.

Even in the absence of overt protein-energy malnutrition, there may be an indication for nutritional support. Medical condition, diagnosis, prognosis, and treatment plans are all factors in the decision to provide medical nutrition therapy. A patient who suffers from multiple chronic conditions is less likely to respond swiftly to an acute insult and may need support through the critical phase. Although oral nutrition is the preferred method of feeding, it may be unreasonable to expect adequate oral nutrient ingestion, particularly since some patients may not be able to eat for extended periods of time because of coma, stroke, head injuries, oral surgery, or gastrointestinal injuries or impairments. Patients who are chronically ill and cannot ingest adequate amounts of nutrients because of anorexia, side effects of drugs such as those used in chemotherapy, or severe limitations on nutrient or fluid intake for therapeutic purposes may be candidates for nutritional support.[26] Having gastrointestinal disease (eg, malabsorption, maldigestion, or motility disorders), surgery, or obstruction may contribute to the need for nutritional support.[27] If the gastrointestinal tract cannot be used, parenteral nutrition may be considered as a viable option.

Even in stable long-term care patients, chronic undernutrition may be a problem, despite the lack of active disease processes. Patients who require long-term care may have inadequate dietary intakes because of dementia[4] or the need for help with feeding.[28,29] The need for help with feeding may be a significant factor for both dependent and apparently independent nursing home patients, not only for adequate energy intake but also for nutrient density.[29,30] For patients who have permanent disabilities that interfere with adequate nutrient ingestion, absorption, or utilization, nutritional support may become a necessity for continued life.

ORAL SUPPLEMENTS

The optimal method for nutritionally supporting patients who are at risk for malnutrition is to feed them a nutritionally dense, well-balanced diet. Patients should be encouraged to eat as much as possible within the limits of their disabilities, oral health status, and medical conditions. If an adequate diet cannot be consumed through standard mealtimes and patterns, consideration should be given to offering multiple small meals or nontraditional meal patterns. If intake can be enhanced by serving breakfast foods for the dinner meal or desserts as between-meal snacks, the opportunity to enrich dietary intake ought to be pursued; there is a great deal to be gained from this approach, and the patient will be the beneficiary.

It has been reported that only 10% of elderly people who have protein-energy malnutrition can ingest nutrients adequate to overcome their nutritional deficits.[28] However, since food is such an important part of life, being the focus of social, cultural, religious, and family gatherings, it is important to encourage elderly individuals to maintain their normal diets as long as they are able.[25]

Unless there is a compelling need or a specific request from the patient, restricting certain nutrients in the diet may contribute to unforeseen problems.[28,29] Many older people have difficulty in discriminating between moderation in eating habits and the elimination of entire groups of food products. Limiting intake of many foods may lead to previously unseen nutritional deficiencies. Liberalizing diet restrictions may lead to a more palatable diet and more interest in food and may not have a negative impact on medical

interventions for chronic disease; it is possible that the patient may enjoy food more and consume a diet that reduces the risk of nutritional problems.[28,29] A thorough dietary history is essential before changes in the diets of patients or clients are initiated.

Dietary Supplements

Many options are available to supplement the diets of individuals who are at risk for malnutrition. Carbohydrate and protein powders are available that can be added to the patient's usual diet to increase the nutrient density without changing the flavor, texture, or color. Vitamin supplements are readily available to compensate for vitamins and minerals that may be lacking in an individual's diet. In a study conducted on elderly Australians, the use of dietary supplements (eg, bran or wheat germ) or vitamin and mineral supplements had no effect on incidence of illness or use of medical resources; however, individuals who used such supplements did have more favorable dietary habits and were more nutritionally aware than those who did not use supplements.[30] Data are inconclusive as to the contribution of supplements to the nutritional value of the diets of elderly Americans.[31-34]

For people who have unpredictable appetite levels, snacks can be prepared in advance to be available as desired. These might include crackers; cheese; hard-cooked eggs; peanut butter; fresh or dried fruit; small meals, such as half a sandwich and a glass of milk or juice; soup; milkshakes or fruit frappes; nutrition bars; or oral liquid nutritional supplements. Commercially available supplements may be nutritionally complete or may provide only a portion of the Recommended Dietary Allowances (RDAs) for adults. Elderly patients who have chewing, swallowing, or feeding problems or gastrointestinal impairments may require either liquid diets or supplemented diets for extended periods of time because of their in ability to ingest adequate nutrients from regular food. Consideration of fluid, mineral, or macronutrient (eg, protein) restrictions is essential to the selection of an appropriate supplement in long-term care patients. Many elderly individuals experience problems with chronic cardiac, renal, pulmonary, and hepatic diseases that contribute to fluid or protein limitations. Careful evaluation of the nutritional profile of supplements is necessary to meet therapeutic guidelines for individual patients.[35]

Many elderly patients, especially African Americans and Hispanics, are lactose deficient or have conditions that temporarily render them lactose deficient (severe malnutrition, sprue, bacterial overgrowth, chemotoxicity); these individuals may need lactose-free nutritional supplements in place of milkshakes, custards, or cream soups.[35]

Commercial Liquid Supplements

Oral supplementation of patients' diets with commercially available liquid formulas has been shown to be efficacious in long-term care patients;[36] patients with bone fractures,[37] infections,[38] cancer;[3,39] surgical patients,[40] and homebound elderly people.[41,42] In a study by Ching and associates,[39] nutritional status was maintained in a group of elderly cancer patients undergoing various cancer treatment modalities through supplementation with commercially available nutritional supplements. Nine long-term care patients benefited from the addition of a nutritional supplement to their diets, in a study reported by Andersson and colleagues.[41] Although the volume of food consumed did not change appreciably in this group of patients, they achieved positive nitrogen balances as a result of increased protein, calorie, and fat intakes. In one study of long-term nursing home patients with a variety of diagnoses (including dementia, diabetes mellitus, pulmonary and urinary tract infections, stroke, and pressure ulcers), oral supplementation with commercial liquid diets contributed to weight gain and improvement in nutritional parameters.[36] In another study, also looking at the effectiveness of oral supplementation in elderly nursing home patients, use of an oral supplement in residents who demonstrated weight loss and poor appetite improved weight with a slow,

steady gain but also improved nutritional profiles in some of these patients.[43]

Volkert and colleagues[42] found that subjects who received oral supplementation in hospital and during a 6-month follow-up period post discharge recovered more effectively than a control group who were not supplemented. In another study of homebound elderly who were dependent on home-delivered meals, the impact of oral nutritional supplements, based on overall nutritional intake, was significant.[44]

Oral nutritional supplements have been shown to improve body weight and fat-free mass.[43] One problem often identified in Alzheimer's disease patients is weight loss, although the mechanism for this weight loss has not been clearly explained—explanations are confounded by a cohort of Alzheimer's patients who gain weight. Nutritional status improved in this group of patients but had no impact on their dementia. A study conducted on free-living, frail elderly failed to show a significant improvement in functional status despite weight gain.[45] Although these investigators did not find a significant improvement in strength or perception of health, they did record a statistically significant difference in the incidence of falls. This may be a meaningful finding for those who care for these individuals.

The composition of oral liquid supplements changes regularly. It is important to obtain current information from industry representatives about available products.

Nutritional intervention can be accomplished successfully by use of oral supplements; however, there are patients who cannot ingest adequate nutrients because of oral and swallowing problems (eg, malignancies, obstructions, wired jaws, lesions associated with chemotherapy or radiation therapy, fungus infections, mucositis); cognitive problems (eg, dementia, coma); functional impairments (eg, due to stroke or head or spinal cord injury); or increased nutrient needs associated with hypermetabolic states, cancer, thermal injuries, malnutrition, or malabsorption. For these patients and others who cannot obtain sufficient nutrients via the oral route, there are alternative methods for providing nutrition to elderly individuals in need of nutritional support. Enteral feeding by tube is the next option to consider, especially if the patient has a functional gastrointestinal tract. A study conducted by Mitchell et al[46] brought a different perspective to the issue of tube feeding elderly, institutionalized people. The report indicates that the likelihood of using a tube to feed elderly, often demented patients is higher among African American, Asian American, and urban residents. This is explained by several factors including the view that tube feeding will prolong life; Medicaid pays for tube feeding but not for the extra help needed to hand feed; lack of living wills, advanced directives, or clear wishes about end of life care; and a feeling among family members that their loved one deserves every aspect of aggressive care.

ENTERAL FEEDING

Aggressive nutritional support via enteral feeding has been shown to be efficacious in restoring nutritional status in individuals who are unable to orally ingest adequate nutrients.[16,47,48] Enteral feeding by tube provides a reasonably safe, cost-effective method of providing protein, calories, vitamins, minerals, trace elements, and fluid while preserving or restoring a functional bowel surface.[49–51] Because most enteral solutions can be prepared in a nonsterile environment or are feeding ready, can be administered without special equipment, and are relatively inexpensive, the choice of enteral solutions for nutritional support of elderly patients is a reasonable one.

Selection of Enteral Feeding Route

Selecting an enteral feeding route is sometimes a challenging decision for a team of health care professionals and the patient or patient representative, such as a family member, an ombudsman, or an individual with power of attorney. Decisions should be made in the context of prognosis, patient autonomy, mental competency, quality of life, and other factors unique

to the patient.[52] When a clinician makes the decision to place a feeding tube in a patient, he or she must consider the option that the tube may, at some time in the future, have to be removed. However, those making the decisions have alternatives to consider; enteral feeding solutions can be effectively delivered to the stomach, duodenum, or jejunum, but relative benefits and risks must be carefully evaluated when selecting an enteral feeding route for a specific patient. Feeding into the stomach via either a nasogastric or a gastrostomy feeding tube takes advantage of the normal physiologic processes of digestion and absorption.

One method of assisted feeding that is somewhat controversial and generally out of practice is syringe feeding. This method, using a feeding syringe with a 30 mL bulb or a piston syringe, has been used with patients who are difficult to feed with standard utensils or who could drink from a cup. This method should only be tried in patients who have intact swallowing function, who are alert, and who can sit upright. This method can be time consuming, since food boluses should be given in small amounts (approximately 1 teaspoon to $\frac{1}{2}$ tablespoon) to avoid aspiration.[53]

Gastric Feeding

The stomach acts to digest food through secretion of acid and hormones, contributes to regulation of pH, and controls release of partially digested meals into the small intestine. Release of liquid food into the small intestine is affected by osmoreceptors in the jejunum that delay emptying of hyperosmolar or hypoosmolar solutions; by acid solutions; by solutions with a high level of fatty acids, with a high nutrient density, or with high or low temperature; and by drugs such as narcotic analgesics and anticholinergic agents.[54]

Although there are many advantages to feeding into the stomach, there are potential risks, primarily associated with aspiration. In elderly patients, the risk of aspiration may be associated with high levels of gastric residuals or an impaired or absent gag reflex.[48]

Nasogastric feeding has been the most commonly used method throughout the history of enteral feeding because of the near normalcy that it evokes.[55] For centuries, the administration of liquid meals through a tube into the stomach provided nutrition to individuals who could not otherwise obtain adequate nutrients.[54] Until the development of the Dobbhoff feeding tube and others like it (all of which are made from new-technology compounds that allow for soft, non-irritating, flexible tubes), the hazards of nasogastric feeding included the development of otitis media and nasopharyngeal lesions, aspiration, and voluntary tube removal. Even with the new materials and advanced technology, risks are still encountered with nasogastric tube feeding. In one case report, difficulty with nasal breathing due to the presence of a nasogastric tube contributed to respiratory failure in an elderly woman who was tube feeding dependent as a result of a stroke.[56] Evaluation of nasal patency is an important step before the insertion of a nasogastric feeding tube.

Placement of a nasogastric tube is the most easily achieved of all tube placements, since it can be accomplished at the bedside, needs a minimal amount of equipment, and can be performed by nurses or other allied health professionals. There are risks associated with the placement of nasogastric tubes that should be prepared for by the individual placing them. Placement of a tube by an inexperienced practitioner can lead to trauma associated with insertion of the tube (eg, esophageal perforation, pneumothorax, pulmonary hemorrhage, pleural effusion, bronchopleural fistula formation, pneumonia) or with aspiration.[56–62] Placement of feeding tubes may lead to other complications that, although uncommon, are potentially dangerous. For example, Lipman and colleagues[61] reported cases of nasopulmonary tube placement that resulted in pneumothorax in one patient and pneumonia and hydrothorax in another.

Despite these potential problems with tube insertion, nasogastric feeding can be used in both acute and chronic care patient settings. Feeding solutions may be administered continuously by using a slow-drip gravity method or an enteral feeding pump that maintains a constant rate of flow. In the acute care setting, nasogastric feeding is a commonly used means of providing short-term enteral nutritional support.[63] However, increasing numbers of long-term care patients are being fed by the enteral tube route; nasogastric feeding can be provided safely for long periods of time[64,65] (Chernoff R, Lipschitz DA, Milton KY. 1988. Unpublished data). Nevertheless, there are reports that indicate that when nursing home patients are admitted to the hospital with an acute illness and then have a feeding tube placed, they appear to have a greater risk of mortality.[66] The focus should be on selecting tube feeding for patients who will have the best outcomes for intervention and will tolerate the tube placement and nutrient solution infusion.

If the indications are that tube feeding will be required for extended periods of time, or if the patient is confused, demented, or combative, leading to inadvertent dislodgment of the feeding tube and putting the patient at serious risk of aspiration or mechanical complications,[58,65,66] the establishment of a permanent gastrostomy should be considered.[52,67–72] Permanent gastrostomies avoid most of the complications associated with nasogastric tube (NG) feeding, but there are some problems that occur with indwelling gastric tubes. Because access is accomplished through an incision in the abdominal wall, complications include intra-abdominal leakage of gastric contents, potentially causing peritonitis; leakage around the catheter insertion site, causing skin excoriation; and migration of the catheter into the abdominal cavity or pylorus.[58,68]

Percutaneous endoscopic gastrostomy (PEG) is an alternate method that may be used with some success in long-term tube-fed patients.[52,67,72–74] Clinicians must carefully evaluate elderly patients for the suitability of this method as part of their care; older patients who are malnourished may have mucosal thinning and skin fragility, which should be considered when placing a gastrostomy tube endoscopically. An organized appraisal of the value of this tube feeding method should be conducted in long-term tube-fed patients to ensure its safety. In most cases, gastrostomy feeding is an efficacious method to use in elderly patients. Ha and Hauge[75] reported on the safety and efficacy of PEG feedings in stroke patients. Within 2 weeks of the stroke, approximately 27% have swallowing recovery; therefore, about 75% have long-term need for enteral feeding support via a tube.

Dwolatzky et al[76] conducted a prospective study comparing the indications and outcomes of enteral feeding via nasogastric tube vs PEG. The subjects were long-term tube feeding dependent elderly patients who were then followed for a minimum of 6 months. Although the subjects receiving feedings via the PEG tubes were older and had a higher incidence of dementia, they had an improved survival, a lower incidence of aspiration, and better tolerated the feedings compared to the NG tube-fed patients. But, as is common when feeding frail elders, others have found disappointing results with PEG tubes.[77]

Jejunal Feeding

Jejunal feedings are usually used when there is an obstruction in the upper gastrointestinal tract or stomach; when there is potential for the exacerbation of gastric disease, such as ulcers; when gastric dysfunction, such as atrophic gastritis or achlorhydria, exists; or when an individual has had surgery that precludes esophageal or gastric feeding.[78] Jejunal access has distinct advantages for patients who cannot be fed via the upper gastrointestinal tract, but it also has some potential risks that must be considered when selecting an enteral feeding route. Jejunostomies reduce the risk of gastroesophageal reflux and aspiration, which is a major consideration in elderly patients. However, jejunostomy tube placement frequently requires surgical procedures, which have their own risks.[78] Jejunostomy feeding should be considered if enteral support will be required for an extended period of time and the upper gastrointestinal tract will not be viable for feeding. Caution must be exercised to avoid inadvertent or purposeful tube dislodgment. Partial extraction of a jejunostomy tube can cause leak-age of formula or intestinal contents into the peritoneum, leading to peritonitis.[79,80] The use of an indwelling jejunostomy tube should be carefully considered for elderly patients who require nutritional support; placement of a jejunal catheter should be seen as a solution for a long-term problem that will necessitate extended enteral nutritional support.

Selection of Enteral Formulas

Many factors must be considered when selecting an enteral feeding formula for an elderly patient.[48,81–83] Some of these factors include an estimation of the duration of tube feeding dependency; the location of the feeding tube; the energy, protein, and micronutrient requirements of the patient; the ability of the patient to digest and absorb nutrients; the need for disease-specific formulas; and the expense and availability of the product to be infused.

In a limited, short-term situation that is characterized by an acute episode, patients probably will be fed nasogastrically, although if the illness required gastrointestinal surgery, an indwelling gastric or jejunal catheter may be in place. In either of these short-term, acute situations, a formula can be selected to meet specific short-term needs. High-protein, high-calorie, predigested, or specially designed nutritional products can be selected to meet unique needs related to the medical condition. Acutely ill individuals may require disease-specific formulas that are part of the treatment plan. Elderly patients who have been undernourished for an extended period may have the additional problem of compromised absorptive capacity, for which a dilute solution or a partially predigested formula may be needed. Whenever enteral feeding is considered for an elderly patient, early feeding protocols should be followed with some caution. It is wise to start with a dilute solution that is infused slowly to ensure tolerance before moving to full strength, full-volume feeding.

The vast majority of elderly patients who are sustained on tube feeding formulas are chronically ill and will be tube feeding dependent for extended periods of time. Selecting a formula for use with long-term tube-fed patients requires consideration of energy, protein, vitamin, mineral, and fluid needs. Although energy needs may be lower related to a decrease in energy output and a slower basal metabolic rate, requirements for other nutrients remain the same, with only small variations. The challenge this represents is that small volumes of formula often do not provide the levels of protein, vitamins, minerals, and trace elements that are needed to maintain nutritional status.

Recent evidence emphasizes the need for careful formula selection for patients who will be dependent on tube feedings for 6 months or longer. Chernoff and colleagues[84] examined serum levels of trace minerals (including zinc and selenium) and trace proteins (carnitine and taurine) in long-term tube-fed elderly patients. They found deficiencies of selenium and low levels of carnitine and taurine in all the subjects who had been maintained on tube feedings for 6 months or longer; these deficiencies were corrected with the substitution of an enteral formula that contained small amounts of these nutrients. These nutrients have important roles in immune function (selenium) and fat metabolism (carnitine and taurine) and are important in long-term nutrition status. These data suggest that use of supplemented formulas should be considered for individuals who will be tube feeding dependent for extended periods of time.

Even with supplemented formulas, adequate volumes must be infused to achieve an adequate intake of all nutrients. Inadequate volumes of enteral solutions may also be a factor in inadequate hydration of chronically tube-fed individuals.

Nutrient levels for tube-fed patients should meet basic needs for protein (approximately 1g/kg of body weight); the RDAs for vitamins, minerals, and trace elements for adults older than 50 years; and fluid requirements of approximately 1500 mL/d. Fluid requirements can be met by providing at least 1 mL/kcal ingested, 30 mL/kg of body weight, or 125% of the volume of the formula. Of particular importance is the fact that the vast majority of enteral formulas require more than 1500 mL or 1500 kcal to meet 100% of the RDAs. Underfeeding of essential nutrients can be a chronic problem in enteral feeding dependent elderly individuals, as described previously.

Consideration must be given to the patient's metabolic status, gastrointestinal function, and diagnosis. Most long-term tube-fed patients can be supported by using a standard, 1 kcal/mL formula that provides the RDA or greater for vitamins and minerals.[47,85] There is rarely a demand for disease-specific, predigested, or nutrient-dense formulation; however, there may be indications for high nitrogen products, such as for pressure ulcer healing.[86,87] Unfortunately, the development of pressure ulcers may be related in part to chronic undernutrition.

Delivery of Enteral Feeding

Enteral Access

The safe and successful provision of enteral nutrition is related to where and in what manner tube feeding is administered. The placement of the feeding tube may be one of the most important factors in minimizing potential complications. For short-term, or initiation of, enteral feeding, nasogastric tubes are frequently used.[63] New generations of nasogastric tubes are comfortable and can remain in place for extended periods of time.

Nasogastric tubes are relatively easy to place, particularly since many tubes have markings that indicate the length for nasogastric or nasoenteric placement.[88] Nasogastric tubes allow the clinician to monitor the viability of the gastrointestinal tract by measuring tube feeding residuals. Although the stomach acts as a reservoir, controlling the release of feeding solutions into the small bowel, the risk of pulmonary aspiration is greater with feedings that remain in the stomach for a time after infusion.[58,89] Individuals who have gastroesophageal reflux, gastroparesis, absent gag reflex, or swallowing dysfunction or who are comatose will be at greater risk for aspiration.[58]

The risk for pulmonary aspiration can be decreased by using a longer tube that permits feeding directly into the small intestine.[58] Nasoenteric tubes that can be passed into the duodenum or jejunum can be used where the risk of aspiration is great. These tubes tend to be small-bored, soft, and weighted so that they remain in place; some come with stylets that act as guidewires to ensure appropriate placement. The small bores that make these tubes comfortable also contribute to the limitation of formula choices that will flow unimpeded through them and the potential collapse of the tube when formula is aspirated to check residuals.[90] Placement of the tube may require the feeding formula be administered in a continuous infusion over 12 to 24 hours, since the reservoir function of the stomach is bypassed by feeding into the proximal small intestine.

For long-term feeding, clinicians often recommend gastric access placement of feeding tubes, usually PEG. Many approaches to direct feeding into the stomach, bypassing the nasal access route, have been used with variable success. These include Janeway, Stamm, and Witzel procedures, all of which require surgery to create a serosal tunnel through which a tube can be inserted. These procedures have had a common problem of gastric acid reflux or leakage around the stoma.[88] Placing a PEG minimizes this complication, is more comfortable for the patient, reduces the problems associated with tube obstruction or blockage, enables feeding of individuals who are unable to voluntarily consume adequate nutrients, and is cosmetically more appealing for the patient and care providers.[52,58,69,91,92]

Patients can be given feedings into the jejunum using the PEG procedure and a gastric jejunal tube. There are both advantages and disadvantages of jejunal feedings that are related to bypassing the digestive processes of the stomach and duodenum.[58] Formulas need to be partially digested and of a thin viscosity to be administered and absorbed with minimal complications.

Enteral Infusion Rate and Volume

The site of tube placement is a major consideration in determining what schedule to establish for enteral feeding. If the infusion site is the stomach, there may be more options because the stomach acts as a natural reservoir, controlling release of nutrient solution into the duodenum. Because the stomach regulates the flow of formula into the small bowel, enteral feedings can be administered by either intermittent or continuous flow without serious concern about osmolarity, nutrient concentration, or formula viscosity. However, if infusion occurs distal to the stomach, either pump-controlled intermittent or continuous feeding is a better choice. Since the reservoir function of the stomach is lost, solutions should not be infused more rapidly than the small bowel can safely absorb. Too rapid infusion or too large a volume may cause problems with poor absorption or diarrhea.[58]

There is considerable diversity of opinion among nutrition professionals about how to infuse tube feeding solutions effectively. The route, formula concentration, and flow rate should be dictated by patient tolerance. In older patients, individual tolerance should be the guide for formula-feeding progression.[69,93] The primary goal should be to provide an adequate volume of formula to meet patient needs while maintaining a safe, tolerable method of infusion.

Complications of Enteral Feeding

There are many risks associated with enteral feeding in elderly patients (Table 19–1); some of these have already been described, but some complications must be addressed more specifically.

It is not uncommon to encounter elderly patients who will not tolerate enteral feeding tubes. Even small-bore, flexible tubes may be uncomfortable; patients are resistant to tube placement and become agitated; and elderly, confused patients may partially dislodge tubes, which can contribute to more serious complications.[4,14,18,63,94–97] Small-bore tubes are susceptible to clogging, kinking, and migration. One of the most frequent causes of clogging is the use of enteral feeding tubes for administering crushed medications. The only medications that should be put into feeding tubes are those that are dissolved in liquid or are in fluid form. The internal diameter of the tube should permit the tube feeding formula of choice

Table 19–1 Potential Enteral Feeding Problems in Elderly Patients

Risk Factor	Problem
Decreased gastric emptying	Gastric retention → aspiration
Hiatal hernia	Gastric reflux → aspiration
Tissue fragility	Esophageal bleeding
Dislocation of tube	Mucosal ulceration
	Pulmonary aspiration and infusion
	Peritonitis
	Gastritis
Altered glucose tolerance	Hyperglycemia → dehydration → altered mental status
Inadequate water	Hypernatremia
	Hyperchloremia
	Azotemia
	Altered mental status
Decreased energy needs	Inadequate intake of nutrients
Decreased bowel motility	Constipation → fecal impaction
Achlorhydria	Increased susceptibility to bacterial contamination
Polypharmacy	Changes in formula osmolarity
	Interference with drug absorption
	Diarrhea
Confusion	Tube dislocation → aspiration

Source: Adapted with permission from J.L. Rombeau and M.D. Caldwell, eds, *Clinical Nutrition: Enteral and Tube Feeding,* p. 394 © 1990, W.B. Saunders Company.

to flow easily; more viscous formulas should only be administered through a moderate-sized tube (eg, 12 French).

Some enteral formulas leave a precipitate on the interior walls of the tube, which eventually leads to clogging. Flushing the tube regularly with liquid, such as water, under pressure minimizes this problem. Since all tube-fed patients require additional free fluid, flushing the tube with water will help to meet this need. Tube feeding formulas are made of nutrients suspended in a liquid medium (water). The volume of the tube feeding is the total water and the displacement of the nutrient sources when dissolved or dispersed in the water. Often the total displacement is close to 25% of the total volume; that amount of free fluid should be provided to the patient either orally, if the patient can swallow, or by tube,

added to the nutrient solution, or used as a tube flush.

Tube location should be monitored at periodic intervals, especially after an episode of vomiting or when there is evidence that the patient has pulled on the tube.[48] Migration of the feeding tube can contribute to complications of aspiration, pulmonary infections, and gastrointestinal dysfunction.[18,98,99] Pulmonary complications are frequently, but not always, related to aspiration. Risk of aspiration can be minimized by always elevating the patient's head or the head of the bed when tube formula is being infused; by using pump-administered feeding; and by using tubes that are placed in the duodenum or jejunum. Particular attention should be paid to patients who have had strokes or neurologic or esophageal diseases that contribute to an impaired gag reflex or swallowing difficulties.[89,96]

Gastrointestinal complications that may be encountered include bloating, nausea, vomiting, diarrhea, and constipation. Frequently these problems can be alleviated by slowing the rate of the enteral infusion; altering the feeding regimen to a slow, controlled, continuous drip; or changing the formula. Diarrhea is the most commonly experienced gastrointestinal problem associated with tube feeding and is most frequently reported in intensive care settings.[97,98] Among elderly persons, residents of nursing homes have the highest incidence of diarrhea. In frail, elderly persons, the consequences of diarrhea may contribute to an increased mortality.[100]

Diarrhea may be related to a number of conditions that affect elderly, hospitalized, or institutionalized patients. In the past, the use of milk-based formulations caused diarrhea, bloating, and gastrointestinal discomfort in lactase-deficient patients. There is now a greater understanding of the extent of this problem, and since the mid-1970s there has been a vast array of lactose-free products from which to choose. Bacterial contamination of tube-feeding formulas appeared to be a cause of diarrhea;[101,102] this problem has also been minimized with the availability of commercially prepared, ready-to-feed products. Homemade formulas were made from blended meats, strained vegetables, cooked cereals, pureed fruit, milk powder, juices, and other ingredients that could be contaminated easily by skin-, air-, and waterborne bacteria.[102]

Diarrhea can be caused by many different kinds of medications; when diarrhea is encountered, it is wise to review the drug profile to identify any drug that might be causing the problem.[98] Diarrhea can also be the result of a too-rapid infusion or a hyperosmolar formulation. Feeding regimens should be slowed to allow the patient time to adapt to the formula. Individuals who have been chronically undernourished may have incompetent bowel surfaces that contribute to malabsorption.[98] Concentrated or hyperosmolar feeding will lead to a watery diarrhea that can be reduced or corrected by diluting the formula and feeding it slowly.

One solution to the problem of diarrhea in tube-fed patients has been the addition of soluble fiber to the enteral feeding products. There is some evidence that fiber may resolve the diarrhea in tube-fed patients.[98,103–105] There have also been investigations that discuss some of the potential problems associated with fiber-supplemented enteral feedings.[106,107] A conservative approach is most appropriate in elderly patients. If diarrhea is present and the cause is not apparent (eg, medications), adding one or two cans (feedings) of a fiber-containing product to the patient's feeding regimen may resolve the problem.

Many other problems unique to older patients require clinical considerations that may not be included in standard enteral feeding protocols. Some of these are itemized in Table 19–2.

Other Issues in Enteral Feeding in the Elderly

Enteral feeding frequently raises some difficult ethical questions when elderly individuals are involved. There are emotional issues that relate to the individuals' medical condition, prognosis, cognitive status, nutritional condition, and patient preference.[108] There is some evidence that many elderly are not familiar with enteral feeding processes or principles and are confused by informed consent materials.[58,104,109,110]

Attention has been brought to the issues surrounding tube feeding and hydration in patients who are cognitively impaired or incompetent or are unable to express their wishes. Certain accepted principles have been decided by the United States Supreme Court and state supreme courts in well-known cases such as those of Karen Quinlan,[111] Claire Conroy, and Nancy Cruzan.[109] The major relevant principle is that nutrition and hydration are medical therapy. While the right to refuse or withhold medical therapy is a personal decision,[111-113] there are many people who categorize nutrition and hydration as symbols of love, caring, and nurturance.[114]

Discussions about advance directives or living wills and durable power of attorney should be held while individuals are still healthy and

Table 19–2 Considerations When Tube-Feeding Elderly People

Clinical Condition	Therapeutic Consideration
Functionally dependent with inadequate nutrient intake	Dental status Ability to feed without assistance Therapeutic restrictions Cost *Consider oral supplements, puddings, snacks*
Protein-energy malnutrition treated by enteral nutrition	Calorie density Protein level Volume tolerance Renal function Cost *Consider high-nitrogen, high-calorie formula until nutritional status is restored, then provide adequate calories, nitrogen*
Diarrhea	Rate/volume of feeding Medication profile Fat content of formula Osmolarity of formula *Consider decrease in rate/volume for brief period, use of fiber-containing formula*
Long-term tube feeding dependency	Placement of tube Adequate caloric intake Availability of pump Cost *Consider gastrostomy feeding with a formula providing complete nutrition*
Pressure ulcers	Calorie level Protein level *Consider high-calorie, high-protein formula*
Constipation	Residue content of diet Fluid intake Medical profile Ambulation *Consider fiber-containing diet with extra free water; increase physical activity if possible*
Intolerance to nasogastric tube	Type of tube Anticipated length of tube dependency Gastrointestinal physiology *Consider soft, pliable, small-bore tube; gastrostomy, jejunostomy*

Source: Adapted with permission from J.L. Rombeau and M.D. Caldwell, eds, *Clinical Nutrition: Enteral and Tube Feeding,* p. 394, © 1990, W.B. Saunders Company.

mentally competent. Every attempt should be made to explain the processes and possible outcomes of enteral nutrition support to ensure that each patient can make the best choices for him- or herself.[109–114] It is equally important that health professionals accept the wishes of the patient even though these may be contrary to the beliefs held by the practitioner.

PARENTERAL NUTRITION

Although enteral nutritional support is the preferred method of nutritional intervention for patients who are unable to ingest adequate nutritional substrate orally, the parenteral route may be used. In fact, some patients, when faced with the option of enteral vs parenteral, will prefer intravenous feeding.[115] The perception is that intravenous feeding will be more comfortable than tube feeding. However, there are very few data, and a great many unanswered questions, about the efficacy and safety of intravenous feeding in elderly patients. A multitude of studies have examined the use of parenteral nutritional support in different populations with assorted diagnoses, but only a few of them have examined the tolerance for parenteral nutrition in elderly individuals.[116,117]

The customary source of calories in parenteral solutions is hypertonic glucose solutions. Standard formulas are often greater than 20% glucose. It is known that glucose tolerance deteriorates with advancing age,[118,119] but the threshold of glucose infusion that can be administered safely to elderly patients has not been thoroughly investigated; the simultaneous infusion of insulin to enhance the absorption of intravenous glucose also warrants more careful study.

The use of intravenous fat emulsions has become a routine part of parenteral nutritional support. Lipid systems may prove to be very effective in elderly patients who are fluid restricted or who have glucose intolerance; however, lipid clearance rates and efficiency are usually not investigated before their use. The ability of elderly patients to adequately tolerate lipid emulsions is an area for further investigation. If lipids are well tolerated and rapidly cleared by older patients, their use in lipid-based peripheral parenteral systems might be very valuable. A combination of peripheral intravenous infusion and oral or enteral feedings might serve to provide an excellent source of nutrition, encourage the patient to take food or fluids by mouth or tube, and preserve gut integrity and function.

Protein solutions should be tolerated equally as well by elderly patients as they are by younger individuals. Limitations of protein infusion in older patients parallel those in younger patients and are usually associated with organ system dysfunction. In a study comparing subcutaneous and intravenous infusion of amino acid solutions in older patients, both routes were equally well-tolerated,[116] opening the possibility of subcutaneous administration of amino acids to replenish protein losses. Since parenteral nutrition solutions are aqueous, patients are usually well hydrated unless there is an excess of electrolytes in the formulation. The maintenance of hydration status in parenteral feeding–dependent patients is essential to a successful course of therapy.

As with other forms of nutritional therapy, adequate vitamins, minerals, and trace elements must be provided in the basic formulation to meet unique nutrition needs. Older patients must be monitored very carefully to ensure adequate hydration; sufficient calories, protein, and micronutrients; maintenance or correction of metabolic status; and positive therapeutic effects. There is some risk, particularly of air emboli, venous thrombosis, and sepsis, associated with parenteral feeding. Many of the complications seen in parenteral feeding are associated with overfeeding,[120,121] which is a threshold easy to reach in frail elderly patients. Parenteral nutrition should be used for the shortest period of time possible. Careful, close monitoring of the elderly, parenterally fed patient is the prudent course.[122]

HOME NUTRITIONAL SUPPORT

It is conceivable that elderly patients may be sent home with nutritional support when their medical condition stabilizes. Because of the management problems associated with the complex administration of parenteral feedings, the most likely method for home nutritional support is enteral feeding. Age-related changes in elderly patients must be considered when deciding to send them home with nutritional support.[123]

Impairments that may have an impact on the success of home nutritional support include alterations of vision; compromised hearing; loss of fine motor skills, coordination, and strength; and cognitive dysfunction. All of these age-related changes limit the patient's ability to understand and follow directions, recognize and correct potential problems, and communicate with caregivers and medical personnel. Successful nutritional support is dependent on the capacity of the patient and caregiver to manage care and obtain advice and guidance when problems arise.

Another factor of major importance is a thorough evaluation of the social circumstances of the patient. The patient's financial situation, including access to private health insurance or Medicare or Medicaid, Social Security benefits, and other sources of support, should be assessed. The availability of other social service systems should be explored as well. The home environment should be surveyed to appraise the availability of space needed for storage and formula preparation. The motivation of both patient and caregiver to undertake the responsibilities associated with home nutritional support must also be evaluated by a professional.

One viable alternative, assuming that Medicare or other health insurance is available, is use of the services of a home nutritional support company. This type of service may be more efficient because it can provide regular formula delivery, minimize the need for storage space, respond rapidly to problems, offer a reliable product, and provide regular monitoring. With careful advance planning, nutritional support can be safely and effectively provided to elderly patients.

CONCLUSION

Nutritional support, whether in the acute, chronic, or home care setting, can be safely and successfully used in elderly patients. Careful attention must be given to gastrointestinal function, unique nutrient needs, tube site location, feeding regimen, and disease-specific requirements. Parenteral, enteral, and oral nutritional support may be used singly or together, as needed. Some caution must be built into the protocols developed for elderly patients; metabolic changes can occur rapidly and must be addressed quickly to avoid serious problems. Nutritional support can be an important component of life-saving or life-sustaining treatments in elderly individuals.

REFERENCES

1. *A Profile of Older Americans: 1997.* Washington, DC: Program Resources Department, American Association of Retired Persons and Administration on Aging, Department of Health and Human Services; 1998.
2. Hanson MJ. How we treat the elderly. *Hastings Cent Rep* 1994;24(5):4–6.
3. Pironi L. Nutritional aspects of elderly cancer patients. *RAYS* 1997;22(1 suppl):42–46.
4. Sheiman SL. Tube feeding the demented nursing home resident. *J Am Geriatr Soc* 1996;44:1268–1270.
5. Martin KI, Sox HC, Krupp JR. Involuntary weight loss: diagnostic and prognostic significance. *Ann Intern Med* 1981;95:568.
6. Rabinovitz M, Pitlik SD, Leifer M, et al. Unintentional weight loss: a retrospective analysis of 154 cases. *Arch Intern Med* 1986;146:186.
7. Olsen-Noll CG, Bosworth MF. Anorexia and weight loss in the elderly. *Postgrad Med* 1989;85:140–144.
8. Sullivan DH. The role of nutrition in increased morbidity and mortality. *Clin Geriatr Med* 1995;11:661–674.
9. Zawada ET. Malnutrition in the elderly. *Postgrad Med* 1996;100:207–225.
10. Morley JE, Silver AJ, Fiatarone M, et al. Geriatric grand rounds: nutrition and the elderly. *J Am Geriatr Soc* 1986;34:823–832.
11. Chapman IM. Endocrinology of anorexia of aging. *Best Pract Res Clin Endocrinol Metabol* 2004;18(3):437–452.
12. Chandra RK. Impact of nutritional status and nutrient supplements on immune responses and incidence of infection in older individuals. *Ageing Res Rev* 2004;3(1):91–104.
13. Harris CL, Fraser C. Malnutrition in the institutionalized elderly: the effects on wound healing. *Ostomy Wound Management* 2004;50(10):54–63.
14. Johnston RE, Chernoff R. Geriatrics. In: Matarese LE, Gottschlich MM, eds. *Contemporary Nutrition Support Practice.* 2nd ed. Philadelphia, PA: WB Saunders; 2003.
15. Constans T, Bacq Y, Berchot J-F, et al. Protein-energy malnutrition in elderly medical patients. *J Am Geriatr Soc* 1992;40:263–268.
16. Mowe M, Bohmer T. The prevalence of undiagnosed protein-calorie undernutrition in a population of hospi-

talized elderly patients. *J Am Geriatr Soc* 1991;39: 1089–1092.

17. Reilly JJ, Hull SF, Albert N, et al. Economic impact of malnutrition: a model system for hospitalized patients. *J Parenter Enter Nutr* 1988;12:371–376.

18. Sullivan DH, Moriarty MS, Chernoff R, et al. Patterns of care: an analysis of the quality of nutritional care routinely provided to elderly hospitalized veterans. *J Parenter Enter Nutr* 1989;13:249–254.

19. Lovat LB. Age related changes in gut physiology and nutritional status. *Gut* 1996;38:306–309.

20. Tierney AJ. Undernutrition and elderly hospital patients: a review. *J Adv Nurs* 1996;23:228–236.

21. Morley JE, Silver AJ. Nutritional issues in nursing home care. *Ann Intern Med* 1995;123:850–859.

22. Posthauer ME, Russell C. Ensuring optimal nutrition in long-term care. *Nutr Clin Pract* 1997;12:247–255.

23. Abassi AA, Rudman D. Observations on the prevalence of protein-calorie undernutrition in VA nursing homes. *J Am Geriatr Soc* 1993;41:117–121.

24. Goodwin JS, Burns EL. Aging, nutrition, and immune function. *Clin Appl Nutr* 1991;1:85–94.

25. Pories WJ. Feeding the elderly patient. *N C Med J* 1988;49:632–635.

26. Nguyen NH, Flint DM, Prinsley DM, et al. Nutrient intakes of dependent and apparently independent nursing home patients. *Hum Nutr Appl Nutr* 1985;39A:333–338.

27. Morley JE. Anorexia in older persons: epidemiology and optimal treatment. *Drugs Aging* 1996;8:134–155.

28. Lipschitz DA, Mitchell CO. The correctability of the nutritional, immune, and hematopoietic manifestations of protein calorie malnutrition in the elderly. *J Am Coll Nutr* 1982;1:17–25.

29. Position of the American Dietetic Association: liberalized diets for older adults in long-term care. *J Am Diet Assoc* 1998;98:201–204.

30. Horwath CC, Worsley A. Dietary supplement use in a randomly selected group of elderly Australians. *J Am Geriatr Soc* 1989;37:689–696.

31. Garry PJ, Goodwin JS, Hunt WC, et al. Nutritional status in a healthy elderly population: dietary and supplemental intakes. *Am J Clin Nutr* 1982;36:319–331.

32. Tripp F. The use of dietary supplements in the elderly: current issues and recommendations. *J Am Diet Assoc* 1997;97(suppl2):S181–S183.

33. O'Hanlon P, Kohrs MB. Dietary studies of older Americans. *Am J Clin Nutr* 1978;31:1257–1269.

34. Gray-Donald K. The frail elderly: meeting the nutritional challenges. *J Am Dietet Assoc* 1995;95:538–540.

35. Bernard MA, Rombeau JL. Nutritional support for the elderly patient. In: Young EA, ed. *Nutrition, Aging and Health.* New York, NY: Alan R Liss Inc; 1986.

36. Johnson LE, Dooley PA, Gleick JB. Oral nutritional supplement use in elderly nursing home patients. *J Am Geriatr Soc* 1993;41:947–952.

37. Delmi M, Rapin CH, Bengoa JM, et al. Dietary supplementation in elderly patients with fractured neck of the femur. *Lancet* 1990;1:1013–1016.

38. Woo J, Ho SC, Mak YT, et al. Nutritional status of elderly patients during recovery from chest infection and the role of nutritional supplementation assessed by a prospective randomized single-blind trial. *Age Ageing* 1994;23:40–48.

39. Ching N, Grossi C, Zurawinsky H, et al. Nutritional deficiencies and nutritional support therapy in geriatric cancer patients. *J Am Geriatr Soc* 1979;27:491–494.

40. Smedley F, Bowling T, James M, Stokes E, Goodger C, O'Connor O, Oldale C, Jones P, Silk D. Randomized clinical trial of the effects of preoperative and postoperative oral nutritional supplements on clinical course and cost of care. *Br J Surg* 2004;91(8):983–990.

41. Andersson H, Falkheden T, Petersson I. A study on liquid diet in geriatric patients. *Aktuel Gerontol* 1979;9: 417–421.

42. Volkert D, Hübsch S, Oster P, et al. Nutritional support and functional status in undernourished geriatric patients during hospitalization and 6-month follow-up. *Aging Clin Exp Res* 1996;8:386–395.

43. Lauque S, Arnaud-Battandier F, Gillette S, Plaze JM, Andrieu S, Cantet C, Vellas B. Improvement of weight and fat-free mass with oral nutritional supplementation in patients with Alzheimer's disease at risk of malnutrition: a prospective randomized study. *J Am Geriatr Soc* 2004;52(10):1702–1707.

44. Lipschitz DA, Mitchell CO, Steele RW, et al. Nutritional evaluation and supplementation of elderly subjects participating in a "Meals on Wheels" program. *J Parenter Enter Nutr* 1985;9:343–347.

45. Gray-Donald K, Payette H, Boutier V. Randomized clinical trial of nutritional supplementation shows little effect on functional status among free-living frail elderly. *J Nutr* 1995;125:2965–2992.

46. Mitchell SL, Teno JM, Roy J, Kabumoto G, Mor V. Clinical and organizational factors associated with feeding tube use among nursing home residents with advanced cognitive impairment. *JAMA* 2003;290:73–80.

47. Allison SP. Cost-effectiveness of nutritional support in the elderly. *Proc Nutr Soc* 1995;54:693–699.

48. Sullivan DH. Nutritional support for elderly patients. In: Morley JE, Glick Z, Rubenstein LZ, eds. *Geriatric Nutrition: A Comprehensive Review.* New York, NY: Raven Press; 1990.

49. Chernoff R, Lipschitz DA. Enteral feeding and the geriatric patient. In: Rombeau JL, Caldwell MD, eds. *Clinical Nutrition: Enteral and Tube Feeding.* 2nd ed. Philadelphia, PA: WB Saunders Co; 1990.

50. Levine GM, Deren JJ, Steiger E, et al. Role of oral intake in maintenance of gut mass and disaccharide activity. *Gastroenterology* 1974;67:975–982.

51. Tilson MD. Pathophysiology and treatment of short bowel syndrome. *Surg Clin North Am* 1980;60:1273–1284.

52. Hasan M, Meara RJ, Bhowmick BK, et al. Percutaneous endoscopic gastrostomy in geriatric patients: attitudes of health care professionals. *Gerontology* 1995;41: 326–331.

53. Soriano R. Syringe feeding: current clinical practice and recommendations. *Geriatr Nurs* 1994;15:85–87.

54. Kelly DG, Fleming CR. Physiology of the gastrointestinal tract: as applied to patients receiving tube enteral nutrition. In: Rombeau JL, Rolandelli RH, eds. *Clinical Nutrition: Enteral and Tube Feeding*. 3rd ed. Philadelphia, PA: WB Saunders Co; 1997.

55. McCamish MA, Bounous G, Geraghty ME. History of enteral feeding: past and present perspectives. In: Rombeau JL, Rolandelli RH, eds. *Clinical Nutrition: Enteral and Tube Feeding*. 3rd ed. Philadelphia, PA: WB Saunders Co; 1997.

56. Hernandez OG, Nelson S, Haponik EF, et al. Obligate nasal breathing in an elderly woman: increased risk of nasogastric tube feeding. *J Parenter Enter Nutr* 1988; 12:531–532.

57. Galindo-Ciocon DJ. Tube feeding: complications among the elderly. *J Gerontol Nurs* June 1993;17–22.

58. Drickamer MA, Cooney LM Jr. A geriatrician's guide to enteral feeding. *J Am Geriatr Soc* 1993;41:272–279.

59. Miller KS, Tomlinson JR, Sahn SA. Pleural pulmonary complications of enteral tube feedings. *Chest* 1985;88: 230–233.

60. Woodall BH, Winfield DF, Bisset GS. Inadvertent tracheobronchial placement of feeding tubes. *Radiology* 1987;165:727–729.

61. Lipman TO, Kessler T, Arabian A. Nasopulmonary intubation with feeding tubes: case reports and review of the literature. *J Parenter Enter Nutr* 1985;9:618–620.

62. McWey RE, Curry NS, Schabel SI, et al. Complications of nasoenteric feeding tubes. *Am J Surg* February 1988; 155:253–257.

63. Rolandelli RH, Ullrich JR. Nutritional support in the frail elderly surgical patient. *Surg Clin North Amer* 1994;74:79–92.

64. Heitkemper MM, Williams S. Prevent problems caused by enteral feeding: know about complications before they arise. *J Gerontal Nurs* 1985;11(7):25–30.

65. Meer JA. Inadvertent dislodgment of nasoenteral feeding tubes: incidence and prevention. *J Parenter Enter Nutr* 1987;11:187–189.

66. Pick N, McDonald A, Bennett N, et al. Pulmonary aspiration in a long-term care setting: clinical and labo-ratory observations and an analysis of risk factors. *J Am Geriatr Soc* 1996;44:763–768.

67. Daly MP, Richardson JP. Geriatrics for the clinician: nutrition in old age. *MD Med J* 1995;44:377–381.

68. Tealey AR. Percutaneous endoscopic gastrostomy in the elderly. *Gastroenterol Nurs* February 1994;151–157.

69. Tokuda Y, Koketsu H. High mortality in hospitalized elderly patients with feeding tube placement. *Intern Med* 2002;41(8):613–616.

70. Sriram K., Palac B. Nasogastric feeding in the elderly. *JAMA* 1984;252:1682.

71. Ciocon JO, Silverstone FA, Graver LM, et al. Tube feedings in elderly patients: indications, benefits, and complications. *Arch Intern Med* 1988;148:429–433.

72. Pomerantz MA, Salomon J, Dunn R. Permanent gastrostomy as a solution to some nutritional problems in the elderly. *J Am Geriatr Soc* 1980;28:104–107.

73. Larson DE, Fleming CR, Ott BJ, et al. Percutaneous endoscopic gastrostomy: simplified access for enteral nutrition. *Mayo Clin Proc* 1983;58:103–107.

74. Miller RE, Kummer BA, Tiszenkel HI, et al. Percutaneous endoscopic gastrostomy: procedure of choice. *Ann Surg* 1986;204:543–545.

75. Ha L, Hauge T. Percutaneous endoscopic gastrostomy (PEG) for enteral nutrition in patients with stroke. *Scand J Gastroenterol* 2003;38(9):962–966.

76. Dwolatzky T, Berezovski S, Friedmann R, Paz J, Clarfield AM, Stessman J, Hamburger R, Jaul E, Friedlander Y, Rosin A, Sonnenblick M. A prospective comparison of the use of nasogastric and percutaneous endoscopic gastrostomy tubes for long-term enteral feeding in older people. *Clin Nutr* 2001;20(6):535–540.

77. Skelly RH. Are we using percutaneous endoscopic gastrostomy appropriately in the elderly? *Curr Opin Clin Nutr Metab Care* 2002;5(1):35–42.

78. DeChicco RS, Matarese LE. Determining the nutrition support regimen. In: Matarese LE, Gottschlich MM, eds. *Contemporary Nutrition Support Practice*. Philadelphia, PA: WB Saunders Company; 1998.

79. Gorman RC, Morris JB. Minimally invasive access to the gastrointestinal tract. In: Rombeau JL, Rolandelli RH, eds. *Clinical Nutrition: Enteral and Tube Feeding*. 3rd ed. Philadelphia, PA: WB Saunders Co; 1997.

80. Lambaise RE, Dorfman GS, Cronan JJ, et al. Percutaneous alternatives in nutritional support: a radiologic perspective. *J Parenter Enter Nutr* 1988;12:513–520.

81. Pasulka PS, Crockett C. Selecting enteral products. In: Borlase BC, Bell SJ, Blackburn GL, Forse RA, eds. *Enteral Nutrition*. New York, NY: Chapman & Hall; 1994.

82. Gottschlich MM, Shronts EP, Hutchins AM. Defined formula diets. In: Rombeau JL, Rolandelli RH, eds.

Clinical Nutrition: Enteral and Tube Feeding. 3rd ed. Philadelphia, PA: WB Saunders Co; 1997.

83. Matarese LE. Rationale and efficacy of specialized enteral and parenteral formulas. In: Matarese LE, Gottschlich MM, eds. *Contemporary Nutrition Support Practice.* 2nd ed, Philadelphia, PA: WB Saunders Co; 2003.

84. Chernoff R, Milton KY, Lipschitz DA. The effect of enteral formula supplementation on carnitine, taurine and selenium status in long-term tube fed patients. *J Parenter Enter Nutr* 1991;15:365.

85. Berner Y, Morse R, Frank O, et al. Vitamin plasma levels in long-term enteral feeding patients. *J Parenter Enter Nutr* 1989;13:525–528.

86. Chernoff R, Milton KY, Lipschitz DA. The effect of a high protein formula (Replete) on decubitus ulcer healing in long term tube fed institutionalized patients. *J Am Diet Assoc* 1990;90(suppl):A130.

87. Finucane TE. Malnutrition, tube feeding, and pressure sores: data are incomplete. *J Am Geriatr Soc* 1995;43: 447–451.

88. Lysen LK, Samour PQ. Enteral equipment. In: Matarese LE, Gottschlich MM, eds. *Contemporary Nutrition Support Practice.* Philadelphia, PA: WB Saunders Co; 1998.

89. Pick N, McDonald A, Bennett N, et al. Pulmonary aspiration in a long-term care setting: clinical and laboratory observations and an analysis of risk factors. *J Am Geriatr Soc* 1996;44:763–768.

90. Powell SK, Marcuard SP, Farrior ES, et al. Aspirating gastric residuals causes occlusion of smallbore feeding tubes. *J Parenter Enter Nutr* 1993;17:243–246.

91. Rees RG, Payne-James JJ, King C, et al. Spontaneous transpyloric passage and performance of "fine bore" polyurethane feeding tubes: a controlled clinical trial. *J Parenter Enter Nutr* 1988;12:469–472.

92. Sloane PD, Rizzolo P. Gastric tube feeding in elderly patients. *Arch Fam Med* 1993;2:927–928.

93. Sullivan DH, Chernoff R, Lipschitz DA. Nutritional support in long-term care facilities. *Nutr Clin Pract* 1987;2(1):6–13.

94. Leff B, Cheuvront N, Russell W. Discontinue feeding tubes in a community nursing home. *Gerontologist* 1994;34(1):130–133.

95. Mitchell SL, Kiely DK, Lipsitz LA. Does artificial enteral nutrition prolong the survival of institutionalized elders with chewing and swallowing problems? *J Gerontol Med Sci* 1998;53A:M207–M213.

96. O'Mahoney D, McIntyre AS. Artificial feeding for elderly patients after stroke. *Age Ageing* 1995;24:533–535.

97. Guenter PA, Settle RG, Perlmutter SG, et al. Tube-feeding related diarrhea in acutely ill patients. *J Parenter Enter Nutr* 1991;15:277–280.

98. Beyer PL. Complications of enteral nutrition. In: Matarese LE, Gottschlich MM, eds. *Contemporary Nutrition Support Practice.* 2nd ed. Philadelphia, PA: WB Saunders Co; 2003.

99. Kamar M, Bar-Dayan A, Zmora O, Ayalon A. Small bowel obstruction from a dislodged feeding tube. *Age Ageing* 2004;33(1):81–82.

100. Bennett RG, Greenough WB III. Approach to acute diarrhea in the elderly. *Gastroenterol Clin North Amer* 1993;22:517–533.

101. Yen PK. Tube feeding safety. *Geriatr Nurs* 1997;18: 40–41.

102. Chernoff R, Bloch AS. Liquid feedings: considerations and alternatives. *J Am Diet Assoc* 1977;70:389–391.

103. Zimmaro DM, Rolandelli RH, Koruda MJ, et al. Isotonic tube feeding formula induces liquid stool in normal subjects: reversal by pectin. *J Parenter Enter Nutr* 1989;13:117.

104. Slavin JL, Nelson NL, McNamara EA, et al. Bowel function of healthy men consuming liquid diets with and without dietary fiber. *J Parenter Enter Nutr* 1985; 9:317–321.

105. Scheppach W, Burghardt W, Bartram P, et al. Addition of dietary fiber to liquid formula diets: the pros and cons. *J Parenter Enter Nutr* 1990;14:204–209.

106. Hart GK, Dobb GJ. Effect of fecal bulking agent on diarrhea during enteral feeding in the critically ill. *J Parenter Enter Nutr* 1988;12:465–468.

107. Heymsfield SB, Roongspisuthipong C, Evert M, et al. Fiber supplementation of enteral formulas: effects on the bioavailability of major nutrients and gastrointestinal tolerance. *J Parenter Enter Nutr* 1988;12:265–273.

108. Hodges MO, Tolle SW. Tube feeding decisions in the elderly. *Clin Geriatr Med* 1994;10:475–487.

109. Krynski MD, Tymchuk AJ, Ouslander JG. How informed can consent be? New light on comprehension among elderly people making decisions about enteral feeding. *Gerontologist* 1994;34(1):36–43.

110. Ouslander JG, Tymchuk AJ, Krynski MD. Decisions about enteral tube feeding among the elderly. *J Am Geriatr Soc* 1993;41:70–77.

111. Ahronheim JC. Nutrition and hydration in the terminal patient. *Clin Geriatr Med* 1996;12:379–391.

112. Meisel A. Barriers to forgoing nutrition and hydration in nursing homes. *Am J Law Med* 1995;21:335–382.

113. Ackerman TF. The moral implications of medical uncertainty: tube feeding demented patients. *J Am Geriatr Soc* 1996;44:1265–1267.

114. Paine CJ. Nursing home patients: can feeding tubes be withheld? *J LA State Med Soc* 1996;148:284.

115. Scolapio JS, Picco MF, Tarrosa VB. Enteral versus parenteral nutrition: the patient's preference. *J Parenter Enteral Nutr* 2002;26(4):248–250.

116. Ferry M, Leverve X, Constans T. Comparison of sub-cutaneous and intravenous administration of a solution of amino acids in older patients. *J Am Geriatr Soc* 1997;45:857–860.

117. Lutz BH. Total parenteral nutrition in the older patient. *Home Healthcare Nurse* 1996;14:123–125.

118. Andres R. Aging and diabetes. *Med Clin North Am* 1971;55:835–846.

119. Hofeldt FD. Diabetes mellitus and dyslipidemia disorders in the elderly. In: Jahnigan DW, Schrier RW, eds. *Geriatric Medicine.* Cambridge, MA: Blackwell Science; 1996.

120. Btaiche IF, Khalidi N. Metabolic complications of parenteral nutrition in adults, part 1. *Am J Health-System Pharm* 2004;61(18):1938–1949.

121. Btaiche IF, Khalidi N. Metabolic complications of parenteral nutrition in adults, part 2. *Am J Health-System Pharm* 2004;61(19):2050–2057.

122. Chernoff R, Lipschitz DA. Total parenteral nutrition: considerations in the elderly. In: Rombeau JL, Caldwell MD, eds. *Clinical Nutrition: Parenteral Nutrition.* Philadelphia, PA: WB Saunders Co; 1986:2.

123. Chernoff R. Home nutrition support in elderly patients. *Clin Nutr* 1987;6(1):36–39.

CHAPTER 20

Continuum of Nutrition Services
for Older Americans

Barbara E. Millen, DPH, RD, FADA,
Lisa S. Brown, MS, RD, and Elyse Levine, PhD, RD

The 21st century will realize an *epidemiological transition* that reflects the progressive aging of the United States population and particular gains in the proportion of persons of very advanced age.[1–3] Average life expectancy in the United States at birth is now about 77 years[4] compared with 47 years in 1900 and those aged 65 years and older, currently estimated at 12% of the overall population, are expected to increase to 20% through the year 2030.[5] Men who reach age 65 years will live an additional 16.3 years on average, women another 19.2 years[6] and the rate of growth in Americans 80 years of age and older over the next three decades is expected to be most dramatic. By 2030, 60.9 million Americans will be 65–84 years of age, 8 million will be 85–99 years, and 381,000 will be centenarians.[7] Despite advancing age, most older Americans perceive their health to be good to excellent[7] and 95% live independently in community-based, noninstitutional settings.[8] In this context, however, the *average* older individual is diagnosed with one or more chronic diseases (notably heart disease, hypertension, diabetes, arthritis, or cancer),[9,10] takes 4 or more prescription medications,[11] and experiences significant disability or reduced quality of life.[7,9,10] Increasingly, the high costs of health care and prescription medications make it difficult for many older Americans to manage their health problems optimally and to access affordable medical, supportive, social, and rehabilitative services.[6] All of these factors threaten the independence of those in advanced age and place their health and quality of well-being at significant risk. Thus, one of the most serious challenges confronting national health policy experts and the medical and public health infrastructures today is to create a continuum of accessible health programs, products, and services for the aging population that promotes health into advanced age and minimizes the adverse consequences associated with aging-related chronic diseases. Key to success with this challenge is the increasing recognition that the achievement of optimal nutritional status in the older population and the availability of preventive nutrition services are key elements of healthful population aging and the management of the prevalent health problems in advanced age.[12]

POPULATION AGING

The phenomenon of population aging emerged for several key reasons. Advances within the 20th century in the prevention and treatment of infectious disease during pregnancy, infancy, and childhood enabled women of childbearing age and their offspring to survive previously ravaging health problems in far greater proportions.[1–3] Enhanced public health measures, including improved food quality, safety, and sanitation, reduced the prevalence of nutrient deficiencies and increased the nutritional well-being of the population.[13,14] Complementing these trends were the technological and clinical advances in the management of the diseases associated with advancing age. The nation's health system was increasingly able to manage acute health events as well as chronic diseases and their severe compli-

477

cations. All of these factors contributed to population aging and allowed older persons to survive into advanced age.[1–3,13,14]

The epidemiological transition is not unique to the United States; indeed, population aging is a global phenomenon.[1–3] Average life expectancy worldwide has increased from 46 years in the 1950s to 65 years in 2002[15] and the gap in life expectancy between all countries narrowed from 25 years in 1955 to 13.3 years in the past decade.[9] Some experts suggest, however, that this gap may be widening once again as a result of the AIDS epidemic, particularly in Africa and other parts of the developing world. Nonetheless, over half of the world's nearly 600 million older persons reside in developing countries and over three-fourths of the projected 1.2 billion persons 60 years and older in the year 2025 will reside in nonindustrialized nations.[15]

These directions in global population aging have brought about dramatic changes in the world's health needs. Murray and Lopez[16] and the World Health Organization[15,17] recently emphasized that chronic diseases, such as heart disease, hypertension and stroke, diabetes, pulmonary disease, and certain cancers are either rapidly emerging or are already established at high rates globally. The chronic diseases associated with aging account for nearly half of population morbidity and mortality in the developing regions of the world and over 80% of all deaths and disability in developed countries.[2,3,15–17] Of particular importance in this chapter is that poor population nutritional status is estimated to account for over twice the estimated "burden of disease" than any other *modifiable* risk factor.[16] Suboptimal nutritional status accounted for about 12% of total deaths and 16% of disability in the world's population (termed disability-adjusted life years [DALY]). Poor nutritional status includes (micro) nutrient deficiencies as well as nutritional imbalances and excesses (particularly high saturated fat intake and calorie intake in excess of needs leading to overweight and obesity). The attributable deaths and DALY for tobacco were 6.0% and 2.6%, respectively; for physical inactivity were 3.9% and 1.0%; and for alcohol

were 1.5% and 3.5%.[10] Clearly, the diagnosis of nutrition-related problems in the older population and the provision of appropriate preventive nutrition services already have important implications in the United States as well as developed and developing nations globally.

Further advances in life expectancy and the quality of life of older Americans have been examined in recent expert panels and public policy statements. Overall, improvements in the health and well-being of older persons will depend on the identification of effective strategies for the prevention and early treatment of diseases or their complications, a better understanding of the aging process, and awareness of methods for life enhancement in older age. Nutritional interventions and related services will play a central role in the promotion of successful aging. As noted by a former United States Surgeon General:[18]

> Sound public education directed toward this group [the older population]—and professional education directed toward individuals who care for older Americans—should focus on dietary means to reduce risk factors for chronic disease, (and) to promote functional independence....

Consistent with these recommendations, the United States National Institute on Aging (National Institutes of Health) also recognized the importance of nutrition in the promotion of elder health and declared nutritional well-being in older Americans a priority research area.[19] *Healthy People 2000* and *Healthy People 2010*,[20,21] the nation's recent health policy directives, emphasized the importance of sound nutrition in advancing age and defined key objectives for reducing nutritional risk in the older population. Among these were the provision of a continuum of nutrition services by qualified professionals in home, community, and institutional settings in order to improve health and well-being and reduce chronic diseases and their complications in older persons. In addition, over 25 professional organizations in the United States joined the Nutrition Screening Initiative (NSI) to urge the development of methods for assessing the prevalence and determinants of nutrition-related problems in elders and the formulation of improved health care delivery standards. The overall intent of NSI was to enhance the nutritional status of older persons and improve the management of chronic diseases of aging.[22] The Institute of Medicine (IOM) also reviewed the role of nutrition in maintaining the health of the nation's elderly and concluded that financing and delivering preventive nutrition services throughout the United States health care and related social service delivery systems was of great importance. Both the original IOM report of 1992[23] and the expert panel report of 2000[12] urged Congress to extend Medicare benefits to reimburse specific nutrition services related to the prevention and treatment of certain diseases including diabetes, pre-dialysis kidney failure, dyslipidemia, hypertension, osteoporosis, and heart failure. As discussed later in this chapter, Medicare began reimbursement of nutrition services for the improved management of diabetes and pre-dialysis kidney failure in 2002.

Globally, in recognition of the serious tolls associated with the chronic diseases of aging, the World Health Organization (WHO) introduced several collaborations involving nations worldwide. The *InterHealth Programme*[2,3] was aimed at reducing risks for chronic diseases at the population level through *integrated* behavioral and policy-level interventions. Among the major features of integrated behavioral risk factor intervention planning was the promotion of sound nutrition practices in a nation's population. Central to *InterHealth* strategies was the understanding that poor nutrition is associated with increased risks for multiple chronic diseases, including coronary heart disease, hypertension, diabetes mellitus, certain forms of cancer, and osteoporosis. Countries participating in *InterHealth*, including the United States, established national policy statements on nutrition for non-communicable disease (NCD) prevention and control and mounted nutrition interventions at the national, community, household, and/or individual levels. In addition, the *InterHealth* collaboration provided a framework for the global sharing of information on methods for implementing interventions for chronic disease risk reduction in populations throughout the developed and developing world.[2,3,24] Similarly, the WHO led members of its European Region in the release of the First Action Plan for Food and Nutrition Policy 2000–2005.[25] It was the intent of this initiative to raise awareness of nutrition policy in the European political agenda by supporting WHO member nations in developing sound food and nutrition policies. The report acknowledged the importance of developing national food and nutrition policies that promote health and reduce the burden of nutrition-related chronic diseases of aging. Multisector approaches, including health care, agriculture, the environment, and the food and mass communications industries, were urged as necessary to place food and nutritional policies high on national health care policy agendas.[25] These global trends and collaborative efforts suggest that nations throughout the world recognize the importance of nutrition in healthful population aging. There is also likely to be keen interest in models that emerge internationally to assess health and nutritional risk in aging adults and to deliver behaviorally based nutrition interventions for elder health promotion and acute and chronic disease risk reduction.

Subsequent sections of this chapter will examine the interrelationships between nutrition, physical functioning, and health with advancing age, including the determinants of nutritional risk in elders. This chapter will also describe major United States policy recommendations and interventions for improving nutritional status in older individuals and enhancing the delivery of nutrition services to the elder population. Furthermore, it will review the nutrition services payment systems, in particular Medicare and Medicaid. Highlights are summarized from the national evaluation of the Elder Nutrition Program (ENP), the largest federally funded mechanism for the delivery of a continuum of home- and community-based nutrition and related health and supportive social services to the older United States adult population. In addition, insights are provided from the Framingham

Study, the longest standing, prospective epidemiological investigation of heart disease and, more recently, other chronic diseases of aging. The Framingham Nutrition Studies have been examining the relationships between population dietary patterns, nutrient intake, and chronic disease risk and outcomes in an aging population for over 15 years. Some of their key findings are highlighted here to offer innovative approaches for the development of targeted, behaviorally based preventive nutrition interventions in aging adult men and women.

NUTRITION, PHYSICAL FUNCTIONING, AND HEALTH IN ADVANCING AGE

Nutritional well-being is an integral component of the health, independence, and quality of life of older individuals.[26,27] Optimal nutrition appears to mitigate existing health problems, improve the management of many chronic diseases, and extend years of healthy living with advancing age.[28] Conversely, the presence of malnutrition increases risk for medical and surgical complications, delays recovery from physical traumas, and is a primary risk factor for recurrent hospitalizations and costly, extended institutionalization.[23] Although the majority of persons aged 65 years and older in the United States consider themselves to be in good to excellent health,[7,27,28] over 75% of noninstitutionalized older persons have one or more chronic health problems that could be improved with proper nutrition and up to half may have clinical evidence of various forms of malnutrition.[10,26,27,29,30]

Myriad nutritional problems exist in the older population and span a broad spectrum ranging from frank nutrient deficiencies, such as protein-energy malnutrition, to evidence of nutritional excesses, including obesity, dyslipidemia, hypertension, and higher than recommended levels of dietary lipids and other nutrients.[26,27,31–36] It is estimated that up to 15% of the free-living older population have demonstrable nutrient deficiencies. Up to 40% of the frail, homebound elderly and a similar proportion of the institutionalized older population may also suffer from protein-

energy malnutrition and frank nutrient deficiencies (such as folate or vitamin B_{12} deficiency).[27,37] In national nutrition studies, low dietary intakes of energy, fiber, calcium, magnesium, antioxidants, certain B vitamins, and other micronutrients are common in older persons.[38–40] As many as one in four older people may consume low levels of nutrients, which results in increased risk for nutrient deficiencies. Micronutrient imbalances may also increase risks for certain nutrition-related chronic diseases, such as diabetes and heart disease, and their complications.[26,37,40]

Factors that increase risk for nutrient deficiencies in the older population are not fully understood. The characteristics that appear to be associated with low nutrient intake are: acute and chronic medical problems, particularly the presence of multiple, coexisting health problems; polypharmacy; losses of functional capacity; advanced age; oral health problems; declines in appetite; reductions in taste and olfactory acuity; social isolation; depression and other psychological disturbances; poverty; lack of nutrition knowledge; and susceptibility to fraud.[41–45] Among the noninstitutionalized elderly, those who are homebound and frail appear to be particularly at risk for nutrient deficiencies.[26,37,43] In addition, there are racial and income disparities in levels of food insecurity and access to food and nutrition services that increase risks for malnutrition in the poor and minority elder populations.[42]

Health problems related to nutritional excesses are also estimated to be quite common and rising in the older population. Dietary patterns that deviate from expert nutrition recommendations and obesity are particular concerns. Up to half of the free-living population 60 years of age and older consume diets with higher than recommended levels of nutrients, such as saturated fat and sodium, which are associated with increased health risk profiles (such as dyslipidemia, hypertension, glucose intolerance, and excess body weight).[26,42,45] It is estimated that in 2002, 70.8% of persons age 60 and older were overweight or obese by accepted clinical standards,[46] an increase of 10% from just a decade earlier.[47]

National prevalence data on overweight and obesity are not available before the 1990s because earlier national health surveys such as the National Health and Nutrition Examination Surveys (NHANES I and II) did not examine persons 75 years and older[47] or particularly high-risk groups such as the homebound, frail elderly. To provide improved estimates in the future, however, NHANES III (1988–94) and the current NHANES (ongoing since 1999) intentionally oversampled black and Mexican American populations 60 years and older and white Americans 60–69, 70–79, and 80 years and older.[47] Contrasts in the prevalence of overweight, obesity, and underweight in American middle-aged and older adults are evident from other cross-sectional and prospective population-based studies including research on the national Elder Nutrition Program (ENP) participants,[48] New England ambulatory and homebound elderly,[28] and an older rural population.[52] Among ENP congregate and home-delivered meal program participants, both underweight and overweight were prevalent. Nearly half (47%) of the frail, homebound ENP participants (those who receive home-delivered meals) were found to be underweight (BMI <22) and about one-third (32%) were overweight (BMI >27). In contrast, the prevalence of under- and overweight in congregate meal participants were 33% and 42%, respectively.[48] In a regionally representative sample of nearly 1200 noninstitutionalized New England elders,[28] 11.5–19.5% of older men and women were underweight (BMI <22) and 40–42% were overweight (>25). Ledikwe et al.[49] found that none of their rural Pennsylvanian elder male and female subjects (66–87 years of age) were underweight (BMI <18.5); 21% were normal weight (BMI 18.5–24.9); 44% were overweight (BMI 25–29); and 35% were obese (BMI >30).

The Framingham Study[50] may offer some of the most interesting prospective information on nutrition risk and health outcomes in aging American adults. These investigations were initiated in the late 1940s in a cohort of 5209 male and female residents of Framingham, Massachusetts. The community was chosen for study because its population mimicked the demographics of a "typical" American community at the study's inception. In 1972, the Framingham Offspring-Spouse (FOS) studies were established with the recruitment of the 5135 offspring of the original Framingham cohort and their spouses. The nutrition-related experiences of these adults over the subsequent 28 years of study are quite dramatic, particularly relating to overweight and obesity (and associated chronic disease).[51] Sixty percent of men who were normal weight at baseline (1972) became overweight or obese over nearly three decades (2001+). On average, all FOS men gained weight into their sixth decade of age, ranging from 10 to 16 pounds depending on baseline BMI status (underweight, normal weight, or overweight). Half of FOS women became overweight or obese, but all women gained on average 8–21 pounds through their seventh decade of life. At the most recent Framingham exam, 81.5% of Framingham men (currently aged 50–97 years), were overweight, including 33.4% who were obese. Some 62% of middle-aged and older Framingham women were overweight, including 27.2% who were obese.

Nutritional excesses, including overweight and obesity, impose increased risks not only for the development of chronic diseases such as hypertension, coronary heart disease, diabetes, and certain forms of cancer, but also for their adverse complications and outcomes including death and physical disabilities.[42,49] Related to this, Framingham research further documented that the rates of overweight and obesity in men and women vary by the habitual dietary patterns found in subgroups of the male and female populations. The identified dietary patterns were also associated with disease risk profiles and health outcomes in Framingham men and women.[50–55] Relationships between dietary patterns, body weight, disease risk, and health outcomes offer new insights into the development of preventive nutrition interventions in the aging adult population.

Little research has characterized the factors that contribute to the development of nutritional excesses and related health problems in the older population. One recent study in a population-based sample of free-living elders in New England[28] suggested that smoking and male gender were associated with nutritional excesses, such as higher than recommended levels of nutrients (particularly dietary lipids). Those elders who continued to smoke were more apt to consume high dietary lipid intake. Older men, compared with elder women, were more likely to comply with recent recommendations for "heart healthy" nutrient intake.[28] Increasing research is focusing on the relationships between dietary behavior, particularly patterns of food and dietary intake, and their relationship to nutritional status and various health outcomes in various adult populations.[49,53–55] In rural Pennsylvania, a low nutrient dense dietary pattern (in comparison with a favorable, high nutrient dense pattern) was associated with an increased risk for obesity (OR 2.03, CI 0.98-4.20). The Framingham Nutrition Studies[50–55,57] have done extensive research on the determinants of nutritional risk from this behavioral perspective. The dietary patterns of Framingham (FOS) men and women have been found to be closely associated with nutrient intake, biological risk factor status, and varying levels of risk for adverse health outcomes over time. Among the health outcomes that have been linked to dietary patterns are overweight and obesity as well as cardiovascular disease risk factors. These findings are summarized here and further details on the Framingham

Nutrition Studies, including complete descriptions of its validated methods for identifying the dietary patterns of aging adult male and female populations, have been published previously.[50–55]

In Framingham, five subgroups of FOS men and five of FOS women were distinguished on the basis of their habitual, unique dietary patterns. It is emphasized that the dietary patterns of men and women were characterized separately and were quite different. The key food and nutrient characteristics of each dietary pattern were identified and used to label each subgroup. In women, the five dietary patterns were: *Heart Healthy*, *Lighter Eating*, *Wine and Moderate Eating*, *High Fat*, and *Empty Calories*. In men, the five dietary patterns were: *Transition to Heart Healthy*, *Higher Starch*, *Average Male*, *Lower Variety*, and *Empty Calories*. The distribution of the dietary patterns in the FOS male and female populations is summarized in Figure 20–1. It is noted that somewhat more equal proportions of FOS men consumed each male dietary pattern whereas considerably more women followed a *Lighter Eating* dietary pattern and smaller proportions of women followed the *Wine and Moderate Eating* and *Empty Calories* dietary patterns. The key distinguishing features of the male and female dietary patterns are summarized in Table 20–1. The baseline (1984–1988) nutrient intakes of Framingham men and women by dietary pattern are compared for compliance with

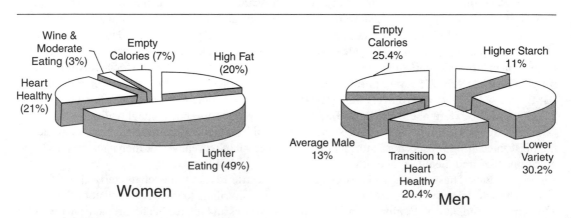

Figure 20-1   Dietary Patterns of Framingham Women and Men

Table 20–1 Key Features of Dietary Patterns Identified among Framingham Women and Men

DIETARY PATTERNS OF WOMEN

Heart Healthy	Higher in fruits, vegetables, low-fat dairy, and other lower-fat foods including whole grains, skinless poultry, and fish; lowest in total and saturated fat content; higher in fiber and micronutrient density (calcium and folate).
Light Eating	Lower in sweets, animal and vegetable fats, and refined grains; lowest in caloric content.
Wine and Moderate Eating	Lower intake of desserts; higher intake of snack foods, eggs, and wine; highest alcohol and dietary cholesterol content with lowest calcium consumption.
High Fat	Higher in sweets, animal and vegetable fats, refined grains and margarine; fewer lower-fat foods; highest in total and saturated fat content.
Empty Calories	Higher in sweetened beverages, red meats, and desserts; lower in fruits and vegetables; high in sugar, total fat, and saturated fat, lower in fiber and micronutrient density (including folate).

DIETARY PATTERNS OF MEN

Transition to Heart Healthy	Higher in fruits, vegetables, and whole grains; lowest in total and saturated fat content, sucrose, and cholesterol; higher in micronutrient density (folate and vitamin E) and lowest in overall nutrient risk score.
Higher Starch	Higher in leaner animal proteins, unsweetened beverages, and firm vegetable fats and relatively higher in grain, fruits, and vegetables; highest in starch, beta carotene, and monounsaturated fat intake.
Average Male	Moderate intakes of most food groups with highest intakes of caffeinated beverages and lowest of unsweetened decaffeinated drinks. Highest protein and lowest carbohydrate (percent energy), lowest calcium, ascorbic acid, and folate.
Lower Variety	Lower intake of most food groups; lowest intake of energy and most micronutrients.
Empty Calories	Highest in refined grains, desserts, animal proteins, sweets, salty snacks, and high-fat dairy products and animal fats; highest in total and saturated fat, carbohydrates (including sucrose), B_{12} and calcium but lowest in beta carotene. Highest overall nutrient risk score.

the expert dietary lipid and sodium nutrition guidelines (the USDA Dietary Guidelines for Americans[56]) in Table 20–2.

In women, the *Heart Healthy* pattern had relatively higher fruit, vegetable, and whole grain intake and lower total and saturated fat intake (more compliant with expert guidelines). However, although this subgroup of women consumed a relatively healthier dietary pattern than other FOS women, it is important to emphasize that they did *not* entirely achieve current expert

recommendations for optimal nutrient intake. The *Lighter Eating* dietary pattern was associated with lower intakes of most food groups including sweets, animal and vegetable fats, and refined grains; these women also consumed the lowest levels of calories. The *Wine and Moderate Eating* female dietary pattern was noteworthy in terms of lower intakes of desserts and higher consumption of snack foods, eggs, and wine. These women had the highest alcohol (as wine) and dietary cholesterol intakes and the lowest calcium

Table 20–2 Age-Adjusted Proportions of Framingham Men and Women by Dietary Pattern Who Meet the USDA Dietary Guidelines[56] Lipid and Sodium Recommendations, 1984–1988

Nutrient Mean % Composition	Men						Women			
	Transition (n = 154)	HS (n = 80)	AM (n = 102)	LV (n = 229)	EC (n = 175)	HH (n = 211)	LE (n = 438)	W & ME (n = 26)	HF (n = 180)	EC (n = 53)
			(95% CI)					(95% CI)		
Cholesterol <300 mg	**62.8**[a]	60.4[a]	58.8[a]	58.2[a]	<u>42.9</u>[b]	**82.0**	78.7	<u>69.7</u>	78.1	76.5
Total Fat ≥30%	**24.2**	<u>14.4</u>	17.0	21.3	16.2	**28.0**[a]	14.4[c]	19.5[abc]	<u>8.1</u>[b]	11.7[ac]
Saturated Fat <10%	**35.5**[a]	15.2[a]	17.4[a]	20.7[b]	<u>14.5</u>[a]	**27.7**[a]	19.8[c]	23.4[ab]	<u>7.1</u>[b]	9.5[ac]
Sodium <2400 mg	**26.2**[a]	<u>10.6</u>[b]	24.3[ac]	26.0[a]	15.7[bc]	<u>45.8</u>	**53.2**	46.8	47.4	48.8
All Four Nutrients	**9.6**	<u>1.1</u>	6.8	6.2	4.5	**13.8**[a]	6.2[c]	3.8[abc]	<u>2.0</u>[b]	3.8[abc]

Men: Transition to Heart Healthy (Transition); High Starch (HS); Average Male (AM); Low Variety (LV); Empty Calories (EC)

Women: Heart Healthy (HH); Lighter Eating (LE); Wine and Moderate Eating (WM); High Fat (HF); Empty Calories (EC)

[abc]Means with different superscripts are significantly different from each other ($p < 0.05$); means that are underlined are lowest; means that are in bold type are highest.

consumption. Women with the *High Fat* dietary pattern had higher intakes of animal and vegetable fats and sweets, refined grains, and margarine; they ate fewer lower-fat foods and had the highest consumption of total and saturated fats. The *Empty Calories* dietary pattern of women was higher in sweetened beverages, red meats, and desserts and lower in fruits and vegetables. It was highest overall in nutritional risk as reflected by high sugar, total and saturated fat consumption, lower micronutrient density (including folate), and poor fiber intake.

It is noteworthy that each female dietary pattern had distinguishing features that could be characterized as relatively *healthy* (such as some level of fruit and vegetable consumption) as well as *less healthy* components (low intakes of whole grains or high consumption of sugar-containing foods). Although none of the habitual eating patterns of women achieved complete compliance with the USDA Dietary Guidelines[57] (Table 20–2) at baseline (1984–1988), 7–82% met the expert standards depending upon the nutrient of interest. There were particularly marked variations in the subgroup's deviations from the dietary guidelines for total and saturated fat among FOS women; there was relatively higher compliance among women with *Heart Healthy* dietary patterns particularly compared to those with the *High Fat* and *Empty Calories* dietary patterns. The presence of both healthful and less healthful aspects of the female dietary patterns and the relative variation in the continuum of nutritional risk associated with these habitual eating practices offers considerable opportunities for preventive nutrition intervention. The ability to characterize the distinguishing features of the habitual dietary patterns of women (and men) enables the identification of specific food and nutrient targets for nutrition education and counseling at the individual and population levels and the formulation of innovative behavioral strategies to promote healthful eating in aging adults.[50–55]

In FOS men, the *Transition to Heart Healthy* dietary pattern was characterized (compared with other male dietary patterns) by higher intakes of fruits, vegetables, and whole grains; higher micronutrient density (in particular, folate and vitamin E) (Table 20–1); the lowest overall nutritional risk; and higher compliance with total and saturated fat and dietary cholesterol guidelines (Table 20–2). Men with the *Higher Starch* dietary pattern consumed leaner animal proteins in greater quantities as well as unsweetened beverages and firm vegetable fats; they had relatively higher intakes of grains, fruits, and vegetables and their intakes were highest in starch, beta carotene, and monounsaturated fat intake. The *Average Male* dietary pattern was distinguished by moderate intakes of most food groups, although these men consumed the highest intakes of caffeinated beverages and the lowest of unsweetened, decaffeinated drinks. They also had the highest protein consumption (percent energy) and lowest carbohydrate, calcium, ascorbic acid, and folate levels. Men with the *Lower Variety* dietary pattern had lower intakes of most food groups including the lowest consumption of energy and selected micronutrients. The *Empty Calories* dietary pattern of FOS men was characterized by the highest intakes of refined grains, desserts, animal proteins, sweets, salty snacks, and high-fat dairy products and animal fats. It was also highest in total and saturated fat, carbohydrates (including sucrose), and vitamin B_{12} and calcium but lowest in beta carotene. These men also had the highest overall nutritional risk.

Only 1% to10% of men in any dietary pattern group were able to achieve all four components of the USDA Dietary Guidelines[57] examined here (Table 20–2). FOS men were most compliant with dietary cholesterol guidelines (43–63% depending upon the dietary pattern). Nonetheless, as observed with the females, dietary patterns, both *healthful* and *less healthful* features of males could be identified (Table 20–1) and these features provide the basis for targeted, behavioral-based preventive nutrition interventions.

It seems important that as innovations are sought to guide preventive nutrition strategies for the aging population that consideration is given to the initial (ie, baseline) identification of the habitual dietary patterns of men and women.

Furthermore, it appears critical that nutrition professionals become skilled in advanced and innovative methods of behaviorally based nutrition interventions to promote healthful dietary patterns and related food and nutrient intake. Such strategies are likely to enhance the prevention and management of chronic diseases and their complications in aging adult men and women.

Each of the FOS male and female dietary patterns can further be contrasted on the basis of a composite nutrient risk profile; the Framingham Nutrient risk score is based upon the comparative intakes of 19 nutrients (Figure 20–2 including footnotes for an explanation). The mean nutritional risk scores of FOS men and women in each dietary pattern subgroup are summarized for 1984–1988 and 1991–1995 in Figure 20–2. Nutritional risk varied by dietary pattern at each time point, and, of key importance, the subgroup contrasts remained consistent over eight years of study. Although slight improvements in food and nutrient intake were observed in the FOS population overall, particularly FOS women, there was a continuum of nutritional risk that enabled the ranking of the dietary pattern subgroups

(Figure 20–2). The further research into the habitual dietary patterns of FOS men and women that is briefly summarized below suggested the dietary patterns of men and women could also be linked to chronic disease risk profiles and a wide variety of health and disease outcomes. Thus, as noted previously, the identification of habitual dietary patterns and preventive interventions directed at their improvement seem important in the promotion of health in the aging adult male and female populations.[50–55]

The cardiovascular disease risk profile of Framingham men and women by dietary pattern, including rates of overweight and obesity, are compared in Figures 20–3 and 20–4. CVD risk varied by dietary pattern; the relatively higher risk profiles of women with the *Empty Calories* pattern compared with others is particularly noteworthy. Nonetheless, the prevalence of CVD risk factors in all women, particularly overweight and obese women, deserves attention. In males, CVD risk profiles were generally higher than those observed in females (except perhaps *High Fat* and *Empty Calories* women) and the rates of overweight and obesity were particularly high. This

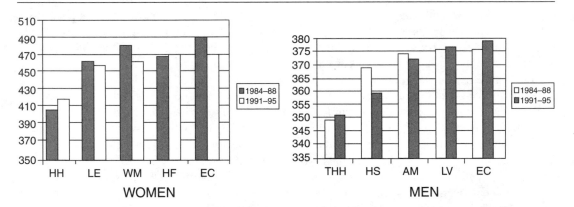

Figure 20–2 Mean Overall Nutrient Risk of Framingham Women and Men by Dietary Pattern 1984–1988 and 1991–1995

Women: HH, Heart Healthy; LE, Light Eating; WM, Wine and Moderate Eating; HF, High Fat; EC, Empty Calories
Men: THH, Transition to Heart Healthy; HS, High Starch; AM, Average Male; LV, Low Variety; EC, Empty Calories
Overall nutrient risk based on scoring of the following 19 nutrients: energy; protein; total fat; monounsaturated, polyunsaturated, and saturated fat; carbohydrate; fiber; alcohol; cholesterol; sodium; calcium; selenium; vitamins C, B_6, B_{12}, and E; folate; and beta carotene.

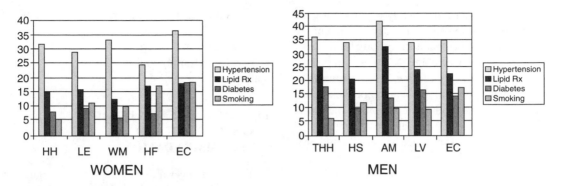

Figure 20–3 Age-Adjusted Proportions (%) of Framingham Men and Women, 30–90 Years, by Dietary Pattern with Selected CVD Risk Factors, 1998–2002
Women: HH, Heart Healthy; LE, Light Eating; WM, Wine and Moderate Eating; HF, High Fat; EC, Empty Calories
Men: THH, Transition to Heart Healthy; HS, High Starch; AM, Average Male; LV, Low Variety; EC, Empty Calories

dimension of Framingham research further suggested that it is not only important to assess the habitual eating patterns of men and women but to combine it with CVD risk factor profiles as *targeted and individualized* preventive nutrition intervention strategies are formulated. The targeting of nutrition interventions specific to the distinct subgroup profiles of aging men and women is now feasible because methods have emerged for the characterization of complex dietary patterns and the related disease risk profiles of men and women as demonstrated here. Further insights into the utilization of the dietary pattern approach to create innovative, targeted behaviorally based preventive nutrition interventions for aging adult men and women will be discussed later in this chapter.

The available literature offers new insights into the levels of nutritional risk in aging populations and the determinants of nutritional risk.

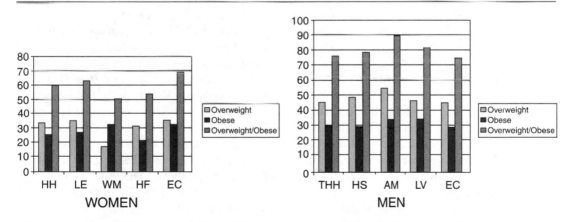

Figure 20–4 Age-Adjusted Proportions (%) of Framingham Men and Women, 30–90 Years Who Are Overweight and Obese by Dietary Pattern, 1998–2002
Women: HH, Heart Healthy; LE, Light Eating; WM, Wine and Moderate Eating; HF, High Fat; EC, Empty Calories
Men: THH, Transition to Heart Healthy; HS, High Starch; AM, Average Male; LV, Low Variety; EC, Empty Calories

Nonetheless, there are clearly significant gaps that continue to exist in our understanding of the etiology and consequences of nutritional risk throughout advancing age. Many existing studies fail to provide *population-based* estimates of the prevalence or etiology of nutritional excesses, deficiencies, and their combinations in older persons. For example, the prevalence of "combined" forms of malnutrition (such as obesity and protein deficiency) have been reported, particularly in the older institutionalized population, but its prevalence and health-related outcomes are underresearched. There is also little known concerning the variation in nutrient requirements with advancing age, particularly in the presence of chronic and acute medical problems or treatment regimens that may alter nutritional status.

Furthermore, the efficacy of behaviorally based nutritional interventions among older individuals in community, home, or institutional settings is poorly understood. Horwath[56] reviewed over 90 studies on diet and nutritional status of older individuals and concluded that the majority were conducted in small, highly selected samples with limited generalizability. A similar conclusion was reached in the IOM reports.[12,23] Little if anything is known about the prevalence of nutritional problems in the oldest-old (those 80 years and older), the impact of chronic diseases and their complications on nutritional status, the health outcomes associated with malnutrition, particularly in the very old population, the directionality of the relationships between nutritional status and health characteristics and outcomes, or optimal methods of nutritional intervention in advanced age. Furthermore, several recent reports have identified the following research areas concerning nutrition and aging as priorities for investigation: the prevalence of nutrition-related problems in the older population, particularly in high-risk older populations such as the frail, homebound elderly; the role of nutritional factors in the etiology and prevention of chronic diseases and age-related impairments in organ system function; the development of guidelines for nutrition interventions that are appropriate for common morbidity

patterns among aging adults; relationships between nutrition, physical functioning, and health; and the nutritional determinants of cognitive and physical functioning and quality of life in older adults.[12,18,20,21,58]

PUBLIC NUTRITION POLICY STATEMENTS AND RECOMMENDATIONS

In the last several decades, growing concern over nutritional risk in the older population has led to the development of key public policy statements to improve the nutritional status of older Americans and to enhance the delivery of nutrition and related health services. Many statements have attempted to provide guidelines and recommendations for optimal food and nutrient intake in advancing age. In addition, both public and private initiatives and programs have emerged to implement these policy directives. Such activities provide elements of a framework for the comprehensive assessment and monitoring of nutrition-related problems in the older population as well as for a network of rational and appropriate nutrition services for elders. The policy statements and dietary recommendations are summarized in Table 20–3 and are discussed below. The recommendations for developing effective nutrition services and interventions are summarized in Table 20–4 and are described in the next section of this chapter.

The nation's most recent health policy statements, *Healthy People 2000* and *Healthy People 2010*,[20,21] outline a set of specific objectives to improve the health status of older Americans. The *Healthy People 2000* goals targeted health status concerns; the need for chronic disease risk reduction activities; and the limited availability of key health promotion and protection services as major priorities. Specifically, the report noted the following goals: reduce morbidity and mortality associated with suicides, motor vehicle accidents, falls, hip fractures, and pneumonia; increase years of healthy and independent living; decrease hearing and visual impairments; improve dental health status; increase abilities to

Table 20–3 Diet-Related Health Recommendations for Healthy Aging

Originating Source, Year	Nutrition and Diet	Health and Related Recommendations
JNC 7, 2003 (ref. 63)	Recommends dietary patterns consistent with the Dietary Approaches to Stop Hypertension (DASH)[64] including 5–9 servings of fruit and vegetables per day, 2–3 servings of reduced-fat dairy, 2–3 servings of nuts and seeds per week, whole grains and low total and saturated fat.	Provides recommendations on lifestyle management of hypertension including increased physical activity and moderation of alcohol intake. Provides specific guidelines on evaluation of hypertension and medication if indicated.
NCEP Adult Treatment Panel III Guidelines, 2001 (ref. 61)	Provide dietary guidance to lower plasma total and LDL cholesterol levels. Recommends both medication and Therapeutic Lifestyle Changes (TLC) that target total and saturated fat and dietary cholesterol intake dietary patterns. High fiber and reduced calories are also recommended. Nutrition recommendations are intended to be prescribed by a health professional and individualized to the patient depending on age, race, gender, comorbidities.	Urges consideration of referral to a Registered Dietitian for all individuals at risk due to elevated cholesterol. Also provides specific guidance on evaluation of cholesterol and recommendations for other lifestyle interventions such as increased physical activity. Provides specific recommendations for medication of high cholesterol if indicated.
DRIs, 1998 (ref. 59)	Levels of recommended nutrient intake (RDAs and AIs) for healthy persons age 51–70 and over 70+ years for calcium, phosphorus, magnesium, vitamin D, fluoride, thiamin, riboflavin, niacin, vitamin B$_6$, folate, vitamin B$_{12}$, pantothenic acid, biotin, and choline Tolerable upper limits and estimated average requirements are also set for certain nutrients. Reference weights are also provided.	
NSI, 1997 (refs. 22, 65–72)	Nutrition guideline specific to the management and prevention of the following diseases and their consequences: cancer, chronic obstructive pulmonary disease, congestive heart failure, coronary heart disease, dementia, diabetes mellitus, failure to thrive, hypertension, osteoporosis, and pneumonia.	Provides guidelines for nutritional screening and assessment. Recommends professional education strategies and includes educational materials.

continues

Table 20–3 continued

Originating Source, Year	Nutrition and Diet	Health and Related Recommendations
NCI, 1996 (ref. 62)	Emphasize 5–9 servings from the fruits and vegetables groups for the promotion of reduced cancer risk.	
Food Guide Pyramid, 1992 (ref. 57)	Outlines recommended daily food intake that is consistent with the Dietary Guidelines: Use fats, oils, and sweets sparingly. Consume 3–5 servings from the milk, yogurt, and cheese group. Consume 2–3 servings from the meat, poultry, fish, dry beans, eggs, and nuts group. Consume 3–5 servings from the vegetable group. Consume 2–4 servings from the fruit group. Consume 6–11 servings from the bread, cereal, rice, and pasta group.	
Dietary Guidelines, 1992 (ref. 57)	Eat a variety of foods. Maintain desirable weight. Avoid too much fat, saturated fat, and cholesterol. Eat foods with adequate starch and fiber. Avoid too much sugar and sodium. If you drink alcohol, do so in moderation.	
Committee on Diet and Health, 1989 (ref. 60)	Reduce total fat intake to 30% of calories or less; saturated fat to less than 10%; cholesterol to less than 300 mg. Eat 5 or more servings of fruits and vegetables per day. Maintain protein intake at moderate levels. Balance food intake and physical activity to maintain appropriate body weight. Alcohol consumption not recommended. Limit sodium chloride intake to 6 g or less. Maintain adequate calcium intake. Avoid supplements in excess of RDAs. Maintain optimal fluoride intake.	Integrate geriatric nutrition curriculum into all professional education. Expand research on nutrition and aging, including research on nutrient requirements, interactions between diet, health, and elders' sociodemographic and functional profiles.

The Surgeon General's Report on Nutrition and Health, 1988 (ref. 18)	Diseases of dietary excesses and imbalances rank as the leading causes of death and disability in the United States including heart disease, atherosclerosis, certain cancers, hypertension and stroke, diabetes mellitus, and cirrhosis. Integrate nutrition services into all health care programs including assessment, nutrition counseling, referral to community-based nutrition and food assistance programs. Increase the use of food labels and food products that promote healthy nutrition.	Reduce consumption of fat, saturated fat and cholesterol. Achieve and maintain desirable body weight. Increase whole grains, cereals, vegetables, and fruits. Reduce sodium intake. Take alcohol only in moderation if at all. Depending on the individual's circumstances, consider fluoride, calcium, and iron needs and the risks associated with sugar intake. Recommend adoption of the *Dietary Guidelines* (49).
Surgeon General's Workshop, 1988 (ref. 58)	Improve quality of life of older Americans and promote autonomy. Promote research on nutrition, chronic diseases, and aging as well as the efficacy of nutrition services in the management of health problems in older persons.	Promote good nutritional status for a high-quality life through physical, psychological, and social mechanisms. In doing so, consider the varying sociodemographic, functional, and physical conditions of elders and their medical care.

Table 20–4 Recommendations for Nutrition Services and Interventions in Older Populations

Originating Source, Year	Clinical/Medical Nutrition Services	Public/Professional Nutrition Education	Food Services
Institute of Medicine Report: *The Role of Nutrition in Maintaining Health in the Nation's Elderly: Evaluating Coverage of Nutrition Services for the Medicare Population, 2000*, (ref. 12)	Recommended Medicare reimbursement for preventative nutrition services to be provided by registered dietitians to individuals referred by their physician for specific medical diagnoses of dyslipidemia, hypertension, pre-dialysis renal disease, heart failure, diabetes, and osteoporosis. As of 2002 Medicare authorized reimbursement for diabetes and pre-dialysis renal disease.	Recognizes registered dietitians as the single identified group with the standardized education, clinical training, continuing education, and national credentialing required to be reimbursed as providers of MNT. Recommends that RDs should be available to serve as consultants to other health professionals in addition to providing direct therapy to Medicare beneficiaries. Recommends increased RD involvement in organized health promotion programs in community and elder service settings. Calls for a task force appointed by the president to devise and execute a program for nutrition education through the mass media. Recommends that laws be strengthened to require public service time on radio and television. Advocates use of mass media for training neighborhood leaders.	Food services, such as congregate and home meals programs, and other social services (like Food Stamps) were acknowledged to address key determinants of appropriate nutrient intake including poverty, poor functional status, and social isolation. Urged increase in home food services to those with impairments and need.
Healthy People 2000, 2010, 1993 (refs. 20,21)	Recommended increased nutrition assessment and counseling by qualified dietitians and nutritionists in primary care settings.	Recommended that nutrition education be part of the continuum of health care for older adults, to be incorporated into all ambulatory, home, and institutional health care service activities.	

Position of the American Dietetic Association, Nutrition, Aging, and the Continuum of Care, 2000 (ref. 26)	Recommended that nutrition services for elders be integrated into institutionally based health care facilities; private or group medical practices; health maintenance organizations; preferred provider practice settings; and ambulatory, home health, and social service settings. Recommends MNT coverage be expanded to cardiovascular disease, osteoporosis, hypertension, and obesity.	Emphasized the need for safe food handling practices to avoid foodborne illnesses. Recommended that all food delivery systems and programs contain some form of nutrition education insofar as possible without hampering the delivery of foods
Institute of Medicine, 1992 (ref. 23)	Recommended nutritional screening, assessment, intervention, and care plans be required in hospitals, nursing homes, and other health care settings that receive federal funding. Promotion of dietary intervention for elders with atherosclerosis, hypertension, diabetes, and osteoporosis.	Encouraged participation in congregate and home-delivered meal programs to support functional independence. Develop and maintain nutrition and food service standards for nursing homes, long-term care facilities, and facilities that receive Medicare and Medicaid reimbursement.
	Promoted self-care and regulation of nutrition fraud. Advocated minimized polypharmacy and further emphasis on adverse drug-nutrient interactions.	

continues

Table 20-4 continued

Originating Source, Year	Clinical/Medical Nutrition Services	Public/Professional Nutrition Education	Food Services
The Surgeon General's Report, 1988 (ref. 19)	Recommended RD delivery of medical nutrition services to be provided within institutional and community-based services for older adults, including homebound elderly.	Called for more research on the efficacy of nutrition interventions and techniques that promote adequate food consumption in elders. Recommended elimination of nutrition-related health fraud.	Noted that those providing food services be required to meet energy and nutrient needs of older clients, including frail and homebound elderly.
Surgeon General's Workshop, 1988 (ref. 58)	Recommended that nutritional assessment be done at admission or enrollment in all institutional or community-based health services for older adults. Recommended employment of RD or credentialed nutrition professionals in policy, planning, administrative, and coordination of aging programs. Addressed needs for health professionals to coordinate community-based services and institutional care. Urged the reimbursement of nutrition services for elders within inpatient, outpatient, and community settings by third-party payers.	Recommended that health-related agencies and associations develop and coordinate messages to meet needs of elderly; utilize advanced communication techniques appropriate to older adults; develop and disseminate successful public/private sector models for health promotion. Recommended the reversal of shortages of knowledgeable personnel in areas of nutrition education, research, and service by training health professionals in nutrition.	Recommended that institutional and community-based food services be evaluated against appropriate nutritional standards for older individuals (RDAs, etc.).

White House Conference on Aging, 1981 (ref. 44)

Committee resolutions recommended reimbursement of nutritional assessment or counseling of elders provided by RDs from Medicaid/Medicare programs.

Called for a task force appointed by the president to devise and execute a program for nutrition education through the mass media. Recommended that laws be strengthened to require public service time on radio and television. Advocated use of mass media to train neighborhood leaders. Recommended that nutrition education be incorporated into all food service delivery systems and programs for older adults.

perform activities of daily living; improve access to and use of supportive social and primary health care services; decrease alcohol and tobacco use; and increase physical activity. In addition, related health objectives were identified for reducing the morbidity and mortality associated with chronic diseases including heart disease, hypertension and stroke, certain cancers, and diabetes. A series of nutrition-related objectives for older persons was also set forth. Primary attention was placed on improvements in dietary intake of older individuals, particularly reducing total and saturated fat and sodium intakes; assuring adequate dietary levels of essential micronutrients; reducing the prevalence of obesity; improving access to food and nutrition services (particularly home-delivered meals and congregate feeding); and promoting the availability of nutrition services, in particular, nutritional assessment, counseling, and education, provided by qualified nutrition professionals to older individuals. *Healthy People 2010* carried forward the objectives of *Healthy People 2000* but was further expanded to place emphasis on closing health-related gaps between minorities and the general population. *Healthy People 2010* also expanded nutrition-related objectives to include prevention of foodborne illnesses.

Although the nation's policy directives provide overall goals for nutrition and related health interventions, they do not establish detailed recommendations for the nutrient-specific goals of behaviorally based dietary interventions in individuals. Such goals and standards for planning have been compiled by the Food and Nutrition Board of the National Academy of Sciences.[59] Its guidelines, termed the Dietary Reference Intakes (DRI), expand and replace the Recommended Dietary Allowances (RDA). They are designed to provide quantitative estimates of nutrient intake for use in many settings, including assessing diets and menu planning, which assures the adequacy of intakes for energy, macronutrients, and selected micronutrients. The DRI include RDA as goals for the intake of individuals; they represent the recommended average daily intake that is sufficient to meet the nutrient needs of nearly all (97–98%) healthy people in a particular age group. They also include three new types of reference values including Adequate Intake (AI), Tolerable Upper Intake Level (UL), and Estimated Average Requirement (EAR). An improvement over the earlier RDAs is the inclusion of two older adult age groups, 51–70 years, and over 70 years. When an RDA cannot be determined, an AI is set as the recommended intake level based upon observational or experimental data on approximated nutrient intake in a group (or groups) of healthy people. The UL is the highest level of daily nutrient intake that is unlikely to pose no health risk in the general population. The EAR is the level of nutrient intake estimated to meet the nutrient needs of half of the healthy people in a group. The EAR is used in determining recommended levels of intake and provides a reference standard for assessing the adequacy of population (group) intake.

Several other groups, including the Office of the Surgeon General,[18,58] the Institute of Medicine,[12,23] the Committee on Diet and Health of the National Research Council,[60] the American Dietetic Association,[26] and the Nutrition Screening Initiative,[22] have also published recommendations for nutrition and healthy aging. They are generally consistent with the *Healthy People 2000* and *Healthy People 2010* and the RDA/DRI guidelines. These reports emphasize the importance of targeting public nutrition education to the older population; the use of individualized and behaviorally based dietary interventions to lower chronic disease risk; the promotion of elder functional independence; and the prevention of adverse consequences from the use of medications that may alter nutritional status.[12,18,26,60] It has been suggested that, as a general measure, population-based recommendations for older persons might include the adoption of dietary patterns that lower total fat and saturated fat; increase complex carbohydrates, fiber, nutrient-rich fruits and vegetables; and reduce sodium intake.[12,23,61]

Furthermore, the development of nutrition interventions for individuals with cognitive and physical impairments were recommended to ensure the consumption of the recommended levels of essential nutrients.[23] These reports point out that population-based dietary guidelines established for the younger adult population appear generally suitable for promoting health and nutritional well-being in the older population. Cited reports include the Food Guide Pyramid and related Dietary Guidelines,[56] the general adult population recommendations set forth by the Committee on Diet and Health,[60] the National Cholesterol Education Program (ATP III),[61] the National Cancer Institute,[62] and the Seventh Report of the Joint National Committee on the Prevention, Detection, Evaluation, and Treatment of High Blood Pressure: The JNC 7 Report (JNC 7).[63] Of particular note is that the JNC 7 Report puts forth a dietary pattern intervention strategy (the DASH diet) that has been formally evaluated in randomized clinical trials of middle-aged and older adults.[64,65]

Additional recommendations set forth by the Nutrition Screening Initiative (NSI) deserve particular attention.[66-72] Although not a governmental body responsible for national health policy, NSI is a collaboration of over 25 professional organizations in the United States that are interested in improving the nutrition and health status of the older population. The initiative is committed to increasing public awareness of the nutritional needs of the older population, promoting optimal nutrition in advancing age, and developing strategies for nutritional risk assessment and intervention planning. Through a consensus-building process and ongoing research, the Nutrition Screening Initiative has developed methods for increasing consumer awareness of nutrition problems and methods for the in-depth detection of nutritional risk among older people.[66-71] Most recently, the initiative published dietary management guidelines for chronic disease care in older individuals.[72] The publication relies on *evidence-based* information, where available, to develop specific recommended strategies for managing the clinical features of various health conditions including cancer, chronic obstructive pulmonary disease,

congestive heart failure, coronary heart disease, dementia, diabetes mellitus, hypertension, failure to thrive, osteoporosis, and pneumonia.

Consensus-based information was used to develop recommendations for dietary intervention where research was more limited or unavailable. Information was also assessed and provided on the expected outcomes of nutrition intervention and the profile of suitable providers of professional nutrition care. The report also highlights the results of several recent research investigations on the cost-effectiveness of nutrition care in older adults in hospital and community settings. It was estimated that the delivery of appropriate nutrition intervention to elders would save up to $1.3 billion in health-related costs by the year 2002.[73] Research of this nature gives us information from which we can draw conclusions concerning the efficacy of nutrition interventions in older adults that were highlighted by the IOM.[12,23]

PROVIDING NUTRITION SERVICES TO OLDER PERSONS

The major recommendations of national government agencies and professional organizations for nutrition services and intervention activities among elders are summarized in Table 20-4. These policy statements and guidelines generally consider that older individuals, particularly those of advanced age or with multiple medical problems, may require a complicated array of nutrition and health-related services. They also acknowledge that services may be provided by various providers in community, home, and institutional settings. Under these circumstances, an urgent need to integrate and coordinate the provision of care to older individuals is recognized. These themes were voiced in the Surgeon General's recommendations regarding public nutrition services for the aging population and were echoed in the 2000 (and earlier) Institute of Medicine report recommending Medicare reimbursement for medical nutrition therapy in ambulatory, institutional, and home-care settings.[12,18]

It was suggested that nutrition services, with particular emphasis on nutritional assessment and "guidance," be offered in institutional health care settings (hospitals, nursing homes, etc.) as well as in community-based health and social service delivery settings (senior centers, congregate nutrition programs, adult day care centers, etc.). It was also recommended that the emerging networks of social and support service providers (home health care providers, managed care networks, etc.) recognize the importance of nutrition in advancing age and arrange for appropriate types of nutrition services for their older clients.

These recommendations are similar to those proposed by Weddle et al.[26] in the American Dietetic Association (ADA) position paper on nutrition and aging. The ADA's positions advocated that nutrition services be included throughout the emerging continuum of long-term health care services for the elderly. The recommended types of nutrition services involved clinical nutrition care (*medical nutrition therapy*), such as *nutritional screening, assessment, monitoring, and evaluation*; individual or family *nutrition education and counseling*; and *enteral or parenteral medical nutrition support*. Other recommended nutrition service activities included the delivery of prepared meals in congregate, institutional, or home settings; the establishment of food pantries or other community resources; related activities that improve access to food (such as transportation, shopping assistance, and Food Stamps); and meal preparation and eating assistance-related activities (such as those carried out by homemakers, home health aides, or occupational therapists).[73,74]

Nutrition screening is described as a focused activity that is designed to identify people who need a particular type of nutrition service or program.[26,27,42,45,66,75] Screening is usually conducted by community agencies, programs, or clinic personnel to identify those with elevated risk for nutritional problems or to determine special considerations in managing an individual's situation (eg, edentulousness, confinement to bed, food allergies or preferences, and therapeutic diet

needs). *Nutritional assessment* determines the individual's nutritional status, identifies significant nutritional problems, and investigates the problems' etiologies and possible solutions. In conducting assessments, trained professionals utilize a relatively complex and comprehensive set of clinical and laboratory techniques. *Nutritional status monitoring* is a process whereby assessments are conducted at predetermined, regular intervals, allowing an assessment of the changes in an individual's or population's nutritional status over time. *Evaluation research*, particularly *outcomes research,* provides a formal mechanism by which to assess the impact of nutrition services on the individual's nutritional status and health. These studies may also include estimates of the costs of providing care and the potential health care cost savings that result from nutritional interventions. *Nutrition education* and *counseling* may occur on an individual level or in small groups with families or clients. (It is noted that population-level nutrition awareness and education activities directed to the older population are important to implement.) Education and counseling are ideally carried out by professionals who are trained to manage behaviorally based, targeted nutrition interventions that clearly address the unique needs of the older population (including subgroups that vary in dietary pattern and disease risk profiles). Nutritional support is a specialized form of clinical nutritional care that involves the planning and management of parenteral and enteral feedings. These services are discussed further by the American Dietetic Association in its publication *Nutrition Services Payment Systems.*[75]

The concept of a health care continuum, as emphasized in the ADA recommendations described above,[26] was first defined in a 1982 California law. It was proposed that there be established "a coordinated continuum of diagnostic, therapeutic, rehabilitative, supportive and maintenance services that addresses the health, social, and personal needs of (older) persons."[76] Posner and Krachenfels[34] presented one of the first models for integrating a continuum of nutrition and health services for older persons within institutional and community-based settings. (Figure 20–5.) As in the most recent ADA statement,[26] it is recognized that older people may receive health care services and related benefits in a variety of settings (at home, in the community, or within institutions) and providers of necessary services may have diverse backgrounds, resources, and orientations. For example, Food Stamps may be handled by community agencies and personnel whose expertise lies in income-related services and programs. Adult day care and home care may be handled by local community social service agencies, which provide a number of benefits (shopping assistance, social services) and refer clients to other programs and services (eg, homemakers and home health aides). The diagnosis and treatment of chronic diseases and the management of terminal illness may be carried out by a network of community-based health and social service providers (eg, health centers, HMOs, ambulatory care centers, private practitioners' offices, or hospices). Institutions (eg, hospitals, rehabilitation centers, and skilled nursing facilities) may provide acute and chronic

care. Increasingly, hospitals are providing short-term care and other community-based and home care providers potentially less costly, alternative care settings, deliver follow-up care.[26,45,77–81] This complex matrix of services, often referred to as the *long-term care system*, presents considerable challenges to those who are attempting to coordinate and monitor service delivery to their older clients.

The integration of nutrition and health care activities for elders is consistent with the recommendations of the Surgeon General, the White House Conference on Aging, the Institute of Medicine, and *Healthy People 2000* and *Healthy People 2010*.[12,18,20,21,23,44] These reports underscore the importance of considering and planning for the nutritional needs of elders, regardless of the setting in which health care services are provided. Several of the reports explicitly recommend that health care reimbursement guidelines cover nutrition services provided by credentialed professionals, particularly RDs, and related food services (congregate and home meals), enteral and parenteral nutrition products, and supplemental feedings.

Health Care Setting along the Continuum of Care	Ambulatory/Community/Home-Based Care/Services	Acute/Skilled Nursing/Long-Term Care/Services
	• Private Practitioners • Health Centers • HMOs • PPOs • Ambulatory Care Centers • Home Health Care Providers • Adult Day Care Centers • Senior Centers	• Hospitals • Rehabilitation Centers • Extended/Skilled Care Facilities • Hospices
Optimal Nutritional Services	• Screening • Assessment • Monitoring & Evaluation • Education & Training • Counseling • Meals/Food Services/Food Access Initiative (Food Stamps, shopping assistance, etc.) • Case Management • Clinical Nutrition Care	

Figure 20–5 Nutrition in the Continuum of Health Services for Older Americans

The NSI has also developed guidelines and recommends methods for screening and in-depth evaluation of nutritional risk in older populations and the designation of appropriate interventions.[22,70,72] The NSI-validated method for assessing warning signs of poor nutritional status in older adults is an easily self-administered 10-item checklist.[66] (Chapter 21) The technique is intended to guide individuals to social service and health care professionals with whom to discuss nutritional concerns and, as needed, to refer those with potential problems to professionals for further assessment and follow-up. At the initial in-depth nutritional assessment of the older individuals, NSI recommends concentrating on changes in body weight, eating habits (ie, dietary patterns), living environment, and functional status that may reflect adverse alterations in nutritional status. More specific diagnostic techniques are considered in later stages of nutritional risk assessment, such as anthropometric measurements, physical observations, laboratory data, cognitive and emotional assessments, detailed questions to evaluate medication use, eating practices, living environment, and functional status. The guidelines and methods are intended to identify those individuals with common nutritional problems such as protein-calorie malnutrition, obesity, or medical conditions (including cognitive impairment or depression), which can have a profound adverse impact on nutritional well-being.[69] NSI has urged clinicians to incorporate nutritional screening as part of routine activities in free-living and institutionalized elderly populations in order to develop appropriate interventions. Several publications provide guidelines for professionals who are involved in nutritional care of older individuals.[66–72]

In summary, there is striking consensus in recent national policy statements and the recommendations of professional groups that nutritional risk assessment and interventions are important components of health care delivery to older persons. There is recognition that the nutritional problems of the elderly span a spectrum from frank nutrient deficiencies, like protein-energy malnutrition, to nutritional excesses, exhibited in obesity, hypercholesterolemia, hypertension, and diabetes. There is also attention given to the importance of assuring that an individual's dietary intake is adequate to meet nutrient requirements, particularly among those who may experience food insecurity for financial, cognitive, functional, or other reasons. As well, these recommendations stress that preventive nutrition is as important among elders as in younger populations. Dietary management for the prevention of the chronic diseases of aging and their adverse complications are likewise evident. Guidelines are provided that promote energy intake to maintain ideal body weight, lower total and saturated fat intake, reduce sodium and sugar intake, and increase fiber-, calcium-, and fluoride-containing foods.

Despite the increasing recognition of the importance of nutrition in assuring the health of elders and emerging consensus on nutrition services and interventions, it is only recently that nutrition services provided by recognized professionals in specific health care settings will be reimbursed under Medicare. Landmark legislation became effective in January 2002 to extend Medicare Part B benefits to cover preventive and therapeutic nutrition services in the treatment of diabetes and renal disease. Details will be described in the following section, but it is noted that significant gaps continue to exist in the provision of a continuum of nutrition services for older adults. At present, there is, at best, a loosely integrated network of health care providers who may or may not consider the nutritional needs of their older clients. Until nutrition services are more broadly addressed in the legislation that covers other health and social services for older Americans, the goals set in the national policy statements for providing frameworks that assure the optimal nutritional status of older Americans will not be met. It is further noted that there are limitations in the existing models for the delivery of individualized or targeted nutrition services to older populations and individuals. Although it is generally recognized that nutrition interventions need to consider the individual's food preferences, the specific health and nutritional risks associated with the individual's pattern of dietary intake, as well as environmental and personal barriers to optimal food and nutrient intake (ie, that they need to be targeted), there are few models for the systematic design and delivery of behaviorally based strategies at either the individual or populations level. Traditionally, nutrition interventions set common goals and offered limited dietary planning options; they tended to focus on the provision of didactic information and often neglected to offer individualized, behaviorally based strategies for changing food and nutrient intake or dietary patterns. These approaches have failed to bring about long-term changes in nutrition behavior and associated health outcomes and have been pinpointed as among the factors which have limited progress in achieving success with certain national health initiatives.[53–55,61]

As noted in the earlier discussion of the Framingham Nutrition Studies (FOS), a new methodology has emerged for more targeted nutritional risk assessment and intervention planning. It centers on the characterization of the dietary patterns of men and women and targets their healthful and less healthful behavioral components. Because the dietary patterns can be characterized, linked to nutritional risk, and chronic disease profiles of adult males and females (Figure 20–4 and Tables 20–1 and 20–2), the dietary pattern approach also offers a framework for planning preventive nutrition interventions at the individual and population levels.[50–55] Health professionals now have new tools to identify informative, behaviorally based dietary patterns that can be used for specific eating behaviors in nutrition interventions aimed at health promotion and chronic disease risk reduction in adult men and women. For each dietary pattern, priorities can be set for changing healthful and less healthful eating practices. It seems quite feasible to guide adult men and women toward gradual improvements in their eating practices from the basis of their habitual dietary patterns. The recognition that dietary patterns are associated with disease risk factor profiles and health outcomes[53–55] provides the important evidence basis for behaviorally

based nutrition interventions in aging men and women to lower chronic disease risk and promote health and well-being.

One should recognize that the dietary pattern approach differs from strategies that advocate uniform diets for all. In contrast, this new method offers a framework for maintaining the *healthful* food intake behaviors, regardless of dietary pattern, while nutrition education and counseling is targeted at promoting gradual changes to modify *less healthful* behaviors and to achieve expert guidelines. The dietary pattern approach, when linked to the individual's biological risk factor profile and medical conditions, further enables the tailoring of relevant and innovative nutrition interventions. At the population level, one would envision that nutrition intervention strategies and communication messages would emerge that are targeted toward the dietary patterns of each subgroup of adult men and women. Thus, formulated, targeted nutrition messages would highlight the favorable and less desirable aspects of each dietary pattern in order to better promote optimal nutritional status in the aging adult population. The importance of individualized and targeted nutrition interventions is increasingly recognized in expert nutrition guideline reports.[61] It is exciting that emerging methods in nutrition epidemiology now allow the formal identification of the dietary patterns of men and women to enable innovative preventive nutrition interventions and health communications (education) campaigns at the individual and population levels. Recommendations and more specific insights into the dietary pattern approach to preventive nutrition intervention are discussed in published Framingham research.[50–55] Future research is needed to extend this work and to explore alternative methodologies for using the dietary pattern approach in clinical nutrition practice and public health promotions.

The following section examines the available federally funded nutrition programs and services, in particular the Elder Nutrition Program and Food Stamps. The primary mechanisms for financing nutrition services for older persons in health care settings, Medicare and Medicaid, are also discussed.

NUTRITION SERVICES FOR OLDER POPULATIONS

Table 20–5 summarizes the features of the major federally funded nutrition programs that are available to elders including the Elder Nutrition Program and Food Stamps. The table also summarizes the major elements of Medicare and Medicaid health care reimbursement systems that can be utilized for providing nutrition services to older individuals. The following sections discuss these programs, their eligibility requirements and service definitions, and their strengths and limitations in assuring a continuum of nutrition services for older people.

FEDERALLY FUNDED NUTRITION PROGRAMS

Community-Based Titles III and VI Nutrition Program for Older Americans

In 1972, Congress amended the Older Americans Act of 1965 (OAA) to establish a national Elder Nutrition Program (ENP). This initiative was established after four years of successful community-based demonstration projects that provided congregate meals (and home meals for the homebound elders) in community-based settings that encouraged social activities and support of noninstitutionalized elders. In the ensuing three decades, ENP has become the largest publicly funded and longest-standing program of coordinated community- and home-based preventive health-related and social services for the nation's elders.[27,44,45,48,80–83] The program responds to evidence of prevalent malnutrition in certain older population segments and emerging evidence of the importance of nutrition in maintaining health and managing medical problems in elders.

ENP distributes funding under Titles of the OAA to states (State Units on Aging [SUAs]) and U.S. territories, and under Title VI to Indian Tribal Organizations (ITOs), for a national network of programs that provide congregate and home-delivered meals for elderly people. ENP funding helps maintain an elaborate infrastructure of Area Agencies on Aging and Nutrition Projects at the regional and local levels, respectively, for the delivery of nutrition and related health and supportive social services to older clients (Figure 20–6). Nutrition programs are required to provide at least one meal a day that meets one-third of the Recommended Dietary Allowances (RDA) and to operate 5 or more days a week.[45] Lesser known, but of great importance, is the role of ENP in administering and/or delivering other health and supportive social services including *access initiatives* (transportation, outreach, information, and referral), *in-home services* (homemaker, home health aide, personal care, and chore assistance), and *community-based health and supportive social activities* (medical screening, case management, legal and financial assistance and counseling, physical fitness programs, rehabilitation services, and social and recreational activities).[42]

ENP maintains two major meal service delivery systems—one which provides community-based congregate (group) and individual services to the ambulatory older population and the other that delivers services to the frail, homebound elderly. ENP services emphasize preventive nutrition, particularly the provision of congregate and home-delivered meals (often called "meals on wheels"), as well as nutrition screening, education, and counseling.

Federal law mandates that ENP be available to all older Americans (those 60 years and older and their spouses regardless of age) and that client contributions (payment) for services be strictly voluntary. Within federal funding limitations, the ENP attempts to strategically place local projects in community facilities that serve those in greatest need: the poor, minority, and frail elderly. Older individuals voluntarily become ENP clients and are referred by health and medical providers (such as hospitals, private physicians, group medical practices, social service agencies, etc.) as well as informal family and social networks.

Table 20–5 Nutrition Programs and Services for Older Adults

Program	Type of Intervention	Funding Source	Eligible/Available Services	Percentage of Older Population Served
FEDERAL NUTRITION PROGRAMS				
Title III and VI Elder Nutrition Program (refs. 84, 88)	Nutrition and socialization intervention. Providing meals, therapeutic diets, access initiatives, and community-based and home health and related supportive social services.	DHHS OHDS AoA	Congregate and home meals; transportation; shopping assistance; outreach; information and referral; nutrition education; case management; homemakers; home health aides; legal and financial counseling; personal care and chore services; fitness and rehabilitation programs; social and recreational activities.	10% to 13% of population 60+ years of age and up to one-third of elder, low-income and minority elders. 50% to 80% of the eligible low-income elderly.
Food Stamps (ref. 93)	Income subsidy	USDA SSA	Coupons for food purchases or cash equivalent	
NUTRITION SERVICES PAYMENT SYSTEMS				
Medicare/ Medicaid (refs. 98, 99)	Third-party payment system: hospital insurance, medical insurance, and extended benefits.	DHHS CMS, SSA	Covers medical and health-related services provided by participating hospitals, HMOs, private medical practices, ambulatory centers, rehabilitation and skilled nursing facilities, home health agencies, and hospice programs. Eligibility for nutrition services varies depending on the setting, reimbursement for care, and their deemed medical necessity. Home meals, enteral/ parenteral nutrition, and weight reduction are particularly limited.	40 million beneficiaries 65 years and older.

AoA   = United States Department of Health and Human Services, Administration on Aging
CMS   = United States Department of Health and Human Services, Centers for Medicare & Medicaid Services formerly known as the Health Care Financing Administration (HCFA)
DHHS   = United States Department of Health and Human Services
HMO   = Health maintenance organization
OHDS   = United States Department of Health and Human Services, Office of Human Development Services
PHS   = United States Department of Health and Human Services, Public Health Services
SSA   = Social Security Administration
USDA   = United States Department of Agriculture

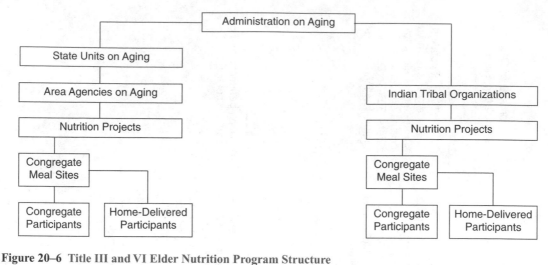

Figure 20–6 Title III and VI Elder Nutrition Program Structure

The Administration on Aging currently distributes about $565 million annually in ENP federal funding to a national network of 57 State and Territorial Units on Aging, 670 Area Agencies on Aging, and over 200 Indian Tribal Organizations (ITOs).[83] It is estimated that ENP provides services to 2.6 million elders through community sites and delivered meals and other in-home services to over 884,000 frail elders.[83,84]

ENP gains additional spending power from a cash/commodity entitlement program supported by the USDA, which expands the resources and meals available through the nutrition program. Federal legislation gives states the option to elect to receive food commodities, cash at a fixed amount per meal served to eligible participants per year, or a flexible combination of food and cash. This support from the USDA exceeds $150 million.[83] Other ENP program revenues are realized from donations from older participants toward meal costs, private or public grant funding or donations, and the value of volunteerism in the program. In 1999 less than half of all ENP resources were from federal funding; 44% of congregate meals and 30% of home-delivered meals were provided through the Administration on Aging.[83]

Many researchers have attempted to determine the impact of ENP on the nutritional well-being and health of older participants.[79,82,85–90] From these reports, it appears that ENP attracts "high-risk" elders, improves food and nutrient intake among participants, and provides beneficial socialization and recreation. Balsam and Rogers[74] found that many NPOA sites were compelled to become innovative in meeting the nutritional needs of its participants. Beyond the congregate and home meals that are required by law, these researchers found that many nutrition programs across the nation provide therapeutic diets; food pantries; ethnic meals; luncheon clubs; breakfast, weekend, and evening meals; and meals for the homeless older population.

Although evaluations of NPOA have demonstrated its effectiveness, design issues limit their generalizability. Most have been conducted in selected, local settings and have not provided a national perspective. Since the last comprehensive national program evaluation more than 10 years ago, ENP has undergone many changes. Since that time, there have been increased numbers of home-delivered meals, targeted services for older persons with the greatest economic or social needs, and the expansion of long-term care activities within the ENP infrastructure to support independent living and functional independence and to reduce risks for premature institutionalization in older clients.[34,82]

For these reasons, in 1992, Congress mandated a comprehensive evaluation of ENP to inform national health policy development. The congressional mandate set forth a set of research questions, several of which are highlighted here:

- Are ENP services well-targeted and reaching elders at greatest health risk?
- Does ENP favorably influence its major mandated health-related outcomes?
- What is the role of ENP in the provision of a continuum of long-term care health and supportive social services to elders?

The ENP evaluation study included a nationally representative sample of the program's ambulatory and homebound clients and a matched comparison sample of eligible elders who do not receive ENP services. Comparison sample elders were drawn from the Health Care Finance Administration (HCFA) now the Center for Medicare and Medicaid Services (CMS) Medicare Beneficiary listings and were individuals who were in the same postal zip code areas as the ENP clients.[79]

Trained field staff conducted in-person interviews and elicited information on subjects' demographic profiles, health status indicators, nutrient intake, and levels of socialization. From a health status perspective, subjects were asked about their current medical conditions, recent hospitalizations and nursing home admissions, and level of physical functioning. Functional status was determined using standardized ADL and IADL inventories.[91] Warning signs of poor nutrition were assessed using the NSI validated checklist and its criteria for interpretation.[66,67,71] Standardized protocols[79] were used to directly measure subjects' heights and weights for the purpose of calculating body mass index (BMI = weight (kg)/height (m^2)). BMIs were compared against clinical standards for older persons to evaluate the prevalence of under- and overweight. Nutrient intake was estimated from 24-hour di-

etary recall interviews that were conducted with validated instruments[92] and standardized protocols. The University of Minnesota Nutrition Coordinating Center nutrient database (Data Collection NDS Version 2.6) was used to estimate nutrient intake of participants and nonparticipants.

The sociodemographic profiles of ambulatory and homebound ENP clients in the Title III and VI programs are compared with the overall United States population in Figure 20–7. Those served by

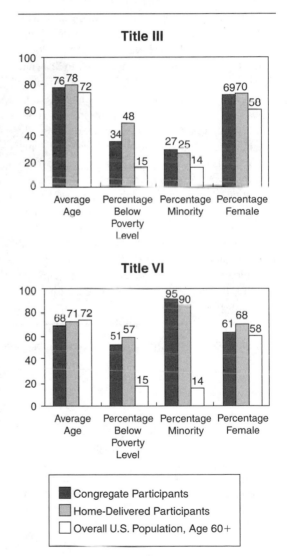

Figure 20–7 Socioeconomic Characteristics of ENP Participants

Title III tend to be older by 4 to 6 years than United States elders overall and include proportionately more females (69–70% of ENP participants are female in contrast with 58% in the population 60 years and older overall). About twice the proportion of minority elders participate in the ENP than are in the older United States population; overall, 25–27% of clients (compared with 14%) are minority older individuals. Some 12–19% of Title III clients are African American and 5–12% are Hispanic minorities. There is more than twice the proportion of impoverished elders being served by Title III than are in the general population. Some 79–90% of ENP clients have incomes below 200% of the DHHS poverty level in contrast to 38% nationally; the proportion of low-income minority elders that receive Title III services is about four times greater than their proportion in the overall older population. Title VI subjects are only slightly younger than United States elders overall (68 and 71 years in the congregate and home-delivered programs). As in Title III, women are more likely to participate in Title VI and there are considerably more impoverished and minority participants than in the United States population overall.

The health characteristics of ambulatory and homebound Title III and VI clients are compared in Table 20–6. On average, ambulatory recipients of Title III services have 2.4 chronic health prob-lems compared with 3.0 in homebound clients; the proportions for Title VI subjects are 2.8 and 2.9, respectively. Some 26–43% of Title III and 30–37% of Title VI participants have been institutionalized (hospitalized or entered nursing homes) in the past year. About one-quarter of ambulatory and 77% of homebound Title III clients and 23% and 44% of Title VI clients, respectively, have difficulty performing one or more activities of daily living, including shopping for food or preparing meals. About two-thirds of both the ambulatory and homebound Title III and VI clients have a weight (as assessed by body mass index) that is outside the healthy range for older persons; however, those who are ambulatory are more likely to be overweight whereas homebound clients are more likely to be underweight.[48,79] From 64–88% of Title III and VI clients reported behaviors or profile characteristics that indicated moderate to high risk for potential nutritional problems by the NSI checklist criteria.

This study emphasized two priority outcomes of ENP that relate directly to overall health and risk of institutionalization in the older population: improvements in participants' levels of nutrient intake and patterns of socialization. The mean daily nutrient intakes of ENP clients, expressed as a percentage of the Recommended

Table 20–6 Health Characteristics of Ambulatory and Homebound Title III and VI Clients

	Title III		Title VI	
	Congregate	Home-Delivered	Congregate	Home-Delivered
Average Diagnosed Chronic Health Conditions (number)	2.4	3.0	2.8	2.9
Hospital/Nursing Home Stays in Previous Year (%)	26	43	30	37
Weight Outside of Health Range (%)	61	64	65	69
Difficulty doing One or More Everyday Tasks (%)	23	77	23	44
Unable to or Have Much Difficulty Preparing Meals (%)	8	41	8	26
Moderate to High Nutritional Risk (%)	64	88	80	78

Dietary Allowances[59] for persons 50 years of age and older, are compared with the matched research comparison group in Figure 20–8. ENP clients' mean daily nutrient intake approached or exceeded the Recommended Dietary Allowances for all nutrients except energy and zinc. For the entire range of essential nutrients studied, ENP clients had consistently higher levels of nutrient

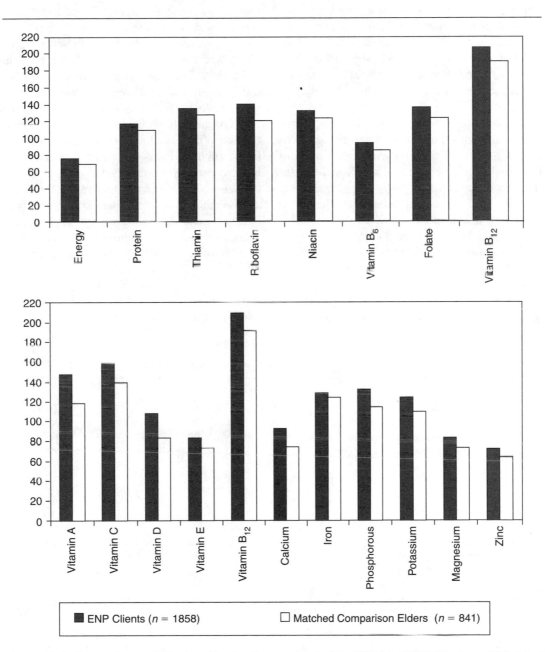

Figure 20–8 Comparisons of Nutrient Intakes (as a percent of the RDA) in ENP Clients and Matched Comparison Elders

intake than matched comparison elders. Intakes of all essential nutrients were significantly higher except for vitamin B_{12} and iron. In addition, mean intakes of dietary fat and cholesterol were not higher among ENP clients compared with nonclients and approached or achieved recommended levels of intake (30% of total energy intake and under 300 mg per day, respectively). The ENP meals were also found to contribute between 30% and 50% of total daily nutrient intake among congregate and homebound program participants.[48,79]

Socialization patterns of ENP clients are compared also with those of matched comparison elders. Results of the ENP evaluation indicate that ENP clients experienced a 17% increase in monthly social contacts.[48,79]

Table 20–7 presents a summary of the long-term care health-related services that are currently offered by Title III and VI programs. Over half of the Title III and VI program sites currently offer their clients information and referral services, recreation and social activities, transportation services to a variety of settings (to meals, health care providers, etc.), and counseling activities. About 7–14% of programs offer homemakers services; fewer provide personal care services and home health aides.

It is important to note that while service provision is relatively high in the ENP sites, the data in Table 20–7 underestimate the role of the ENP infrastructure in the delivery of long-term care services. As part of the ENP evaluation, various levels of the ENP program administrative structure were evaluated concerning their roles in long-term care. It was quite clear from comprehensive interviews conducted in the State Units on Aging, the ITO administrative units, and the Area Agencies on Aging that most are involved in the administration, coordination, and direct delivery of home- and community-based long-term care services.[48,79] This aspect of ENP activities is

Table 20–7 Nutrition Projects Offering Various Types of Nonnutrition Services (Percentages)

Services Provided	Congregate Participants	Participants Home-Delivered
Title III		
Information and Referral	85	84
Recreation and Social Activities	69	NA
Transportation to and from Meal Site	68	NA
Other Assisted and Nonassisted Transportation	57	58
Other Counseling	53	55
Home Services	12	14
Personal Care Services	4	5
Home Health Aide Services	5	6
Title VI		
Information and Referral	89	86
Recreation and Social Activities	75	NA
Transportation to and from Meal Site	83	NA
Other Assisted and Unassisted Transportation	77	81
Other Counseling	49	52
Home Services	7	7
Personal Care Services	7	7
Home Health Aide Services	4	4

NA= Not applicable

important to underscore since ENP is often viewed strictly as a nutrition program. This evaluation documented the major role these programs have in attempting to provide a coordinated continuum of care for their elder clients.

The ENP evaluation demonstrates that the program is well-targeted, efficient, and effective in providing health-related and supportive social services to the elders at greater health risk, in particular low-income and minority elders. The study underscores the emerging role of ENP in the coordination of long-term care activities for homebound and ambulatory elders in community settings. It is intriguing that the coordination of this care evolved from the long-standing activities of community providers in the delivery of meals to needy elders. Once again, this serves to emphasize the importance of nutrition and its central role in maintaining the health and independence of elders. The ENP offers a model framework for the coordination of a continuum of health and related supportive, social services to elders, particularly the low-income and minority elder populations.

Food Stamps

The USDA Food Stamp program, which was authorized by the 1964 Food Stamp Act, provides an income supplement to low-income households in the form of coupons or electronic benefit transfer (EBT) cards used to purchase food. About 2 million American households headed by older people, or between 40% and 80% of eligible elders, currently participate in the Food Stamp program.[93] Reasons cited for nonparticipation by eligible older people include the "stigma of welfare" associated with the program's income means test, lack of information on program availability, and the perceived complexity of the application process.[94] In recognition of low participation rates in the Food Stamp program (FSP) by low-income, elderly individuals, USDA implemented the Elderly Nutrition Demonstration in six states (Arizona, Connecticut, Florida, Maine, Michigan, and North Carolina) in 2002. Three strategies to increase participation were tested: simplifying the

eligibility requirements for elderly individuals, directly assisting them with completing the application process, or offering them the option of receiving packages of commodities each month instead of getting benefits through an electronic benefits transfer card. Preliminary analysis indicates that FSP participation by the elderly rose substantially after the test programs started. In Arizona, Florida, Maine, and North Carolina, participation grew significantly more in intervention counties than in nonintervention counties.

Results concerning the impact of food stamps on the nutritional status of participating households have been inconclusive. Butler et al.[95] and Lee and Frongillo[96] concluded that elderly food stamp participants consumed levels of nutrients that were similar to those of nonparticipants who had otherwise similar characteristics. They suggested that food stamps act as an effective income supplement but may not be a mechanism to improve the nutrient intake of older individuals. In contrast, Akin and colleagues[97] found that food stamp participants consumed higher levels of many nutrients than did members of nonparticipating households with similar incomes.

Further research is needed to resolve these conflicting findings. In particular, it is important to assess the specific role and impact of food stamps in the continuum of nutrition services and interventions involving older persons.

NUTRITION SERVICES PAYMENT SYSTEMS

In addition to federally funded mechanisms for the provision of congregate and home meals and related services to elder populations (under ENP) and the provision of income subsidies in the form of food stamps to eligible elders, the major mechanism for providing nutrition services to elder clients is the third-party payment system, notably Medicare and Medicaid. These programs provide guidelines for the reimbursement of health-related services in institutional, community, and home settings. A summary of the general guidelines that determine the nature and extent of coverage for nutrition services within Medicare and Medicaid is found in Table 20–5. The following discussion provides an overview of general policies and procedures that affect reimbursement of nutrition services within Medicare and Medicaid. Further details are provided by the ADA on policies for nutrition care services coverage and reimbursement under Medicare and Medicaid;[98] and the ADA's published procedures for implementing a Nutrition Services Payment System,[75] including service definitions and documentation, fee setting, billing, and patient monitoring procedures.

Medicare

The Medicare program receives its statutory authority under Title XVIII of the 1965 Social Security Act and is administered by the Centers for Medicare and Medicaid Services (CMS), formerly known as the Health Care Financing Administration (HCFA), of the United States Department of Health and Human Services. Medicare is a national health insurance program for persons 65 years and older, certain younger disabled persons, and those with kidney failure. HCFA forms partnerships with thousands of health care providers (hospitals, nursing homes, home health agencies, physicians, medical equipment suppliers, labs, and managed care plans such as HMOs) to provide reimbursement for services to over 40 million Medicare beneficiaries (ie, eligible people aged 65 years and older and disabled of all ages).[99] The Medicare program consists of four parts: part A (hospital insurance), part B (medical insurance), part C (Medicare + Choice), and part D (supplementary prescription drug plan). Part A covers inpatient hospital care, skilled nursing facility care, home health care, and hospice care. Part B provides reimbursement for "medical and other services" not covered by part A including outpatient physicians' services and hospital services, laboratory services, durable medical equipment, and other clinical, therapeutic, or rehabilitative professional services deemed to be "incident to the provision of medical care." These include physical and speech therapy and nutrition services (as determined

to be appropriate) and other items and services as specified by Medicare. Part C was established as part of the Balanced Budget Act of 1997 and is intended to enable Medicare enrollees to elect alternative health care (beyond the traditional fee-for-service plans) such as HMOs, preferred provider organizations, provider-sponsored organizations, and medical savings accounts. Medicare enrollees are required to pay deductible and coinsurance costs. They can also elect to purchase supplemental insurance, called Medigap insurance, a private insurance that is intended to help pay Medicare cost-sharing amounts.

Part A: Medicare Hospital Insurance

Medicare part A provides reimbursement for all covered costs of care in hospitals and skilled nursing facilities during defined "benefit periods." Medicare beneficiaries are responsible for hospital deductibles and coinsurance costs during their stays. Part A pays for a semiprivate room, meals, regular nursing services, drugs, medical supplies, lab tests, X-rays, and the use of operating and recovery rooms, intensive care and coronary care units, and other defined "medically necessary care." During hospital stays, Medicare does not pay for the use of phones, televisions, private duty nurses, or extra charges unless they are medically necessary.

While Medicare patients are in skilled nursing facilities, Medicare part A pays for semiprivate rooms, skilled nursing and rehabilitative services, and other defined services and supplies. Medicare provides full payment for skilled nursing facility care for up to 20 days, adjusted rates of payment from 21–100 days, and nothing after 100 days. Medicare part A provides payments for unlimited home health care as long as the patient requirements for "defined need" are met. Part A home health care benefits include part-time or nursing care, home health aide services, durable medical equipment (some beneficiary co-payment is required) and supplies, and other defined services. Hospice care is covered under Medicare part A as long as a physician certifies a beneficiary's need. Reimbursed care includes pain relief, symptom management, support services for the terminally ill person, and respite services.

Part B: Medicare Medical Insurance

Medicare part B helps pay doctors bills and a wide range of medical services and supplies in both in-patient and out-patient settings. Reimbursed medical expenses include physician fees; surgical services and supplies; physical, occupational, and speech therapy (when provided by therapists of the approved Medicare facility); mental health services; clinical services of psychologists and social workers; clinical laboratory services, prosthetic devices; braces; diagnostic tests and durable medical equipment (wheel chairs, etc.); and medical supplies (surgical dressings, ostomy bags, etc.). Part B also helps pay for ambulance transportation and certain preventive services such as flu shots, Pap smears, and mammography. Part B will also pay for home health care if beneficiaries do not have Medicare part A coverage. In January 2002, Medicare part B began reimbursement of Medical Nutrition Therapy (MNT) for beneficiaries with diabetes and non-dialysis kidney disease.

The new policy stated that Medical Nutrition Therapy must include nutritional diagnostic, therapeutic, and counseling services provided by a Registered Dietitian upon referral by a doctor. Services are covered based on calendar year and are limited to a certain number of hours of coverage. In preparation for MNT, the American Dietetic Association created Evidence-Based Nutrition Practice Guidelines/Protocols, which are utilized by most RDs who receive reimbursement under MNT. These protocols lay out a schedule of visits and the activities that should take place during each visit. For diabetes, five visits are recommended in the protocol, but the Medicare act allows for more if the referring physician believes it is necessary. In this case, the physician needs to write another referral for MNT and needs to document the order and change of condition in the patient's chart. The Centers for Medicare and Medicaid Services (CMS) paid approximately $800,000 in 2002 for MNT services delivered to approximately 10,000 individuals. There are currently no plans to expand this coverage to other conditions, but it is hoped that with the recent recognition of obesity as a medical condition, Medicare will cover obesity and related diseases in the near future.

Coverage of MNT and addition of preventative coverage to Medicare remains a dynamic topic. When Congress passed H.R. 1, the Medicare Prescription Drug, Improvement and Modernization Act in 2003, it included a provision that, for the first time, provides new preventive services to Medicare beneficiaries. Beginning January 1, 2005, Medicare pays for an initial preventive physical examination designed to determine the physical condition of new beneficiaries as they become eligible for Medicare. The bill provides for screening and other preventive services that include among other things, Medical Nutrition Therapy services provided by a Registered Dietitian (as defined by the current eligibility for providing MNT to diabetes and renal patients).

The second recently adopted expansion of MNT relates to the management of chronic diseases. The conference report establishes a voluntary chronic disease management program within the traditional Medicare program. The bill defines chronic diseases as "congestive heart failure, diabetes, chronic obstructive pulmonary disease, or other diseases or conditions, as selected by the Secretary [of Health and Human Services]." This provision went into effect January 1, 2006, and will be phased in over a period of three to five years. The program will require HHS to enter into agreements with chronic care improvement organizations (such as disease management organizations, health insurers, integrated delivery systems, physician group practices or other entities approved by HHS). During phase one, the program will cover at least 10% of Medicare beneficiaries. Phase two will evaluate how well the program functions and its cost-effectiveness before the program is expanded to cover all Medicare beneficiaries. Each individual chronic care management plan will (to the extent appropriate) include self-care education through approaches such as disease management or medical nutrition therapy and education for primary caregivers and family members.

Consistent with this approach is the targeted, behaviorally based framework of nutrition intervention that is discussed in the context of the Framingham studies in this chapter. Language in the conference report relating to medical nutrition therapy strongly indicates that it is the intent of Congress that Registered Dietitians will provide the MNT under this section of the bill. It should be noted that these new measures do not constitute a continuum of care and political and professional groups must continue to push progress forward if a true continuum is to develop. As with part A, Medicare part B beneficiaries are responsible for certain co-payments and deductibles. There are many medical services and items not covered by Medicare including routine physical exams, most dental care and dentures, routine foot care, hearing aids, most prescription drugs, and eyeglasses except if needed after cataract surgery.

Nutrition Services Reimbursement Conditions of Participation

The rates of Medicare reimbursement *to hospitals* for costs incurred in patient care are fixed and based on 470 diagnosis-related groups (DRGs). There is a flat reimbursement rate for each DRG regardless of the services that a patient receives. There is only limited flexibility within the Medicare reimbursement guidelines to adjust hospital reimbursement rates for patients who have unusually long hospital stays or multiple, complicated diagnoses. As a consequence, the DRG-based fixed payment system creates an incentive for hospitals that are able to limit patients' lengths of stay and encourages early patient discharge.

The Medicare program sets specific "conditions of participation" that must be met in order for the hospital to receive Medicare funding. Several of these conditions pertain to nutrition. A hospital that receives Medicare payments must have an organized dietary department. The guidelines, however, do not specify that it be headed by a Registered Dietitian. A consulting dietitian must be available to meet with medical and nursing staff and instruct patients on diet modifications, write diet histories, and participate in ward rounds and conferences. Diets must be recorded on patients' charts, and orders for therapeutic diets must appear there as well. Meals must be consistent with diet orders and must meet the National Research Council's RDA.[59] Although these guidelines provide general criteria for hospital nutrition services, they leave considerable latitude for determining the type and organization of these services and the availability of nutrition professionals for the provision of clinical nutrition care.

An additional factor that may determine the availability of nutrition services in the hospital setting is a voluntary hospital accreditation process that is carried out by the Joint Commission on Accreditation of Healthcare Organizations (JCAHO). Hospitals that participate in this process, including about 5200 of the 6700 hospitals that participate in Medicare,[34] are required to maintain a set of basic nutrition care services, including routine dietary screening; nutritional assessment of individual patients; clinical nutrition care (including the availability of both enteral and parenteral nutrition); dietary counseling; and the administration of safe, appropriate, and sanitary food service operations. The Joint Commission guidelines further emphasize the availability of qualified nutrition professionals in the provision of both food service and clinical nutrition care activities. There appears to be specific wording in the Medicare policy that denies separate coverage for nutritional supplements such as enteral feedings in the hospital setting; supplements are considered to be "self-administered drugs" and ineligible for coverage.

Hospitals consider the services necessary for Medicare and JCAHO participation and how to balance quality of care against cost efficiency. Under this system, the extent to which nutrition services are provided will, in part, depend on how they are perceived within the institutional framework. Nutrition services that are perceived as increasing the hospital's cost of providing care may be limited or not provided. Those nutrition services that are perceived as improving patients' rates of recovery or reducing hospital stays for a given diagnosis may be incorporated into the hospital's "core services."[80] This decision is made at the institutional level and is not regulated by the third-party payers. When provided, nutrition services are not reimbursed separately but are covered as part of the hospital's routine or administrative costs.

Special Considerations in Providing Nutrition Services under Medicare Ambulatory Settings

In addition to coverage of Medical Nutrition Therapy for diabetes and pre-dialysis renal disease, Medicare part B may cover nutrition services provided in hospital ambulatory centers or private physicians' offices if they are deemed "incident to medical care." Guidelines concerning nutrition services carried out in the hospital ambulatory center require that the nutrition professional be an employee of the hospital. Nutrition services provided in a private practice must be carried out by a professional who is an employee of the physician, rather than a private contractor; the physician must also be present to supervise the nutrition care. Unless specifically covered as MNT for diabetes or pre-dialysis renal disease, nutrition services in hospital-based ambulatory centers and private practice settings are billed by the hospital or medical practice as a medical visit and are reimbursed as such.

Health Maintenance Organizations

An HMO participating in the Medicare program must offer its Medicare beneficiaries the full range of services that are available to all HMO clients. The HMO legislation does include nutrition education and counseling as an allowable service but does not specify that these services be carried out by a professional with a specific background. Cost-containment concerns guide the development of the available services of HMOs, similar to the hospital setting. For these reasons, the profiles of nutrition services paid for by HMOs differ considerably across the nation. Since the adoption in 2002 of reimbursement for Medical Nutrition Therapy for diabetes and pre-dialysis renal disease some HMOs are following suit and also reimbursing for selected diagnoses.

Home Health Agencies

Home health agency services may be reimbursed under both Medicare parts A and B. To qualify, a patient or beneficiary must be homebound, under a physician's care, and in need of skilled nursing or speech or physical therapy. There are no limits to the number of home visits a person can receive and, unlike institution-based skilled nursing or rehabilitative care, the beneficiary need not have been hospitalized prior to receiving home care. Home services that are considered appropriate for reimbursement are generally those that would be provided under hospital-based care. Home meals, however, are specifically excluded since they are not a component of hospital care.

Home health agencies are reimbursed on a "reasonable cost" basis for visits; these rates include the administrative component of arranging care. In addition, the home health agency receives a negotiated overhead rate. Conditions for participation require that, as part of administrative overhead, the agency must develop a treatment plan for each client, including his or her diet. Therefore, nutrition services are allowable under the agency's administrative costs. Home visits by nutrition professionals are generally not allowed as separate visits; rather, the nutrition professionals' time is likely to be reflected in administrative costs and their level of effort reflective of the agency's case load. Parenteral and enteral nutrition products can be reimbursed under Medicare part B but must not be billed separately (ie, they are also included as an administrative cost).

Hospice Care

Medicare part A covers hospice care services, but guidelines specify limits on the length of allowable coverage and set ceilings on the total cost of service reimbursement per client. Many hospice programs across the country elect not to participate in the Medicare program because of these ceilings. Unlike other settings of care, dietary counseling is reimbursed directly. However, nutrition professionals are not designated as preferred providers of these services.

Medicaid

Medicaid is a publicly funded health insurance program for persons who meet certain low to moderate income eligibility guidelines. Medicaid is funded under Title XIX of the Social Security Act. It is difficult to generalize about the Medicaid program since each state determines the types of covered services, based on its resources and the needs of its population. However, Medicaid "conditions of participation" by settings of care are generally identical to those under the Medicare program. With regard to nutrition services, they may be covered if considered "incident to" ongoing medical care (as in hospital ambulatory care or private medical practice settings) or are part of service packages (as in the case of HMOs). Certain Medicaid programs may also specify guidelines for adult day care and personal care services provided to older people. These may exceed guidelines for services provided under Medicare. Despite similarities in participation guidelines, Medicaid coverage for services is generally considered more restricted than Medicare.

Summary

Public policy statements on nutrition and aging increasingly recognize the importance of nutrition in promoting the health of older populations and have begun to influence the Medicare and Medicaid programs toward expanded coverage for professional nutrition services along the continuum of health care for older persons. Going forward, it is important to advocate for the expansion of coverage for appropriate nutrition services relating to a broader range of chronic conditions associated with nutritional risk, in particular dyslipidemia, hypertension, osteoporosis,

overweight and obesity, and certain forms of cancer. No other set of activities would more effectively change the panorama of nutrition service options for aging American adults regardless of the settings in which health care and related services are provided.

CONCLUSION

The health and nutrition status of middle-aged and older adults have improved in this and the last century, but significant numbers of elder individuals have elevated nutritional risk and unmet needs for nutritional services. The most prevalent nutritional problems of those 60 years and older are the nutrition-related chronic diseases of aging, including coronary heart disease, hypertension, diabetes, certain cancers, overweight and obesity, and osteoporosis. These affect many, if not most, older people. There are also distinct subgroups of the older population, notably those who are socially isolated, racial and ethnic minorities, very old and frail, and poor, who are particularly at greatest nutritional risk (including nutritional excesses, imbalances, and deficiencies). The factors and personal characteristics that influence the nutritional status of older populations are better but inadequately understood. Considerable future research, of both a basic and applied nature, is needed to resolve these information deficits and to provide the evidence basis for improving the nutritional status of older Americans and providing appropriate nutrition programs and services throughout the continuum of health care.

The Elder Nutrition Program offers a model framework for the delivery of nutrition and related health and supportive social services to elders in home and community settings. The recent national evaluation provides strong evidence of its success and favorable impacts on nutrition and socialization of elder participants. There is also emerging evidence that the agencies involved in the delivery of ENP have evolved into an infrastructure that is increasingly involved in case management and the delivery of a continuum of services (beyond simply congregate or home-delivered meals) that support the independent living of older clients. These emerging roles of the ENP network are not well understood by those in institutional and ambulatory health care settings. Further integration of the community, home, and community-based health care settings is needed to coordinate a continuum of services that promote health and well-being in the older United States population.

The Medicare and Medicaid programs are changing in a direction that more clearly supports the delivery of preventive nutrition services and Medical Nutrition Therapy (MNT) by qualified professionals in the wide range of participating health care settings. Consistent with the emergence of Medicare/Medicaid funding, new, innovative, and evidence-based models are emerging from the Framingham Nutrition Studies, the Nutrition Screening Initiative, and others for comprehensive nutritional risk assessment and intervention planning. Among the most innovative techniques emerging from the field of nutrition epidemiology is the identification of the distinct dietary patterns of adult men and women that are associated with nutrient intake, compliance with expert dietary guidelines, and chronic disease risk. The dietary pattern approach offers new insights into the assessment of nutritional risk and the development of behaviorally based nutrition education and counseling activities in the aging population. Further advocacy and research in such areas are needed, particularly on the efficacy of nutrition interventions and services for older adults at the individual and population levels. Such efforts will enable the more complete realization of the goals set forth in our nation's public policy statements for the development of a coordinated continuum of preventive nutrition and related health programs and services for the older population.

The Framingham Nutrition Studies are supported by the National Heart, Lung, and Blood Institute grants R01-HL-60700 and R01-HL-54776. The Framingham Study is supported by NIH/NHLBI N01-HC-25195, Bethesda, MD, and Boston University, Boston, MA.

REFERENCES

1. Omran AR. A century of epidemiologic transition in the United States. *Prev Med* 1977;6:30–51.
2. Millen Posner B, Quatromoni PA, Franz M. Nutrition policies and intervention for chronic disease risk reduction in international settings: the *InterHealth* Nutrition Initiative. *Nutr Rev* 1994;52:179–187.
3. Millen Posner B, Franz M, Quatromoni P, InterHealth Steering Committee. Nutrition and the global risk for chronic diseases: the *InterHealth* nutrition initiative. *Nutr Rev* 1994;52:201–207.
4. National Vital Statistics Report. *Estimated Life Expectancy at Birth in Years, by race and sex.* Vol 52 No 14, Feb 18, 2004 http://www.cdc.gov/nchs/data/dvs/nvsr52_14t12.pdf.
5. Bureau of the Census. *Aging in the United States—Past, Present, and Future.* Current Populations Report No. P25-1130, Washington, DC; 1996. http://www.census.gov/ipc/prod/97agewc.pdf.
6. Administration on Aging. *A Profile of Older Americans: 2002.* Washington, DC: US Department of Health and Human Services. http://research.aarp.org/general/profile_2002.pdf
7. Federal Interagency Forum on Aging-Related Statistics, *Older Americans 2000: Key Indicators of Well-Being.* Federal Interagency Forum on Aging-Related Statistics, 2000. http://www.agingstats.gov/chartbook2000/population.html#Indicator%201.
8. Hetzel L, Smith A. *The 65 and Over Population: 2000, Census 2000 Brief.* Issued October 2001. http://www.census.gov/prod/2001pubs/c2kbr01-10.pdf.
9. Administration on Aging. *A Profile of Older Americans: 2003.* http://www.aoa.gov/prof/Statistics/profile/2003/15.asp.
10. Current Population Reports. *Americans with Disabilities, 1997.* P70 73, February 2001
11. FDA Consumer Magazine. *Medications and Older People* September–October, 1997. Pub No. FDA 03-1315C. http://www.fda.gov/fdac/features/1997/697_old.html.
12. Committee on Nutrition Services for Medicare Beneficiaries, Food and Nutrition Board. *The Role of Nutrition in Maintaining Health in the Nation's Elderly: Evaluating Coverage of Nutrition Services for the Medicare Population.* Institute of Medicine, 2000. http://www.iom.edu/report.asp?id=5565.
13. Caldwell JC. Population health in transition. *Bulletin of the World Health Organization* 2001;79(2):159–160.
14. Drewnowski A. Nutrition transition and the global dietary trends. *Nutrition* 2000;16:486–487.
15. World Health Organization. *The World Health Report 2003: Shaping the Future: A Vision for Global Health*

World Health Organization. 1211 Geneva 27, Switzerland. http://www.who.int/whr/2003/overview/en/index3.html.

16. Murray CJL, Lopez AD. *The Global Burden of Disease.* Geneva: World Health Organization; 1996.

17. *Diet, Nutrition and the Prevention of Chronic Disease.* Report of a WHO Study Group. Technical report series 797. Geneva: World Health Organization; 1990. http://www.who.int/hpr/NPH/docs/who_fao_expert_report.pdf.

18. US Department of Health and Human Services, Public Health Service. Aging. In: *The Surgeon General's Report on Nutrition and Health.* Washington, DC: US Government Printing Office; DHHS (PHS) Publication No. 88-50210; 1988.

19. National Institutes of Health. National Institutes on Aging. *Malnutrition in Older Persons.* PA-94-088. 1994.

20. U.S. Department of Health and Human Services, Public Health Service. *Healthy People 2000: National Health Promotion and Disease Prevention Objectives. Full Report, with Commentary.* Boston, MA: Jones and Bartlett Publishers; 1992.

21. U.S. Department of Health and Human Services. *Healthy People 2010.* 2nd ed. With Understanding and Improving Health and Objectives for Improving Health. 2 vols. Washington, DC: United States Government Printing Office; November 2000.

22. Dwyer JT. *Screening Older Americans' Nutritional Health: Current Practices and Future Possibilities.* Washington, DC: The Nutrition Screening Initiative; 1991.

23. Berg RL, Cassells JS, eds. *The Second Fifty Years. Promoting Health and Preventing Disability.* Institute of Medicine, Division of Health Promotion and Disease Prevention. Washington, DC: National Academy Press; 1992.

24. *Guidelines for Protocols for Local Demonstration Projects.* Division of Noncommunicable Diseases and Health Technology. INTERHEALTH. Geneva: World Health Organization; 1990.

25. The First Action Plan for Food and Nutrition Policy. WHO European Region, 2001.

26. Weddle DO, Fanelli-Kuczmarski M. Position of the American Dietetic Association: Nutrition, aging and the continuum of health care. *J Am Diet Assoc* 2000;100: 580–595.

27. Posner BM, Levine EL. Nutrition services for older Americans. In: Chernoff R, ed. *Geriatric Nutrition: A Health Professional's Handbook.* Gaithersburg, MD: Aspen Publishers; 1991.

28. Posner BM, Jette A, Smigelski C, Miller D, Mitchell P. Nutritional Risk in New England Elders. *J Gerontol: Med Sci* 1994;49:M123–132.

29. The Nutrition Screening Initiative. *Incorporating Nutrition Screening and Interventions into Medical Practice.*

A Monograph for Physicians. Washington, DC: The Nutrition Screening Initiative; 1994.

30. Agency for Healthcare Research and Quality. *Preventing Disability in the Elderly with Chronic Disease.* April 2002.

31. Dwyer JT. Nutrition concerns and problems of the aged. In: Satin D, ed. *Clinical Care of the Aged Person.* New York, NY: Oxford University Press; 1993.

32. Goodwin JS. Social, psychological and physical factors affecting the nutritional status of elderly subjects: Separating cause and effect. *Am J Clin Nutr* 1989;50:1201–1209.

33. Hutchinson M, Munro HN. *Nutrition and Aging.* New York, NY: Academic Press; 1986.

34. Posner BM, Krachenfels MM. Nutrition services in the continuum of care. *Clin Geriatr Med* 1987;3:261–274.

35. Carroll MD, Abraham S, Dresser CM, eds. *Dietary Intake Source Data: United States, 1976–80, NHANES I, II.* Hyattsville, MD: National Center for Health Statistics; 1983.

36. Food Research and Action Center. *A National Survey of Nutritional Risk Among the Elderly.* Washington, DC: Food Research and Action Center; 1987.

37. Bailey LB. Vitamin B_{12} status of elderly persons from urban low-income households. *J Am Geriatr Soc* 1980; 28:276–278.

38. Morley JE. Nutritional status of the elderly. *Am J Med* 1986;81:679–695.

39. U.S. Department of Health and Human Services, U.S. Department of Agriculture. *Nutrition Monitoring in the United States: A Report from the Joint Nutrition Monitoring Evaluation Committee.* Washington, DC: US Government Printing Office; US Public Health Service; USDHHS publ. PHS 86-1255; 1986.

40. Posner BM, Smigelski CG, Krachenfels MM. Dietary characteristics and nutrient intake in an urban homebound population. *J Am Diet Assoc* 1987;87:452–456.

41. House Select Committee on Aging, Subcommittee on Health and Long-Term Care. *Quackery: A $10 Billion Scandal.* Washington, DC: US Government Printing Office; Publication No. 98-435; 1984.

42. Millen BE, Nason CA. Creating a Continuum of Nutrition Services for the Older Population. Totowa, NJ: Humana Press; 2004.

43. Vaughan LA, Manore MM. Dietary patterns and nutritional status of low income, free-living elderly. *Food Nutr News* 1988;60:27–30.

44. White House Conference on Aging. *Final Report of the 1981 White House Conference on Aging: A National Policy on Aging.* Washington, DC: US Government Printing Office; 1981.

45. Torres-Gil FM, Lloyd JL, Carlin J. Role of elderly nutrition in home and community-based care. *Persp Appl Nutr* 1995;2:9–15.

46. Hedley AA, Ogden CL, Johnson CL, Carroll MD, Curtin LR, Flegal KM. Prevalence of overweight and obesity among US children, adolescents, and adults, 1999–2002. *JAMA* 2004;291:2847–2850.

47. Burt VL, Harris T. The Third National Health and Nutrition Examination Survey: contributing data on aging and health. *Gerontologist* 1994;34:486–490.

48. Millen BE, Ohls JC, Ponza M, McCool AC. An effective national framework for preventive nutrition interventions. The Elderly Nutrition Program. *J Am Diet Assoc* 2002;102: 234–240.

49. Ledikwe JH, Smiciklas-Wright H, Mitchell DC, Miller CK, Jensen GL. Dietary patterns of rural older adults are associated with weight and nutritional status. *J Am Geriatr Soc* 2004; Apr;52(4):589–595.

50. Millen BE, Quatromoni PA. Nutritional Research within the Framingham Heart Study. *J Nutr Hlth Aging* Special Issue: Nutrition and Cardiovascular Disease. 2001;5: 139–143.

51. Millen BE. The Framingham Nutrition Studies: Insights on Dietary Patterns and Obesity Prevention and Risk Reduction. National Heart, Lung and Blood Institute. Workshop on Predictors of Obesity,Weight Gain, Diet, and Obesity. Bethesda, MD; August 4–5, 2004

52. Quatromoni PA, Copenhafer DL, D'Agostino RB, Poole C, Millen BE. Dietary patterns predict the development of overweight in women. The Framingham Nutrition Studies. *J Am Diet Assoc* 2002;102(9):1240–1246.

53. Millen BE, Quatromoni PA, Nam BH, O'Horo CE, Polak JF, D'Agostino RB. Dietary patterns and the odds of carotid atherosclerosis in women. The Framingham Nutrition Studies. *Prev Med* 2002;6:540–547.

54. Millen BE, Quatromoni PA, Gagnon DR, Cupples LA, Franz M, D'Agostino RB. Dietary patterns of men and women suggest targets for health promotion: The Framingham Nutrition Studies. *Am J Hlth Promo* 1996;11(1):42–52.

55. Millen BE, Quatromoni PA, Nam BH, Kozak W, Pierce D, D'Agostino RB. Unique dietary patterns and chronic disease risk profiles of adult men. The Framingham Nutrition Studies. In press.

56. Horwath CC. Dietary intake studies in elderly people. *World Rev Nutr Diet* 1989;59:1–70.

57. U.S. Department of Agriculture. *The Food Guide Pyramid*. Home and Garden Bulletin No. 252. Hyattsville, MD: Human Nutrition Information Service; 1992.

58. *Surgeon General's Workshop on Health Promotion and Aging*. Washington, DC: US Government Printing Office; Publication No. 1988–201–875/83669.

59. Yates AA. National nutrition and public health policies: issues related to bioavailability of nutrients when developing dietary reference intakes. *J Nutr* 2001; Apr 131(4 suppl):1331S–1334S.

60. National Research Council. *Diet and Health. Implications for Reducing Chronic Disease Risk*. Washington, DC: National Academy Press; 1989.

61. Expert Panel on Detection, Evaluation, and Treatment of High Blood Cholesterol in Adults. Executive Summary of the Third Report of the National Cholesterol Education Program (NCEP) Expert Panel on Detection, Evaluation, and Treatment of High Blood Cholesterol in Adults (Adult Treatment Panel III). *JAMA* 2001; May 16;285(19):2486–2497.

62. Heimendinger J, Van Duyn MA, Chapelsky D, Foerster S, Stables G. The national 5 A Day for Better Health Program: a large-scale nutrition intervention. *J Public Health Manag Pract* 1996;Spring;2(2):27–35.

63. Chobanian, AV, Bakris GL, Black HR, Cushman WC, et al. The Seventh Report of the Joint National Committee on Prevention, Detection, Evaluation, and Treatment of High Blood Pressure: the JNC 7 report. *JAMA* 2003; May 21;289(19):2560–2572.

64. Harsha DW, Lin PH, Obarzanek E, Karanja NM, Moore TJ, Caballero B. Dietary Approaches to Stop Hypertension: a summary of study results. DASH Collaborative Research Group. *J Am Diet Assoc* 1999; Aug;99 (8 suppl):S35–39.

65. Whelton, PK, Appel LJ, Espeland MA, Applegate WB, et al. Sodium reduction and weight loss in the treatment of hypertension in older persons: a randomized controlled trial of nonpharmacologic interventions in the elderly (TONE). TONE Collaborative Research Group. *JAMA* 1998; Mar 18;279(11):839–846.

66. White JV, Dwyer JT, Millen Posner B, et al. Nutrition Screening Initiative: Development and implementation of the Public Awareness Checklist and screening tools. *J Am Diet Assoc* 1992;92:163–167.

67. Posner BM, Jette AM, Smith KW, Miller DR. Nutrition and health risks in the elderly: the Nutrition Screening Initiative. *Am J Public Health*. 1993;83:972–978.

68. White JV, Ham RJ, Lipschitz DA, Dwyer JT,Wellman NS. Consensus of the Nutrition Screening Initiative: risk factors and indicators of poor nutritional status in older Americans. *J Am Diet Assoc* 1991;91:783–787.

69. Nutrition Screening Initiative. *Nutrition Screening Manual for Professionals Caring for Older Americans*. Washington, DC: Nutrition Screening Initiative; 1991.

70. Nutrition Screening Initiative. *Nutrition Interventions Manual for Professionals Caring for Older Americans*. Washington, DC: Nutrition Screening Initiative; 1992.

71. Nutrition Screening Initiative. *Incorporating Nutrition Screening and Interventions into Medical Practice. A Monograph for Physicians*. Washington, DC: Nutrition Screening Initiative; 1994.

72. White JV, ed. *The Role of Nutrition in Chronic Disease Care*. Washington DC: The Nutrition Screening Initiative; 1997.

73. Disbrow DD. The costs and benefits of nutrition services: a literature review. *J Am Diet Assoc* 1989;89(4suppl).

74. Balsam AL, Rogers BL. *Service Innovations in the Elderly Nutrition Program: Strategies for Meeting Unmet Needs.* Boston, MA: Tufts University School of Nutrition; 1988.

75. American Dietetic Association. *Nutrition Services Payment Systems: Guidelines for implementation.* Chicago, IL: American Dietetic Association; 1985.

76. Monteith M. Role of nutritionists in community-based long term care. Presented at the Annual Meeting of the American Dietetic Association; September 15, 1983; Anaheim, CA.

77. Rubin DC. Waxing of the gray, waning of the green. In: Committee on an Aging Society, Institute of Medicine and the National Research Council, eds. *America's Aging: Health in an Older Society.* Washington, DC: National Academy Press; 1985.

78. Bezold C, Carlson RJ, Peck IC. *The Future of Work and Health.* Dover, MA: Auburn House Publication Co; 1986.

79. Ponza M, Ohls JC, Millen BE; *Serving Elders at Risk. The Older Americans Act Nutrition Programs. National Evaluation of the Elderly Nutrition Program, 1993–1995.* Washington, DC: US Department of Health and Human Services, Office of the Assistant Secretary for Aging, Office of the Assistant Secretary for Planning and Evaluation; 1996.

80. U.S. Department of Health and Human Services, Public Health Service. *Prevention 86/87, Federal Programs and Progress.* Washington, DC: Public Health Service, OHDS; 1987.

81. National Association of Nutrition and Aging Services Programs. *The Aging Networks Guide to USDA.* Grand Rapids, MI: National Association of Nutrition and Aging; 1988.

82. Caliendo MA, Smith J. Factors influencing the nutrition knowledge and dietary intake of participants in the Title III-c meal program. *J Nutr Elderly* 1981;1:65–77.

83. Food Research and Action Center. Elderly Nutrition Program Fact Sheet. http://www.frac.org/pdf/ENPfactsheet.PDF.

84. Ohls JC, Ponza M, Chu D. *Serving Elders at Risk. The Older American Act Nutrition Programs:National Evaluation of the Elderly Nutrition Program. 1993–1995. Volume III: Methodology and Appendices.* Princeton, NJ: Mathematica Policy Research Inc; 1996.

85. Kirschner Associates Inc, Opinion Research Corporation. *Longitudinal Evaluation of the National Nutrition Program for the Elderly.* Washington, DC: Administration on Aging; US Department of Health, Education, and Welfare Publ. no. 80-20249; 1980.

86. Kohrs MB, O'Hanlon P, Eklund D. Title VII nutrition program for the elderly, I: contribution to one day's dietary intake. *J Am Diet Assoc.* 1978;72:487–492.

87. Kohrs MB. Association of participation in a nutritional program for the elderly with nutritional status. *Am J Clin Nutr* 1980;33:2643–2656.

88. LeClerc H, Thornbury ME. Dietary intakes of Title III meal program recipients and nonrecipients: *J Am Diet Assoc* 1983;83:573–577.

89. Nestle M, Lee PR, Fullarton JE. *Nutrition and the Elderly: A Working Paper for the Administration on Aging.* Policy Paper No. 2. San Francisco: Aging Health Policy Center, University of California; 1983.

90. Zandt SV, Fox H. Nutritional impact of congregate meals programs. *J Nutr Elderly* 1986;5:31–43.

91. Reuben DB, Siu AL. An objective measure of physical function of elderly outpatients: the physical performance test. *J Am Geriatr Soc* 1990;38:1105–1112.

92. Millen Posner B, Smigelski C, Duggal A, et al. Validation of two-dimensional models for estimation of portion size in nutrition research. *J Am Dietet Assoc* 1992;92: 738–741.

93. U.S. Department of Agriculture. Elderly Participation and the Minimum Benefit. November. http://www.fns.usda.gov/oane/MENU/Published/FSP/FILES/Participation/ ElderlyPartRates.pdf.

94. U.S. Senate Special Committee on Aging. *Developments in Aging: 1986. A Report of the Special Committee on Aging.* Washington, DC: US Government Printing Office ASI No. 25144.3; 1987.

95. Butler JS, Ohls JC, Posner BM. The effect of the Food Stamp program on the nutrient intake of the eligible elderly. *J Hum Resources* 1985;20:405–419.

96. Lee JS, Frongillo EA Jr. Nutritional and health consequences are associated with food insecurity among United States elderly persons. *J Nutr* 2001;131(5): 1503–1509.

97. Akin JS, Guilkey DK, Popkin BM, et al. The impact of federal transfer programs on the nutrient intake of elderly individuals. *J Hum Resources* 1985;20:382–404.

98. The Medicare Program and Nutrition Services. June 1997. http://www.eatright.org.med.html. The American Dietetic Association; 1998.

99. U.S. Department of Health and Human Services, Health Care Financing Administration. *Your Medicare Handbook 1997.* Washington, DC: US Government Printing Office, 552–158; 1997.

CHAPTER 21

Health Promotion and Disease Prevention in the Elderly

Beverly J. McCabe, PhD, RD and
Ruth E. Johnston, MS, RD

In the decade and a half since the 1988 Surgeon General's Workshop on Health Promotion and Disease Prevention and the 1989 United States Preventive Services Task Force (USPSTF) report entitled *Guide to Preventive Services,* dramatic changes have occurred in the health care system in the United States.[1-6] Important scientific studies, lay interest, government policy, disease-related activities by private organizations, food industry advertising, and health professionals' practices all have added new luster to health promotion and disease prevention across the life span. The field of nutrition has moved from a focus on the prevention of nutrient deficiency diseases to a focus on the role of nutrition in the prevention of chronic diseases.[7-10] The value of exercise is no longer confined to children and young adults. Its value is being recognized among all geriatric populations including those with chronic diseases such as rheumatoid arthritis.[11-14] The importance of community-based, culturally sensitive interventions also has been recognized.[15-25] Strategies for health promotion and disease prevention have evolved from a single plan applied in many communities to the use of focus groups to develop a local plan that directly involves the participants in decision making, implementation, and evaluation of the interventions.[15-18,26] Large intervention trials such as the Multiple Risk Factors Intervention Trial (MRFIT) program planned with the best of scientific methods have demonstrated only small changes.[17]

Others note that health promotion and disease prevention have undergone two important shifts: (1) from a focus on the individual to the focus on the community; and (2) from the expert biomedical model to the global health movement including the public or patient participation as central to health care.[27] Within the focus on the community, the impact of the built environment and other factors on physical activity have become hot topics.[24,28-35]

Although scientific support for the benefits of health promotion has grown along with increased public awareness, the funding for intervention programs has not kept pace.[36] The lack of funding is due to several factors. In the United States, expensive health care for end-stage diseases consumes the bulk of resources (ie, hospital stays, nursing home care, physician services, nursing care, medications, and other services).[36,37] The last year, and especially the last months of life, cost nearly 30% of Medicare dollars compared with only 3% for prevention.[36,37] A consensus is building that more resources need to be spent on prevention if future health care costs are to be contained. A new theme among health promotion interventions is sustainability.[38] Thus, a new requirement for intervention research is not only efficacy but also sustainability, sometimes described as long-term maintenance of seven years or more. Short-term funding of three years or less may make sustainability difficult to demonstrate.

A major obstacle to funding decisions for prevention programs, especially for elderly people, has been the lack of research to define the effectiveness of the prevention strategy.[39] Important questions include how, when, where, and by whom health promotion interventions are best provided.[39,40] Research is needed to determine if strategies and methods used successfully in the young apply to the old.[41] The presence of comorbidity may well modify success with a particular approach.[42]

Research to support both the efficacy and economic benefits of health promotion among the elderly is growing, especially in the benefits of physical activity, not only on disease management as in diabetes, but also in the promotion of mental health and the prevention of dementia. Two recent major studies provide strong evidence of the value of physical activity on mental health among both men[43] and women.[44] The major unexpected difference was that women in the Nurses Health Study appear to benefit from less than two hours of walking a week compared to daily walking of greater than one hour for men.

DEFINITIONS

Health promotion, wellness, and disease prevention may have different meanings to different health professionals. For some, wellness is defined as aerobic exercise while others see wellness and health promotion as smoking cessation, immunization, weight control, sanitation, and changes in any number of other individual health behaviors. Several government reports use a working definition of health promotion originally coined by Green in 1979[45] as "any combination of educational, organization, economic, and environmental supports for behavior and conditions of living conducive to health."

Thus, health promotion focuses on personal health behavior while disease prevention is seen in the aggregate. Disease prevention is generally assigned to one of three levels: primary, secondary, or tertiary. Primary prevention interventions involve healthy people (eg, programs such as influenza vaccination or the Five-A-Day fruits and vegetables consumption program), while secondary prevention measures involve individuals

with a risk factor but whose disease is not apparent (eg, interventions such as a Pap smear or weight control efforts with a family history of type 2 diabetes mellitus). Tertiary prevention measures apply to individuals with an overt disease (eg, antibiotic therapy after injury or instruction on good food sources of potassium when diuretics are ordered).[3,5]

The World Health Organization (WHO) has proposed five principles of health promotion: (1) health promotion involves the population within the context of everyday life and without a focus on people at risk for specific disease; (2) health promotion directs action on the determinants or causes of health; (3) health promotion involves diverse but complimentary approaches; (4) health promotion elicits effective and concrete public participation; and (5) Primary health care by health professionals aims to nurture and enable health promotion.[46]

Aging has been described as a series of processes that increase vulnerability to challenges that can result in increased risk for disability and death.[47] Health promotion and disease prevention activities in elderly people aim to interrupt or slow the process of aging. Risk factors for the elderly may not be the same as those for the young or for a mature adult. For example, weight loss and low serum cholesterol may be greater risk factors than mild obesity and moderately high (greater than 250 mg/dL) serum cholesterol in elderly people.[41]

Successful aging is likely to become increasingly important to American business as the aging population lives longer, retirement age is likely to be pushed back by 5–10 more years as Social Security benefit-eligible age is pushed back toward 70 years. With concern over an increasing national debt and uncertainty of maintenance of current Social Security benefits, many are choosing to remain employed longer. Businesses are increasingly recruiting retired individuals into part-time work in the service areas. A recent paper by Shephard[48] highlighted the need to consider the older worker in worksite health promotion as older workers are drawn to multimodal programs that focus on improving health and fitness, minimize risk of physical injury, and are designed to meet the special needs of older workers. In young people, motivational factors of competition, rapid movement, and social contacts are not primary motivators of older men.[48]

In elderly adults, primary health prevention measures involve healthy lifestyle and good medical care with greater emphasis on eliminating or minimizing preexisting conditions (secondary prevention) or minimizing discomfort, disability, and dependency caused by established disease even if life cannot be saved (tertiary prevention). The goal of preventive medicine in older people should be not only the prevention of premature morbidity and mortality but also the preservation of function, independence (autonomy), and quality of life.[28] In general, the older the person, the less value primary prevention measures have.[39,49–53]

Quality of life has been characterized as an elusive phenomenon, encompassing biological, psychological, interpersonal, social, economic, and cultural dimensions.[31] The growth in life expectancy has greatly outpaced society's planning for the social economics and health care needs of older adults. The formulation of health care policy needs to encompass these multiple dimensions.[53] If prolonging life also prolongs disability at the end of life, then it is not optimizing the quality of life.[39] A recent review of health screening and health promotion programs for the elderly by Drewnowski et al.[35] calls for the maintenance of health-related quality of life (HR-QOL) as a key goal for all nutrition and physical activity programs targeted toward elders.[35] They note that nutrition screening and evaluation tools focus almost exclusively on biomedical measures and overlook the quality of life measures that might identify the impact of race, ethnicity, education, and access to economic and social resources on nutritional status.[35] Increasingly, health-related quality of life for patients with long-term medical conditions are being examined. For example, Widar et al.[54] examined health-related quality of life in persons with long-term pain after a stroke. Focht et al.[55] examined the

contribution of daily experiences and acute exercise to fluctuations in daily feeling states among older, obese adults with knee osteoarthritis. They note that improvements in feeling uplift from exercise in younger, more physically active individuals are not observed with older, sedentary individuals.[55]

Many determinants of health have little to do with medical care. Lifestyle, genetics, and environment contribute significantly to health and to quality of life. Lifestyle and behavior of individuals involve nutrition, substance abuse, use of protective devices, and physical activity. The environment includes education, literacy, income, housing, and exposure to toxins and pollutants.[53] Sandison et al[56] in a survey of 320 older English women found that women at high risk for osteoporosis had inadequate calcium intake and were the least likely to have made lifestyle changes. Results of the PREMIER clinical trial support the effects of comprehensive lifestyle modifications on blood pressure control.[57]

Thus, effective health promotion must encompass individual behaviors, population-based initiatives, and physician actions. Decisions to include health promotion activities into clinical practice should be well-grounded in scientific evidence.[52] A review of the literature by Patterson and Feightner[52] summarized recommendations that meet these criteria. A recent review by Taylor et al[32] critically examined the health benefits and effectiveness of interventions.

Two additional terms used in health promotion in the elderly have been recently defined by Hazzard[58] as preventive gerontology and preventive geriatrics. Hazzard distinguishes between the two by defining preventive gerontology as prevention occurring before old age and preventive geriatrics as prevention occurring in old age. Preventive gerontology is further defined as preventive measures taken before old age to retard processes that lead to premature morbidity and mortality. Interventions such as diet, exercise, controlled exposure to toxic substances, and limited adverse environmental exposure must be practiced on a long-term basis, requiring considerable personal choice and discipline. Should preventive gerontology be applied broadly, then Hazzard[58] sees geriatric medicine as becoming largely a field of caring for the frail elderly. Preventive geriatrics would focus on those interventions that are short term and yield a shorter return.

Although the benefits of health promotion are well documented in the general population, much less research has examined the benefits in the elderly population. "Early in the 21st century a fifth of the US population will be 65 years of age or older, and one third of the American life span will likely be spent in retirement." Similarly, nearly 25% of the Canadian population will be over 65 years of age.[52] McPhee and Johnson[59] recently surveyed assisted-living residents in a comparison of health status and healthy habits. They concluded that the acquisition of a physical health condition induced the practice of healthier habits and noted that physical exercise and recreational activity related to greater practice of all other healthy habits.[59] Jenkins[60] examined data from the Asset and Health Dynamics Among the Oldest Old (AHEAD) survey to determine if obese older adults are more likely to experience the onset of functional impairment and how health behaviors and health conditions may explain the relationship between obesity and functional impairment. Her findings support active treatment of weight problems in older adults.[60]

Because of the increase in both absolute numbers and percentages of the population who will be classified as elderly, the importance of promoting "successful" and "healthy" aging becomes critical if health care costs are to be contained.[58,61] With few exceptions, Medicare, designed to cover the cost of acute illness, has not covered the cost of health promotion.[62] The Health Care Financing Administration (HCFA) funded a series of demonstration programs to evaluate the impact of providing health promotion and preventive services to Medicare recipients. Questions under consideration included whether health promotion would produce significant improvements in the health of older Americans, whether money would be saved, and

whether the elderly would participate in such services.[63–67] Other issues included whether such programs would simply delay the onset of disability or prolong the period of disability.

The aging of America, the longer life expectancy, the question as to whether the U.S. government can afford to deliver all the benefits currently available to older Americans are impacting on retirement plans. Many older adults are opting to remain in the work force well past the traditional retirement age of 65 years of age.

Currently, women live almost 7 years longer than men but they have almost twice as many years of disability prior to death.[63] The diseases in women that account for death and the consumption of health care resources, are also diseases that are major contributors to disability. Interventions that affect heart disease, cancer, stroke, fracture, pneumonia, osteoarthritis, and cataracts would impact elderly women's health most.[66]

In a study in rural Pennsylvania, 41% of elderly participants were identified as eligible for a nutrition program, 11% for a smoking cessation program, 2% for alcohol counseling, and 7% for dementia and depression evaluations.[11,14] Participants not only varied across the type of program but also within programs by gender, education, and group assignment (hospital-based versus physician-based). Use of service was higher by participants with more education and physician-based programs. Participation was greater in programs involving a single intervention (eg, immunization) than programs requiring more sessions and more participant action (eg, weight loss). Attendance was best in the five-session cholesterol-lowering program. Sixty-seven percent of the participants attended 75% or more of the sessions compared with 39% of participants attending at least 50% of the eight smoking cessation sessions, and 40% attending at least 50% of the 16 weight loss sessions. Overall, at least one session was attended by 44.8% of those eligible for nutrition intervention, 17% for smoking cessation, and 57.5% for immunizations. Thus, rural Americans will use health promotion services if covered by Medicare.[62,63]

A small sample of Canadian elderly perceived differing benefits from individualized counseling and group wellness sessions.[32] Subjects described group sessions as a means to get general information about life and lifestyle choices but that some services are best provided to meet individualized needs.[53] In a survey of a wide range of health behaviors and preventive care activities among a representative sample of 17,454 older Canadians, Newsom et al[67] found a substantial proportion lead relatively inactive lives and fail to follow recommended standards of preventive care and screening care; about two-thirds had made no effort in the previous years to improve their health and thought no changes were needed.[67]

In California, 237 study participants over the age of 60 were randomly assigned to either a treatment or a control group after a standardized assessment.[68] The assessment included a health history, nutritional evaluation, and limited physical assessment by a nurse. The treatment group received a written personal health plan and counseling, while the control group received only the health assessment, risk identification, and limited verbal health plan counseling. The treatment group completed significantly ($p <$ .001) more preventive referrals and health behavior changes upon reassessment 1 year later. The results support the conclusion that a client-centered process with supportive counseling by public health nurses combined with written health plans can significantly increase the prevention activities of older adults.[69] For example, Kulp et al[70] evaluated the effectiveness of an educational video in a gynecological waiting room on increasing osteoporosis knowledge and preventive health behaviors immediately and three months later. The intervention group exhibited both increased knowledge ($p <$ .001) and reported starting calcium and vitamin D supplements usage ($p <$ .001).

These studies suggest that elderly Americans will participate in health promotion interventions if offered and that the referral of physicians will significantly improve participation. Guidelines for preventive services have been outlined by several expert panels.[3,10,45] The question is whether physicians and other health professionals will follow such guidelines to reduce morbidity and mortality.

Eleven urban hospitals and 46 primary care practitioners consented to a survey of 1800 patients between the ages of 52 and 77 who had been followed by these physicians for at least 2 years.[71] Study physicians were primarily family or general practitioners (61%), general internists (34%), and others (6%). Surveys were returned by 1457 (81%) patients who were mostly female (59%), white (87%), with an income of $40,000 or less (75%), who possessed a high school education or more (78%), and who had health insurance (98%) with 51% Medicare and 20% health maintenance plan (HMP) coverage.

Of the 215 smokers, 93% had been told the health risks of smoking, 87% had been advised to stop smoking, 66% had been counseled, and 36% had been referred to a smoking cessation program. Physicians were least likely to discuss or ask about alcohol use (15%) or to advise the use of seat belts (17%).

Seventy-nine percent of the physicians recommended regular checkups, 73% asked about regular exercise, 72% discussed eating a healthy diet, 68% asked about smoking, and 67% recommended a flu shot. Physicians less frequently asked patients younger than age 60 about family history of early heart disease (56%), breast cancer (53%), or colon cancer (46%). At least 50% of the patients were offered and had a screening test within the past 2 years, regardless of the frequency of expert recommendations. When grouped, age trends were noted in increased likelihood of sigmoidoscopy ($p <$ .001) and fecal occult blood tests ($p <$ .002). While men were increasingly likely to be screened for prostate cancer ($p <$ .001), women were decreasingly likely to receive most screening tests, particularly mammograms ($p <$ .001) and Pap smear tests ($p <$ .02). Patients with a positive family history were not more likely to receive screening than patients without the family history.[71]

COSTS VERSUS BENEFITS

If the benefits of health promotion in the elderly are demonstrated, if elderly clients will participate in health promotion interventions, and if physicians appear to be using age more than risk to order screening tests, an important question is: At what age do the costs of intervention begin to outweigh the benefits? In 1980, a noted rheumatologist predicted that by the middle of the 21st century, the average human longevity would become stable at 85 years of age.[69] This prediction, coupled with limited data on benefits of preventive screening beyond the age of 85, has supported age 85 as a general cutoff range for conventional screening.[34,36,71] The risks-benefits and costs of preventive gerontology with its long-term, low-cost, low-risk interventions partnered with individualized short-term, low-risk secondary prevention may yet demonstrate a maximal longevity of high quality for individuals and populations. That age has yet to be determined.[58]

The failure to use low-cost, low-risk screening tests such as mammograms in elderly women is disturbing in that breast cancer is among the leading causes of disability in the elderly.[72] As the benefits of exercise intervention (even in the frail elderly) and nutrition programs such as home-delivered meals and decreasing length of stay in hospitals become well documented, the assumption that health promotion interventions should cease at age 85 will likely be challenged.

NUTRITION IN GENERAL HEALTH PROMOTION AND DISEASE PREVENTION

Although interest in diet and nutrition as means of chronic disease prevention has grown steadily since the 1960s, it was not until three important reports were issued in 1988 and 1989 that a concerted effort began to help Americans translate dietary recommendations into a pattern that would emphasize chronic disease prevention over nutrient deficiency prevention.[72–75] A number of other government agencies assisted in the process of revamping recommendations for American eating patterns.[75,76] The United States Congress established the National Nutrition Monitoring and Related Research (NNMRR) Act of 1990, which directed that the Department of Health and Human Services (DHHS) and the United States Department of Agriculture (USDA) share responsibility for implementing the program and contract with a scientific body such as the National Academy of Sciences (NAS) or the Federation of American Societies for Experimental Biology (FASEB) to interpret available data analyses and publish a report on the dietary, nutritional, and health-related status of the American people and the nutritional quality of food consumed in the United States at least once every 5 years.[75,76] The three reports issued under NNMRR provide five measurement components:[45]

- Nutrition and related health measurements
- Food and nutrient consumption
- Knowledge, attitudes, and behavior assessments
- Food composition and nutrient databases
- Food supply determinants

Another important development was the 1990 Nutrition Labeling and Education Act (NLEA). It simplified the nutrition information provided on a label and required listing only those nutrients associated with chronic disease risks.[71,77–79] A new book from the Institute of Medicine provides updated guiding principles for nutrition labeling and fortification within the framework of the new Dietary Reference Intakes (DRIs).[80] The 1990 NLEA act also allowed food manufacturers to petition the Food and Drug Administration (FDA) for approval of health claims by providing data to demonstrate the validity of the claim. This significant change in food policy enabled food advertisements to provide messages about the role of nutrients and food constituents in health promotion and disease prevention.[77,78]

The USDA and DHHS released two important food guides for Americans in 1990.[79] The fourth edition of the USDA dietary guidelines assists in the selection of a diet that decreases dietary risks for chronic diseases while providing adequate nutrients and energy.[79] These seven revised guidelines are:

- Eat a variety of foods.
- Balance the food you eat with physical activity. Maintain or improve your weight.
- Choose a diet low in fat, saturated fat, and cholesterol.
- Choose a diet with plenty of vegetables, fruits, and grain products.
- Choose a diet moderate in salt and sodium.
- Choose a diet moderate in sugars.
- Drink alcoholic beverages in moderation if you choose to drink.

In order to assist individuals in translating these dietary guidelines into appropriate food choices, the USDA replaced the Basic Four recommendations with the Food Guide Pyramid in 1990.[79,10] The pyramid recommends that the daily diet contain 6–11 portions of grain products, 2–4 servings of fruit, 3–5 servings of vegetables, 2–3 servings of meats or meat substitutes, and 2–3 servings of dairy products.

The National Cancer Institute developed the "5-A-Day" campaign to encourage the public to consume five servings of fruits and vegetables daily to promote diets that meet the Food Guide Pyramid guidelines.[10] More recently, the American Cancer Society convened an Advisory Committee on Diet, Nutrition, and Cancer Prevention to update the 1991 guidelines for cancer prevention.[10] These 1996 recommendations are to:

- Choose most of the foods you eat from plant sources. Eat five or more servings of fruits and vegetables each day. Choose green and dark yellow or cabbage-family vegetables. Use soy products and legumes. Eat other plant source foods including breads, cereals, grain products, rice, pasta, and beans several times each day. Choose whole grains in preference to refined grains. Choose beans as a replacement for meats.
- Limit your intake of high-fat foods, particularly from animal sources. Choose foods low in fat. Prepare foods with little or no fat.

Bake or broil meats and vegetables rather than fry foods. Choose nonfat and low-fat milk and dairy products. Eat smaller portions of high-fat dishes. Select low-fat food items when snacking or eating in restaurants. Limit meat intake, especially high-fat meats. Use lean meat more as a condiment and less as an entree. Choose seafood, poultry, or beans over beef, pork, and lamb.

- Be physically active. Achieve and maintain a healthy weight. Be active for at least 30 minutes several times a week. Control caloric intake. Be within your healthy weight range.
- Limit consumption of alcoholic beverages, if you drink at all. Limit alcoholic beverages to two or less drinks a day. Do not combine the use of tobacco and alcohol.

Table 21–1 lists the committee's best advice on how to reduce the risk of various types of cancer.[10]

The public's awareness of the role of diet and nutrition in the prevention of cancer continues to grow. So too is the scientific evidence of the importance of food and nutrients in cancer protection, and good news is coming from the American Cancer Society. In 1997, 1,382,400 new cases of cancer were projected for calendar year 1997.[81] A midyear adjustment reduced the estimate to 1,257,800, a decrease of 9%.[82] Landis and colleagues[83] predicted 1,228,600 new cases (an additional decrease of 2%) for the calendar year 1998. Overall, this figure represents a 1% decrease over the original 1997 protection, largely due to fewer cases of prostate cancer. These figures reflect the first downward trend in cancer cases since record keeping began in the 1930s.[83,84]

In addition, 5-year relative survival rates also are improving but not equally well in all population groups and all specific cancer sites. Death rates in men have declined more than in women, largely due to increased death rates in women from lung cancer. Survival rates among African American men and women have improved, but to a lesser degree than those for whites.[84]

Table 21–1 Advice on Risk Reduction for Various Types of Cancer

Dietary Advice	Type of Cancer						
	Breast	Colorectal	Endometrial	Lung	Oral/Esophageal	Prostate	Stomach
Limit alcohol	X				XX		
Eat vegetables/fruits		XX		XX	XX		XX
Be physically active	X	X	X				
Avoid obesity	X	X	X				
Consume less high-fat foods/saturated fats		X			X		
Eat grains		X					
Limit red meat		X				X	
Avoid tobacco				XX	XX		
Eat fresh foods					X		X

Source: Data from American Cancer Society 1996, Advisory Committee on Diet, Nutrition, and Cancer Prevention, Reducing the Risk of Cancer with Healthy Food Choices and Physical Activities, CA: *A Cancer Journal of Clinicians*, Vol. 46, pp. 326–339, © 1996.

To better assess the overall diet quality and to monitor the compliance of Americans to the Food Guide Pyramid and the Dietary Guidelines, the Healthy Eating Index (HEI) was first computed using 1989 data from the Continuing Survey of Food Intakes by Individuals (CSFII).[85,86] The CSFII survey is a nationally representative survey containing information on people's consumption of foods and nutrients.[85,86] The HEI is the sum of 10 components, each representing different aspects of a healthful diet. Figure 21–1 illustrates the distribution of these components into a score of 100.[86]

The first five components measure the degree to which a person's diet complies with the recommendations for the five major food groups of the Food Guide Pyramid: grains, vegetables, fruits, meats, and milk. The percentage of total kilocalories from fat is the sixth component, while percentage from saturated fat is the seventh, total cholesterol intake is the eighth component, total sodium intake is the ninth component, and variety in the diet is the tenth component. An HEI score of over 80 is considered a "good" diet, an HEI score between 51 and 80 indicates a diet that needs improvement, and

an HEI score below 51 is considered to be a "poor" diet.[86,87]

The Healthy Eating Index 1994–1996 provides a comparison of diet quality from 1989 to 1996.[85,87] Between 1989 and 1996 the overall HEI score improved from 61.5 to 63.8, a small but significant increase. In 1996 older females (51 years and above) had a better overall score than older men (67.5 and 65.2, respectively). Likewise women 19–50 scored higher than men in the same age group (62.7 and 60.6, respectively).[85]

The release of the first set of Dietary Reference Intakes (DRIs) in 1997 enlarged the concept of the single-value Recommended Dietary Allowances (RDA) to a range of values designed to go beyond the prevention of deficiency diseases and to include current concepts of the role of nutrients and food components in long-term health.[1–9,18,88–91] Although the RDA is still included in this set, its purpose has been limited to that of being a goal for individuals.[7,8,90,91] For all other purposes, the three other reference values should be selected: the Adequate Intake (AI), the Tolerable Upper Intake Level (UL), and the Estimated Average Requirement (EAR).[6] Exhibit 21–1 presents the definitions of the DRIs.

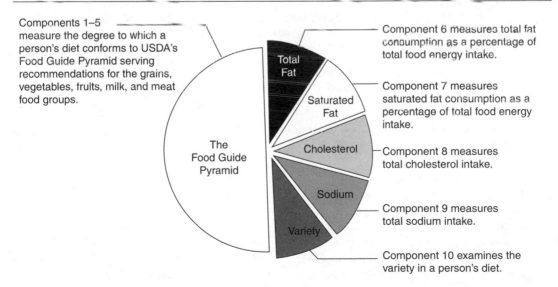

Figure 21–1 Components of the Healthy Eating Index
Source: Reprinted from *Healthy Eating Index 1994–1996*, United States Department of Agriculture, Center for Nutrition Policy and Promotion, CNPP-5.

Exhibit 21–1 Definitions of Terms Used in the 1997–1998 Dietary Reference Intakes

Requirement. The lowest continuing intake level of a nutrient that, for a specified indicator of adequacy, will maintain a defined level of nutriture in an individual.

Basal Requirement. The level of intake needed to prevent pathologically relevant and clinically detectable signs of a dietary inadequacy.

Estimated Average Requirement (EAR). The daily intake estimated to meet the requirement, as defined by the specific indicator of adequacy, in 50% of the individuals in a life-stage or gender group. The EAR is used to determine the RDA.

Recommended Dietary Allowance (RDA). The daily intake that is sufficient to meet the daily nutrient requirements of most individuals in a specific life-stage and gender group. If the variation in requirements is well defined, the RDA is set at 2 standard deviations (SDs) above the EAR.

$$RDA = EAR + 2\ SDS_{EAR}$$

If the variation is not well defined or available, a standard estimate of variance is applied. A coefficient of variation of 10% and equal to 1 SD is assumed for most nutrients.

$$RDA = 1.2 \times EAR$$

If the coefficient of variation is greater than 10% as it is with niacin (15%), then the RDA formula would be adjusted accordingly.

$$Niacin\ RDA = 1.3 \times EAR$$

Adequate Intake (AI). The recommended daily intake based on observed or experimentally determined approximations of the average nutrient intake by a defined population or subgroup that appears to sustain a defined nutritional state. The AI is used when scientific data are insufficient to determine an EAR and consequently the RDA.

Tolerable Upper Intake Level (UL). The highest daily intake level that is unlikely to pose a risk of adverse health effects in almost all individuals in the specified life-stage and gender group. The UL is used to examine the potential fortification of foods and the use of dietary supplements. The UL is not intended as a recommended level of intake. The UL is based on a risk assessment model developed specifically for nutrients from careful literature review with systematic scientific considerations and judgments. The model is based on the lowest levels at which no observed adverse effects are found. Lack of data on adverse effects has limited the number of nutrients for which ULs have been set.

Source: Reprinted with permission from Institute of Medicine's *Dietary Reference Intakes: Calcium, Phosphorus, Magnesium, Vitamin D, and Fluoride,* pp. S1–S7, ©1997, National Academy Press.

The uses and preferred values to which the DRIs can be put include four primary areas:

- assessing intakes of individuals for which the EAR would be used to examine potential for inadequacy and for which the UL would be used to examine for overconsumption;
- assessing intakes of population groups for which the EAR would be used to examine prevalence of inadequate intakes within a group;
- planning diets for individuals for which the RDA would be the target value if available;

otherwise, the AI would be the target value (the UL would be used as a guide to limit intake of individuals on a chronic basis but not as a target intake); and

- planning diets for groups for which the EAR would be used to set goals for the mean intake of a specified population.

An estimate of the variability of the group's intake would be required to set realistic goals. Thus, the appropriate use of the DRIs requires dietetic and other health professionals to invest time and effort in understanding how to use the

DRIs and in collecting baseline data (eg, a group's intake of nutrients with which to use these tools most effectively).[7]

In addition, DRIs for many other nutrients and food components are being developed. The DRI project has been divided into at least seven nutrient groups and two areas of general concern by the Food and Nutrition Board's Standing Committee on the Scientific Evaluation of Dietary Reference Intakes. The first two groups, calcium and related nutrients, and folate and other B vitamins, were released in 1997 and 1998.[8,9] The third group, antioxidants (eg, vitamins C and E, selenium), was released in 2000;[92] additional sets of DRIs in 2002; trace elements (ie, iron, zinc) in 2003; and electrolytes and water in 2004.[93–95]

The order and timelines for studying the nutrients are being determined by the interests of those funding the studies and by the availability of funds. If DRIs are not available for a nutrient, the 1989 RDAs remain the best available guidelines for assessing and planning diets.[88,90]

NUTRITION IN GERIATRIC HEALTH PROMOTION AND DISEASE PREVENTION

Nutrition Screening Initiative

The Nutrition Screening Initiative (NSI) was established in early 1990 to promote nutrition screening and better nutritional care for the elderly in the United States.[96–98] This multifaceted effort was a direct response to the 1988 Surgeon General's Workshop on Health Promotion and Aging and the DHHS call for nutrition screening. This project involved the American Academy of Family Physicians (AAFP), the American Dietetic Association (ADA), and the National Council on the Aging (NCOA) with advisors from medicine, health, nutrition, and aging.[96–98] The NSI Technical Review Committee provided the technical expertise and directions that produced the DETERMINE Your Nutritional Health Checklist and the Level I and Level II Nutrition Screening tools.[98–99]

More than 235,000 checklists and 22,500 screening manuals were distributed nationwide in the first 2 years.[100] These tools are being used in meal programs, senior citizen and adult day care centers, home services programs, physicians' offices, hospitals, and nursing homes to identify the nutrition risks of older Americans. The use of the checklist or Level I screen is usually the first step in screening individuals at high risk for poor nutrition status in order to identify who will benefit from nutrition interventions.[65] The Level II screen provides more specific diagnostic information. As more caregivers have recognized those at nutritional risk, interest in advice on nutrition has increased.[100]

Nutrition Strategies

The NSI Technical Review Committee identified specific strategies to improve the nutritional status of older Americans.[99] These strategies include:

- Place higher priority on nutrition screening and care in senior centers, congregate meal sites, physicians' offices, and hospitals.
- Establish interdisciplinary, community-based models for nutrition care.
- Integrate the use of foods and medical nutritional products for special dietary and medical purposes into nutrition counseling and support.
- Provide a range of practical therapeutic options.
- Develop highly structured practice protocols that measure outcomes in several ways.
- Reshape third-party reimbursement schedules to include nutrition screening and services.
- Offer continuing medical education with hands-on training to develop skills in nutrition diagnosis and treatment.
- Educate the public about the importance of nutrition status to overall health and quality of life and on ways to improve nutrition health.
- Stimulate partnerships and volunteer efforts in cooperation with a variety of lay people and professionals.[61]

In 1992, the Intervention Roundtable of the NSI involved 30 professionals who came to a consensus on recommendations in six areas of nutrition intervention: social services, oral health, mental health, medication use, nutrition education and counseling, and nutrition support.[98] In 1994, the NSI began to distribute a continuing education program for physicians, *Incorporating Nutrition Screening and Interventions into Medical Practices: A Monograph for Physicians*.[100] This monograph identifies ways to incorporate nutrition screening and intervention into quality preventive care for the geriatric patient.[100]

Nutrition screening differentiates individuals who are at high risk of nutritional problems and those who already have poor nutritional status. Screening begins with the DETERMINE Your Nutritional Health Checklist (Exhibit 21–2). There are 10 items on this checklist. If the score is 0–2, the respondent is categorized as having good nutritional health; if the score is 3–5, they are at moderate nutritional risk; and if the checklist yields a score of 6+, the individual is deemed at high nutritional risk.[96–100] The acronym of the DETERMINE checklist outlines nine warning signs for nutritional risk (Exhibit 21–3). The checklist was validated in both retrospective and prospective protocols to predict nutrition-related problems in elderly individuals. Although it is not a diagnostic device, this instrument provides a valid measure of potential nutrition risks. It can be used by anyone, including a geriatric client or a caregiver.[100]

The next step, the Level I screen (Exhibit 21–4) differentiates those individuals who need further assessment and possibly nutrition intervention by calculation of body mass index (BMI) and change in body weight and evaluation of eating habits, living environment, and functional status. This tool can be used by a wide range of health care professionals. If an individual has a documented, significant, involuntary weight change or has a BMI above 27 or below 22, a referral to a physician or nurse for further detailed screening is warranted. For those individuals who have other risk factors, referral for preventive interventions such as dietary counseling, shopping assistance, meal delivery, or nutrition support is appropriate.[99,100]

The Level II screen (Exhibit 21–5) needs a more skilled administrator as this tool confirms the Level I screen and expands to include more anthropometric measurements; laboratory tests; and evaluation of drug use, clinical features, eating habits, living environment, functional status, and mental/cognitive status. This tool also identifies major and minor indicators of poor nutritional status as shown in Exhibit 21–5.[64] Patients exhibiting one or more major indicators require immediate medical attention. Patients with less quantifiable but multiple minor indicators should be referred to other health care or social service providers, as appropriate.[100]

Intervention-specific screening tools also are available for oral health, feeding difficulties, drug-nutrient interactions, and nutrition counseling. In addition, the NSI monograph also includes a social service intervention contact guide, an algorithm for nutrition support route selection, and a schematic diagram providing tips on how to incorporate nutrition screening and intervention into an office practice.[99–100]

Social service interventions can help improve the nutritional status of older Americans. Social isolation, poverty, and dependency and disability intervention programs include:

- Food Stamp program
- Congregate nutrition and home-delivered meal programs
- Social Security
- Supplemental Security Income
- Medicare/Medicaid
- Federally assisted housing programs
- Employment training programs
- Adult day care services
- Transportation services
- Older Americans volunteer programs
- Case management services
- In-home health aide and personal care services
- Respite and caregiver support services[66]

A prospective study of newly hospitalized elderly patients found that 30 recipients of home-delivered meals had only half the length of stay of 30 nonrecipient controls matched by diagnosis,

Exhibit 21–2 DETERMINE Your Nutritional Health Checklist

The warning signs of poor nutritional health are often overlooked. Use this checklist to find out if you or someone you know is at nutritional risk. Read the statements below. Circle the number in the yes column for those that apply to you or someone you know. For each yes answer, score the number. Total your nutritional score.

	Yes
I have an illness or condition that made me change the kind and/or amount of food I eat.	2
I eat fewer than two meals per day.	3
I eat few fruits or vegetables or milk products.	2
I have three or more drinks of beer, liquor, or wine almost every day.	2
I have tooth or mouth problems that make it hard for me to eat.	2
I don't always have enough money to buy the food I need.	4
I eat alone most of the time.	1
I take three or more different prescribed or over-the-counter drugs a day.	1
Without wanting to, I have lost or gained 10 pounds in the last 6 months.	2
I am not always physically able to shop, cook, and/or feed myself.	2
Total	

Total Your Nutritional Score. If It Is

0–2   Good! Recheck your nutritional score in 6 months.

3–5   You are at moderate nutritional risk. See what can be done to improve your eating habits and lifestyle. Your office on aging, senior nutrition program, senior citizens center, or health department can help. Recheck your nutritional score in 3 months.

6 or more   You are at high nutritional risk. Bring this checklist the next time you see your physician, dietitian, or other qualified health or social service professional. Talk with them about any problems you may have. Ask for help to improve your nutritional health.

Source: Reprinted with permission by the Nutrition Screening Initiative, a project of the American Academy of Family Physicians, the American Dietetic Association, and the National Council on the Aging, Inc., and funded by a grant from Ross Products Division, Abbott Laboratories, Inc.

age, gender, and other factors.[101] In most states the cost of feeding one meal a day to an elderly person over a year's time was less than the price of one day's stay in a hospital.[102] The relatively low cost of nutrition interventions that yield positive health costs savings is increasingly being documented.[102,103]

The NSI also has prepared two additional manuals to encourage health professionals in managed care practices and organizations and in

Exhibit 21–3 Remembering the Warning Signs

The nutrition checklist is based on the warning signs described below. Use the word DETERMINE *to remind you of the warning signs.*

- **Disease.** Any disease, illness, or chronic condition that causes you to change the way you eat, or makes it hard for you to eat, puts your nutritional health at risk. Four out of five adults have chronic diseases that are affected by diet. Confusion or memory loss that keeps getting worse is estimated to affect one out of five or more of older adults. This can make it hard to remember what, when, or if you've eaten. Feeling sad or depressed, which happens to about one in eight older adults, can cause big changes in appetite, digestion, energy level, weight, and well-being.

- **Eating poorly.** Eating too little and eating too much both lead to poor health. Eating the same foods day after day or not eating fruits, vegetables, and milk products daily also will cause poor nutritional health. One in five adults skips meals daily. Only 13% of adults eat the minimum amount of fruits and vegetables needed. One in four older adults drinks too much alcohol. Many health problems become worse if you drink more than one or two alcoholic beverages per day.

- **Tooth loss/mouth pain.** A healthy mouth, teeth, and gums are needed to eat. Missing, loose, or rotten teeth or dentures that don't fit well or cause mouth sores make it hard to eat.

- **Economic hardship.** As many as 40% of older Americans have incomes of less than $6,000 per year. Having less, or choosing to spend less, than $25 to $30 per week for food makes it very hard to get the foods you need to stay healthy.

- **Reduced social contact.** One third of all older people live alone. Being with people daily has a positive effect on morale, well-being, and eating.

- **Multiple medicines.** Many older Americans must take medicines for health problems. Almost half of older Americans take multiple medicines daily. Growing old may change the way we respond to drugs. The more medicines you take, the greater the chance for side effects such as increased or decreased appetite, change in taste, constipation, weakness, drowsiness, diarrhea, nausea, and others. Vitamins or minerals taken in large doses can act like drugs and can cause harm. Alert your physician to everything you take.

- **Involuntary weight loss/gain.** Losing or gaining a lot of weight when you are not trying to do so is an important warning sign that must not be ignored. Being overweight or underweight also increases your chance of poor health.

- **Needs assistance in self-care.** Although most older people are able to eat, one of every five has trouble walking, shopping, and buying and cooking food, especially as they get older.

- **Elder years above age 80.** Most older people lead full and productive lives. But as age increases, risk of frailty and health problems increases. Checking your nutritional health regularly makes good sense.

Source: Reprinted with permission by the Nutrition Screening Initiative, a project of the American Academy of Family Physicians, the American Dietetic Association, and the National Council on the Aging, Inc., and funded by a grant from Ross Products Division, Abbott Laboratories, Inc.

home health agencies to incorporate nutrition screening and intervention processes.[103,104] These scientifically based manuals provide general guidelines on how to set up a nutrition screening and intervention program and how to incorporate the program into current services.[103,104] The manuals' algorithms provide visual summaries, while the graphs present data on the cost savings accrued through medical nutrition therapy.[103,104] Profiles and case studies provide materials for

Exhibit 21–4 Level I Screen

Body Weight

Measure height to the nearest inch and weight to the nearest pound. Record the values below and mark them on the body mass index (BMI) scale to the right. Then use a straight edge (ruler) to connect the two points and circle the spot where this straight line crosses the center line (body mass index). Record the number below. Healthy older adults should have a BMI between 24 and 27.

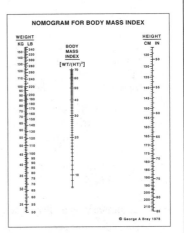

Height (in):

Weight (lbs):

Body mass index: (number from center column) Check any boxes that are true for the individual:

☐ Has lost or gained 10 pounds (or more) in the past 6 months

☐ Body mass index <24

☐ Body mass index >27

For the remaining sections, please ask the individual which of the statements (if any) is true for him or her and place a check by each that applies.

Eating Habits

☐ Does not have enough food to eat each day

☐ Usually eats alone

☐ Does not eat anything on one or more days each month

☐ Has poor appetite

☐ Is on a special diet

☐ Eats vegetables two or fewer times daily

☐ Eats milk or milk products once or not at all daily

☐ Eats fruit or drinks fruit juice once or not at all daily

☐ Eats breads, cereals, pasta, rice or other grains five or fewer times daily

☐ Has difficulty chewing or swallowing

☐ Has more than one alcoholic drink per day (if woman); more than two drinks per day (if man)

☐ Has pain in mouth, teeth, or gums

Living Environment

☐ Lives on an income of less than $6000 per year (per individual in the household)

☐ Lives alone

☐ Is housebound

☐ Is concerned about home security

☐ Lives in a home with inadequate cooling or heating system

☐ Does not have a stove and/or refrigerator

☐ Is unable or prefers not to spend money on food (<$25–$30 per person spent on food each week)

Functional Status

Usually or always needs assistance with (check each that applies):

☐ Bathing

☐ Dressing

☐ Grooming

continues

Exhibit 21–4 continued

☐ Toileting
☐ Eating
☐ Walking or moving about
☐ Traveling (outside the home)
☐ Preparing food
☐ Shopping for food or other necessities

If you have checked one or more statements on this screen, the individual you have interviewed may be at risk for poor nutritional status. Please refer this individual to the appropriate health care or social service professional in your area. For example, a dietitian should be contacted for problems with selecting, preparing, or eating a healthy diet, or a dentist if the individual experiences pain or difficulty when chewing or swallowing. Those individuals whose income, lifestyle, or functional status may endanger their nutritional and overall health should be referred to available community services: home-delivered meals, congregate meal programs, transportation services, counseling services (alcohol abuse, depression, bereavement, etc.), home health care agencies, day care programs, etc.

    Please repeat this screen at least once each year—sooner if the individual has a major change in his or her health, income, immediate family (eg, spouse dies), or functional status.

Source: Reprinted with permission by the Nutrition Screening Initiative, a project of the American Academy of Family Physicians, the American Dietetic Association, and the National Council on the Aging, Inc., and funded by a grant from Ross Products Division, Abbott Laboratories, Inc.

---

training staff. For example, one mnemonic device used is the NSI "Three Rs":

- **Remind.** Post charts to remind health care professionals and staff of the nutrition screening and intervention process.
- **Reach.** Keep references on procedures, risk factors, and interventions readily accessible.
- **Reinforce.** Communicate with all involved. Let them know what a valuable role they play. Keep them posted on the program's progress.[103]

In 1999 the NSI released long-term care nutrition screening and intervention practice guidelines with five objectives:

- Define the roles and responsibilities of the members of the interdisciplinary care team.
- Provide guidance for the front-line care providers on how to conduct nutrition screening and assessment.
- Distinguish different approaches to geriatric case management based on nutrition risk stratification of nursing facility residents.

- Provide protocols for nutrition screening interventions to enhance nursing home staff that already use the HCFA Minimum Data Set and select resident assessment protocols to identify residents in need of medical nutrition therapies.
- Advise on ways to develop and implement a nutrition care plan including follow-up nutrition assessment and interventions to maintain nutritional health.

Today, NSI publications are jointly sponsored by the American Dietetic Association and the American Academy of Family Practice and are available on the website http://www.aafp.org/PreBuilt/NSI_neworderforma.pdf.[104] The latest NSI publication is *A Physician's Guide to Nutrition in Chronic Disease Management* and is available in print and on a CD.

NUTRITION AND HEALTH FOR OLDER AMERICANS

Analysis of the HEI results suggested some modification in the recommended number of servings in the Food Guide Pyramid for older

Exhibit 21–5 Indicators of Nutritional Status

Complete the following screen by interviewing the patient directly and/or by referring to the patient chart. If you do not routinely perform all of the described tests or ask all of the listed questions, please consider including them but do not be concerned if the entire screen is not completed. Please try to conduct a minimal screen on as many older patients as possible, and please try to collect serial measurements, which are extremely valuable in monitoring nutritional status.

Anthropometrics

Measure height to the nearest inch and weight to the nearest pound. Record the values below and mark them on the body mass index (BMI) scale. Then use a straight edge (paper, ruler) to connect the two points and circle the spot where this straight line crosses the center line (body mass index). Record the number below; healthy older adults should have a BMI between 24 and 27; check the appropriate box to flag an abnormally high or low value.

Height (in):   Weight (lbs):   Body mass index (weight/height^2):

Please place a check by any statement regarding BMI and recent weight loss that is true for the patient.

☐ Body mass index <24
☐ Body mass index >27
☐ Has lost or gained 10 pounds (or more) of body weight in the past 6 months

Record the measurement of mid-arm circumference to the nearest 0.1 centimeter and of triceps skinfold to the nearest 2 millimeters.

Mid-arm circumference (cm): ___
Triceps skinfold (mm): __
Mid-arm muscle circumference (cm): __

Refer to the table and check any abnormal values:

☐ Mid-arm muscle circumference < 10th percentile
☐ Triceps skinfold <10th percentile
☐ Triceps skinfold >95th percentile

Note: Mid-arm circumference (cm) − [0.314 × triceps skinfold (mm)] = Mid-arm muscle circumference (cm)

For the remaining sections, please place a check by any statements that are true for the patient.

Laboratory Data

☐ Serum albumin below 3.5 g/dL
☐ Serum cholesterol below 160 mg/dL
☐ Serum cholesterol above 240 mg/dL

Drug Use

☐ Three or more prescription drugs, over-the-counter medications, and/or vitamin/mineral supplements daily

Clinical Features

Presence of (check each that applies):

☐ Problems with mouth, teeth, or gums
☐ Difficulty chewing
☐ Difficulty swallowing
☐ Angular stomatitis
☐ Glossitis
☐ History of bone pain
☐ History of bone fractures
☐ Skin changes (dry, loose, nonspecific lesions, edema)

continues

Exhibit 21–5 continued

Eating Habits
☐ Does not have enough food to eat each day
☐ Usually eats alone
☐ Does not eat anything on one or more days each month
☐ Has poor appetite
☐ Is on a special diet
☐ Eats vegetables two or fewer times daily
☐ Eats milk or milk products once or not at all daily
☐ Eats fruit or drinks fruit juice once or not at all daily
☐ Eats breads, cereals, pasta, rice, or other grains five or fewer times daily
☐ Has more than one alcoholic drink per day (if a woman); more than two drinks per day (if a man)

Living Environment
☐ Lives on an income of less than $6,000 per year (per individual in the household)
☐ Lives alone
☐ Is housebound
☐ Is concerned about home security
☐ Lives in a home with inadequate heating or cooling
☐ Does not have a stove and/or refrigerator
☐ Is unable or prefers not to spend money on food (<$25–$30 per person spent on food each week)

Functional Status
Usually or always needs assistance with
(check each that applies):
☐ Bathing
☐ Dressing
☐ Grooming
☐ Toileting
☐ Eating
☐ Walking or moving about
☐ Traveling (outside the home)
☐ Preparing food
☐ Shopping for food or other necessities

Mental/Cognitive Status
☐ Clinical evidence of impairment (eg, Folstein < 26)
☐ Clinical evidence of depressive illness (eg, Beck Depression Inventory > 15, Geriatric Depression Scale > 5)

Patients in whom you have identified one or more major indicators of poor nutritional status require immediate medical attention; if minor indicators are found, ensure that they are known to a health professional or to the patient's own care or social service professional (dietitian, nurse, dentist, case manager, etc.).

Source: Reprinted with permission by the Nutrition Screening Initiative, a project of the American Academy of Family Physicians, the American Dietetic Association, and the National Council on the Aging, Inc., and funded by a grant from Ross Products Division, Abbott Laboratories, Inc.

adults due to the lowered energy requirements. (Table 21–2). Dietary Guidelines for Americans are currently undergoing review and a new version is anticipated in the near future. Minutes of the meetings of the Dietary Guidelines Committee are posted on the USDA website.

Table 21–2 Recommended Number of Food Guide Pyramid Servings per Day for Older Adults

Gender/ Age	Energy (k/cals)	Grain (servings)	Vegetables (servings)	Fruits (servings)	Milk (cups)	Meat (oz)
Females 25–50	2,200	9	4	3	2	6.00
Males 25–50	2,900	11	5	4	2	7.00
51 +	2,300	9.1	4.2	3.2	2	6.25

Source: Data from *The Healthy Eating Index 1994–96,* United States Department of Agriculture, Center for Nutrition Policy and Promotion.

The Expert Committee of Nutrition and Health for Older Americans has developed a Food Guide Pyramid for older adults.[105] This pyramid focuses on the recommended food guides for older adults and includes one unique feature. The base of this pyramid rests on water to emphasize the critical importance of fluid intake and the prevention of dehydration and its sequelae to the elderly with impaired thirst mechanisms and less reserve capacity for recovering from fluid deprivation.[105] This committee also has developed another important guide, the Exercise Guide for Older Adults.[105]

Nutrition and Heart Disease

Heart disease remains the leading cause of death in the United States, accounting for 32.8% of all deaths.[106] Among elderly people, the number of deaths from circulatory diseases, ischemic heart disease, and cerebrovascular diseases has declined since their peak in 1970.[51,73] The decline from the 1950 death rates has been the greatest for cerebrovascular diseases among those 70 to 74 years of age; the 1990 death rate was only 26.2% of the 1950 value, and only 44.3% among those 85 to 89 years of age. This change may be partially due to the implementation of Medicare, but a similar value of 28.8% of the 1950 value also was noted among those 45 to 49 years of age, who are not recipients of Medicare benefits.[13] The availability of medical treatment has undoubtedly played a significant role in this de-

cline in all age groups. For the other two categories, circulatory diseases and ischemic heart diseases, a much greater decline in death rates has occurred among those 45 to 49 years old than among those 70 to 74 years and 85 to 89 years old. Among those 45 to 49 years old, the 1990 value was only one-third of the 1950 rate while the decline was only about one-half of the 1950 death rates in the two older age groups.

Hypertension remains a substantial problem in elderly people. In the National Health and Nutrition Examination Survey (NHANES III), prevalence was higher in females. About 75% of females 80 years of age had elevated blood pressure compared with 60% of males in the same age group.[106] Table 21–3 presents data on the prevalence of hypertension by age, sex, and race/ethnicity as found in NHANES III, 1988–1991. The clinical trials with the Dietary Approaches to Stop Hypertension (DASH) diet have provided evidence of effective treatment through lifestyle changes without requiring extensive medications.[57] Black[107] presents a summary of risk stratification and treatment of older patients based on blood pressure stages from the Sixth Report of the Joint National Committee on Prevention, Detection, Evaluation, and Treatment of High Blood Pressure (JNC-VI). Groups A and B should receive lifestyle modifications treatment along with drug therapy.[107] Tsang et al[108] conducted a retrospective study of 1160 patients with a first cardiovascular (CV) event to determine if echocardiography would enhance prediction of first

Table 21–3 Percentage of People 50 Years of Age and Older Who Have Hypertension Distributed by Sex, Age, and Race/Ethnicity

Sex/Age (years)	All Groups	White	Non-Hispanic African American	Mexican American
Males				
50–59	42.2	1.8	55.9	36.0
60–69	52.1	51.3	63.6	53.8
70–79	60.7	60.3	68.0	52.1
80+	60.5	60.3	62.4	70.5
Females				
50–59	38.8	36.8	47.9	33.5
60–69	53.5	50.9	77.8	59.3
70–79	67.6	66.9	72.6	67.0
80+	74.7	74.3	80.5	71.0

Source: Adapted from Third Report of NNMRRP.

age-related CV event. They concluded that echocardiography can enhance prediction of the first event.[108] Referrals to dietitians for lifestyle modifications based on echocardiography might well be an earlier intervention to prevent disability from a serious CV event.

High serum cholesterol is a major risk factor for coronary heart disease. Since 1970 public awareness of the relationship between diet and serum cholesterol has increased, but only 50% of American adults reported having had their serum cholesterol checked in the NHANES III survey.[75] Of those who had a serum cholesterol check, 85% reported being told by a physician or other health professional to change their diet; 54% were told to exercise; 47% were told to lose weight; and 20% were told to take medications; 89% reported they were currently following advice to change their diet compared with 70% who were trying to lose weight, exercise, and/or take medications.[45] Despite widespread education efforts by government and private agencies, only 60% of American adults were aware that "saturated fats" are more likely to raise "blood" cholesterol levels than "polyunsaturated fatty acids."[75] (Note: Quotation marks indicate specific terms used in survey items.) More people are aware of the relationship between dietary

cholesterol and health than of the relationship between dietary "fat," "saturated fat," and health. People who were African American, over 60 years of age, less educated, and from lower income levels were less aware than white, middle-aged, more educated people from higher income levels.[75] Only when nutrition policy changes allowed health claim advertisements and specially designed programs for minority populations did increases in diet knowledge begin to emerge among lower income, less educated, nonwhite populations.[78]

More recently, research interest has grown in potential risk factors other than serum cholesterol including the hypothesized relationship between vitamin intake and coronary heart disease secondary to hyperhomocysteinemia.[109–112] Subsequently 1160 surviving elderly members of the Framingham Study cohorts were examined for their blood levels and dietary intakes of vitamin B_{12}, B_6, and folate compared with their serum homocysteine levels.[109] Homocysteine increased with both age and lower B vitamin intakes. Selhub and colleagues[110] suggest that a substantial majority of the cases of high homocysteine in elderly subjects may be due to vitamin status. In a later investigation of 70 participants between the ages of 54 and 81 years (the Boston Veterans

Affairs Normative Aging Study), vitamin status and homocysteine levels were used to predict vascular disease status and cognitive performance.[110] Homocysteine levels did not appear to predict clinical diagnosis of vascular disease in this sample. No significant relationship was observed between plasma concentration of the B vitamins or homocysteine and age or years of education. Plasma folate and vitamin B_{12} concentrations were, however, negatively correlated with plasma homocysteine levels.[110]

In a review of over 75 studies involving more than 15,000 subjects, Parnetti and associates[112] concluded that homocysteine is an independent risk factor for cardiovascular diseases, especially for extracranial carotid atherosclerosis. They suggest that homocysteine may represent a metabolic link in the pathogenesis of atherosclerotic vascular disease and old-age dementias.[112] Ebly and colleagues[113] found low serum folate to be a significant explanatory variable for stroke and all types of dementias in 1171 subjects in the Canadian Study of Health and Aging (CSHA). Several epidemiological and animal studies have suggested that vitamin E may play a significant role in the prevention of cardiovascular disease, but clinical trials now in progress will help shape any specific recommendations about the use of vitamin E in the prevention of cardiovascular disease.[114]

In a sample of 150 elderly people in Spain, the number of meals eaten was inversely related to serum cholesterol levels, very-low-density lipoprotein (VLDL) cholesterol, and triacylglycerol levels.[115] As the number of meals increased, subjects came closer to meeting the recommended intake of energy and other nutrients (protein, fiber, vitamin C, thiamin, riboflavin, calcium, magnesium, and iodine).[115] Institutionalized subjects ($n = 58$) were less likely to eat four meals a day than noninstitutionalized subjects ($n = 92$).[115]

Nutrition and Cancer

Cancer rates second among leading causes of all deaths in the United States, accounting for 23.4% of deaths in 1993.[116] Between 1950 and 1990, the death rate from all cancers rose among those over 70 years of age while falling nearly 20% among those 45 to 49 years old. Among those age 70 to 74, the 1990 death rate was 192.5% and for those age 85 to 89 the 1990 death rate was 172.8% of the 1950 death rates.[81] However, a new trend is evident in the 1997 and 1998 cancer statistics, which show a decline in the number of new cases and death rates.[81–84] This trend may be due to prevention, early detection, or aggressive therapy.[10] Whatever the primary cause, efforts in all areas need to be encouraged.[116]

In a review of 206 human epidemiological studies and 22 animal studies on diet and cancer prevention, the consumption of vegetables and fruits was most favorable toward cancer prevention.[113] The evidence is particularly strong for cancers of the gastrointestinal and respiratory tracts; it is less strong for prevention of cancers related to hormones (eg, breast and prostate cancers).[10] The types of vegetables and fruits that are most often cited as protective include raw vegetables, allium vegetables (onion and garlic), carrots, green vegetables, cruciferous (cabbage family) vegetables, tomatoes, soy proteins, and legumes.[10,116] This protective effect is not limited to the value of vitamins such as beta carotene and minerals such as selenium but appears to include many other food constituents that are not classified as nutrients.[10,116] Examples of potential protective substances are fibers, phytochemicals such as flavonoids, terpenes, sterols, indoles, and phenols that are of plant origin.[10]

Elderly people tend to reduce their overall consumption of food due to multiple factors (eg, dental problems, limited access to shopping, loss of appetite, early satiety, indigestion. fatigue, and bone pain).[47,49,117] Many studies[109,116–118] document an intake of vegetables and fruits well below recommended levels. The NHANES III data reported older women averaged four servings of fruits and vegetables compared with the seven servings a day recommended by the Food Guide Pyramid and the Five-A-Day program advocated by the National Cancer Institute.[10,85–87] Moreover, women living in rural east Tennessee public housing reported mean intakes for all vegetables as 15.1 ± 9.7 servings/week and for all fruit and juice as 9.9 ± 9.8 with a mean intake of 1377 ± 594 kilocalories.[118] Even correcting for an underreporting of energy intake of 10% to 30% as reported in various studies comparing dietary intake data with energy expenditures measured by doubly labeled water, these intakes would fall short of recommended intakes for many women, including the elderly.[118–122]

In a study of elderly Illinois women using a 7-day food record to estimate energy intake and doubly labeled water to estimate energy expenditure over a 6-day span, there was an underreporting of approximately 10% for a total energy intake of 1599 ± 126 compared with a total energy expenditure of 1,782 ± 253.[120] Mares-Perlman and associates[121] using a modification of the Block Food Frequency Questionnaire estimated the dietary intake of middle-aged (43 to 64 years of age) men and women and of elderly (65 to 84 years of age) men and women in Wisconsin during the Beaver Dam Eye Study. Older men and women consumed less protein, fat, cholesterol, niacin, riboflavin, calcium, iron, zinc, and lycopene.[121] Less energy came from protein and alcohol and more came from carbohydrates. The evaluation of the impact of dietary supplements on median intakes was greatest for vitamins A, C, E, riboflavin, and calcium, but as previously noted, the use of supplements was less among those with a poor diet.[121]

Although diet plays a critical role in the health and well-being of older adults, the health promotion strategies to incorporate nutrient-dense foods into their diets have not often resulted in behavior change. Bell et al[20] have suggested that the focus on specific nutrients rather than on the overall pattern of food consumption is a potential explanation.

Using three 24-hour recalls, Sharkey et al[123–126] examined the dietary intake of homebound elders from several perspectives. Although regularly receiving home-delivered meals providing one-third of the DRIs, the participants still had suboptimal intake of several nutrients.[124–126] In reviewing the dietary intake data categorized by diuretic users vs. nondiuretic users, dietary intake of selected nutrients indicated significant differences. Inadequate dietary intake of B vitamins among diuretic users was strongly predicted by non-breakfast consumption.[127,128]

Nutrition and Osteoporosis

Osteoporosis affects more than 25 million Americans. It is the major underlying cause of bone fractures in elderly and postmenopausal women (Chapter 14). The 1.5 million fractures a year cost $10 billion in direct health care costs.[129,130]

The 1988–1994 NHANES III survey used dual-energy X-ray absorptiometry (DEXA) scanning of the proximal femur to assess the prevalence of bone mass density indicative of osteoporosis in 14,646 men and women aged 20 years or older who underwent direct standardized physical examinations and household interviews.[129] The prevalence of osteoporosis in the 1249 women over 64 years of age was 29.3% by bone density findings, but only 6.3% of these women reported being told they had osteoporosis. These cross-sectional data suggest that over 90% of women with osteoporosis are unaware of their condition.[98] Women with higher education, living in urban areas, who had seen a physician in the last 6 months were more likely to self-report osteoporosis.[129]

Institutionalized elderly women are more likely to have lower bone density than non-institutionalized controls.[130] Reduced peripheral fat was significantly associated with the lower bone density found in these institutionalized women.[128] Sharkey et al[126] developed a "musculoskeletal nutrient" index of calcium, vitamin D, magnesium, and phosphorus and compared the index to lower-extremity physical performance in homebound older men and women. Poorer dietary intake of the four nutrients was associated with poorer physical performance.[126]

Bone health is dependent on many factors.[131] Thin, small, white or Asian women are at greater risk for the development of osteoporosis. African American women and men also may develop osteoporosis given long-term presence of lifestyle choices of a diet deficient in calcium, vitamin D, phosphorus, magnesium, or fluoride; lack of weight-bearing exercise; cigarette smoking; excessive alcohol intake; family history of osteoporosis; and use of some medications.[132,133] Long-term use of glucocorticoids, anticonvulsants, loop diuretics, anti-mitotics, cyclosporine, heparin, cholestyramine, thyroid hormones, and aluminum-containing antacids has been associated with osteoporosis.[128,132] The elderly may have limited sunlight exposure and may produce less cholecalciferol, have less renal ability to convert cholecalciferol to its active form, and may have a decreased ability to absorb calcium, thereby leading to a higher requirement for dietary vitamin D.[8]

A review paper summarized the evidence that vitamin K may play a role in bone metabolism as well as in coagulation synthesis.[134] Because the overall data for an association between diet and osteoporosis were so strong and the average intake of calcium by older women was less than 600 mg/day, nutrition policy about health claims was revised to allow claims to be made in food advertising.[77,78] The FDA began to approve the fortification of more foods with calcium and to allow claims on nutrition labels. For example, the fortification of orange juice, which was not previously considered a good source of calcium, has made it an important source of calcium for those individuals who cannot or will not consume dairy products. As noted in the 1994 National Institutes of Health (NIH) consensus conference, calcium intake in men and women older than 65 years is commonly less than 600 mg.[129] An analysis of calcium intake drawn from the 1994–1996 CSFII by McCabe and coworkers[135] yielded mean intakes and standard deviations of 578 ± 290 mg and 768 ± 397 mg for females and males 55 to 60 years of age, respectively. The mean intakes and standard deviations were 579 ± 290 mg and 720 ± 356 mg for females and males 75 to 80 years of age, respectively.[135]

The addition of three servings of a food fortified to become an excellent source of calcium would be needed to raise the mean intake to the AI of 1000 to 1500 mg recommended for older women.[1,96] (For a food to be labeled an excellent or high source of calcium, a serving must provide 200 mg.)[80] For older individuals at the 90th percentile of calcium intake, 955 mg for women and 1240 mg for men ages 55 to 60, three calcium-fortified products a day would be well below the Tolerable Upper Intake Level of 2500 mg calcium.[8,135] Thus, foods fortified with calcium could play a significant role in assisting elderly people attain these new recommended intakes of calcium.

Even with menopausal hormone therapy (MHT), an adequate intake of calcium remains essential.[129,130] The use of MHT reduces the recommended daily calcium intake from 1500 mg to 1000 mg per day.[133] Moreover, the CSFII data suggest that the elderly are increasing their intakes of calcium and that many are using calcium supplements.[8,121,134] The average multiple vitamin and mineral supplement, however, does not provide sufficient calcium to move the current intake of elderly people to the recommended level of 1000 to 1500 mg per day.

Nutrition, Hypertension, Obesity, and Diabetes

Hypertension, obesity, and diabetes share many common relationships and treatment strategies. They also are recognized as risk factors for the same diseases; the literature becomes somewhat repetitious when viewed separately.

Hypertension remains a major health problem among elderly people, particularly in the southern United States and among African Americans.[136–142] The incidence of hypertension increases with age and is a major risk factor for both heart disease and stroke. Clinical trials of antihypertensive medication therapy have shown a reduction in these disease risks.[136,137] More recently, interest has grown in alternative approaches due to the potential for adverse effects of the drugs, drug-drug interactions, and the high cost of the drugs.[138] Obesity and dietary salt intake have been suggested as contributors to the development of hypertension. Weight loss and reduction of dietary sodium have been recommended for older persons based on clinical trials in middle-aged adults.[138–142]

A recent, randomized, controlled trial (TONE) of nonpharmacological interventions in the elderly in 875 men and women aged 60 to 80 years demonstrated that reduced sodium intake and weight loss are effective and safe therapies for hypertension in older persons upon withdrawal from antihypertensive drugs.[140] Obese subjects were randomized to weight loss, reduced sodium intake, both, or usual care. Antihypertensive drugs were withdrawn after 3 months of intervention. The combined weight loss-low sodium intake regimen yielded the best outcome measures.[140] Although this study did not offer other interventions such as increased physical activity, increased potassium intake, or other diet modifications, these approaches might offer additional benefits. This study did demonstrate that older subjects are both able to make and sustain lifestyle changes.[140]

Among the elderly, hypertension brings morbid effects such as cognitive impairment in the otherwise healthy individual and loss of mobility in community-dwelling persons.[136] The antihypertensive drug regimens and public education programs have proven effective overall, but less so in some populations.[74,78,136]

Older African Americans in the southeast United States present a stubborn public health problem.[138] In a study of 6473 elderly South Carolinians, age was shown to be negatively related to lifestyle changes.[136] Social participation was identified as an important factor in willingness to change diet or exercise practices. The presence of comorbidities such as heart attack, stroke, kidney disease, atherosclerosis, and diabetes appears to be a relatively unimportant influence on lifestyle changes.[136] One possible explanation for this surprising finding is that the primary disease is being treated without providing health education for lifestyle change.[136] Increasingly, faith-based interventions are being conducted for African American churches. Dietary interventions such as "Body and Soul" delivered collaboratively by community volunteers and a health-related agency can reach middle-aged and older African Americans to promote increased fruit and vegetable consumption.[140,141]

Low-income, unmarried African American males were less likely to report changes; this group may need to be targeted differently than other groups of African American elderly. Extensive outreach initiatives, such as rides, meals, and fellowship, would appear to be justified for this hard-to-reach group.[136] In addition, socialization and feeding programs such as congregate meals and home-delivered meals can have positive impacts on health care costs.[101] A prospective observational study of newly hospitalized patients found that 30 recipients of home-delivered meals had only half the lengths of stay of 30 nonrecipients matched by diagnosis, age, gender, and other factors.[101] Outcome studies are beginning to be documented more frequently.[141,142]

Indeed, older men are more difficult to reach with health interventions because they appear to value health less, participate less frequently in health screenings, experience poorer health, have shorter life expectancies, and wait longer to consult a doctor about an illness.[143] Promoting self-motivation may be the key to increasing older men's participation in health promotion activities. Men who perceive themselves as healthy and having healthy lifestyles appear to have greater intrinsic motivation.[143]

Obesity is widely accepted as a major risk factor for several diseases, particularly hypertension, heart disease, and type 2 diabetes mellitus, and as an aggravating problem for other chronic diseases such as osteoarthritis.[144–154] Obesity is a heterogeneous group of disorders characterized by an accumulation of excess body fat. The prevalence of overweight increases with age up to 50 years for men and up to 70 years for women.[148] A logistic regression of body weight health behaviors and health conditions revealed a much higher odds ratio of obesity than any other factor.[60]

Clinical trials have established the benefits of weight loss and low-fat diets in obese middle-aged and older men reducing the cardiovascular risk factors and in premenopausal women with diet or diet and exercise programs.[144] Brach et al.[28] report that participants in 20–30 minutes of moderate intensity exercise on most days of the week have better physical function than older persons who are simply active each day or who are sedentary.[28] For older women, the benefits of weight loss in reducing the risks of cardiovascular disease have not been demonstrated.[145] Weight loss through reduced daily energy intake and moderate endurance exercise has been the primary strategy in reducing cardiovascular risk factors in the obese based on clinical trials in younger adults. Fox and colleagues[145] demonstrated that weight loss in moderately obese older women was feasible but no effects on reducing common cardiovascular risk factors such as lipid lowering was observed with the weight loss. When considering the effects of brisk walking speed on body composition, Parise et al.[146] asked participants to self-report time, speed, and intensity of walking. Self-reported brisk walking in older adults was reported.

A consensus exists about the health risks of overweight (BMI ≥ 25 kg/m²) and obesity (BMI ≥ 30 kg/m²).[146-148] No consensus exists, however, about the management of these conditions, especially in special groups such as the elderly. In order to evaluate published data and to determine the most appropriate treatment strategies, the National Heart, Lung, and Blood Institute and the Diabetes and Digestive and Kidney Diseases Institute joined in convening the Expert Panel on the Identification, Evaluation, and Treatment of Overweight in Adults. The panel recently released a set of clinical guidelines based on a systematic review of scientific literature from 1980 through 1997.[147,148] The guidelines present classifications of overweight and obesity by BMI, waist circumference, and associated disease risks. The general goals of weight loss and weight management are to prevent further weight gain, to reduce body weight, and to maintain a lower body weight. An algorithm summarizes the assessment and decision steps in the overall strategy for these goals.

The guidelines present the needs of special treatment groups including older adults.[147,148] They note that randomized clinical trials suggest that weight loss has a favorable effect on older adults in reducing heart disease risks. A caution

is issued that food restrictions in elderly patients can result in inadequate intake of some nutrients. Another risk is that involuntary weight loss due to occult disease might appear to be successful voluntary weight loss.[147] The summary statement offers the following guidance:

> A clinical decision to forgo obesity treatment in older adults should be guided by an evaluation of the potential benefits of weight reduction for day-to-day functioning and reduction of the risk of future cardiovascular events, as well as the patient's motivation for weight reduction. Care must be taken to ensure that any weight reduction program minimizes the likelihood of adverse effects on bone health or other aspects of nutritional status.[147]

The precautions above are well taken. The reduction of cardiovascular risk in middle-aged and older men is likely, but after menopause, cardiovascular disease is more common in women. This later onset in women and the finding of greater abdominal obesity in older women suggest that cardiovascular risk reduction should be gender and age specific. In a study of 41 healthy, moderately obese (120% to 140% of ideal body weight) postmenopausal women over the age of 80 years, the loss of body weight did not result in improved lipid levels.[145] Abdominal fat may be more of a risk than body fatness in other areas, and older women do not readily lose this fat.

In other chronic diseases and disabilities, body fatness in elderly women may be protective or it may be predictive of increased risk. In a study of 22 institutionalized, but independent, Italian women (age range, 66 to 88 years), the experimental group was matched with 22 controls who were independent but not institutionalized. The institutionalized women had a lower bone density, and reduced peripheral body fat was found to be significantly associated with low bone mineral density.[131]

High body fat, however, is predictive of disability in older Americans.[149] In the Cardiovascular Health Study, an ongoing, population-based observational study of 5201 older men and women (aged 65 to 100 years) in four states, a baseline prevalence for disability was 26.5% of the women and 16.98% of the men.[149] In a 3-year follow-up of those who had originally reported no disability, 20.3% of the women and 14.8% of the men reported onset of disability.[150] This increase in disability was not explained by age, physical activity, chronic disease, or other potential confounders. High body fatness, but not low fat-free mass, was predictive of disability.[150] This study used the simple, inexpensive and clinically feasible method of bioelectrical impedance to evaluate body composition.[150] Although not considered the most rigorous method of estimating body composition, the results achieved with this approach equaled those obtained by the same investigators using the more sophisticated, expensive, and less clinically available DEXA method.[148,149]

Another chronic disease commonly found in the obese older adult is type 2 diabetes mellitus. Diabetes in the elderly is a major public health problem in the United States with a threefold or greater risk of hospitalization and institutionalization in nursing homes for people over the age of 65 who have diabetes compared with those who do not have the disease.[151] Estimates of the prevalence of diabetes in the elderly range from 18% at 65 years of age to 40% at 80 years of age. Among African American women older than age 55, one in four is estimated to have diabetes.[152] African American women also have a higher prevalence of risk factors for diabetes and complications from diabetes.[152,154] Low-income African American women are less likely to have private health insurance and a regular source of medical care.[152]

Diabetes is an expensive and time-consuming disease to manage.[151–155] Acute and chronic stress have been found to affect insulin resistance and blood glucose control adversely.[153] Inexpensive, fat-filled, low-nutrient-density foods are common in African American communities with a high consumption of high-fat pork products such as sausage, luncheon meats, and bacon, and a low consumption of fruits, vegetables, dietary fiber, and calcium.[156]

Other populations at high risk for diabetes are Hispanics and American Indians, who have not only a higher prevalence of type 2 diabetes but also poorer outcomes from treatment.[1,152,154] In a study of 51 Mexican Americans attending patient education trials, about half ($n = 24$) were judged in "good" glucose control and the other half ($n = 26$) were judged in "fair" or "poor" control.[154] None of the patients completely followed treatment plans.[154]

Four key factors influenced the multiple treatment decisions they faced each day: (1) belief in the power of modern medicine; (2) desire to act and feel "normal"; (3) desire to avoid physical symptoms; and (4) limited economic resources.[157] Patients preferred the quieter risk of hyperglycemia symptoms to the physical distress of hypoglycemic symptoms. Due to limited resources, the subjects were concerned about the greater costs of fresh fruits and vegetables not usually in the diets of their families. Some patients did eat correctly when they had the money but less appropriately when they were short on cash.[152]

Subjects reported taking medicine instead of making other behavioral changes. This over-reliance on medications may partially result from physicians emphasizing medications during patient visits. The economic and social barriers are important factors in self-care by patients.[153,154] Care providers should avoid presuming that poor outcomes are due to ignorance or lack of motivation.[154]

The general nutrition guidelines for older adults with diabetes are no different than those for other type 2 diabetes patients.[157] Special problems may exist due to functional limitations that impact patient ability to shop for or prepare foods.[154] In a cross-sectional study of those over the age of 85 years, 26% were unable to prepare meals and 34% were unable to shop.[150] Older and obese diabetics are less likely to be able to shop and prepare foods than their nondiabetic cohorts.

Another hindrance to compliance with current recommendations is the ingrained belief that older diabetics simply need to avoid foods with sugar. Many elderly patients adhere to this belief and report that they cannot afford sugar-free foods.[156] Older, obese women were more likely to consume sugar-free foods such as sugar-free candies, cookies, and cakes and have lower quality diets than those who used both reduced-fat and reduced-sugar foods.

The American Diabetes Association revised its recommendation that carbohydrates in the diabetic diet could be increased up to 60% of total kilocalories and lifted the prohibition against sucrose-containing foods.[151] Another important modification was the substitution of the goal of "reasonable" body weight for ideal body weight.[151] Improvement in diabetes control has been noted with a weight loss of 5 to 10 kg without achievement of "desirable" or ideal body weight.[157]

Very few studies have examined the effect of diet interventions in the elderly. Caloric restriction, while a cornerstone of weight loss in the obese, may result in malnutrition.[154] Only recently has the effect of nutritional risks on quality of life been reported.[158] A field-based, cross-sectional study of participants who received congregate meals or home-delivered meals assessed their quality of life. Quality of life was positively correlated with quality of health and negatively correlated with nutrition risk indicators, food insecurity, decreased enjoyment of food, depression, and impaired functional status.[158]

Dietary Supplements

While evidence of a relationship between diet and disease has grown steadily, largely from human epidemiological and animal studies, the use of dietary supplements has grown even more.[10,121,159–161] With the possible exception of folic acid supplementation, clinical trials of individual nutrients in prospective studies have not yet documented benefits unless dietary intakes were inadequate or specific diseases (eg, pernicious anemia) were present. Thus, the American Dietetic Association recommends that use of vitamin and mineral supplementation be based on individual assessment.[159,160] Over a 10-year period, the supplement use nearly doubled in a sample of older Wisconsin adults. The increase was the greatest among individuals 65 to 84 years of age, with the major increase coming in regular use compared with occasional use. Approximately half of all females reported current use of supplements; 31% of males aged 43 to 64 years and 42% of males aged 65 to 81 years reported current use.[121]

In another study of supplement use among community-dwelling elderly aged 60 to 69 ($n = 89$), 80 to 89 ($n = 90$), and 100 and older ($n = 76$) in Georgia, usage was similar in all age groups.[161] Women were twice as likely to be current users. Subjects who were physically active, had stomach problems, used arthritis medications, and had healthier diets were more likely to use supplements. Healthier diets were defined as being lower in fat, higher in protein and fiber, and containing yogurt and whole-grain products.[161] Physically active elders were more likely to take calcium supplements and vitamin C than their sedentary counterparts.[121,161] Thus, supplement use does appear to be one among a cluster of health behaviors. Dietary intake studies of the elderly have shown both adequate and inadequate intakes.[121,157,161] In studying the effects of supplement use on disease, control for both dietary intakes and physical activity is essential.[162]

A number of studies have looked at the vitamin status and supplement use of one or more nutrients. Epidemiological, animal, and observational studies suggest that supplementing vitamin E beyond the amount normally consumed in a diet may be protective against cardiovascular diseases. Clinical trials are currently in progress that may demonstrate a reduction in cardiovascular events.[115]

While a high prevalence of vitamin B_{12} deficiency in the older population has been established on the basis of low serum cobalamin concentrations, newer research[163,164] suggests this prevalence is underestimated. Anemia occurs in only the most severely B_{12}-depleted individuals.[164] In an examination of 548 Framingham subjects aged 67 to 96 years, the prevalence of cobalamin deficiency was established at 12% based on elevated serum concentrations of methylmalonic acid (MMA) and serum homocysteine (Hcys).[164] These two metabolites are considered highly sensitive indicators of tissue deficiency of cobalamin.[163] Thus, many elderly people are metabolically deficient in cobalamin while appearing to have "normal" serum values.[163] More widespread use of MMA and Hcys tests could potentially prevent irreversible central nervous system damage and vitamin-dependency dementias.

In a placebo-controlled, double-blind trial of daily low-to-moderate micronutrient supplements, subjects aged 59 to 85 years showed significant increases in mean serum levels of ascorbate, β- carotene, folate, vitamin B_6, and α-tocopherol.[165] Improved delayed hypersensitivity skin test responses also were found in these healthy, independently living older adults.[164] Other studies in the elderly have suggested an association between enhanced immune responsiveness and vitamin E. Recommending vitamin E supplementation awaits further definition of the mechanisms between nutrition and immunity.[165]

Since the 1960s, folic acid deficiencies have been increasingly recognized in the presence of disease, polypharmacy, and poverty.[160,166–167] From 11% to 28% of the elderly have been estimated to have folic acid deficiency, largely from poor dietary intake.[166] A low red cell folate suggests a long-term dietary inadequacy.[167]

Dietary folate varies greatly in bioavailability and may also be destroyed in prolonged food preparation. When increased food folate intake did not lead to significant increases in folate status, attention turned to food fortification.[167] Ready-to-eat cereals were fortified with folate, and then flour was fortified with folate to provide additional folate to women of child-bearing age as a means to prevent neural tube defects.[167] Cereals and breads, however, are consumed in limited amounts by some elderly, who also are at increased risk of folate deficiency.

Institutionalized elderly are more likely to have low serum folate.[166] Milk was selected as a vehicle for folic acid supplementation in a prospective clinical trial. Forty-nine subjects received the fortified milk for at least 6 months and 40 controls received unfortified milk. The experimental group had a mean serum folate of 5.81 μg/L compared with 2.16 μg/L for the control (p < .0001); thus, fortified milk appears to be a feasible and effective vehicle for elderly subjects to receive folic acid supplementation.[166]

Three large trials of β-carotene, vitamin A, and α-tocopherol failed to duplicate the protection against cancer that had been associated with fruits and vegetables.[168] An increased risk for lung cancer occurred in smokers who received β-carotene supplements in the Alpha-Tocopherol-Beta-Carotene (ATBC) study.[169] Follow-up data on the ATBC subjects suggest that supplemental β-carotene is risky for smokers. Combined with the lack of benefits for nonsmokers in any of the other large trials, β-carotene supplementation is not recommended.[168]

Other supplements such as selenium, vitamin B_6, and iron also may have toxic or adverse effects in some individuals or in excess amounts.[170–172] The elderly are at special risk of iron overload because they have few mechanisms by which to excrete excess iron.[170] A number of clinical conditions that occur more frequently in the elderly promote blood loss such as gastrointestinal ulceration, aspirin-induced bleeding, ulcerative colitis, and colonic neoplasia.[170] Iron overload also can be iatrogenic. In infections, iron is bound to lactoferrin and transferrin to withhold iron from microorganisms. If the patient is mistakenly diagnosed as iron deficient and given iron supplements, the benefits of this natural defense mechanism of the immune system are lost.[170] To avoid iron overload, Mertz[171] proposes that nutritional supplements be made in two forms, one with and the other without iron.

Another potential cause of toxicity of dietary supplements in the elderly is chronic disease states.[172] Kidney and liver diseases raise the potential for nutrient toxicity such as for vitamin A.[172] Vitamin and mineral supplementation are not recommended for elderly patients with renal or liver disease.[170] The risk of nutrient toxicity reinforces the importance of individual assessment before recommending supplementation.[159]

Other "dietary" supplements include herbs, herbal medicines, and herbal teas. In 1996 herb sales were estimated to be in excess of $12 billion.[121] Americans are rapidly increasing their use of herbal remedies either in conjunction with, or as a substitute for, traditional medicine. Physicians and other health care providers need to ask direct questions about patient use of such products.

A major change in the marketing of herbs occurred when the Dietary Supplements Health and Education Act of 1994 (DSHEA) allowed herbal manufacturers to make structure or function claims on their labels without approval from the FDA.[173] Four guidelines for claims are: (1) claims must be truthful and not misleading; (2) claims cannot be for cure, treatment, or prevention of disease; (3) a disclaimer must appear stating that the claim has not undergone FDA evaluation; and (4) claims must be based on scientific evidence that is kept in the manufacturer's files.[174] The manufacturer does not have to demonstrate compliance; the FDA must prove lack of compliance. The biggest problem with American herbal products is the lack of quality control. Products may be contaminated, may not contain the actual herbs listed, and may vary in strength.[175]

Outside the United States, careful evaluation and regulation of herbal medicine may be maintained. In Germany about 70% of primary care physicians prescribe herbal products.[174] In order to evaluate safety and efficacy of various herbs, the Federal Institute for Drugs and Medical Devices, commonly called Commission E, was established. The results of the first 300 evaluations have been translated and published in English.[174] Approximately 100 of the herbs were judged to lack safety, but the other 200 were seen to have some efficacy. This book provides additional information that can supplement previous American texts on pharmacognosy.[174] Herb-herb interactions can occur as with other medications and treatments; drug-herb interactions can happen as well.[175] No specific information has been published on food-herb interactions but the likelihood exists that they may occur.

FOOD SAFETY

Increased incidence, severity, and risk of death from many foodborne illnesses occur in elderly people.[176] Susceptibility to foodborne infections appears to be age dependent.[175] Moreover, several clinical disease states appear to create these increased risks. As gastric acidity, intestinal mi-

croflora, intestinal mucus, mucosal epithelium, intestinal motility, and granulocyte function decline with age, the likelihood of serious infection increases.[177] Death rates for diarrheal diseases are five times greater in adults over the age of 74 years.[176] Part of this increased incidence and risk may be related to the previously unrecognized presence of other gastrointestinal diseases in the elderly.[177]

In the past, foodborne outbreaks occurred more frequently due to improperly cooked or stored chicken, eggs, milk, cheese products, and seafood. Increasingly, more fresh fruits and vegetables are being identified as the source of outbreaks, especially in the presence of inadequate washing and preparation.[178-182] In one case, imported raspberries were responsible for an outbreak of cyclosporiasis, a parasite.[178] In another case, unwashed green onions were identified as the source of an outbreak of cryptosporidium, another parasite.[179] The number of cases of foodborne illness related to fresh sprouts such as raw alfalfa sprouts led the United States Food and Drug Administration to advise older adults and other individuals with compromised immune systems to not consume raw alfalfa sprouts.[181]

The marketing of fresh, unprocessed fruit juices as healthier than conventionally processed juices also has contributed to the problem.[182] Unpasteurized, fresh-pressed apple juice was responsible for several outbreaks of *Escherichia coli 0157.H7* and cryptosporidium.[182,183] The usual procedures for food sanitation become even more critical in group living situations for the elderly and in restaurants with a large elderly clientele.

An expert consortium has developed 18 recommendations that provide guidance on food safety policies and procedures. These recommendations may be readily accessed at http://www. cast-science.org.[183] The recommendations for education on food safety include:

- Educate the general public and food handlers relative to safe food preparation and handling.
- Identify high-risk populations and provide food safety education.

- Provide risk information relative to food choices to persons with enhanced disease susceptibility.
- Use and evaluate food labeling to communicate safe food preparation and storage practices to food preparers.[183]

PREVENTION OF FRAILTY, DISABILITY, AND FALLS

Although no precise scientific definition of frailty exists, a practical definition is the diminished ability to carry out the important practical and social activities of daily living (ADLs) and little reserve capacity to tolerate stresses of life.[184–188] The Assessment of Frailty Scale measures 21 practical items, 9 social activities, and 5 reserve capacity items.[188] This model converges physical, social, and environmental factors and allows the dynamic state of frailty to be identified.[187]

The importance of preventing frailty is evident when its association with physical and cognitive impairment, falls, morbidity, institutionalization, and mortality is considered.[186] Frailty has been linked to physical inactivity, heavy alcohol intake, visual and hearing impairment, psychotropic drugs, depression, impaired strength in the extremities, and gait/balance disturbances.[187] Although a disabling disease may not be cured or prevented, many of the physiological decline factors can be overcome. For example, one study[189] found balance and strength to be the primary predictors between frail and nonfrail elderly. It is therefore important to maintain balance and strength during aging. Taylor et al[32] found that the level of activity among older adults, especially those living in care homes, was well below the level thought to be needed to benefit health, especially among those living in care homes or those over the age of 75.[32] Walking appears to be the favorite form of exercise and the most amenable to change. Others concur with the findings of Taylor.[28,140,189–191]

Dzewaltowski et al[192] believe there is a gap between physical activity intervention research and the delivery of evidence-based programs in practice. They propose the Reach, Efficacy/ Effectiveness, Adoption, Implementation, and Maintenance (RE-AIM) as a useful framework of organizing and reporting the translation of research into health promotion practice.[192]

Several studies have investigated the most effective form of exercise for improving strength and balance in the elderly. Elderly people involved in regular, high-intensity resistance training appear to have the greatest increase in strength when compared with elderly subjects using low to moderate resistance training.[192] If weights and machinery are not available, other methods can be considered. One such approach is Tai Chi. Small clinical trials have suggested that older people derive improved confidence in balance and movement along with a sense of well-being from Tai Chi.[193]

Only recently has exercise been advocated for elderly persons with diseases such as rheumatoid arthritis (RA).[193–201] The loss of lean body mass common to RA may be slowed by resistance training. Likewise, resistance training may reduce pain and improve function in people with RA, osteoarthritis, and fibromyalgia.[193] Another study by Cardinal et al.[202] addressed the exercise behavior of adults with physical disabilities.

To begin an exercise program, the patient with arthritis should first visit his or her physician. Selection of an exercise place with a warm indoor pool is ideal because water-based exercises strengthen muscles, tone the cardiovascular system, and put less stress on the joints. Resistance machines place less stress on hand joints than do hand weights.[193]

Environmental hazards can be an aggravating factor for the frail elder. Because frailty is a primary cause of falls, removing environmental risks in the home can greatly benefit the individual. The following steps are recommended to reduce the risks of falls:

- Provide proper lighting.
- Install handrails on stairs and steps.
- Remove loose throw rugs or frayed carpeting.
- Install bars and/or adhesive strips in baths and showers.

- Eliminate trailing electrical cords, sharp corners, slippery floors, and storage locales that require a stool to access.
- Place the bed and other furniture at an easily accessible height.
- Choose footwear with appropriate traction (ie, thin soles allow a better feel of the floor surface than thick sports soles).[201]

Physiological loss can have many causes; therefore, it is important to identify persons at risk. One important assessment tool may be the patient's self-report of health or perceived health or ADLs he or she can perform without assistance.[185,197] Regular clinical assessment of gait and balance, as well as vision tests, can identify risk factors before they contribute to a fall or a disability that may result from a fall.[184–187]

AGING VERSUS PATHOLOGY

Differentiating age-related from age-dependent disorders challenges clinicians and researchers. Age-related diseases and disorders have specific temporal patterns. They display incidence peaks and then decline in frequency with advancing age. Ulcerative colitis, gout, peptic ulcers, and some cancers are age-related diseases. If the initiating factors can be determined and prevented or treated, the disease might never appear in the older person.[198] Evidence is growing that persons with lower health risk not only live longer but also have a later onset and shorter period of disability.[199]

Age-dependent diseases are directly correlated with age and closely related to the usual aging processes. Coronary heart disease, adult-onset diabetes, and Alzheimer's disease are examples of age-dependent diseases. Most disability of old age is increasingly being associated with these age-dependent conditions, which ultimately are the primary causes of death and disability in persons over age 65.[38,52,73] Nonetheless, some diseases may be more or less dependent on age than previously thought. For example, an increase in type 2 diabetes mellitus is occurring more frequently in children and young adults. About one-third of new cases of celiac disease (gluten enteropathy), once labeled a pediatric disease, is now being diagnosed in the seventh decade of life or above.[177] Adult celiac disease is associated with neurological complications and insulin-dependent diabetes mellitus and may be asymptomatic for years before diagnosis.[157]

STRATEGIES FOR DISEASE PREVENTION AND HEALTH PROMOTION IN OLD AGE

Many studies[62–64,66,68] document the finding that the elderly will participate in health promotion programs if offered the opportunity. Most demonstrated improved attention to simple preventive measures such as having an annual checkup and obtaining immunizations.[62] Less success was noted in lifestyle changes that involve everyday activities such as weight control and smoking cessation.[13,62]

Yarcheski et al.[199] conducted a meta-analysis of predictors of positive health practices in 37 articles and 14 predictors. They found eight predictors with moderate effect sizes (loneliness, social support, perceived health status, self-efficacy, future time perspective, self-esteem, hope, and depression) and six predictors with small effect sizes (stress, education, marital status, age, income, and gender). Nevertheless, elderly women are now eating more servings of vegetables a day than any other group of adults, and they score higher on the Healthy Eating Index than other adults.[75–77,121,122,203] In general, women are using more reduced-fat and reduced-sugar products and more supplements.[121,156]

Certain hard-to-reach groups need special targeting such as minorities who have been provided less health education and have less access to health care and who now experience much higher rates of chronic diseases such as hypertension and diabetes.[136,152] Community interventions require greater involvement of participants in planning and implementation if success is to be optimized. Moreover, a broader view of theoretical models needs to be considered in planning

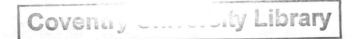

assessments and interventions. Quality-of-life issues are likely to become even more important in obtaining resources, cooperation, and successful outcomes in health promotion intervention programs. Health professionals need to recognize the cohort of the clients in a program and the stresses that are present in order to interact more effectively.[194–202]

TRAINING OF HEALTH PROFESSIONALS

Training of health professionals practicing in a wide variety of settings can be assisted by expert-compiled manuals published by the Nutrition Screening Initiative and by other practitioners with specialized interest and experience in gerontology.[102,103,200,204,205] Haber[206] presents five best practice principles that provide a summary background for health professional training in health promotion for the older population.

CONCLUSION

Providing disease prevention and health promotion advice to older people presents a new challenge for health professionals. Recent research has begun to document the benefits of smoking cessation, diet modification, increased exercise, and limited intake of alcohol and drugs for older as well as younger adults. Health promotion strategies can improve function as well as reduce the risk of morbidity and premature death. Greater consideration of quality of life and lifestyle factors are important to nutritionists providing optimal nutrition care to older adults.

For those over age 50, health promotion is less about preventing the symptoms of disease and more about preserving function and maintaining independence, productivity, and personal fulfillment. Reasons for geriatric health promotion and disease prevention activities include the following:

- Aging is a lifelong phenomenon consisting of physiological, psychological, and behavioral processes.

- Aging occurs at different rates in different people; thus biological age may not be equal to chronological age.
- Most disabilities of old age are not inevitable, universal, or irreversible.

Effective health promotion and disease prevention messages should be directed toward all older people when knowledge justifies such recommendations. Additional guidance and health interventions should be based on individual assessments of health status for those identified as being at high risk for disease or disability.

A geriatric assessment should be included as a regular part of health monitoring of older people, in addition to chronic disease screening. Nutrition screening and intervention can and should be a major part of any geriatric assessment.

REFERENCES

1. *Healthy People: The Surgeon General's Workshop on Health Promotion and Disease Prevention.* Washington, DC: US Dept of Health, Education and Welfare. HEW publication 79-55071; 1979.
2. Koop CE. Keynote address, March 20–23,1988. In: *Surgeon General's Workshop on Health Promotion and Aging.* Washington, DC: US Dept of Health and Human Services; 1988:1–4.
3. US Preventive Services Task Force. *Guide to Preventive Services.* Baltimore, MD: Williams & Wilkins; 1989.
4. US Public Health Service. *Healthy People 2000: National Health Promotion and Disease Prevention Objectives.* Washington, DC: US Dept of Health and Human Services: DHHS publication (PHS) 91-50212 ; 1991.
5. Woolf SH, Jonas S, Lawrence RS, eds. *Health Promotion and Disease Prevention in Clinical Practice.* Baltimore, MD: Williams & Wilkins; 1996.
6. Fishman P. Healthy People 2000: what progress toward better nutrition? *Geriatrics* 1996;51:38–42.
7. Yates AA, Schlicker SA, Suitor CW. Dietary reference intakes: the new bases for recommendations for calcium and related nutrients, B vitamins, and choline. *J Am Diet Assoc* 1998;98:699–707.
8. Institute of Medicine, Food and Nutrition Board. *Dietary Reference Intakes for Calcium, Phosphorus, Magnesium, Vitamin D, and Fluoride.* Washington, DC: National Academy Press; 1997.

9. Institute of Medicine, Food and Nutrition Board. *Dietary Reference Intakes for Thiamin, Riboflavin, Niacin, Vitamin B-6, Folate, Vitamin B-12, Pantothenic Acid, Biotin, and Choline.* Washington, DC: National Academy Press; 1998.

10. American Cancer Society, Advisory Committee on Diet, Nutrition and Cancer Prevention. Reducing the risk of cancer with healthy food choices and physical activities. *CA Cancer J Clin* 1996;46:325–341.

11. Lee I-M, Paffenbarger RS, Hennekens CH. Physical activity, physical fitness, and longevity. *Aging(Milano)* 1997;9:2–11.

12. Jones J, Jones KD. Promoting physical activity in the senior years. *Gerontol Nurs* 1997;23:40–48.

13. Buchner DM. Preserving mobility in older adults. *West J Med* 1997;167:258–264.

14. Rooks DS, Kiel DP, Parsons C, Hayes WC. Self paced resistance training and walking exercise in community-dwelling older adults: effects on neuromotor performance. *J Gerontol A Biol Sci Med Sci* 1997;52:M161–M168.

15. Powell RA, Single HM. Focus groups. *Int J Qual Health Care* 1996;8:499–504.

16. Gulanick M, Keough V. Focus groups: an exciting approach to clinical nursing research. *Prog Cardiovasc Nurs* 1997;12:24–29.

17. Hiatt RA. Where have we been? An overview. Paper presented at the American College of Epidemiology Annual Meeting; Sept 26–28, 1998; San Francisco, CA.

18. Ockene JK. Community-based interventions. Smoking trials as an example. Paper presented at the American College of Epidemiology Annual Meeting; Sept 26–28,1998; San Francisco, CA.

19. Belza B, Walwick J, Shin-Thornton S, Schwartz S, Taylor M, LoGerfo J. Older adults perspectives on physical activity and exercise: voices from multiple cultures. *Preventing Chronic Disease* [serial online], 2004. Oct. Accessed October 11, 2004. Available from: http://www.cdc.ped/issues/2004/oct/04_0028.htm.

20. Bell RA, Quandt SA, Vitolina MZ, Arcury TA. Dietary patterns of older adults in a rural, tri-ethnic community: a factor analysis approach. *Nutr Res* 2003;23:1379–1390.

21. Sennott-Miller L, May KM, Miller JLL. Demographic and health status indicators to guide health promotion for Hispanic and Anglo rural elderly. *Patient Educ Counseling* 1998;33:13–23.

22. de Rekeneire N, Rooks RN, Simonsick EM, Shorr RI, Kuller LH, Schwarta AV, Harris TB. Racial differences in glycemic control in a well-functioning older diabetic population: findings from the health, aging and body composition study. *Diabetes Care* 2003;26:1986–1992.

23. Kim S, Koniak-Griffin D, Flaskerud JH, Guarnero PA. The impact of lay health advisors on cardiovascular health promotion using a community-based participatory approach. *J Cardiovas Nursing* 2004;19:192–199.

24. Cunningham GO, Michael YL.Concepts guiding the study of the impact of the built environment on physical activity for older adults: a review of the literature. *Am J Health Promot* 2004;18:435–443.

25. Nunez DE, Armbruster C, Phillips WT, Gale BJ. Community-based senior health promotion program using a collaborative practice model: the Escalante health partnerships. *Public Health Nursing* 2003;20:25–32.

26. Stevens PE. Focus groups: collecting aggregate level data to understand community health phenomena. *Public Health Nurs* 1996;13:170–176.

27. Falk-Rafael AR, Ward-Griffin C, Laforet-Fliessner Y, Beynon C. Teaching nursing students to promote the health of communities: a partnership approach. *Nurse Educator* 2004;29:63–67.

28. Brach JS, Simonsick EM, Kritchevsky S, Yaffe K, Newman AB. The association between physical function and lifestyle activity and exercise in the Health, Aging and Body Composition Study. *J Am Geriatr Soc* 2004;52:502–509).

29. Levy SS, Cardinal BJ. Effects of a self-determination theory-based mail-mediated intervention on adults' exercise behavior. *Am Health Promot* 2004;18:345–349.

30. Cohen-Mansfield J, Marx MS, Biddison JR, Guralnik JM. Socio-environmental exercise preferences among older adults. *Prev Med* 2004;38:804–811.

31. Estabrooks PA, Munroe KJ, Fox EH, Gyuresik NC, Hill JI, Lyon R, Rosenkranz S, Shannon VR. Leadership in physical activity groups for older adults: a qualitative analysis. *J Aging Physical Activity* 2003;12:232–245.

32. Taylor AH, Cable NT, Faulkner G, Hillsdon M, Narici M, Van Der Bij AK. Physical activity and older adults: a review of health benefits and the effectiveness of interventions. *J Sports Sci* 2004;22:703–725.

33. Delechuse C, Colman V, Roelants M, Verschueren S, Derave W, Ceux T, Eijnde BO, Seghers J, Pardaens K, Brumagne S, Goris M, Buchers MI, Spaepen A, Swinnen S, Stijnen V. Exercise programs for older men: mode and intensity to induce the highest possible health-related benefits. *Prev Med* 2004;39:823–833.

34. Crombie IK, Irvine L, Williams B, McGinnis AR, Slane PW, Alder EM, McMurdo MET. Why older people do not participate in leisure time physical activity: a survey of activity levels, beliefs, and deterrents. *Age and Ageing* 2004;33:287–292.

35. Drewnowski A, Monsen E, Birkett D, Gunther S, Vandeland S, Su J, Marshalol G. Health screening and health promotion programs for the elderly. *Dis Manage Health Outcomes* 2003;11:299–309.

36. US Centers for Disease Control and Prevention. Estimated national spending on prevention—United States, 1988. *MMWR* 1992;41:529–531.

37. Lubitz JD, Riley GF. Trends in Medicare payments in the last year of life. *N Engl J Med* 1993;328:1092–1096.

38. Swerissen H, Crisp BH. The sustainability of health promotion intervention for different levels of social organization. *Health Promot Int* 2004;19:123–130.

39. Hickey T, Stilwell DL. Health promotion for older people. All is not well. *Gerontologist* 1991;31:822–829.

40. Fox PJ, Breuner W, Wright JA. Effects of a health promotion program in sustaining health behaviors in older adults. *Am J Prev Med* 1997;13:257–264.

41. Resnick B. Measurement tools: do they apply equally to older adults? *J Gerontol Nurs* 1995;21:18–22.

42. Schneider G, Driesch G, Kruse A, Wachter M, Nehen H-G, Heuft G. What influences self-perception of health in the elderly? The role of objective health condition, subjective well-being and sense of coherence. *Arch Gerontol Geriatrics* 2004;39:227–237.

43. Abbott RD, White LR, Ross GW, Masaki KH, Curb JD, Petrovitch H. Walking and dementia in physically capable elderly men. *JAMA* 2004;292:1447–1453.

44. Weuve J, Kang JH, Manson JAE, Breteier MB, Ware JH, Grodstein F. Physical activity, including walking and cognitive function in obese women. *JAMA* 2004; 292:1454–1461.

45. Green LW. National policy in the promotion of health. *Int J Health Educ* 1979;22:161–168.

46. Catford J. Health promotion's record card: how principled are we 20 years on? *Health Promot Int* 2004;19: 1–4.

47. Bogden JB, Louria DB. Micronutrients and immunity in older people. In: Bendich A, Deckelbaum RJ, eds. *Preventive Nutrition: The Comprehensive Guide for Health Professionals.* Totowa, NJ: Humana Press; 1998.

48. Shepherd RJ. Worksite health promotion and the older worker. *Int J Industrial Ergonomics* 2000; 25:465–475.

49. Chernoff R. Nutrition. In: Jahnigen D, Schrier R, eds. *Geriatric Medicine.* 2nd ed. Cambridge, MA: Blackwell Scientific Publications; 1996:196–200.

50. Goldberg TH, Chavin SI. Preventive medicine and screening in older adults. *J Am Geriatr Soc* 1997;45: 344–354.

51. Pizzi ER, Wolf ZR. Health risks and health promotion of older women: utility of a health promotion diary. *Holist Nurs Pract* 1998;12:62–72.

52. Patterson C, Feightner J. Promoting the health of senior citizens. *Can Med Assoc J* 1997;157:1107–1113.

53. Keister KJ, Blixen CE. Quality of life and aging. *J Gerontol Nurs* 1998;24:22–28.

54. Widar M, Ahlstrom G, Ek AC. Health-related quality of life in persons with long-term pain after a stroke. *J Clin Nursing* 2004;13:497–505.

55. Focht BC, Gauvin L, Rejeskei WJ. The contribution of daily experiences and acute exercise to fluctuations in daily feeling states among older, obese adults with knee osteoarthritis. *J Behav Med* 2003;27:101–121.

56. Sandison R, Gray M, Reid DM. Lifestyle factors for promoting bone health in older women. *J Adv Nursing* 2004;45:603–610.

57. Writing Group of the PREMIER Collaborative Research Group. Effects of comprehensive lifestyle modification on blood pressure control. *JAMA* 2003; 289:2083–2093.

58. Hazzard WR. Ways to make "usual" and "successful" aging synonymous: preventive gerontology. *West J Med* 1997;167:206–215.

59. McPhee SD, Johnson TR. Comparing health status with healthy habits in elderly assisted-living residents. *Community Health* 2004;27:158–169.

60. Jenkins KR. Obesity's effects on onset of functional impairment among older adults. *The Gerontologist* 2004; 44:206–218.

61. Fried LP, Freedman M, Endres TE, Wasik B. Building communities that promote successful aging. *West J Med* 1997;167:216–219.

62. Lave JR, Ives DG, Traven ND, Kuller LH. Participation in health promotion programs by the rural elderly. *Am J Prev Med* 1995;11:46–53.

63. Lave JR, Ives DG, Traven ND, Kuller LH. Evaluation of a health promotion demonstration program for the rural elderly. *Health Serv Res* 1996;31:261–281.

64. Viverais-Dresler GA, Bakker DA, Vance RJ. Elderly clients perception: individual health counseling and group sessions. *Can J Public Health* 1995;86:234–237.

65. US Preventive Services Task Force. *Guide to Clinical Preventive Services.* 2nd ed. Baltimore, MD: Williams & Wilkins; 1997.

66. LaCroix AZ, Newton KM, Leveille SG, Wallace J. Healthy aging: a woman's issue. *West J Med* 1997;167: 220–232.

67. Newsom JT, Kaplan MS, Huguer N, McFarland BH. Health behaviors in a representative sample of older Canadians: prevalence, reported change, motivation to change, and perceived barriers. *The Gerontologist* 2004; 44:193–205.

68. Love RR, Davis JE, Mundlt M, Clark C. Health promotion and screening services reported by older adult patients of urban primary care physicians. *J Fam Pract* 1997;45:142–150.

69. Fries JF. Aging, natural death, and the compression of morbidity. *N Engl J Med* 1980;3031:130–133.

70. Kulp JL, Rane S, Bachmann G. Impact of preventive osteoporosis education on patient behavior: immediate and 3-month follow-up. *Menopause* 2004;11:116–119.

71. Elder JP, Williams SJ, Drew JA, Wright BL, Boulan TE. Longitudinal effects of preventive services on health behaviors among the elderly cohort. *Am J Prev Med* 1995; 11:354–359.

72. *US Surgeon General's Report on Nutrition and Health.* Washington, DC: Government Printing Office. DHHS publication (PHS) 88-50210; 1988.

73. National Research Council, Food and Nutrition Board. *Diet and Health: Implications for Reducing Chronic Disease.* Washington, DC: National Academy Press; 1989.

74. Burt VL, Cutler JA, Higgings M, et al. Trends in prevalence, awareness, and treatment and control of hypertension in the adult US population: data from the heart examination surveys, 1960 to 1991. *Hypertension* 1995; 26:60–69.

75. Interagency Board for Nutrition Monitoring and Related Research, Life Sciences Research Office, FASEB. *Third Report on Nutrition Monitoring in the United States: Executive Summary.* Washington, DC: Government Printing Office; 1995.

76. Interagency Board for Nutrition Monitoring and Related Research. *Nutrition Monitoring in the United States: The Directory of Federal and State Nutrition Monitoring Activities, 1992.* Hyattsville, MD: Human Nutrition Information Services. DHHS publication (PHS92-1255-1361); 1992.

77. Mackey MA, Hill BP. Health claims regulations and new food concepts. In: Kotsonis FN, Mackey MA, eds. *Nutrition in the 90's: Current Controversies and Analysis.* New York, NY: Marcel Dekker; 1994:2.

78. Ippolito PM, Mathios AD. *Information and Advertising Policy: A Study of Fat and Cholesterol Consumption in the United States, 1977–1990.* Bureau of Economics Staff Report. Washington, DC: Federal Trade Commission; 1996.

79. USDA, USDHHS. *Nutrition and Your Health: Dietary Guidelines for Americans.* 4th ed. Washington, DC: Government Printing Office, Home and Garden Bulletin 232; 1995.

80. Institute of Medicine, Food and Nutrition Board. *Dietary Reference Intakes: Guiding Principles for Nutrition Labeling and Fortification, Institute of Medicine.* Washington, DC: National Academy Press; 2003.

81. Parker SL, Tong T, Bolden S, et al. Cancer statistics, 1997. *CA Cancer J Clin* 1997;47:5–27.

82. Wingo PA, Landis S, Ries LAG. An adjustment to the 1997 estimate for new prostate cancer cases. *CA Cancer J Clin* 1997;47:239–242.

83. Landis SH, Murray T, Bolden S, et al. Cancer statistics, 1998. *CA Cancer J Clin* 1998;48:6–29.

84. Rosenthal DS. Changing trends. *CA Cancer J Clin* 1998;48:3–5.

85. Bowman SA, Lino M, Gerior SA, Basiotis PP. *The Healthy Eating Index 1994–96.* Hyattsville, MD: Human Nutrition Information Services CNPP-5; 1998.

86. Kennedy ET, Ohls J, Carlson S, Feming K. The healthy eating index: design and applications. *J Am Diet Assoc* 1995;95:1103–1108.

87. USDA Center for Nutrition Policy and Promotion. *The Healthy Eating Index.* Hyattsville, MD: Human Nutrition Information Services CNPP-1; 1995.

88. Sims LS. Uses of the recommended dietary allowances: a commentary. *J Am Diet Assoc* 1996;96:659–662.

89. Most frequently asked questions ... about the 1997 Dietary Reference Intakes (DRIs). *Nutr Today* 1997;32: 189–190.

90. National Research Council Subcommittee on the 10th Edition of the RDAs, Food and Nutrition Board, Commission on Life Sciences. *Recommended Dietary Allowances.* 10th ed. Washington, DC: National Academy Press; 1994.

91. Yates AA. Process and development of dietary reference intakes: basis, need, and application of recommended dietary allowances. *Nutr Rev* 1998;56:55–S9.

92. Institute of Medicine, Food and Nutrition Board. *Dietary Reference Intakes for vitamin C, vitamin E, selenium, and carotenoids.* Washington, DC: National Academy Press; 2000.

93. Institute of Medicine, Food and Nutrition Board. *Dietary Reference Intakes for Vitamin A, Vitamin K, Arsenic, Boron, Chromium, Copper, Iodine, Iron, Manganese, Molybdenum, Nickel, Vanadium, and Zinc.* Washington, DC: National Academy Press; 2003.

94. Institute of Medicine, Food and Nutrition Board. *Dietary Reference Intakes for Energy, Carbohydrates, Fiber, Fat, Fatty Acids, Cholesterol, Protein, and Amino Acids.* Washington, DC: National Academy Press; 2003.

95. Institute of Medicine, Food and Nutrition Board. *Dietary Reference Intakes for Water, Potassium, Sodium, Chloride, and Sulfate.* Washington DC: National Academy Press; 2004.

96. Nutrition Screening Initiative Technical Review Committee. *Report of Nutrition Screening I: Toward a Common View.* Washington, DC: Nutrition Screening Initiative; 1991.

97. Dwyer JT. *Screening Older Americans' Nutritional Health: Current Practices and Future Possibilities.* Washington, DC: Nutrition Screening Initiative; 1991.

98. White JV, Ham RJ, Lipschitz DA, Dwyer JT, Wellman NS. Consensus of the Nutrition Screening Initiative:

risk factors and indicators of poor nutritional status in older Americans. *J Am Diet Assoc* 1991;91:783–787.

99. Nutrition Screening Initiative Technical Review Committee. *Nutrition Interventions Manual for Professionals Caring for Older Americans.* Washington, DC: Nutrition Screening Initiative; 1992.

100. Nutrition Screening Initiative Technical Review Committee. *Incorporating Nutrition Screening and Interventions into Medical Practices: A Monograph for Physicians.* Washington, DC: Nutrition Screening Initiative; 1994.

101. Adams TL, Chernoff R, Winger RM, Hosig KW, McCabe BJ. The effect of home-delivered meals on length of hospital stay. *J Am Diet Assoc* 1998;98:A12.

102. Nutrition Screening Initiative Technical Review Committee. *Keeping Older Americans Healthy at Home: Guidelines for Nutrition Programs in Home Health Care.* Washington, DC: Nutrition Screening Initiative; 1996.

103. Nutrition Screening Initiative Technical Review Committee. *Managing Nutrition Care in Health Plans: A Guide to the Incorporation of Nutrition Screening Interventions in Managed Care.* Washington, DC: Nutrition Screening Initiative; 1996.

104. Nutrition Screening Initiative. A physician's guide to nutrition in chronic disease management. 2004. Available from http://www.aafp.org/PreBuilt/NSI_new orderforma.pdf.

105. Expert Committee of Nutrition and Health for Older Americans. *Nutrition and Health for Older Americans—A Campaign of the American Dietetic Association. Food Guide for Older Adults.* Chicago: American Dietetic Association; 1998.

106. Smith DWE. Changing causes of death of elderly people in the United States, 1950–1990. *Gerontology* 1998; 44:331–335.

107. Black HR. Risk stratification of older patients. *AJH* 2002;15:77S–81S.

108. Tsang TSM, Barnes ME, Gersh BJ, Takemoto Y, Rosales AG, Bailey KR, Seward JB. Prediction of risk for first age-related cardiovascular events in an elderly population: the incremental value of echocardiography *J Am Coll Cardiol* 2003;42:1199–1205.

109. Clarke R, Daly L, Robinson K, et al. Hyperhomocysteinemia: an independent risk factor for vascular disease. *N Engl J Med* 1991;324:1149–1155.

110. Selhub J, Facques PF, Wilson PFW, Rush D, Rosenberg IH. Vitamin status and intake as primary determinants of homocysteinemia in an elderly population. *JAMA* 1993;270:2693–2698.

111. Riggs KM, Spiro A, Tucher K, Rush D. Relations of vitamin B-12, vitamin B-6, folate and homocysteine to cognitive performance in the Normative Aging Study. *Am J Clin Nutr* 1996;63:306–314.

112. Pametti L, Bottiglieri T, Lowenthal D. Role of homocysteine in age-related vascular and non-vascular diseases. *Aging (Milano)* 1997;9:241–257.

113. Ebly EM, Schaefer JP, Campbell NRC, Hogan DB. Folate status, vascular disease and cognition in elderly Canadians. *Age Aging* 1998;27:485–491.

114. Tangney CC. Vitamin E and cardiovascular disease. *Nutr Today* 1997;32:13–22.

115. Rodondo MR, Ortega RM, Zamora MJ, et al. Influence of the number of meals taken per day on cardiovascular risk factors and the energy and nutrient intakes of a group of elderly people. *Int J Vitamin Nutr Res* 1997; 67:176–182.

116. Steinmetz KA, Potter JD. Vegetables, fruits and cancer prevention: a review. *J Am Diet Assoc* 1996;96: 1027–1039.

117. Morley JE. Anorexia in older persons: epidemiology and optimal treatment. *Drugs Aging* 1996;8:134–155.

118. Knol LL, Haughton B. Fruit and juice intake associated with higher dietary status index in rural East Tennessee women living in public housing. *J Am Diet Assoc* 1998; 98:576–579.

119. Johnson RK. In-person vs telephone collection of dietary intake data in children and women: validation with doubly labeled water. Paper presented at What We Eat in America: Research and Results Survey Conference; Sept 14–17, 1998; Rockville, MD.

120. Johnson RK, Soultanakis RP, Matthews DE. Literacy and body fatness are associated with underreporting of energy intake in U.S. low-income women using multiple-pass 24-hour recall: a doubly labeled water study. *J Am Diet Assoc* 1998;98:1136–1140.

121. Mares-Perlman JA, Klein BEK, Klein R, Ritter LL, Freudenhelm JL, Luby MH. Nutrient supplements contribute to the dietary intake of middle- and older-aged adult residents of Beaver Dam, Wisconsin. *J Nutr* 1993; 123:176–188.

122. Gretebeck RJ, Boileau RA. Self reported energy intake and energy expenditure in elderly women. *J Am Diet Assoc* 1998;98:574–576.

123. Sharkey JR. Risk and presence of food insufficiency are associated with low nutrient intakes and multimorbidity among homebound women who receive home-delivered meals. *J Nutr* 2003;133:348S–349S.

124. Sharkey JR Nutrition risk assessment of homebound older persons. In: *Abstracts and Proceedings of the Nutrition and Aging XVIII Conference, Obesity in Older Adults:* Sept 17, 2003; Little Rock, AR.

125. Sharkey JR Branch LG, Schoori N, et al. Inadequate nutrient intake among homebound older adults in the community and its correlation with individual characteristics and health-related factors. *Am J Clin Nutr* 2002; 76:1435–1446.

126. Sharkey JR, Guiliani C, Haines PS, et al. A summary measure of dietary intake of musculoskeletal nutrients (calcium, vitamin D, magnesium, and phosphorus) is associated with lower-extremity physical performance in homebound older men and women. *Am J Clin Nutr* 2003;77:837–856.

127. McCabe BJ, Sharkey JR, Bogle ML. Diuretic therapy use increases the risk for low thiamin intake in homebound elders. *FASEB J* 2004;18:A95.

128. McCabe BJ, Sharkey JR. Do older adults need closer monitoring of dietary B vitamin needed? *J Am Diet Assoc* 2004;104:A11.

129. NIH Consensus Development Panel on Optimal Intake. NIH Consensus. Optimal calcium intake. *JAMA* 1994; 272:1942–1948.

130. Division of Health Examination Statistics, National Center for Health Statistics, CDC. Osteoporosis among estrogen-deficient women—United States, 1988–1994. *MMWR* 1998;47:969–973.

131. del Puente A, Postiglione A, Esposito-del Puenta A, Carpinelli A, Roman M, Oriente P. Peripheral body fat has a protective role in bone mineral density in elderly women. *Eur J Clin Nutr* 1998;52:690–693

132. Bidlack WR. Interrelationships of food, nutrition, diet and health: the National Association of State Universities and Land Grant Colleges white papers. *J Am Coll Nutr* 1996;15:422–433.

133. Drugay M. Breaking the silence: a health promotion approach to osteoporosis. *J Gerontol Nurs* 1999;23: 36–43.

134. Weber P. Management of osteoporosis: is there a role for vitamin K? *Int J Vitam Nutr Res* 1997;67:350–356.

135. McCabe BJ, Champagne CM, Allen HR. Calcium intake of selected age and gender groups from CSFII. 1994–96. Unpublished data. 1998.

136. Ciesla JR, Piane G, Rubens AJ. Hypertension in community-dwelling elders from a statewide study: implications for nonpharmacological therapy. *J Health Care Poor Underserved* 1998;9:62–75.

137. SHEP Cooperative Research Group. Prevention of stroke by antihypertensive drug treatment in older persons with isolated systolic hypertension: final results of the Systolic Hypertension in the Elderly Populations (SHEP). *JAMA* 1991;265:3255–3264.

138. National High Blood Pressure Education Program Working Group. National High Blood Pressure Education Program working group report on hypertension in the elderly. *Hypertension* 1994;23:275–285.

139. The Sixth Report of the Joint National Committee on Prevention, Detection, Evaluation and Treatment of High Blood Pressure. *Arch Intern Med* 1997;157: 2413–2446.

140. Whelton PK, Appel LJ, Espeland MA, et al. Sodium reduction and weight loss in the treatment of hyperten-sion in older persons: a randomized controlled trial of nonpharmacologic interventions in the elderly *(TONE). JAMA* 1998;299:839–846.

141. Resnicow K, Campbell MK, Carr C, McCarty F, Wang T, Periasamy S, Rahotep S, Doyle C, Williams A, Stables G. Body and Soul: a dietary intervention con-ducted through African-American churches. *Am J Prev Med* 2004;27:97–105.

142. Barents Group of Peat Marwick. *The Clinical and Cost Effectiveness of Medical Nutritional Therapy: Evidence and Estimates of Potential Medicare Savings from the Use of Selected Nutrition Interventions.* Washington, DC: Nutrition Screening Initiative; 1996.

143. Loeb SJ. Older men's health: motivation, self-ratings and behaviors. *Nursing Res* 2004;53:198–206.

144. Dengel JL, Katzel LI, Goldberg AP. Effects of an American Heart Association diet with or without weight loss on lipids in obese middle-aged and older men. *Am J Clin Nutr* 1995;62:715–721.

145. Fox AA, Thompson JL, Butterfield GE, Gylfadottir U, Moynihan S, Spiller G. Effects of diet and exercise on common cardiovascular disease risk factors in moderately obese older women. *Am J Clin Nutr* 1996;63:225–233.

146. Parise C, Sternfeld B, Samuels S, Tager IB. Brisk walk-ing speed in older adults who walk for exercise. *JAGS* 2004;52:411–416.

147. The National Heart, Lung, and Blood Institute Expert Panel on the Identification, Evaluation and Treatment of Overweight and Obesity. Clinical guidelines on the identification, evaluation, and treatment of obesity in adults: executive summary. *J Am Diet Assoc* 1998;98: 1178–1191.

148. Expert Panel on the Identification, Evaluation, and Treatment of Overweight in Adults. Clinical guidelines on the identification, evaluation and treatment of over-weight in adults: executive summary. *Am J Clin Nutr* 1998;68:899–917.

149. Visser M, Langlois J, Guralnik JM, et al. High body fat-ness but not low fat-free mass predicts disability in older men and women: the Cardiovascular Health Study. *Am J Clin Nutr* 1998;68:584–590.

150. Visser M, Harris TB, Langlois J, et al. Body fat and skeletal muscle mass in relation to physical disability in very old men and women of the Framingham Heart Study. *J Gerontol A Biol Sci Med Sci* 1998;53: M214–M221.

151. Fonseca V, Wall J. Diet and diabetes in the elderly. *Clin Geriatr Med* 1995;11:613–624.

152. Rajaram SS, Vinson V. African American women and diabetes: a sociocultural context. *J Health Care Poor Underserved* 1998;9:236–244.

153. Hunt LM, Pugh J, Valenzuela M. How patient adapt self care recommendations in everyday life. *J Fam Pract* 1998;46:207–215.

154. Carter JS, Pugh JA, Monterrosa A. Non-insulin de-pendent diabetes mellitus and ethnic minorities: the double jeopardy. *Ann Intern Med* 1996;125:221–232.

155. Havlik RJ, Liu BM, Lovar MC. *Health Statistics on Older Persons*. US Vital and Health Statistic Services 3, No. 25. Washington, DC: Government Printing Office National Center for Health Statistics; DHSS publication (PHS) 87-1409; 1987.

156. Georgiou C, Goldman J, Anderson E. Reduced fat and reduced-sugar foods: Americans who use them and their diet quality. Paper presented at What We Eat in America: Research and Result, Survey Conference; Sept 14–17, 1998; Rockville, MD.

157. Franz MJ, Horton ES, Bantle JP, et al. Nutrition princi-ples for the management of diabetes and related com-plications. *Diabetes Care* 1994;17:490–518.

158. Vailas LI, Nitze SA, Becker M, Gast J. Risk indicators for malnutrition are associated inversely with quality of life for participants in meal programs for older adults. *J Am Diet Assoc* 1998:98:548

159. Position of the American Dietetic Association. Vitamin and mineral supplementation. *J Am Diet Assoc* 1996;96: 73–77.

160. Tripp F. The use of dietary supplements in the elderly: current issues and recommendations. *J Am Diet Assoc* 1997;97:S181–S183.

161. Houston DK, Johnson MA, Daniel TD, Poon LW. Health and dietary characteristics of supplement users in an elderly populations. *Int J Vitam Nutr Res* 1997;67: 18:–191.

162. Morley JE, Flood HM, Perry HM, Kumar VB. Peptides, memory, food intake and aging. *Aging (Milano)* 1997; 9:17–18.

163. Allen LH, Casterline J. Vitamin B-12 deficiency in eld-erly individuals: diagnosis and requirements. *Am J Clin Nutr* 1994;60:12–14.

164. Lindenbaum J, Rosenberg IH, Wilson PWF, Stabler SP, Allen RH. Prevalence of cobalamin deficiency in the Framingham elderly population. *Am J Clin Nutr* 1994;60:2–11.

165. Bogden JD, Bendich A, Kemp FW, et al. Daily mi-cronutrient supplements enhance delayed hypersensi-tivity skin test responses in older people. *Am J Clin Nutr* 1994;60:437–447.

166. Keane EM, O'Broin S, Kelleher B, Coakley D, Walsh JB. Use of folic acid-fortified milk in the elderly pop-ulation. *Gerontology* 1998;44:336–339.

167. Cuskelly GJ, McNulty H, Scott JM. Effect of increasing dietary folate on red cell folate: implications for preven-tion of neural tube defects. *Lancet* 1996;349:657–659.

168. Omenn GS. An assessment of the scientific basis for at-tempting to define the dietary reference intakes for beta carotene. *J Am Diet Assoc* 1998;98:1406–1409.

169. Alpha-Tocopherol, Beta-Carotene Cancer Prevention Study Group. The effect of vitamin E and beta carotene in the incidence of lung cancer and other cancers in male smokers. *N Engl J Med* 1994;330:1029–1035.

170. Connor JR, Beard JL. Dietary iron supplements in the elderly: to use or not to use. *Nutr Today* 1997;32: 102–109.

171. Mertz W. Food fortification in the United States. *Nutr Rev* 1997;55:44–49.

172. Russell RM. The impact of disease states as a modify-ing factor for nutrition toxicity. *Nutr Rev* 1997;55: 50–53.

173. Spaulding-Albright N. A review of some herbal and re-lated products commonly used in cancer patients. *J Am Diet Assoc* 1997;97:S208–S215.

174. Blumenthal M, Busse WH, Goldberg A, et al., eds. *The Complete German Commission E Monographs: Thera-peutic Guide to Herbal Medicine*. Boston, MA: Integrative Medicine Communications; 1998.

175. Gurley BJ, Hagan DW. Herbal and dietary supplements with drugs. In: McCabe BJ, Frankel EH, Wolfe JJ, eds. *Handbook of Food-Drug Interactions*, Boca Raton, FL: CRC Press; 2003.

176. Klontz KC, Adler WE, Potter M. Age-dependent re-sistance factors in the pathogenesis of foodborne infec-tious disease. *Aging (Milano)* 1997;9:320–326.

177. Beaumont DM, Mian MS. Celiac disease in old age: "a catch in the rye." *Age Ageing* 1998;27:535–538.

178. Caceres VM, Ball RT, Somerfeldt SS, et al. A food-borne outbreak of cyclosporiasis caused by imported raspberries. *J Fam Pract* 1998;47:231234.

179. Quinn K, Baldwin G, Stepak P, et al. Foodborne out-break of cryptosporidiosis—Spokane, WA, 1997. *MMWR* 1998;47:565–567.

180. Millard PS, Gensheimer KF, Addiss DG, et al. An out-break of cryptosporidiosis from fresh-pressed apple cider. *JAMA* 1994;272:1592–1596.

181. FDA Statement. Consumers in Oregon area advised of risks associated with raw sprouts. US Food and Drug Administration News Release, November 26, 2003. Available at: http://www.fda.gov. Accessed December 12, 2003.

182. Centers for Disease Control. Outbreaks of *Escherichia coli* 0157:H7 infection and cryptosporidiosis associated with drinking unpasteurized apple cider—Connecticut and New York, October 1996. *MMWR* 1997;46:4–8.

183. Council for Agricultural Science and Technology (CAST). Foodborne pathogens: review of recommen-dations. Available at: http://www.cast-science.org. Accessed January 8, 1999.

184. Buchner DM, Wagner EH. Preventing frail health. *Clin Geriatr Med* 1992;8:1–16.

185. Dayoff NE, Suhrheinrich J, Wigglesworth J, Topp R, Moore S. Balance and muscle strength as predictors of frailty among older adults. *J Gerontol Nurs* 1998;24: 18–27.

186. Raphael D, Cava M, Brown I, et al. Frailty: a public health perspective. *Can J Public Health* 1995;86: 224–227.

187. Brown I, Renwich R, Raphael D. Frailty: constructing a common meaning definition and conceptual framework. *Int J Rehabil Res* 1995;18:93–102.

188. Guralnik JM, Simonsick EM. Physical disability in older Americans. *J Am Geriatr Soc* 1993;48:310.

189. Sullivan D. Exercise in the frail elderly. Paper presented at Nutrition, Exercise and Aging. Nutrition and Aging XIII; Sept 16–17, 1998; Little Rock, AR.

190. O'Grady M. Exercise and fall prevention. Paper presented at Nutrition, Exercise and Aging. Nutrition and Aging XIII; Sept 16–17, 1998; Little Rock, AR.

191. Brassinton GS, Atienza AA, Perezek RE, DiLorenzo TM, King AC. Intervention-related cognitive versus social mediators of exercise adherence in the elderly. *Am J Prev Med* 2002;23:80–86.

192. Dzewaltowski DA, Estrabrooks PA, Glasgow RE. The future of physical activity behavior change research: what is needed to improve the translation of research into health promotion practice. *Exerc Sport Sci Rev* 2004;32:57–63.

193. Roubenoff R. Exercise for people with arthritis: can you and should you? Paper presented at Nutrition, Exercise and Aging. Nutrition and Aging XIII; Sept 16–17,1998; Little Rock, AR.

194. Borgenicht K, Carty E, Fergenbaum L. Community resources for frail older patients. *West J Med* 1997;167: 291–294.

195. Rall LC, Rosen CJ, Dolnikowski G, et al. Protein metabolism in rheumatoid arthritis and aging. *Arthritis Rheum* 1996;39:1115–1124.

196. Colbert LH, Visser M, Simonsick EM, Tracy RP, Newman AB, Kritchevsky SB, Pahor M, Taafee DR, Brach J, Rubin S, Harris TB. Physical activity, exercise, and inflammatory markers in older adults: findings from the health, aging and body composition study. *JAGS* 2004;52:1098–1104.

197. Haber D. *Health Promotion and Aging.* New York, NY: Springer Publishing; 1994.

198. Wagner EH. Preventing decline in function: evidence from randomized trials around the world. *West J Med* 1997;167:276–284.

199. Yarcheski A, Mahon NE, Yarcheski TJ, Cannella BL. A meta-analysis of predictors of positive health practices. *J Nurs Scholarship* 2004:36:102–108.

200. Vita AJ, Terry RB, Hubert HB, Fries JF. Aging, health risks, and cumulative disability. *N Engl J Med* 1998; 338:1035–1041.

201. Williams SJ, Elder JP, Seidman RL, Mayer J. 1. Preventive services in a Medicare managed *care* environment. *J Community Health* 1997;22:417–433.

202. Cardinal BJ, Kosma M, McCubbin JA. Factors influencing the exercise behavior of adults with physical disabilities. *Med Sci Sports Exerc* 2004;36:868–875

203. Gilbride JA, Amella EJ, Breiner EB, Mariano C, Mezey M. Nutrition and health status of community dwelling elderly in New York City: a pilot study. *J Am Diet Assoc* 1998;98:554–557.

204. Nutrition Screening Initiative Technical Review Committee. NSI update. *Nutr Screening Initiative Newsletter* 1998;25:3–4.

205. Kniedert KC, Domer B, Gerwick C, Posthauer ME, Sichterman C, eds. *Nutritional Care for the Older Adult.* Chicago, IL: American Dietetic Association; 1998.

206. Haber D. Serving older adults with health promotion. *Art of Health Promot* 2004;1:1–5.

Index

Note: The italicized *f* or *t* following a page number denotes a figure or table on that page. The italicized *ff* or *tt* following a page number denotes multiple figures or tables on that page